# COLOR ATLAS AND SYNOPSIS OF VASCULAR DISEASES

## NOTICE

Medicine is an ever-changing science. As new research and clinical experience broaden our knowledge, changes in treatment and drug therapy are required. The authors and the publisher of this work have checked with sources believed to be reliable in their efforts to provide information that is complete and generally in accord with the standards accepted at the time of publication. However, in view of the possibility of human error or changes in medical sciences, neither the authors nor the publisher nor any other party who has been involved in the preparation or publication of this work warrants that the information contained herein is in every respect accurate or complete, and they disclaim all responsibility for any errors or omissions or for the results obtained from use of the information contained in this work. Readers are encouraged to confirm the information contained herein with other sources. For example and in particular, readers are advised to check the product information sheet included in the package of each drug they plan to administer to be certain that the information contained in this work is accurate and that changes have not been made in the recommended dose or in the contraindications for administration. This recommendation is of particular importance in connection with new or infrequently used drugs.

# COLOR ATLAS AND SYNOPSIS OF VASCULAR DISEASES

## EDITORS

### Steven M. Dean, DO, FACP, RPVI, FSVM

Associate Professor of Internal Medicine
Division of Cardiovascular Medicine
Director, Vascular Medicine Program
The Ohio University Wexner Medical Center
Columbus, Ohio

### Bhagwan Satiani, MD, MBA, RPVI, FACS

Professor of Clinical Surgery
Division of Vascular Diseases & Surgery
Department of Surgery
Director, FAME Faculty Leadership Institute
Director, Vascular Labs
The Ohio State University Wexner Medical Center

## SERIES EDITOR

### William T. Abraham, MD, FACP, FACC, FAHA, FESC

Professor of Medicine, Physiology, and Cell Biology
Chair of Excellence in Cardiovascular Medicine
Director, Division of Cardiovascular Medicine
Deputy Director, Davis Heart and Lung Research Institute
The Ohio State University
Columbus, Ohio

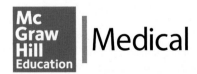

New York   Chicago   San Francisco   Athens   London   Madrid   Mexico City
Milan   New Delhi   Singapore   Sydney   Toronto

**Color Atlas and Synopsis of Vascular Diseases**

1 2 3 4 5 6 7 8 9 0   CTP/CTP   18 17 16 15 14 13

Set ISBN 978-0-07-174954-1; Set MHID 0-07-174954-3;
Book ISBN 978-0-07-174951-0; Book MHID 0-07-174951-9
DVD ISBN 978-0-07-174952-7; DVD MHID 0-07-174952-7

This book was set in Perpetua by Cenveo® Publisher Services.
The editors were Christine Diedrich and Regina Y. Brown.
The production supervisor was Catherine H. Saggese.
Production management was provided by Sapna Rastogi.
China Translation & Printing Services Ltd. was printer and binder.

This book is printed on acid-free paper.

**Library of Congress Cataloging-in-Publication Data**

Color atlas and synopsis of vascular diseases/editors, Steven Dean,
Bhagwan Satiani.
            p. ; cm.
    Includes bibliographical references.
    ISBN-13: 978-0-07-174954-1 (alk. paper)
    ISBN-10: 0-07-174954-3
    I. Dean, Steven (Steven M.)    II. Satiani, Bhagwan.
    [DNLM:   1.   Vascular Diseases—diagnosis—Atlases.   2.   Vascular
Diseases—therapy—Atlases.   WG 17]
    RC694
    616.1'3100222—dc23
                                        2013004370

# DEDICATION

I would like to dedicate this book to my wonderful family. First of all, never-ending gratitude is owed to my wife, Jenny and daughter, Annie. They have been incredibly understanding and supportive of all the time I've invested in editing this book as well as my profession. To my brother, Michael. Thanks as you've made life more fun! Finally, my career in medicine would not have been possible without the initial support of my parents, Merrell and Sherma. I love you all.

Steven M. Dean

To my best friend and wife Mira. To the land of the free and home of the brave, the most blessed place on earth for immigrants.

Bhagwan Satiani

# CONTENTS

Contributors . . . . . . . . . . . . . . . . . . . . . . . . . . . . . . ix
Preface . . . . . . . . . . . . . . . . . . . . . . . . . . . . . . . . . . xv
Acknowledgments. . . . . . . . . . . . . . . . . . . . . . . . . . xvii

## PART 1

## LOWER EXTREMITIES: MISCELLANEOUS DISEASES

1   Aortoiliac Disease: Occlusion. . . . . . . . . . . . . . .2
2   Aortoiliac Occlusive Disease: Treatment With Stenting. . . . . .6
3   Femoral Popliteal Disease: Bypass. . . . . . . . . . .11
4   Femoral Popliteal Disease: PTA and Stenting . . . . . . . . . . 14
5   Tibioperoneal Occlusive Disease . . . . . . . . . . . . 18
6   Limb Gangrene and Amputation. . . . . . . . . . . . . 22
7   Extra-Anatomic Bypass Grafts . . . . . . . . . . . . . 25
8   Blue Toe Syndrome (Atheromatous Embolization) . . . . . . . 29

## PART 2

## AORTIC AND UPPER EXTREMITY ARTERIAL DISEASE

9   Atherosclerotic Arch Vessel Disease . . . . . . . . . . . . 34
10  Thoracic Aortic Dissection. . . . . . . . . . . . . . . . . 42
11  Innominate and Subclavian Artery Peripheral Arterial Disease . . . . . . . . . . . . . . . . . . . . . . . . . 46
12  Upper Extremity Ischemia: Access Site Complications. . . . . . 49
13  Thoracic Outlet Syndrome and Arterial Aneurysm of Upper Extremity . . . . . . . . . . . . . . . . . . . . . 54
14  Arterial Thoracic Outlet Syndrome. . . . . . . . . . . . 57
15  Vertebrobasilar Insufficiency: Subclavian Steal Syndrome . . . . . . . . . . . . . . . . . . . . . . . . 62
16  Subclavian Coronary Steal . . . . . . . . . . . . . . . . 67
17  Congenital Vascular Anomalies of the Upper Extremity . . . . . . . . . . . . . . . . . . . . . 71
18  Allen Test and Evaluation of the Palmar Arch . . . . . . . . . 79
19  Hypothenar Hammer Syndrome. . . . . . . . . . . . . . 82
20  Hand Ischemia After Placement of Hemodialysis Access. . . . . 84

## PART 3

## CAROTID ARTERY OCCLUSIVE DISEASE

21  Arteriosclerotic Carotid Occlusive Disease: Surgical . . . . . . .88
22  Arteriosclerotic Carotid Occlusive Disease: Stent . . . . . . . .92
23  Arteriosclerotic Carotid Occlusive Disease: Ulcerative . . . . .97
24  Arteriosclerotic Carotid Occlusive Disease: Occlusion . . . . .99
25  Carotid Artery Fibromuscular Dysplasia . . . . . . . . . 102
26  Carotid Artery Dissection . . . . . . . . . . . . . . . . 105
27  Carotid Artery Aneurysm . . . . . . . . . . . . . . . . 108
28  Carotid Artery Traumatic Injuries. . . . . . . . . . . . . 111

## PART 4

## ANEURYSMAL DISEASE

29  Endovascular Aneurysm Repair . . . . . . . . . . . . . . . . .118
30  Endovascular Abdominal Aortic Aneurysm Repair for Ruptured Abdominal Aortic Aneurysm . . . . . . . . . . . . . 122
31  Thoracic and Thoracoabdominal Aneurysms: Open Repair . . . . . . . . . . . . . . . . . . . . . . . . .125
32  Thoracic Endovascular Aneurysm Repair . . . . . . . . . . .130
33  Femoropopliteal Aneurysms . . . . . . . . . . . . . . . 133
34  Arterial Pseudoaneurysms . . . . . . . . . . . . . . . . 137
35  Mycotic Aneurysmal Disease . . . . . . . . . . . . . . . 141
36  Vascular Ehlers-Danlos Syndrome. . . . . . . . . . . . . 144
37  Marfan Syndrome . . . . . . . . . . . . . . . . . . . . 149
38  Loeys Dietz Syndrome and Related Disorders . . . . . . . . 155

## PART 5

## NON-ATHEROSCLEROTIC DISORDERS

39  Popliteal Artery Entrapment Syndrome. . . . . . . . . . . . 160
40  Iliac Artery Endofibrosis . . . . . . . . . . . . . . . . . 163
41  Klippel-Trenaunay Syndrome. . . . . . . . . . . . . . . 168
42  Congenital Arteriovenous Malformations. . . . . . . . . . . 172

## PART 6

## ARTERIAL & VENOUS VISCERAL DISEASE

43  Atherosclerotic Renal Artery Stenosis . . . . . . . . . . . . 182
44  Fibromuscular Dysplasia–Associated Renal Artery Stenosis . . . . . . . . . . . . . . . . . . 187
45  Acute Mesenteric Ischemia . . . . . . . . . . . . . . . . 193
46  Celiac Axis Compression Syndrome . . . . . . . . . . . . 199
47  Chronic Mesenteric Ischemia . . . . . . . . . . . . . . . 202
48  Budd-Chiari Syndrome . . . . . . . . . . . . . . . . . 212
49  Splenic Vein Thrombosis . . . . . . . . . . . . . . . . . 215
50  Mesenteric Venous Thrombosis . . . . . . . . . . . . . . 219

## PART 7

## VENOUS DISEASES

51  Acute Superficial Venous Thrombosis: Evaluation and Treatment . . . . . . . . . . . . . . . . . . . 226
52  Evaluation and Treatment of Calf Vein Thrombosis. . . . . . 230
53  Medical Management of Femoropopliteal Deep Venous Thrombosis . . . . . . . . . . . . . . . . . . . 235
54  Percutaneous Endovenous Intervention in Femoropopliteal Deep Venous Thrombosis . . . . . . . . . . 243
55  May-Thurner Syndrome . . . . . . . . . . . . . . . . . 251
56  Paget-Schroetter Syndrome . . . . . . . . . . . . . . . . 255
57  Benign Acute Blue Finger . . . . . . . . . . . . . . . . . 259

# CONTENTS

58 Phlegmasia Cerulea Dolens . . . . . . . . . . . . . . . . . . . . . 263

59 Panniculitis . . . . . . . . . . . . . . . . . . . . . . . . . . . . . . . . 269

60 Stasis Dermatitis. . . . . . . . . . . . . . . . . . . . . . . . . . . . . 275

61 Pseudo-Kaposi Sarcoma (Acroangiodermatitis). . . . . . . . 279

62 Heparin-, Low–Molecular Weight Heparin–,
and Warfarin-Induced Skin Necrosis . . . . . . . . . . . . . . . 283

63 Overview of Spider, Reticular, and Varicose Veins . . . . . . 288

64 Sclerotherapy. . . . . . . . . . . . . . . . . . . . . . . . . . . . . . . . 293

65 Endovenous Laser Ablation for Varicose Veins . . . . . . . . . 296

## PART 8

## LIMB SWELLING

66 Primary and Secondary Lymphedema . . . . . . . . . . . . . . . 302

67 Lower Extremity Cellulitis . . . . . . . . . . . . . . . . . . . . . . 307

68 Leg Swelling Secondary to Muscle Rupture . . . . . . . . . . . 312

69 Pretibial Myxedema . . . . . . . . . . . . . . . . . . . . . . . . . . . 316

70 Lipedema . . . . . . . . . . . . . . . . . . . . . . . . . . . . . . . . . . 321

71 Lipolymphedema . . . . . . . . . . . . . . . . . . . . . . . . . . . . 327

72 Phlebolymphedema . . . . . . . . . . . . . . . . . . . . . . . . . . . 333

73 Factitial Edema. . . . . . . . . . . . . . . . . . . . . . . . . . . . . . 337

## PART 9

## VASOSPASTIC AND VASCULITIC DISEASES

74 Raynaud Phenomenon. . . . . . . . . . . . . . . . . . . . . . . . . 342

75 Livedo Reticularis and Livedo Racemosa . . . . . . . . . . . . . 348

76 Acrocyanosis . . . . . . . . . . . . . . . . . . . . . . . . . . . . . . . 353

77 ANCA-Negative Small Vessel Vasculitis. . . . . . . . . . . . . . 358

78 Granulomatosis with Polyangiitis (Wegener) . . . . . . . . . . 364

79 Microscopic Polyangiitis . . . . . . . . . . . . . . . . . . . . . . . 368

80 Churg-Strauss Syndrome (Eosinophilic Granulomatosis
with Polyangiitis) . . . . . . . . . . . . . . . . . . . . . . . . . . . . 372

81 Polyarteritis Nodosa . . . . . . . . . . . . . . . . . . . . . . . . . . 376

82 Thromboangiitis Obliterans (Buerger Disease) . . . . . . . . . 381

83 Giant Cell and Takayasu Arteritis . . . . . . . . . . . . . . . . . 384

84 Behçet Syndrome . . . . . . . . . . . . . . . . . . . . . . . . . . . . 391

85 Nephrogenic Systemic Fibrosis . . . . . . . . . . . . . . . . . . . 398

## PART 10

## ENVIRONMENTAL DISEASES

86 Frostbite . . . . . . . . . . . . . . . . . . . . . . . . . . . . . . . . . . 404

87 Pernio. . . . . . . . . . . . . . . . . . . . . . . . . . . . . . . . . . . . 407

88 Immersion Foot Syndrome . . . . . . . . . . . . . . . . . . . . . . 410

89 Erythromelalgia . . . . . . . . . . . . . . . . . . . . . . . . . . . . . 414

90 Erythema AB Igne . . . . . . . . . . . . . . . . . . . . . . . . . . . . 418

## PART 11

## LIMB ULCERATIONS

91 Venous Stasis Ulceration . . . . . . . . . . . . . . . . . . . . . . . 422

92 Arterial Ulcerations . . . . . . . . . . . . . . . . . . . . . . . . . . . 425

93 Neuropathic Ulceration. . . . . . . . . . . . . . . . . . . . . . . . 430

94 Pyoderma Gangrenosum . . . . . . . . . . . . . . . . . . . . . . . 435

95 Necrobiosis Lipoidica and Diabetic Dermopathy . . . . . . . 440

96 Calciphylaxis . . . . . . . . . . . . . . . . . . . . . . . . . . . . . . . 445

Appendix. . . . . . . . . . . . . . . . . . . . . . . . . . . . . . . . . . . . . 449

Index. . . . . . . . . . . . . . . . . . . . . . . . . . . . . . . . . . . . . . . . 455

**Scott P. Albert, MD**
Assistant Professor of Surgery
Department of Surgery
Division of Hepatobiliary Surgery
Upstate Medical University
Syracuse, NY

**Lana Alghothani, MD**
Department of Internal Medicine
The Ohio State University Wexner Medical Center
Columbus, OH

**Georgann Anetakis Poulos, MD**
Fellow
Department of Dermatology
University of Pittsburgh Medical Center
Pittsburgh, PA

**A. George Akingba, MD, PhD**
Assistant Professor
Surgery and Biomedical Engineering Department of Surgery
Division of Vascular Surgery
Indiana University School of Medicine
Indianapolis, IN

**Clint Allred, MD**
Department of Internal Medicine
The Ohio State University Wexner Medical Center
Columbus, OH

**Stacy P. Ardoin, MD, MS**
Division of Rheumatology and Immunology
The Ohio State University Wexner Medical Center
Columbus, OH

**W. David Arnold, MD**
Assistant Professor
Departments of Neurology and PM&R
Division of Neuromuscular Medicine
The Ohio State University Wexner Medical Center
Columbus, OH

**Benjamin J. Aumiller, MS, MD**
Section of Vascular Surgery
Indiana University School of Medicine
IU-Methodist Hospital
Indianapolis, IN

**Faisal Aziz, MD, RVT, RPVI**
Assistant Professor
Department of Surgery
Division of Vascular Surgery
Pennsylvania State University College of Medicine
Hershey, PA

**Shalene Badhan, MD**
Division of Rheumatology and Immunology
The Ohio State University Wexner Medical Center
Columbus, OH

**John R. Bartholomew, MD, FACC, MSVM**
Professor of Medicine, Cleveland Clinic Lerner College of Medicine
Section Head, Vascular Medicine
Robert and Suzanne Tomsich Department of Cardiovascular
    Medicine
Cleveland Clinic
Cleveland, OH

**Joshua A. Beckman, MD, MS**
Cardiovascular Division Brigham and Women's Hospital
Harvard Medical School
Boston, MA

**Peter M. Bittenbender, MD**
Department of Internal Medicine
Division of Cardiovascular Medicine
The Ohio State University Wexner Medical Center
Columbus, OH

**Mark Bloomston, MD**
Associate Professor of Surgery
Department of Surgery
Division of Surgical Oncology
The Ohio State University Wexner Medical Center
Columbus, OH

**Thomas E. Brothers, MD**
Department of Surgery
Medical University of South Carolina
Charleston, SC

**Nicole C. Bundy, MD, MPH**
Division of Rheumatology
Department of Internal Medicine
The Ohio State University Wexner Medical Center
Columbus, OH

**Teresa L. Carman, MD**
Department of Medicine
Division of Cardiovascular Medicine
University Hospitals Case Medical Center
Assistant Professor of Medicine
Case Western Reserve University School of Medicine
Cleveland, OH

**Marissa J. Carter, MA, PhD**
President
Strategic Solutions, Inc.
Cody, WY

**Ana Casanegra, MD**
Assistant Professor
Vascular Medicine Program
Cardiovascular Section
Department of Internal Medicine
University of Oklahoma Health Sciences Center
Oklahoma City, OK

**Stephen L. Chastain, MD, RVT**
Medicine Fellow
Greenville Hospital System Vascular Health Alliance
Greenville, SC

**Shane Clark, MD**
Dermatology Resident
The Ohio State University Wexner Medical Center
Gahanna, OH

**Mark Crandall, MD**
Department of Internal Medicine
Department of Cardiovascular Medicine
The Ohio State University Wexner Medical Center
Columbus, OH

**Kevin P. Cohoon, DO, MSc**
Department of Internal Medicine
Fellow, Division of Cardiovascular Disease
Mayo Clinic
Rochester, MN

**Anthony J. Comerota, MD, FACS, FACC**
Director, Jobst Vascular Institute
Toledo, OH
Adjunct Professor of Surgery
University of Michigan
Ann Arbor, MI

**Michael C. Dalsing, MD**
E. Dale and Susan E. Habegger Professor of Surgery
Director of Vascular Surgery
Division of Vascular Surgery
Department of Surgery
Indiana University School of Medicine
Indianapolis, IN

**Michael Davis, MD, FSVM**
Assistant Professor of Internal Medicine
Department of Internal Medicine
Division of Cardiovascular Medicine
The Ohio State University Wexner Medical Center
Columbus, OH

**Steven M. Dean, DO, FACP, RPVI**
Associate Professor of Clinical Medicine
The Ohio State University Wexner Medical Center
Columbus, OH

**Sapan S. Desai, MD, PhD**
Assistant Professor
Department of Surgery
Duke University Medical Center
Durham, NC

**Essa M. Essa, MBBS**
Department of Internal Medicine
Division of Cardiovascular Medicine
The Ohio State University Wexner Medical Center
Columbus, OH

**Borzoo Farhang, DO, MS**
Clinical Instructor
University of Vermont School of Medicine
Fletcher Allen Medical Center
Department of Anesthesiology
Fletcher Allen Health Care
Burlington, VT

**Caroline E. Fife, MD**
Medical Director
St. Luke's Wound Center
The Woodlands, TX

**John H. Fish III, MD, FSVM, RPVI**
Aurora Cardiovascular Services
The Vascular Center at St. Luke's Medical Center
Milwaukee, WI

**Jonathan Forquer, DO**
Department of Internal Medicine
Division of Cardiovascular Medicine
University of Cincinnati
Cincinnati, OH

**Miriam L. Freimer, MD**
Associate Professor and Clinical Vice Chair
Department of Neurology
The Ohio State University Wexner Medical Center
Columbus, OH

**Nitin Garg, MBSS, MPH**
Department of Surgery & Radiology
Division of Vascular Surgery
Medical University of South Carolina
Ralph H. Johnson VA Medical Center
Charleston, SC

**Michael R. Go, MD**
Assistant Professor of Surgery
Department of Surgery
Division of Vascular Diseases and Surgery
The Ohio State University Wexner Medical Center
Columbus, OH

**Christopher J. Goltz, MD**
Vascular Surgery Fellow
Department of Surgery
Division of Vascular Surgery
Indiana University School of Medicine
Indianapolis, IN

**NavYash Gupta, MD, FACS**
Chief, Division of Vascular Surgery
NorthShore University HealthSystem
Clinical Associate Professor, Department of Surgery
University of Chicago Pritzker School of Medicine
Skokie, IL

**Joseph Habib, MD**
Vascular Surgery Fellow
Division of Vascular Diseases and Surgery
Department of Surgery
The Ohio State University Wexner Medical Center
Columbus, OH

**Rula A. Hajj-Ali, MD**
Assistant Professor of Medicine
Department of Rheumatic and Immunologic Diseases
Center for Vasculitis Care and Research
Cleveland Clinic, OH

**Katya L. Harfmann, MD**
Resident
Department of Internal Medicine
Division of Dermatology
The Ohio State University College of Medicine
Columbus, OH

**Mounir J. Haurani, MD**
Assistant Professor of Clinical Surgery
Division of Vascular Diseases and Surgery
Department of Surgery
The Ohio State University Wexner Medical Center
Columbus, OH

**Travis Hubbuch, DPM**
Resident, Department of Orthopedic Surgery
Cleveland Clinic
Cleveland, OH

**Stephanie Jacks, MD**
Dermatology Resident
The Ohio State University Wexner Medical Center
Gahanna, OH

**Michael R. Jaff, DO**
Department of Vascular Medicine
Division of Cardiovascular Medicine
Massachusetts General Hospital
Boston, MA

**Wael N. Jarjour, MD, FACP**
Associate Professor of Medicine
Division of Rheumatology and Immunology
The Ohio State University Wexner Medical Center
Columbus, OH

**Benjamin H. Kaffenberger, MD**
Chief Resident
Division of Dermatology
The Ohio State University Wexner Medical Center
Columbus, OH

**Vikram S. Kashyap, MD**
Professor of Surgery
Case Western Reserve University School of Medicine
Chief, Division of Vascular Surgery and Endovascular Therapy
Department of Surgery
University Hospitals Case Medical Center
Cleveland, OH

**Tanaz A. Kermani, MD, MS**
Assistant Clinical Professor
David Geffen School of Medicine
Department of Medicine
Division of Rheumatology
University of California
Los Angeles, CA

**Raghu Kolluri, MD, FACP, FSVM**
Director, Vascular Medicine and Vascular Laboratories
Prairie Cardiovascular Consultants
Springfield, IL

**Andrew K. Kurklinsky, MD, RPVI, FSVM**
Assistant Professor of Medicine
Division of Cardiovascular Medicine
Mayo Clinic
Jacksonville, FL

**James Laredo, MD, PhD**
Associate Professor
Department of Surgery
Division of Vascular Surgery
George Washington University Medical Center
Washington, DC

**Byung Boong Lee, MD, PhD**
Clinical Professor
Department of Surgery
Division of Vascular Surgery
George Washington University Medical Center
Washington, DC

**Gary W. Lemmon, MD**
Professor of Surgery
Department of Surgery
Division of Vascular Surgery
Indiana University School of Medicine
Indianapolis, IN

**Maria E. Litzendorf, MD**
Assistant Professor of Surgery
Division of Vascular Diseases and Surgery
The Ohio State University Wexner Medical Center
Columbus, OH

**Robert Lookstein, MD, FSIR, FAHA**
Associate Professor of Radiology and Surgery
Chief, Division of Interventional Radiology
Mount Sinai Medical Center
New York, NY

**Michael Maier, DPM**
Department of Cardiovascular Medicine
Division of Vascular Medicine
Cleveland Clinic
Cleveland, OH

**Ashima Makol, MD**
Division of Rheumatology,
Mayo Clinic,
Rochester, MN

**Julie E. Mangino, MD**
Professor of Internal Medicine
Medical Director, Department of Clinical Epidemiology
Division of Infectious Diseases
The Ohio State University Wexner Medical Center
Columbus, OH

**Angela H. Martin, MD**
General Surgery Resident
Department of General Surgery
Indiana University School of Medicine
Indianapolis, IN

**Sheryl Mascarenhas, MD**
Division of Rheumatology and Immunology
The Ohio State University Wexner Medical Center
Columbus, OH

**Ali Mehdi, MD**
Department of Internal Medicine
Cleveland Clinic, OH

**Ari J. Mintz, DO**
Resident
Department of Internal Medicine
Clinical Associate in Medicine
Tufts University School of Medicine
Lahey Hospital and Medical Center
Burlington, MA

**Bruce Mintz, DO, FSVM**
Clinical Associate Professor
Internal Medicine
Rutgers New Jersey Medical School
Director Vascular Technology Training Program
Newark , NJ

**Rocio Moran, MD, FACMG**
Medical Director, General Genetics Clinics
Center for Personalized Genetic Healthcare
Genomic Medicine Institute
Cleveland Clinic Foundation
Cleveland, OH

**Raghu Motaganahalli, MD, FRCS, FACS**
Assistant Professor-Program Director
Department of Surgery
Section of Vascular Surgery
Indiana University School of Medicine
Indianapolis, IN

**Eric Mowatt-Larssen, MD**
Assistant Professor
Division of Vascular Surgery
Duke University Medical Center
Durham, NC

**Alan Nadour, MD, FSVM**
Prairie Cardiovascular Consultants
Springfield, IL

**John Anthony O'Dea, MD**
Department of Medicine
Division of Vascular Medicine and Intervention
Massachusett's General Hospital
Boston, MA

**Luigi Pascarella, MD**
Department of Surgery
Division of Vascular Surgery
Duke University Medical Center
Durham, NC

**David H. Pfizenmaier II, MD, DPM**
Consultant, Vascular Medicine
Cardiovascular Diseases
Mayo Clinic
Rochester, MN

**Jason Prosek, MD**
Clinical Instructor/House Staff
Department of Internal Medicine
Division of Nephrology
The Ohio State University Wexner Medical Center
Columbus, OH

**Daniel J. Reddy, MD**
Professor of Surgery, Wayne State University
J.D. Dingell VA Medical Center
Detroit, MI

**Suman Rathbun, MD**
Professor
Vascular Medicine Program
Cardiovascular Section
Department of Internal Medicine
University of Oklahoma Health Sciences Center
Oklahoma City, OK

**Christina Rigelsky, MS, CGC**
Certified Genetic Counselor
Genomic Medicine Institute
Lerner Research Institute
Cleveland Clinic
Cleveland, OH

**Thom W. Rooke, MD, FSVM**
Department of Vascular Medicine
Division of Cardiovascular Diseases
Mayo Clinic
Rochester, MN

Irving L. Rosenberg, MD
Department of Internal Medicine
Division of Rheumatology and Immunology
The Ohio State University Wexner Medical Center
Columbus, OH

Jean M. Ruddy, MD
Department of Surgery
Medical University of South Carolina
Charleston, SC

Satish K. Sarvepalli, MD, MPH
Fellow
Department of Internal Medicine
Division of Infectious Diseases
The Ohio State University Wexner Medical Center
Columbus, OH

Bhagwan Satiani, MD, MBA, RPVI, FACS
Professor of Clinical Surgery
Medical Director, Vascular Laboratories, OSU Heart &
    Vascular Center
Director Faculty Leadership Institute
Division of Vascular Diseases & Surgery
Department of Surgery
The Ohio State University Wexner Medical Center
Columbus, OH

Adil Sattar, MD
Department of Internal Medicine
SIU School of Medicine
Residency Office
Springfield, IL

Robert M. Schainfeld, DO, FSVM, FSCAI
Department of Vascular Medicine
Division of Cardiovascular Medicine
Massachusetts General Hospital
Boston, MA

Irina Shakhnovich, MD
Department of Surgery
Division of Vascular Surgery
Medical College of Wisconsin
Milwaukee, WI

Mohsen Sharifi, MD, FACC, FSCAI, FSVM
Director, Arizona Cardiovascular Consultants & Vein Clinic
Adjunct Professor, A.T.Still University
Mesa, AZ

Aditya M. Sharma, MD, RPVI
Assistant Professor of Medicine
Cardiovascular Division
University of Virginia School of Medicine
Charlottesville, VA

Sachin Sheth, MD
Clinical Fellow
Division of Interventional Radiology
Mount Sinai Medical Center
New York, NY

Lawrence A. Shirley, MD
Surgical Oncology Fellow
Department of Surgery
Division of Surgical Oncology
The Ohio State University Wexner Medical Center
Columbus, OH

Cynthia K. Shortell, MD, FACS
Department of Surgery
Division of Vascular Surgery
Duke University Medical Center
Durham, NC

Mitchell Silver, DO, FACC, FSVM
Director, Center for Critical Limb Care
Riverside Methodist Hospital
Columbus, OH

Marcus D. Stanbro, DO, FSVM, RPVI
Assistant Professor of Clinical Surgery
Department of Surgery
Division of Vascular Surgery
Greenville Health System
Greenville, SC

Jean Starr, MD, FACS, RPVI
Associate Professor of Clinical Surgery
Division of Vascular Diseases and Surgery
Department of Surgery
The Ohio State University Wexner Medical Center
Columbus, OH

Shankar M. Sundaram, MD, FACS, FCCP
Harrison Health Partners
Thoracic and Vascular Surgery
Bremerton, WA

Axel Thors, DO
Department of Surgery
Division of Vascular Diseases and Surgery
The Ohio State University Wexner Medical Center
Columbus, OH

Nikos Tsekouras, MD
Jobst Vascular Institute
Toledo, OH

Christopher Valentine, MD
Assistant Professor of Clinical Medicine
Department of Internal Medicine
Division of Nephrology
The Ohio State University Wexner Medical Center
Columbus, OH

# CONTRIBUTORS

**Marcelo P. Villa-Forte Gomes, MD, FSVM**
Program Director, Vascular Medicine Fellowship
Department of Cardiovascular Medicine
Division of Vascular Medicine
Cleveland Clinic
Cleveland, OH

**John C. Wang, MD, MSc**
Assistant Professor of Surgery
Case Western Reserve University School of Medicine
Department of Surgery
Division of Vascular Surgery and Endovascular Therapy
University Hospitals Case Medical Center
Cleveland, OH

**Kenneth J Warrington, MD**
Associate Professor of Medicine
Department of Medicine
Division of Rheumatology
Mayo Clinic
Rochester, MN

**Ido Weinberg, MD**
Department of Vascular Medicine
Division of Cardiovascular Medicine
Massachusetts General Hospital
Boston, MA

Vascular diseases involving the arterial, venous, and lymphatic systems are becoming increasingly common commensurate with the aging population. Inexplicably, the proper identification and therapy of these myriad disease states is unfortunately not typically included in the education of neither the medical student nor the resident. Thus, most practicing physicians are not prepared to accurately diagnose and manage affected patients.

Consequently, we have constructed the *Color Atlas and Synopsis of Vascular Diseases* to enable medical students, postgraduate physician trainees, and practicing clinicians to rapidly assimilate information on a wide variety of vascular-related topics. The book integrates the fields of vascular medicine, vascular surgery, and endovascular therapy in an "easy to learn" fashion. Ninety-six chapters are presented in a unique format of succinct, bulleted teaching points combined with multiple singular photographs of vascular pathology. When appropriate, vivid arteriographic and ultrasonographic images are included as well.

Since the text is clinically oriented, concise, and current, we feel that you will not only derive practical and useful knowledge, but also thoroughly enjoy perusing this compilation.

Steven M. Dean and Bhagwan Satiani

I'd like to acknowledge the following people who either directly or indirectly assisted in bringing this book to fruition: My former mentors at the Cleveland Clinic Foundation (Drs Jess Young, Jeff Olin, John Bartholomew, and William Ruschhaupt) for their incredible teaching of the principles of Vascular Medicine; my co-editor Dr. Bhagwan Satiani—he is both a true scholar and friend; proof editor Sapna Rastogi as she somehow consistently managed to keep this project on time and accurately edited; my good friends and colleagues (Thompson, Baldwin, Vasquez, Olminator, Stanbro, and DTY) at Readership Central for their daily wisdom and unbelievable wit; the Series Editor, Dr. Bill Abraham—thanks for allowing me to complete this project and for your unyielding support!

Steven M. Dean

Thanks are due to my friend and hard-working co-editor Steven M. Dean, my faculty in the Division of Vascular Diseases and Surgery at Ohio State for contributing immensely to the atlas, to all the authors who submitted their excellent work on time and to the folks at McGraw-Hill and the very persistent Sapna Rastogi!

Bhagwan Satiani

## PART 1

# LOWER EXTREMITIES: MISCELLANEOUS DISEASES

# 1 AORTOILIAC DISEASE: OCCLUSION

Mounir J. Haurani, MD

## PATIENT STORY

A 60-year-old woman with hypertension and a 40 pack-year smoking history presented to the emergency department with acute onset of right leg numbness and pallor. She also related long-standing burning and cramping in her hips and buttocks after walking about 50 yd. She had difficulty climbing stairs because she felt extremely weak after walking up 2 to 3 stairs.

On examination she had no palpable pulses in her lower extremities, including the femoral arteries. She had monophasic signals via a Doppler probe in her femoral and pedal arteries. Her skin envelope over both feet was intact, and she had normal motor function in both feet. Her right foot was slightly cooler than the left. She was started on heparin and admitted for further management of her acute and chronic presentation of peripheral vascular disease.

## EPIDEMIOLOGY

### Aortoiliac Occlusive Disease

*   Often found in conjunction with multilevel disease involving the femoropopliteal or infrageniculate arteries.
*   Patients with isolated aortoiliac occlusive disease (AIOD) tend to be younger with a significant smoking history and hypercholesterolemia.[1]
*   Patients with multilevel disease are older, diabetic, and hypertensive.[1]
*   A particularly aggressive form of AIOD is seen in younger female patients who are smokers, in that they have not only the occlusive disease but small or hypoplastic aortoiliac segments. These patients tend to fare worse because the durability of their repair is compromised due to the small arteries.[2]

## ETIOLOGY AND PATHOLOGY

AIOD, like many other forms of vascular disease, begins at branch points where the laminar flow is disrupted and turbulence arises.

*   This occurs at the aortic bifurcation and origins of the common iliac arteries.
*   Thrombosis or extension of the disease typically progresses in retrograde fashion into the aorta and the contralateral iliac.[3]

It is rare for patients with multilevel disease to have involvement of the visceral segment of the aorta or the renal arteries, and simultaneous procedures are rarely needed during lower extremity revascularization.

If the onset of thrombosis is gradual, collateralization is possible, and therefore the limb ischemia symptoms are not as dramatic as those with acute aortoiliac occlusion. Sources of collateralization include

*   Lumbar arteries via the circumflex iliac into the femoral, and profunda arteries (Figure 1-1).

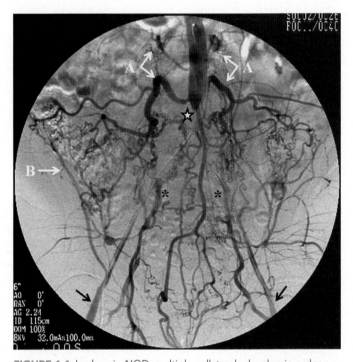

**FIGURE 1-1** In chronic AIOD, multiple collaterals develop in order to provide perfusion to the lower extremities. In this patient there is occlusion of the aorta and bilateral common iliac arteries just below a pair of large lumbar arteries (A). The superior pair of lumbar arteries is normal sized compared to the inferior pair. Collaterals from the lumbar arteries are one of many that provide blood flow to the lower extremities in AIOD (B). The black arrows designate the common femoral arteries as they are reconstituted by collaterals, and the asterisks (∗) indicate the origins of the internal iliac artery. These are filled in a retrograde fashion from the collateral flow in the femoral arteries as well as by pelvic collaterals from the IMA (white star) and lumbar arteries.

- Internal mammary artery, which continues as the inferior epigastric artery into the femoral artery.
- Superior mesenteric artery continues into the inferior mesenteric artery (IMA) and hemorrhoidal artery pathway via the arc of Riolan and the meandering mesenteric artery.
- All of these collaterals are important sources of flow to the lower extremity and should be preserved during interventions[4] (Figure 1-2).

## DIAGNOSIS

History and physical examination in a patient with vascular risk factors who complains of hip, buttock, and thigh claudication should raise suspicion. The physical examination finding of absent femoral pulses all but confirms the diagnosis. However, the symptoms associated with arthritis or degenerative lumbar disk disease or spinal stenosis can sometimes present in a similar fashion. In practice it is not always easy to separate these patients from patients with AIOD. Patients with combined AIOD and infrainguinal disease may present exclusively with calf claudication. In addition, without complete occlusion, palpable femoral and even pedal pulses may be detectable at rest and only become diminished after exercise.

Noninvasive physiologic arterial testing or segmental systolic blood pressure measurements and pulse volume recordings can confirm the disease. A greater than 20 to 30 mm Hg difference between the brachial pressure and the high thigh measurement may suggest the presence of AIOD. Because patients with disabling symptoms occasionally demonstrate ankle-brachial indices (ABIs) close to normal, it is important to repeat the pressure measurements following treadmill exercise test.

## IMAGING

### Duplex Ultrasound

- Is time-consuming and requires a dedicated vascular laboratory technician in order to obtain useful information.
- In patients with renal insufficiency it may be a useful definitive diagnostic test in order to avoid contrast use.
- In the absence of vascular laboratory experience in this technique, it is difficult to plan an operative approach based on duplex ultrasound alone.

### Axial Imaging With CT Scan or MRA

- Is highly sensitive and produces adequate data in order to plan the level and extent of repair.
- Axial imaging has replaced conventional angiography in many hospitals.
- Catheter-directed arteriography continues to play an important role in AIOD because it is useful for diagnosis and can also allow for treatment.

## TREATMENT OPTIONS

### Open Repair

Open repair involves replacement of the diseased portion of the aorta. This can be done in an end-to-end fashion or an end-to-side

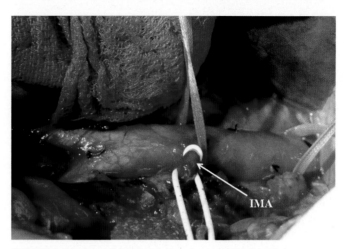

**FIGURE 1-2** A large inferior mesenteric artery (IMA) is often encountered in patients with chronic AIOD. Notice that the aortic bifurcation is whitish colored in comparison to the more proximal (right side of image) aorta due to the heavy calcification.

fashion. Iliac stenting and endovascular repair options will be discussed in a separate chapter.

### End-to-End Anastomosis

- Allows for thromboendarterectomy of the proximal stump and in-line flow.
- This approach is needed when there is a concurrent aneurysm of the aorta allowing for replacement of the aneurysm as well as treatment of the AIOD.

### End-to-Side Anastomosis (Figure 1-3)

- Advantageous when the external iliac arteries are occluded but there is flow into the internal iliac arteries, thus preserving pelvic circulation.
- Large IMAs can be preserved in this configuration as an important source of collateral flow (Figure 1-2).

In either repair, the distal anastomosis is made onto the common femoral artery and onto the origin of the profunda femoral artery. This improves graft patency because the profunda femoral arteries are an important outflow source and provide collaterals to the popliteal artery even if there is concurrent superficial femoral artery (SFA) occlusion (Figure 1-4).

### RESULTS

Both the short- and long-term results of aortobifemoral (ABF) grafting are excellent. Several large series demonstrate 5-year patency rates of 95% and 10-year rates between 85% and 90%. Perioperative mortality rates have been reported to be as low as 1%, and 30-day mortality rates are 1% to 4%.

### EARLY COMPLICATIONS

Morbidity rates range from 17% to 32%.

- Cardiac complications are the most common cause of morbidity resulting from fluid shifts during the postoperative period. About 1% to 5% of patients will have a myocardial infarction.
- Risk factors for pulmonary complications (pneumonia) include elderly age, chronic obstructive pulmonary disease (COPD), smoking history, and poor preoperative nutritional status. These complications may be prevented with adequate postoperative pulmonary toilet and diuresis. Pneumonia occurs in fewer than 7% of patients.
- Other complications include hemorrhage (1%-2%), renal failure (<5%), acute limb ischemia (1%-3%), bowel ischemia (2%), wound complications (3%-15%), sexual dysfunction (≤25%), ureteral injury (<1%), and spinal cord ischemia (0.25%).

### LATE COMPLICATIONS

Late complications are rare, with graft thrombosis being the most common in 5% to 30% of patients. It is rare for the entire graft to occlude, and usually it is a limb. It is most easily diagnosed by loss of a femoral pulse in the affected side with return of symptoms in that leg.

Other complications that may occur include

- Graft infection (0.5%-3%), diagnosed by CT scan or nuclear imaging. The groin is the usual source of infection. Explantation is almost always required.

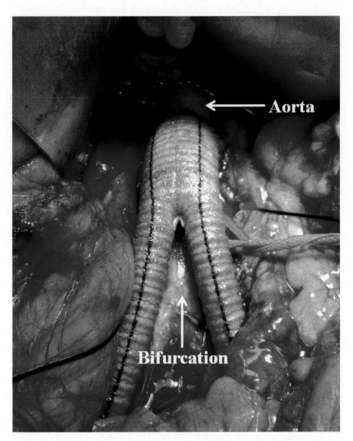

FIGURE 1-3 In patients with patent internal iliac arteries or a large IMA and lumbar arteries with collaterals to the lower extremities, an end-to-side anastomosis, as shown in the figure, is preferable. It allows for retrograde filling of the pelvic arteries as well as preservation of collaterals important for perfusing the lower extremities.

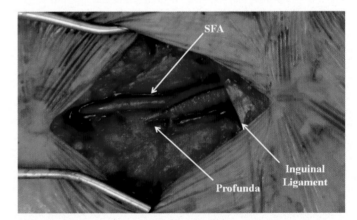

FIGURE 1-4 The distal anastomosis of the bypass graft is fashioned so that it tunnels beneath the inguinal ligament. The hood of the graft is sewn to the common femoral artery and terminates onto the profunda femoral artery as depicted in the figure.

- Aortoenteric fistula (<3%) most commonly involves erosion of the proximal aortic suture line through the third or fourth portion of the duodenum. It may also present as erosion of the iliac anastomosis into the small bowel or colon. The diagnosis is made with a combination of CT scanning, endoscopy, and angiography. Practitioners need to be wary of the self-limited "herald bleed." Treatment is essentially the same as that for infected grafts and requires explantation.

- Anastomotic pseudoaneurysms (1%-5%) are less commonly seen in the modern era as different suture materials have been used. They are most likely related to progression of atherosclerosis, infection, or weakening of the suture lines or graft material. Treatment with debridement and replacement of the graft is indicated for those that are greater than 2 cm in the groin, or greater than 50% of the graft diameter in the aortic portion.

## FOLLOW-UP

- There are no standardized practice guidelines for patient follow-up after ABF bypass. Patients are usually discharged when they are ambulatory and tolerating a diet.

- They are seen at 2 to 3 weeks for suture removal and a wound check. At that time the physical examination is the most useful tool in the diagnosis of complications.

- The patient should be followed yearly thereafter with an ABI and physical examination to assess for femoral pulses.

- History will reveal if there is any recurrence of symptoms indicative of either worsening of infrainguinal disease or stenosis of the femoral anastomosis.

- Return of symptoms or a decrease in the ABIs is an indication for repeat angiography or axial imaging.

## REFERENCES

1. Darling RC, Brewster DC, Hallett JW, Jr., Darling RC, 3rd. Aorto-iliac reconstruction. *Surg Clin North Am.* Aug 1979;59(4): 565-579.

2. Cronenwett JL, Davis JT, Jr., Gooch JB, Garrett HE. Aortoiliac occlusive disease in women. *Surgery.* Dec 1980;88(6):775-784.

3. Leriche R, Morel A. The syndrome of thrombotic obliteration of the aortic bifurcation. *Ann Surg.* Feb 1948;127(2):193-206.

4. Krupski WC, Sumchai A, Effeney DJ, Ehrenfeld WK. The importance of abdominal wall collateral blood vessels. Planning incisions and obtaining arteriography. *Arch Surg.* Jul 1984;119(7):854-857.

# 2 AORTOILIAC OCCLUSIVE DISEASE: TREATMENT WITH STENTING

Jean Starr, MD, FACS, RPVI

## PATIENT STORY

A 67-year-old man presented with a history of right hip and buttock claudication at one block distance for the past year. Over the past several days, however, he had new onset of numbness in the right foot. There was no right femoral pulse on physical examination, but he had normal motor and sensory function. He was actively smoking with a history of hypertension and coronary artery disease. An ankle-brachial index (ABI) with waveforms was performed; it showed a monophasic right ankle waveform with an ABI of 0.56 (Figure 2-1).

An angiogram was performed that illustrated a right common iliac occlusion with reconstitution of the external iliac artery (Trans-Atlantic Intersociety Consensus [TASC] class B lesion) (Figure 2-2) at the takeoff of the internal iliac artery (Figure 2-3). It was believed to be an acute occlusion of a chronic stenosis. The lesion was crossed using an antegrade and retrograde approach (Figure 2-4), and primary stenting was completed (Figure 2-5). The patient symptomatically improved immediately, as did his noninvasive testing results (Figure 2-6), and his claudication had resolved by his follow-up visit.

**PREPROCEDURE ABI**

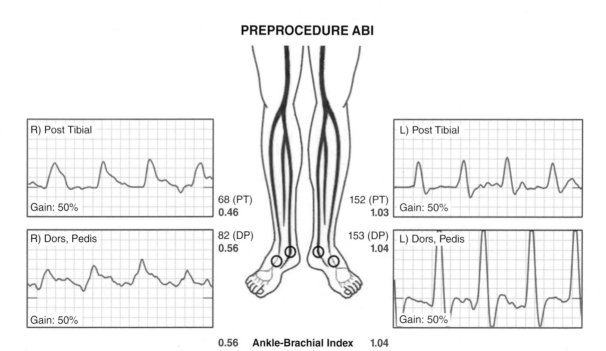

| R) Post Tibial | | 68 (PT) | 152 (PT) | L) Post Tibial |
| Gain: 50% | | **0.46** | **1.03** | Gain: 50% |
| R) Dors, Pedis | | 82 (DP) | 153 (DP) | L) Dors, Pedis |
| Gain: 50% | | **0.56** | **1.04** | Gain: 50% |

0.56    **Ankle-Brachial Index**    1.04

**FIGURE 2-1** Preprocedure ankle-brachial index with monophasic right ankle waveform.

| Type A lesions | • Unilateral or bilateral stenosis of CIA<br>• Unilateral or bilateral single short (<3 cm) stenosis of EIA |
|---|---|
| Type B lesions | • Short (<3 cm) stenosis of infrarenal aorta<br>• Unilateral CIA occlusion<br>• Single or multiple stenoses totaling 3–10 cm involving the EIA, not extending into the CFA<br>• Unilateral EIA occlusion not involving the origins of internal iliac or CFA |
| Type C lesions | • Bilateral CIA occlusions<br>• Bilateral EIA stenosis 3–10 cm long not extending into the CFA<br>• Unilateral EIA stenosis extending into the CFA<br>• Unilateral EIA occlusion that involves the origins of the internal iliac and/or CFA<br>• Heavily calcified unilateral EIA occlusion with or without involvement of origins of internal iliac and/or CFA |
| Type D lesions | • Infrarenal aortoiliac occlusion<br>• Diffuse disease involving the aorta and both iliac arteries, requiring treatment<br>• Diffuse multiple stenoses involving the unilateral CIA, EIA, and CFA<br>• Unilateral occlusions of both CIA and EIA |

**FIGURE 2-2** TASC II classification for aortoiliac occlusive disease from TASC II Working Group.[1] CFA, common femoral artery; CIA, common iliac artery; EIA, external iliac artery.

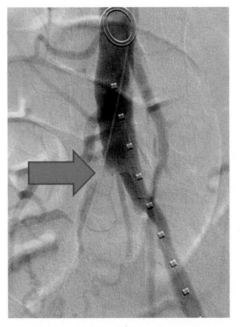 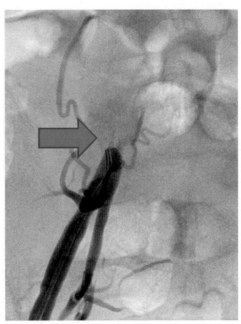

**FIGURE 2-3** Angiogram indicating right iliac artery occlusion. Image on the left shows location of occlusion (blue arrow). Image on the right shows the common iliac artery where the occlusion ends (blue arrow) and reconstitution of the distal common iliac artery.

## EPIDEMIOLOGY

- Aortoiliac occlusive disease (AIOD) is just one manifestation of peripheral arterial disease (PAD) that affects 8 to 12 million Americans. Almost half of patients with PAD are asymptomatic.

- If claudication exists, the prognosis is generally good since 70% to 80% of patients' claudication remains stable over a 10-year time period.[2]

- Unfortunately, the risk of stroke, myocardial infarction, and cardiovascular death is increased in patients with PAD.

- Men tend to be more commonly affected than women.

- Risk factors include those that are risks for coronary artery disease: hypertension, tobacco use, diabetes, hyperlipidemia, advanced age, and family history of PAD or coronary artery disease.

## ETIOLOGY OR PATHOPHYSIOLOGY

The chief causative factor for AIOD disease is atherosclerosis. Other less common mechanisms include embolic phenomenon, fibromuscular dysplasia, dissection, vasculitis, and congenital lesions.

## CLINICAL FEATURES

- Patients with AIOD may present with a variety of symptoms, including claudication, rest pain, and tissue loss. A significant portion may be asymptomatic, especially if they are not active enough to experience claudication.

- Claudication symptoms tend to be in the more proximal muscle groups, including the buttock, hip, and thigh. If severe enough, patients may begin to manifest calf claudication as well.

- Typically the claudication is reproducible and is relieved with standing still. There are usually no symptoms at rest and a burning/tingling sensation is not a prominent symptom.

## DIFFERENTIAL DIAGNOSIS OF AIOD

- Spinal canal stenosis
- Peripheral neuropathy
- Radicular nerve pain
  ○ Herniated disk impinging on sciatic nerve
- Osteoarthritis of the hip
- Venous claudication
- Muscle spasms or cramps

## DIAGNOSTIC STUDIES

- Physical examination, followed by noninvasive studies, can help to differentiate arterial claudication from other causes of leg pain, especially if a decreased or absent femoral pulse is appreciated. Lower extremity arterial noninvasive studies typically will show a diminished ABI, but also a flattened femoral waveform.

- Arterial duplex imaging can be a reliable way of planning an intervention before the procedure.[3]

## MANAGEMENT OR INTERVENTION OPTIONS

- The goals of any therapy for PAD include improvement in quality of life and reduction of cardiovascular adverse events. These may

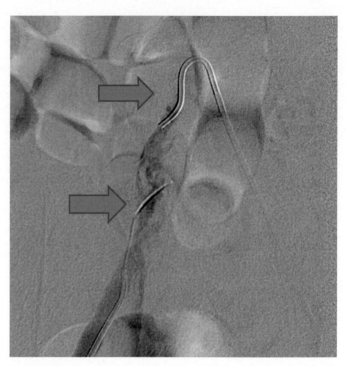

**FIGURE 2-4** Lesion crossing using antegrade and retrograde approach (blue arrows).

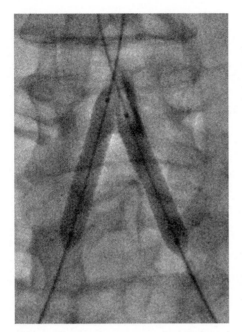 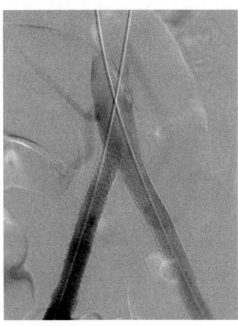

**FIGURE 2-5** Stenting of iliac occlusion. The image on the left shows both dilated balloons ("kissing balloons") in place. The right image shows both iliac stents in place.

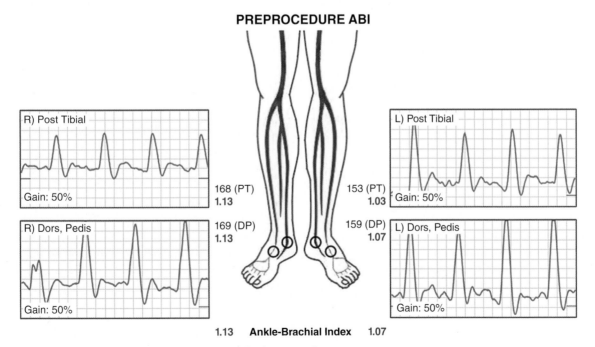

**FIGURE 2-6** Postprocedure improvement in ABI back to normal.

include medical management of diabetes, blood pressure, and hyperlipidemia, as well as smoking cessation. A trial of cilostazol along with a walking program may be a good option in some patients, although this is not as successful in AIOD patients as in those with infrainguinal disease. If conservative therapy is neither successful nor indicated, then a decision regarding open surgical versus endovascular revascularization should be made.

- Endovascular therapeutic options include balloon angioplasty (plain, cutting/scoring, and drug delivered), atherectomy, and stent placement (self-expanding, balloon expandable, drug coated, and covered), although not all devices are approved for all indications. Chronic total occlusions can be crossed with wire/catheter combinations, laser catheters, and other specialized crossing devices. Bilateral common iliac lesions often require "kissing" stents, which are juxtaposed in each iliac artery orifice.

- TASC A lesions represent those that yield excellent results from, and should be treated by, endovascular means, and B lesions offer sufficiently good results with endovascular methods that this approach is still preferred first, unless an open revascularization is required for other associated lesions in the same anatomic area. Open surgical revascularization techniques are generally preferred for TASC C lesions and produce superior enough long-term results with open revascularization that endovascular methods should be used only in patients at high risk for open repair, and D lesions do not yield good enough results with endovascular methods to justify them as primary treatment.[1]

## COMPLICATIONS

- A review of 19 nonrandomized studies revealed a complication rate between 3% and 45%, including access site hematomas, distal embolization, pseudoaneurysms, arterial ruptures, and dissections.[4]

- Treatment of iliac artery occlusions versus iliac stenotic lesions by endovascular means was found to be similar in regard to procedural complications, reintervention rates, and primary and secondary patency.[5]

- A recent meta-analysis suggested that primary patency at 12 months was almost 90% for TASC C lesions and 87% for TASC D lesions. This was comparable to all lesions.[6]

- There are conflicting reports assessing outcomes of open aortobifemoral (ABF) bypass versus endovascular treatment of AIOD. Some suggest a greater increase in ABI after ABF,[7] whereas others find them to be equivalent.[8] These studies also differ in short- and long-term patency results as well. There has been a decrease in the volume of open procedures over the past few years.

- Endovascular treatment of total aortic occlusions is feasible with reasonable midterm patency rates but is associated with a significant periprocedural complication rate, including spinal cord ischemia, distal embolization, and artery rupture.[9]

## PATIENT EDUCATION AND FOLLOW-UP

- Patients should be carefully instructed on early signs of revascularization (impending) failure and what to do if this occurs.

- Recurrent symptoms should not be ignored, even if occurring early.

- All patients should be started on best medical therapy, which includes risk factor modification and antiplatelet therapy, regardless of which approach is taken.

## REFERENCES

1. Norgren L, Hiatt WR, Dormandy JA, Nehler MR, Harris KA, Fowkes FG. TASC II Working Group Inter-Society Consensus for the Management of Peripheral Arterial Disease (TASC II). *J Vasc Surg.* Jan 2007;45(suppl S):S5-S67.

2. Olin JW, Sealove BA. Peripheral artery disease: current insight into the disease and its diagnosis and management. *Mayo Clin Proc.* Jul 2010;85(7):678-692.

3. Fontcuberta J, Flores A, Orgaz A, et al. Reliability of preoperative duplex scanning in designing a therapeutic strategy for chronic lower limb ischemia. *Ann Vasc Surg.* Sep-Oct 2009;23(5):577-582.

4. Jongkind V, Akkersdijk GJ, Yeung KK, Wisselink W. A systematic review of endovascular treatment of extensive aortoiliac occlusive disease. *J Vasc Surg.* Nov 2010;52(5):1376-1383.

5. Pulli R, Dorigo W, Fargion A, et al. Early and long-term comparison of endovascular treatment of iliac artery occlusions and stenosis. *J Vasc Surg.* Jan 2011;53(1):92-98.

6. Ye W, Liu CW, Ricco JB, Mani K, Zeng R, Jiang J. Early and late outcomes of percutaneous treatment of Trans-Atlantic Inter-Society Consensus class C and D aorto-iliac lesions. *J Vasc Surg.* Jun 2011;53(6):1728-1737. http://www.ncbi.nlm.nih.gov/pubmed?Db=pubmed&DbFrom=pubmed&Cmd=Link&LinkName=pubmed_pubmed&IdsFromResult=203073807. Accessed April 29, 2013.

7. Burke CR, Henke PK, Hernandez R, et al. A contemporary comparison of aortofemoral bypass and aortoiliac stenting in the treatment of aortoiliac occlusive disease. *Ann Vasc Surg.* Jan 2010;24(1):4-13.

8. Kashyap VS, Pavkov ML, Bena JF, et al. The management of severe aortoiliac occlusive disease: endovascular therapy rivals open reconstruction. *J Vasc Surg.* Dec 2008;48(6):1451-1457, 1457, e1-3.

9. Kim TH, Ko YG, Kim U, et al. Outcomes of endovascular treatment of chronic total occlusion of the infrarenal aorta. *J Vasc Surg.* Jun 2011;53(6):1542-1549.

# 3 FEMORAL POPLITEAL DISEASE: BYPASS

Axel Thors, DO

## PATIENT STORY

A 61-year-old man was referred to vascular surgery for a several-year history of bilateral lower extremity calf claudication at two blocks. His claudication symptoms were described as significantly lifestyle limiting. Peripheral vascular risk factors included hypertension (HTN), hyperlipidemia, and tobacco abuse (20 pack-years). The patient denied symptoms of rest pain and did not have any evidence of tissue loss. His pedal pulses were not palpable but were heard with a Doppler bilaterally. After discussing options, the patient agreed to a 3-month trial of a supervised exercise program with an oral phosphodiesterase inhibitor (cilostazol) and tobacco cessation.

At the return office visit, the patient reported minimal improvement and he was unable to quit smoking. At this time, the patient wished to proceed with noninvasive vascular laboratory studies and aortography with possible intervention.

Aortogram findings indicated an occlusion of the left superficial femoral artery (SFA) (Figure 3-1) with reconstitution of the popliteal artery above the knee (Figure 3-2), with two-vessel runoff to the foot (Figure 3-3). The patient's right side showed a diffusely diseased but patent SFA with two-vessel runoff to the foot.

An endovascular attempt to re-establish flow in the left SFA was unsuccessful using a chronic total occlusion (CTO) device. Consequently, the patient decided to proceed with a femoral to popliteal bypass.

## EPIDEMIOLOGY

### Peripheral Arterial Disease

- Progressive narrowing of the arteries due to atherosclerosis.[1]

- Mostly silent in early stages until luminal narrowing exceeds 50% vessel diameter.[2]

- Prevalence of peripheral arterial disease (PAD) in adults over 40 years in the United States is approximately 4%.

- Prevalence of PAD in adults over 70 years in the Unites States is approximately 15%.

- 20% to 25% of patients will require revascularization.[2]

- Approximately 5% of patients will progress to critical limb ischemia.[2]

- Patients with limb loss have 30% to 40% mortality in the first 24 months.[2]

## ETIOLOGY AND PATHOPHYSIOLOGY

### Peripheral Arterial Disease

- Global arterial tree inflammation accounts for atherogenesis and participates in local, myocardial, and systemic complications of atherosclerosis.[3]

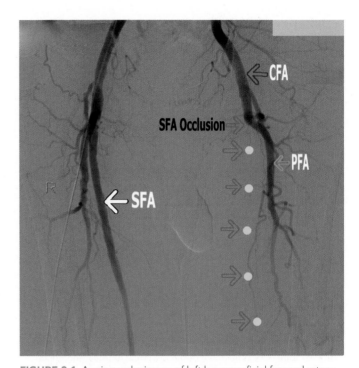

**FIGURE 3-1** Angiography image of left leg superficial femoral artery (SFA) occlusion. White arrow marks contralateral right SFA, which is patent. Red arrows and yellow dots depict estimated course of left SFA. Orange arrow marks profunda femoral artery (PFA). Blue arrow indicates the common femoral artery (CFA).

- Vascular risk factors including diabetes, HTN, hyperlipidemia, and tobacco abuse augment cell adhesion molecules, which promote leukocyte binding to the arterial cell wall. This process perpetuates, causing remodeling of the arterial wall and lipid deposition within the tunica media, followed by narrowing of the lumen and eventually calcification of the arterial wall.[3]

## OPERATIVE PLANNING

### Imaging

- Inflow, outflow, and runoff vessels must be determined in all patients with symptomatic PAD.
- Angiography remains the gold standard for evaluating the arterial tree.
- Computed tomography angiography (CTA) is readily available in most hospitals; it is rapid and is an excellent modality to evaluate the aorta and its branches. CTA is limited in evaluating tibial arteries due to their small size and calcification.
- Magnetic resonance angiography (MRA) continues to improve as an imaging modality for peripheral vascular bypass.[4]
- Duplex arterial mapping is another noninvasive method for evaluating bypass targets.[5]

### Conduit

- Autogenous vein conduits are the best option for infrainguinal bypass if the vein is structurally normal and the diameter is greater than or equal to 3 mm.[6]
- A search for a usable vein should be undertaken before intervention by duplex vein mapping of the lower extremities and upper extremities if necessary.
- Polytetrafluoroethylene (PTFE) and heparin-bonded PTFE (ePTFE) are the most common synthetic conduits for infrainguinal bypass. Hemashield (Dacron) woven polyester grafts are also a viable option for bypass graft.
- Infrageniculate PTFE anastomotic sites should be modified with vein cuff, patch, or vein boot technique whenever vein conduit is unavailable.[7,8]
- Cryopreserved vein grafts are another option primarily for use in the setting of infection.[9]

## OPERATIVE TECHNIQUE

- Reversed vein bypass technique, where the vein is harvested and reversed to avoid venous valve lysis. The vein can be tunneled in anatomic or subcutaneous plane.
- In situ vein bypass technique, where the vein is exposed proximally and distally. The valves are then lysed using a valvulotome device followed by careful ligation of venous tributaries along the length of the vein.
- Prosthetic conduit tunneled anatomically or in the subcutaneous tissue.

## RESULTS

- In general, reversed vein and in situ bypass techniques have similar patency rates: 70% to 80% at 3 years for above- or below-knee popliteal bypasses.[10,11]

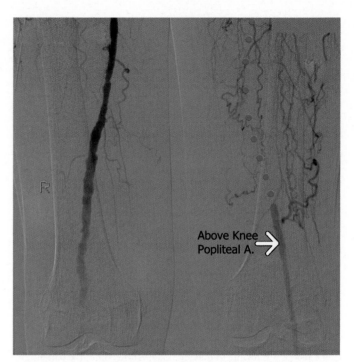

**FIGURE 3-2** Angiography image of the left leg SFA occlusion with reconstitution of the above-knee popliteal artery (white arrow). Red dots depict estimated course of occluded SFA. Diffusely diseased but patent right SFA is seen.

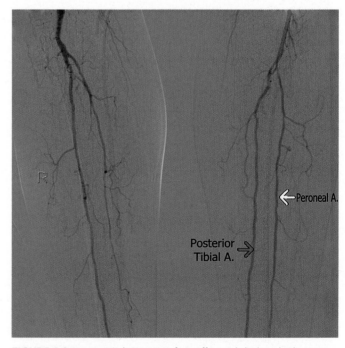

**FIGURE 3-3** Angiography image of runoff vessels below the knee. Red arrow indicates the posterior tibial artery. White arrow denotes the peroneal artery.

- PTFE above-knee bypass has patency of 79% at 1 year and 60% at 4 years.[10,11]
- PTFE below-knee bypass has patency of 68% at 1 year and 48% at 4 years.[10,11]

## POSTOPERATIVE MANAGEMENT

- Antiplatelet therapy with aspirin or clopidogrel is indicated for most patients with infrainguinal bypass.[12]
- In general, warfarin therapy should not be used for infrainguinal bypass unless the bypass is high risk. A high-risk bypass is defined as poor arterial runoff, suboptimal vein graft, or reoperative cases.[13]
- Optimization of peripheral arterial disease should be aggressively pursued including HTN, diabetes, hyperlipidemia, congestive heart failure, and smoking cessation.

## COMPLICATIONS

- Early: Death (2.7%), myocardial infarction (4.7%), major amputation (1.8%), graft occlusion (5.2%), major wound complications (4.8%), and graft hemorrhage (0.4%).[14]
- Late: Lymphedema, graft infection, graft aneurysm, and graft stenosis.[14]

## PATIENT FOLLOW-UP

- ABI testing and duplex graft surveillance prior to discharge to establish postoperative baseline.[15]
- ABI and duplex graft surveillance repeated every 3 months for 1 year, every 6 months for an additional 2 years, and annually thereafter.[15]

## REFERENCES

1. Selvin E, Erlinger TP. Prevalence of and risk factors for peripheral arterial disease in the United States: results from the national health and nutrition examination survey, 1999-2000. *Circulation.* 2004;110:738-743.

2. Garcia LA. Epidemiology and pathophysiology of lower extremity peripheral arterial disease. *J Endovasc Ther.* 2006;13(suppl II): II-3-II-9.

3. Libby P, Theroux P. Pathophysiology of coronary artery disease. *Circulation.* 2005;111:3481-3488.

4. Dorweiler B, Neufang A, Kreitner KF, et al. Magnetic resonance angiography unmasks reliable target vessels for pedal bypass grafting in patients with diabetes mellitus. *J Vasc Surg.* 2002;35: 766-772.

5. Mazzariol F, Ascher E, Hingorani A, et al. Lower-extremity revascularization without preoperative contrast arteriography in 185 cases: lessons learned with duplex ultrasound arterial mapping. *Eur J Vasc Endovasc Surg.* 2000;19:509-515.

6. Donaldson MC, Whittemore AD, Mannick JA. Further experience with all-autogenous tissue policy for infrainguinal reconstruction. *J Vasc Surg.* 1993;18(1):41-48.

7. Stonebridge PA, Prescott RJ, Ruckley CV. Randomized trial comparing infrainguinal polytetrafluoroethylene bypass grafting with and without vein interposition cuff at the distal anastomosis. The joint vascular research group. *J Vasc Surg.* 1997;26(4): 543-550.

8. Yeung KK, Mills JL, Hughes JD, et al. Improved patency of infrainguinal polytetrafluoroethylene bypass grafts using a distal Taylor vein patch. *Am J Surg.* 2001;182(6):578-583.

9. Farber A, Major K, Wagner WH, et al. Cryopreserved saphenous vein allografts in infrainguinal revascularization: analysis of 240 grafts. *J Vasc Surg.* Jul 2003;38(1):15-21.

10. Harris PL, Veith FJ, Shanik GD, et al. Prospective randomized comparison of in situ and reversed infrapopliteal vein grafts. *Br J Surg.* Feb 1993;80(2):173-176.

11. Comparative evaluation of prosthetic, reversed, and in situ vein bypass grafts in distal popliteal and tibial-peroneal revascularization. Veterans Administration Cooperative Study Group 141. *Arch Surg.* Apr 1988;123(4):434-438.

12. Collaborative overview of randomized trials of antiplatelet therapy—II: maintenance of vascular graft or arterial patency by antiplatelet therapy. Antiplatelet Trialists' Collaboration. *BMJ.* Jan 15 1994;308(6922):159-168.

13. Johnson WC, Williford WO. Benefits, morbidity, and mortality associated with long-term administration of oral anticoagulant therapy to patients with peripheral arterial bypass procedures: a prospective randomized study. *J Vasc Surg.* Mar 2002;35(3): 413-421.

14. Conte MS, Bandyk DF, Clowes AW, et al. Results of PREVENT III: a multicenter, randomized trial of edifoligide for the prevention of vein graft failure in lower extremity bypass surgery. *J Vasc Surg.* Apr 2006;43(4):742-751.

15. Davies AH, Hawdon AJ, Sydes MR, et al. Is duplex surveillance of value after leg vein bypass grafting? Principal results of the Vein Graft Surveillance Randomised Trial (VGST). *Circulation.* Sep 2005;112(13):1985-1991.

# 4 FEMORAL POPLITEAL DISEASE: PTA AND STENTING

Axel Thors, DO

## PATIENT STORY

A 70-year-old man was referred to vascular surgery for a several-year history of bilateral lower extremity calf claudication at one block. His claudication symptoms were described as significantly lifestyle limiting with the right leg worse than the left. The patient had previous bilateral iliac artery stenting 2 years prior to presentation (Figure 4-1). His peripheral vascular risk factors include hypertension (HTN), hyperlipidemia, and tobacco abuse (30 pack-years). The patient denied symptoms of rest pain and did not have any evidence of tissue loss. His pedal pulses were palpable bilaterally. After discussing options, the patient agreed to a 3-month trial of a supervised exercise program with an oral phosphodiesterase inhibitor (cilostazol) and tobacco cessation.

At the return office visit, the patient reported minimal improvement. The patient was unable to quit smoking. Ankle-brachial index (ABI) and segmental lower extremity pressures revealed diminished blood flow bilaterally with a significant drop postexercise. The patient subsequently underwent an angiogram with bilateral lower extremity runoff.

Angiogram findings indicated a 70% stenosis of the right above-knee popliteal artery (Figure 4-2) and 80% stenosis of the popliteal-tibial artery junction (Figure 4-3).

The patient subsequently underwent percutaneous transluminal angioplasty (PTA) of both lesions with a cryoplasty balloon. This achieved a good angiographic result (Figure 4-4). He was maintained on daily antiplatelet therapy (clopidogrel).

### EPIDEMIOLOGY

#### Peripheral Arterial Disease

- Progressive narrowing of the arteries due to atherosclerosis.[1]

- Mostly silent in early stages until luminal narrowing exceeds 50% vessel diameter.[2]

- Prevalence of peripheral arterial disease (PAD) in adults over 40 years in the United States is approximately 4%.[2]

- Prevalence of PAD in adults over 70 years in the United States is approximately 15%.[2]

- 20% to 25% of patients will require revascularization.[2]

- Approximately 5% of patients will progress to critical limb ischemia.[2]

- Patients with limb loss have 30% to 40% mortality in the first 24 months.[2]

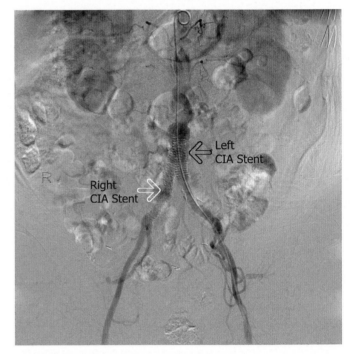

**FIGURE 4-1** Abdominal aortogram showing previous iliac artery stents on both sides (arrows).

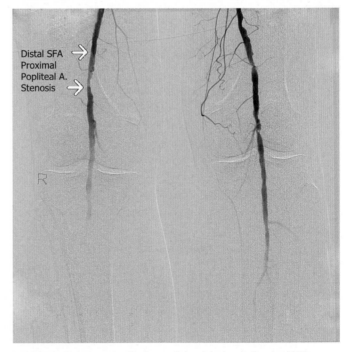

**FIGURE 4-2** Angiogram findings of the right leg indicating 70% stenosis of the right above-knee popliteal artery (two arrows).

## ETIOLOGY AND PATHOPHYSIOLOGY

### Peripheral Arterial Disease

- Global arterial tree inflammation accounts for atherogenesis and participates in local, myocardial, and systemic complications of atherosclerosis.[3]

- Vascular risk factors including diabetes, HTN, hyperlipidemia, and tobacco abuse augment cell adhesion molecules, which promote leukocyte binding to the arterial cell wall. This process perpetuates, causing remodeling of the arterial wall and lipid deposition within the tunica media. This process continues and begins to narrow the vessel lumen, eventually causing calcification of the arterial wall.[3]

## PROCEDURE PLANNING

### Imaging

- Angiography remains the gold standard for evaluating the arterial tree.

- Computed tomography angiography (CTA) is readily available in most hospitals; it is rapid and is an excellent modality to evaluate the aorta and its branches. CTA is limited in evaluating tibial vessels due to their small size and calcification.

- Magnetic resonance angiography (MRA) continues to improve as an imaging modality for peripheral vascular intervention.[4] Higher-strength magnetic fields generally improve imaging results and diminish motion artifact.

- Duplex ultrasound arterial mapping is another noninvasive method for evaluating peripheral arterial lesions, particularly superficial femoral and popliteal disease.[5]

## DETERMINANTS OF ENDOVASCULAR OUTCOME

### Location

- Endovascular treatment (ET) of large proximal arteries (aortic and iliac) has improved patency compared to infrainguinal lesions.[6]

### Disease Pattern

- Treatment of stenotic lesions versus totally occluded vessels yields improved immediate and long-term results.[7,8]

- The length of a treated stenosis or occlusion is inversely related to technical success, limb salvage, symptom resolution, and patency.[9] (Long lesion equals worse outcome.)

- Treatment of focal disease has better outcome than multifocal disease.[10]

- Treatment of multilevel disease has worse outcomes with endovascular therapy versus surgery. Treatment with a combined approach (hybrid) has shown favorable outcomes.[11]

- Patients with compromised runoff vessels (tibial vessels) have worse results with endovascular therapy and open surgery.[12]

## INDICATION FOR INTERVENTION

- Treatment of patients with critical limb ischemia (CLI) versus claudication has consistently shown worse outcomes due to multilevel disease, medical comorbidities, and lesion characteristics.[13]

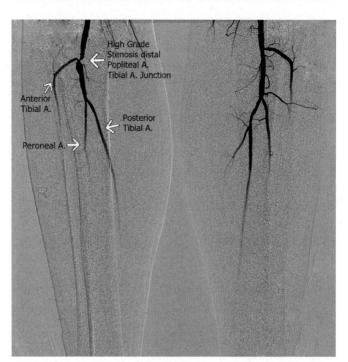

FIGURE 4-3 Angiogram of the right lower leg showing 80% stenosis of the popliteal-tibial artery junction (large arrow) and the three tibial arteries (small arrows).

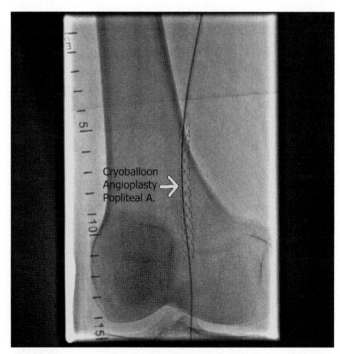

FIGURE 4-4 Angiogram of the right leg showing a good angiographic result after percutaneous transluminal angioplasty (PTA) of both lesions with a cryoplasty balloon.

## POSTPROCEDURAL FACTORS

- Improvement in postprocedural ABI has been shown to improve short-term and long-term outcomes.[14]

## RESULTS

### Femoropopliteal Angioplasty or Stenting

- Patency is variable and is dependent on the above patient factors. Muradin et al. reported 3-year patency rates as 61% for claudicants, 48% for occlusions in claudicants, 43% for stenosis in CLI patients, and 30% for occlusions in CLI patients.[15]
- Angioplasty and selective stenting demonstrates 3-year patency rates ranging from 63% to 66%.[15]
- Drug-eluting stents in the peripheral vasculature have not shown improved efficacy to date; however, continued trials are under way.[16,17,18]
- Stent grafts created to replicate the open femoral-popliteal bypass (endoconduit) have shown short-term patency rates similar to those with open surgery.[19]

## POSTOPERATIVE MANAGEMENT

- Control of peripheral vascular risk factors including tobacco abuse, obesity, hyperlipidemia, HTN, diabetes, and antiplatelet therapy.[20]
- Dual antiplatelet therapy with aspirin and clopidogrel has not been shown to be superior to aspirin alone with regard to stroke, vascular death, or myocardial infarction.[21]

## COMPLICATIONS

- Local complications including bleeding, pseudoaneurysm, or arteriovenous fistula occur in 0.3% to 3% of patients.[22]
- Angioplasty site vessel rupture or thrombosis occurs in 0.3% to 3% of patients, respectively.[22]
- Distal vessel dissection or embolization after angioplasty occurs in 0.4% to 2% of patients, respectively.[22]
- Renal failure or fatal myocardial infarction occurs in 0.2% of patients.[22]

## PATIENT FOLLOW-UP

- ABI testing and duplex graft surveillance prior to discharge to establish postoperative baseline.[16]
- ABI and duplex graft surveillance repeated every 1, 3, 6, 9, and 12 months, and then yearly if testing remains stable.[14]

## REFERENCES

1. Selvin E, Erlinger TP. Prevalence of and risk factors for peripheral arterial disease in the United States: results from the national health and nutrition examination survey, 1999-2000. *Circulation*. 2004;110:738-743.

2. Garcia LA. Epidemiology and pathophysiology of lower extremity peripheral arterial disease. *J Endovasc Ther*. 2006;13(suppl II): II-3-II-9.

3. Libby P, Theroux P. Pathophysiology of coronary artery disease. *Circulation*. 2005;111:3481-3488.

4. Dorweiler B, Neufang A, Kreitner KF, et al. Magnetic resonance angiography unmasks reliable target vessels for pedal bypass grafting in patients with diabetes mellitus. *J Vasc Surg*. 2002;35: 766-772.

5. Mazzariol F, Ascher E, Hingorani A, et al. Lower-extremity revascularization without preoperative contrast arteriography in 185 cases: lessons learned with duplex ultrasound arterial mapping. *Eur J Vasc Endovasc Surg*. 2000;19:509-515.

6. Ruef J, Hofmann M, Haase J. Endovascular interventions in iliac and infrainguinal occlusive artery disease. *J Interv Cardiol*. 2004;17:427-435.

7. Johnston KW. Factors that influence the outcome of aortoiliac and femoropopliteal percutaneous transluminal angioplasty. *Surg Clin North Am*. 1992;72:843-850.

8. Norgren L, Hiatt WR, Dormandy JA, Nehler MR, Harris KA, Fowkes FG. TASC II Working Group: inter-society consensus for the management of peripheral arterial disease (TASC II). *J Vasc Surg*. 2007;45S:S5-S67.

9. Stanley B, Teague B, Raptis S, et al. Efficacy of balloon angioplasty of the superficial femoral artery and popliteal artery in the relief of leg ischemia. *J Vasc Surg*. 1996;23:679-685.

10. Jorgensen B, Tonnesen KH, Holstein P. Late hemodynamic failure following percutaneous transluminal angioplasty for long and multifocal femoropopliteal stenoses. *Cardiovasc Intervent Radiol*. 1991;14:290-292.

11. Cotroneo AR, Iezzi R, Marano G, et al. Hybrid therapy in patients with complex peripheral multifocal steno-obstructive vascular disease: two-year results. *Cardiovasc Intervent Radiol*. 2007;30:355-361.

12. DeRubertis BG, Pierce M, Chaer RA, et al. Lesion severity and treatment complexity are associated with outcome after percutaneous infra-inguinal intervention. *J Vasc Surg*. 2007;46:709-716.

13. Jeans WD, Armstrong S, Cole SE, et al. Fate of patients undergoing transluminal angioplasty for lower-limb ischemia. *Radiology*. 1990;177:559-564.

14. Rutherford RB, Baker JD, Ernst C, et al. Recommended standards for reports dealing with lower extremity ischemia: revised version. *J Vasc Surg*. 1997;26:517-538.

15. Muradin GS, Bosch JL, Stijnen T, Hunink MG. Balloon dilation and stent implantation for treatment of femoropopliteal arterial disease: meta-analysis. *Radiology*. 2001;221:137-145.

16. Duda SH, Pusich B, Richter G, et al. Sirolimus-eluting stents for the treatment of obstructive superficial femoral artery disease: six-month results. *Circulation*. 2002;106:1505-1509.

17. Duda SH, Bosiers M, Lammer J, et al. Sirolimus-eluting versus bare nitinol stent for obstructive superficial femoral artery disease: the SIROCCO II trial. *J Vasc Interv Radiol*. 2005;16: 331-338.

18. Katzen B. Zilver Stent trial update. International Symposium on Endovascular Therapy. Miami Beach, FL; 2006. http://www.netsymposium.com/index.php?select=conference&data=193. Accessed April 29, 2013.

19. Kedora J, Hohmann S, Garrett W, et al. Randomized comparison of percutaneous Viabahn stent grafts vs prosthetic femoral-popliteal bypass in the treatment of superficial femoral arterial occlusive disease. *J Vasc Surg*. 2007;45:10-16.

20. Yusuf S, Sleight P, Pogue J, et al. Effects of an angiotensin-converting-enzyme inhibitor, ramipril, on cardiovascular events in high-risk patients. The Heart Outcomes Prevention Evaluation Study Investigators. *N Engl J Med*. 2000;342:145-153.

21. Bhatt DL, Fox KA, Hacke W, et al. Clopidogrel and aspirin versus aspirin alone for the prevention of atherothrombotic events. *N Engl J Med*. 2006;354:1706-1717.

22. Pentecost MJ, Criqui MH, Dorros G, et al. Guidelines for peripheral percutaneous transluminal angioplasty of the abdominal aorta and lower extremity vessels. A statement for health professionals from a special writing group of the Councils on Cardiovascular Radiology, Arteriosclerosis, Cardio-Thoracic and Vascular Surgery, Clinical Cardiology, and Epidemiology and Prevention, the American Heart Association. *Circulation*. 1994;89:511-531.

# 5 TIBIOPERONEAL OCCLUSIVE DISEASE

Jean Starr, MD, FACS, RPVI

## PATIENT STORY

An 80-year-old man presented with a nonhealing foot ulcer over the base of the left first metatarsal head (Figure 5-1). It had been present for several months and appeared after he wore a new pair of shoes. He had a history of diabetes and hypertension. There was no previous history of claudication.

Lower extremity arterial Doppler studies were completed and showed bilateral ankle-brachial indices (ABIs) greater than 1.2 with triphasic femoral and popliteal waveforms and monophasic tibial waveforms (Figure 5-2).

Surgical intervention and endovascular procedures were discussed with him. An angiogram was performed that showed no significant occlusive disease above the knee and severe tibial occlusive disease below the knee (Figure 5-3).

Balloon angioplasty was performed on the anterior tibial and peroneal arteries (Figure 5-4), and there was resultant improvement in angiographic results (Figure 5-5).

Ulcer healing was complete approximately 1 month after the procedure.

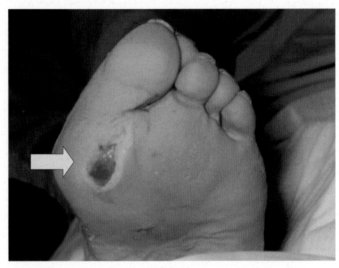

**FIGURE 5-1** Diabetic foot ulcer (arrow), noted to be over a bony prominence with callused edges and unhealthy-appearing base.

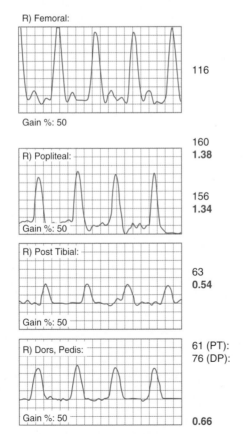

R) Femoral:

116

Gain %: 50

160
**1.38**

R) Popliteal:

156
**1.34**

Gain %: 50

R) Post Tibial:

63
**0.54**

Gain %: 50

R) Dors, Pedis:

61 (PT):
76 (DP):

Gain %: 50

**0.66**

| | | Index |
|---|---|---|
| Brachial: | 116 | |
| High Thigh: | 160 | 1.38 |
| Low Thigh: | 156 | 1.34 |
| Calf: | 63 | 0.54 |
| Ankle (PT): | 61 | 0.53 |
| Ankle (DP): | 76 | 0.66 |

**FIGURE 5-2** Left lower extremity noninvasive arterial waveform study showing normal femoral and popliteal pressures and diminished pedal waveforms.

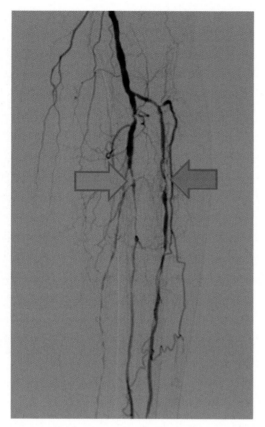
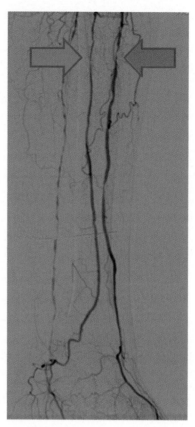

FIGURE 5-3 Initial angiogram with blue arrows highlighting peroneal disease and red arrows indicating anterior tibial artery disease.

## EPIDEMIOLOGY

- Lower extremity peripheral arterial disease (PAD) affects 8 to 10 million Americans and the incidence increases as the population ages, affecting 12% to 15% of people over the age of 65 years.[1] PAD is a main cause of lower extremity amputation, other cardio-vascular morbidity, decreased quality of life, and cost to our health care system.

- Occlusive disease isolated to the tibial or peroneal arterial bed typically occurs in patients with diabetes. Ulceration and gangrene in this patient population is often multifactorial and difficult to treat.

- Factors contributing to poor healing wounds include tissue ischemia, renal failure, soft tissue or underlying bone infection, excessive pressure, poor glucose control, and inappropriate or inadequate wound care.

- Prevention of tissue loss is a prime objective in these patients.

## ETIOLOGY OR PATHOPHYSIOLOGY

- A study of lower extremity amputation segments showed that atherosclerosis and vessel wall medial calcification was prominent in diabetic patients.[2] There was also an increased occurrence of severe atherosclerosis in older patients and those with hypertension. Medial calcification was also significant in younger patients less than 70 years of age.

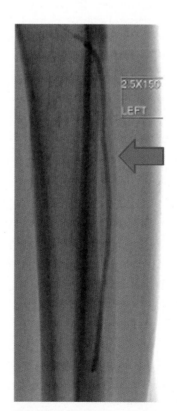
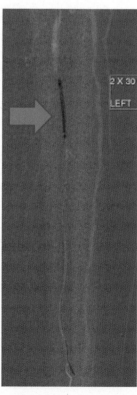

FIGURE 5-4 Balloon angioplasty procedure with the blue arrow indicating the peroneal and red arrow representing the anterior tibial artery balloon.

- Arteriography in diabetic patients with chronic limb ischemia found that 74% had disease below the knee and 66% of these were occlusions.[3] Diabetics were found to have more diffuse atherosclerotic disease with greater severity in the tibial vessels and higher occurrence of long-segment occlusions.

- Calcification within the vessel wall tends to increase in the more distal tibial distribution of the arterial tree. This was not found to be related to any clinical factors.[4]

## CLINICAL FEATURES

- Tibial occlusive disease may often be asymptomatic until tissue loss occurs. Claudication is not a common manifestation unless there coexists more proximal occlusive disease as well.

- Neuropathy may be a prominent symptom in these patients, especially when diabetes is present.

- Tissue breakdown often occurs at pressure points over bony prominences and with ill-fitting footwear.

## DIFFERENTIAL DIAGNOSIS

The etiology of pedal ulcerations can be multifactorial, and in addition to atherosclerotic occlusive disease, other contributors are poorly controlled diabetes, renal failure, neuropathy, inappropriate pressure, infection, and trauma.

## DIAGNOSTIC STUDIES

- Noninvasive imaging studies are the best tests to start with to gauge the degree of arterial insufficiency and to try to localize disease location. This may include ABIs, waveform analysis at multiple levels, and color duplex ultrasonography (DUS) of arterial segments. The ABI may be falsely elevated in patients with diabetes due to medial calcinosis causing stiff, incompressible vessel walls. This makes waveform analysis invaluable for determining degree of ischemia. In addition, digit pressures and plethysmographic waveforms are valuable in these patients.

- DUS has been found to be very good compared to digital subtraction angiography, but not as accurate in delineating the more distal tibial vessels.[5] It can, however, be an initial good, noninvasive test to use for therapeutic planning purposes.

- More in-depth anatomic information can be gleaned with contrast computed tomography angiography (CTA) and magnetic resonance angiography (MRA) studies.[6] Advantages are the lack of invasiveness, but the disadvantages include contrast administration and exposure to radiation, as well as the inability to treat the disease within the same setting. MRA has limited application in patients with renal failure due to the possibility of nephrogenic systemic fibrosis. CTA may falsely interpret the anatomy of calcified lesions.

- Catheter-based angiography with concomitant endovascular intervention offers the most expedient approach to improving flow to an ischemic limb.[6] It may also provide better imaging quality and spatial resolution, especially in the face of extensive calcification. Acute thrombus may also be better identified.

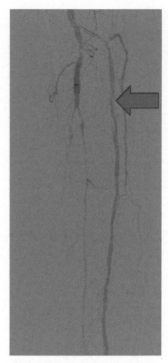
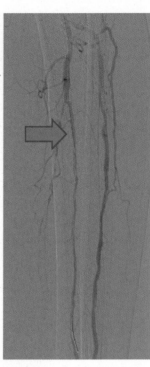

FIGURE 5-5 Final angioplasty demonstrates improved results with the blue arrow pointing to the peroneal and red arrow to the anterior tibial artery.

## MANAGEMENT OR INTERVENTION OPTIONS

- Various endovascular options exist, including balloon angioplasty, cryoplasty, stenting, and atherectomy. No single approach truly surpasses the others in terms of results, but these minimally invasive approaches have challenged traditional open surgical revascularization procedures.

- Surgical options included distal bypass with prosthetic or autogenous graft, endarterectomy with patch angioplasty, and primary amputation.

- The BASIL trial showed that outcomes were generally similar for patients with critical limb ischemia who were candidates for both surgery and an endovascular approach.[7] Surgery was found to be more expensive over the first-year follow-up period. This study, however, was not stratified to examine patients with femoral-popliteal versus tibial occlusive disease.

## COMPLICATIONS OR OUTCOMES

- Surgical complications include infection, early and late graft occlusion, and medical problems, especially those cardiac in nature. Endovascular complications can include short- and long-term recurrence or occlusion, access site problems, and medical issues.

- Endovascular tibial interventions have been found to have acceptable limb salvage and wound healing rates, but have a higher rate of reintervention.[8] Patients with renal failure, poor pedal flow, and isolated peroneal runoff had worse outcomes.

- Patients expected to live less than 2 years may be better served with angioplasty first as they may not reap the long-term patency benefit from surgical revascularization.[9] Patients who have a reasonable 2-year life expectancy are appropriate surgical candidates, and those with autogenous vein are better treated first with open bypass.

## PATIENT EDUCATION AND FOLLOW-UP

- Patients should have regular follow-up after endovascular or surgical revascularization to assess patency and success of the procedure.

- They should be advised about the warning signs of recurrent disease, for which they should notify their physician.

- Wounds should also be closely followed until completely healed.

- Patients should be advised about risk factor modification, including smoking cessation, blood pressure control, lipid management, glucose control, weight loss, and appropriate foot care.

- Avoidance of future tissue loss is the main target of future medical management of these patients.

## REFERENCES

1. Hirsch AT, Hartman L, Town RJ, Virnig BA. National health care costs of peripheral arterial disease in the Medicare population. *Vasc Med*. Aug 2008;13(3):209-215.

2. Soor GS, Vukin I, Leong SW, Oreopoulos G, Butany J. Peripheral vascular disease: who gets it and why? A histomorphological analysis of 261 arterial segments from 58 cases. *Pathology*. Jun 2008;40(4):385-391.

3. Graziani L, Silvestro A, Bertone V, et al. Vascular involvement in diabetic subjects with ischemic foot ulcer: a new morphologic categorization of disease severity. *Eur J Vasc Endovasc Surg*. Apr 2007;33(4):453-460.

4. Bishop PD, Feiten LE, Ouriel K, et al. Arterial calcification increases in distal arteries in patients with peripheral arterial disease. *Ann Vasc Surg*. Nov 2008;22(6):799-805.

5. Eiberg JP, Grønvall Rasmussen JB, Hansen MA, Schroeder TV. Duplex ultrasound scanning of peripheral arterial disease of the lower limb. *Eur J Vasc Endovasc Surg*. Oct 2010;40(4):507-512.

6. Pomposelli F. Arterial imaging in patients with lower extremity ischemia and diabetes mellitus. *J Vasc Surg*. Sep 2010;52(suppl 3): S81-S91.

7. Adam DJ, Beard JD, Cleveland T, et al. BASIL trial participants. Bypass versus angioplasty in severe ischaemia of the leg (BASIL): multicentre randomised controlled trial. *Lancet*. Dec 3 2005;366(9501):1925-1934.

8. Fernandez N, McEnaney R, Marone LK, et al. Predictors of failure and success of tibial interventions for critical limb ischemia. *J Vasc Surg*. Oct 2010;52(4):834-842.

9. Bradbury AW, Adam DJ, Bell J, et al. Multicentre randomised controlled trial of the clinical and cost-effectiveness of a bypass-surgery-first versus a balloon-angioplasty-first revascularisation strategy for severe limb ischaemia due to infrainguinal disease. The Bypass versus Angioplasty in Severe Ischaemia of the Leg (BASIL) trial. *Health Technol Assess*. Mar 2010;14(14):1-210, iii-iv.

# 6  LIMB GANGRENE AND AMPUTATION

Axel Thors, DO

## PATIENT STORY

A 60-year-old man with past medical history significant for diabetes presented with a several-week history of a left-foot wound. The patient stated that a small ulcer developed on the plantar surface of his foot, which gradually progressed to erythema with tracking streaks to above the ankle. Despite having baseline mild neuropathy, he described significant pain across the forefoot and noticed increasing dark discoloration across the forefoot and plantar surface. The patient also admitted to subjective fevers and chills.

On examination the patient's temperature was 101.9°F, pulse 110, and blood pressure was normal. He had proximal and pedal pulses in both lower extremities. The left foot was malodorous, edematous, and erythematous, with dark gangrenous changes along the third to fifth toes and plantar surface (Figures 6-1 to 6-3). Subcutaneous crepitance could also be appreciated along the forefoot extending to just below the ankle.

Given these findings, a necrotizing diabetic foot infection was suspected. The patient was started on broad-spectrum intravenous antibiotics with coverage for clostridium and group B streptococcal species.

The patient was subsequently taken for operative wound exploration with finding of extensive tracking necrotizing infection along all fascial planes. A guillotine amputation above the ankle was performed with the wound left open.

After 3 days of antibiotics the patient was subsequently taken for conversion to a planned below-knee amputation.

### EPIDEMIOLOGY

- Diabetes and peripheral arterial disease (PAD) account for the vast majority of amputations worldwide.[1]
- Patients with diabetes have a 10-fold higher risk of amputation than nondiabetic patients, secondary to the higher incidence of PAD in diabetic patients.[2]
- Treatment of critical limb ischemia (CLI) differs significantly among regions due to surgeon specialty training, experience, and case volume, with low volume centers having higher amputation rates.[1]
- Regional, socioeconomic, racial, and ethnic disparities have been shown to affect amputation rates.[3]
- Earlier endovascular and open bypass procedures have decreased the national amputation rate to approximately 15%.[4,5]

### INDICATIONS FOR AMPUTATION

- CLI with failed revascularization
- Extensive pedal gangrene
- Nonreconstructible arterial anatomy

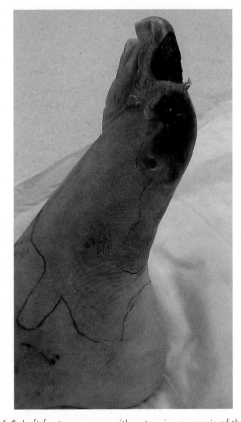

**FIGURE 6-1** Left-foot gangrene with extensive necrosis of the plantar surface and the first toe. Tracking cellulitis, outlined with pen markings, extends above the medial malleolus.

- Overwhelming pedal sepsis
- Excessive surgical risk
- Nonambulatory status

## PREOPERATIVE MANAGEMENT

- Standard evaluation of patient comorbidities should be performed to determine anesthetic strategy (general vs regional block).

- Aggressive cardiac evaluation is not necessary in the absence of active cardiac symptoms, evidence of congestive heart failure, or acute changes on electrocardiogram.[6]

- Beta-blockade has been shown to be beneficial in the general vascular surgery population and should be given unless contraindicated.[7]

- The high incidence of perioperative deep venous thrombosis (DVT) and pulmonary embolism (PE), upwards of 17%, emphasizes the need for aggressive prophylaxis in this patient population.[8]

- Aggressive control of infection should be instituted with surgical debridement, antibiotics, and guillotine amputation if necessary, with staged reconstruction.[9]

- Determination of amputation level should consider remaining blood flow, extent of nonviable tissue, ambulatory status, and rehabilitation potential including use of prosthetic limb postoperatively.

- Below-knee amputees require 10% to 40% more energy expenditure versus above-knee amputees, who require 50% to 70% more to ambulate with a prosthesis.[8]

## POSTOPERATIVE MANAGEMENT

- Multidisciplinary rehabilitation facilities which include physical medicine and rehabilitation physicians, physical and occupational therapists, psychiatrists, nutritionists, prosthetic specialists, and social workers are crucial for returning the patient to maximal mobility following amputation.

- Careful wound evaluation should be undertaken in the postoperative period so further tissue loss can be minimized.

## COMPLICATIONS

- Operative mortality is generally low for major extremity amputation (4%-9%).[4]

- Above-knee amputation carries increased mortality (11%-17%) in comparison to below-knee amputation (3%-9%), which is a correlation with more significant cardiovascular disease in the former.[10]

- The rate of significant postoperative bleeding ranges from 3% to 9%.[11]

- Stump infection is variable and is dependent on multiple factors including residual blood supply, diabetes, nutrition status, socioeconomic class, and presence or absence of foreign body in wound (graft material, stents, etc).[12]

- Flexion contractures at the hip or knee occur in 3% to 9% of patients and can prohibit prosthetic limb use with as little as 15 degrees of flexion.[13]

- Myocardial infarction is the most common cause of death following major amputation.[11]

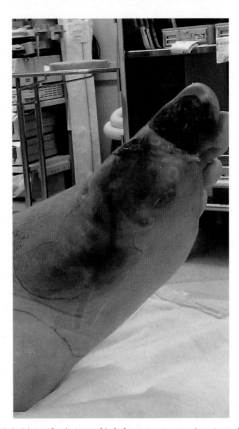

FIGURE 6-2 Magnified view of left-foot gangrene showing plantar extension. The tissue was boggy with subcutaneous crepitance indicating gas-forming necrotizing infection.

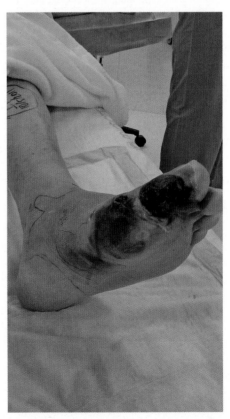

FIGURE 6-3 Left-foot gangrene depicting extent of cellulitis. Despite appearing localized externally, all fascial planes of the foot and ankle were extensively necrotic.

- The majority of major amputees have chronic pain, which must be managed via multimodality therapy. Phantom limb pain is described in most amputees; however, it is difficult to separate from other causes of pain. Medications must be multifocal in this regard.[14]

## PATIENT FOLLOW-UP

- Patients are typically seen for staple removal at 3 to 4 weeks. If wound is healed well, then routine follow-up is recommended.

- Referral to a licensed prosthetist can generally be performed postoperatively 4 to 6 weeks following surgery, and is dependent on the patient's physical and medical condition.

## REFERENCES

1. Group TG. Epidemiology of lower extremity amputation in centers in Europe, North America and East Asia. The Global Lower Extremity Amputation Study Group. *Br J Surg*. 2000;87:328.

2. Feinglass J, Brown JL, LoSasso A, et al. Rates of lower-extremity amputation and arterial reconstruction in the United States, 1979 to 1996. *Am J Public Health*. 1999;89:1222.

3. Huber TS, Wang JG, Wheeler KG, et al. Impact of race on the treatment for peripheral arterial occlusive disease. *J Vasc Surg*. 1999;30:417.

4. Nowygrod R, Egorova N, Greco G, et al. Trends, complications, and mortality in peripheral vascular surgery. *J Vasc Surg*. 2006;43:205.

5. Abou-Zamzam AM, Gomez NR, Molkara A, et al. A prospective analysis of critical limb ischemia: factors leading to major primary amputation versus revascularization. *Ann Vasc Surg*. 2007;21:458.

6. Krupski WC, Nehler MR, Whitehill TA, et al. Negative impact of cardiac evaluation before vascular surgery. *Vasc Med*. 2000;5:3.

7. Fleisher LA, Beckman JA, Brown KA, et al. ACC/AHA 2007 Guidelines on Perioperative Cardiovascular Evaluation and Care for Noncardiac Surgery: executive summary: a report of the American College of Cardiology/American Heart Association Task Force on Practice Guidelines (Writing Committee to Revise the 2002 Guidelines on Perioperative Cardiovascular Evaluation for Noncardiac Surgery): developed in collaboration with the American Society of Echocardiography, American Society of Nuclear Cardiology, Heart Rhythm Society, Society of Cardiovascular Anesthesiologists, Society for Cardiovascular Angiography and Interventions, Society for Vascular Medicine and Biology, and Society for Vascular Surgery. *Circulation*. 2007;116:1971.

8. DeFrang RD, Taylor LM, Porter JM. Basic data related to amputations. *Ann Vasc Surg*. 1991;5:202.

9. Fisher, DF, Jr., Clagett GP, Fry RE, et al. One-stage versus two-stage amputation for wet gangrene of the lower extremity: a randomized study. *J Vasc Surg*. 1988;8:428.

10. Sandnes DK, Sobel M, Flum DR. Survival after lower-extremity amputation. *J Am Coll Surg*. 2004;199:394-402.

11. Nehler MR, Coll JR, Hiatt WR, et al. Functional outcome in a contemporary series of major lower extremity amputations. *J Vasc Surg*. 2003;38:7-14.

12. Rubin JR, Marmen C, Rhodes RS. Management of failed prosthetic grafts at the time of major lower extremity amputation. *J Vasc Surg*. 1988;7:673-676.

13. Wasiak K, Paczkowski P, Garlicki J. Surgical results of leg amputation according to Ghormley's technique in the treatment of chronic lower limb ischaemia. *Acta Chir Belg*. 2006;106:52-54.

14. Ephraim PL, Wegener ST, MacKenzie EJ, et al. Phantom pain, residual limb pain, and back pain in amputees: results of a national survey. *Arch Phys Med Rehabil*. 2005;86:1910-1919.

# 7 EXTRA-ANATOMIC BYPASS GRAFTS

Irina Shakhnovich, MD

## PATIENT STORY

A 61-year-old man presented to his primary care physician complaining of worsening intermittent claudication of the right hip, buttock, and calf while trying to walk half a block. Upon further questioning the patient also admitted waking up in the middle of the night because of throbbing pain in his right toes. Significant findings on physical examination were absence of femoral and distal pulses of the right lower extremity. He also had evidence of muscle atrophy of the right calf. The left lower extremity had a normal palpable femoral pulse.

Ankle-brachial indices (ABIs) confirmed the presence of severe ischemia of right lower extremity with index of 0.4. Computed tomographic arteriogram (CTA) confirmed occlusion of the right common iliac and the right external iliac artery (Figure 7-1).

This patient was seen by a vascular surgeon and because of severe claudication and developing rest pain, an extra-anatomic femoral–femoral artery bypass surgery was recommended.

He underwent uneventful left to right femorofemoral bypass surgery, during which blood flow from his left iliac artery was redirected to the right lower extremity (Figure 7-2).

## GENERAL CONCEPTS

- Aortofemoral bypass remains the standard against which all extra-anatomic bypass surgeries' methods of reconstruction for distal aortic occlusion and iliac artery occlusion must be measured.[1]

- The term *extra-anatomic bypass* applies to any bypass graft that is placed in a site different from that of the native arterial segment being bypassed. While many common vascular procedures such as femorotibial bypass might be considered extra-anatomic, this term specifically describes procedures addressing diseases of the aortoiliac and femoral arteries.[1]

- Common extra-anatomic bypasses include axillofemoral and femorofemoral bypasses. Less common and more complex bypasses include obturator, thoracofemoral, and supraceliac-to-iliofemoral bypasses.

- Historically, extra-anatomic procedures were developed to treat high-risk patients with severe medical comorbidities or with "hostile" abdomens. "Hostile" abdomen refers to patients with prior multiple abdominal operations that result in adhesions ("frozen" abdomen) or patients with active intra-abdominal infections (including "mycotic" aortic aneurysms, infected aortic prostheses, aortoenteric fistulae). "Hostile" groin refers to patients with infected femoral artery aneurysm, prosthetic graft groin infection, history of groin radiation, and malignancies involving the groin or femoral vessels.

- Extra-anatomic bypasses require a long, subcutaneously placed prosthetic graft. These grafts are often externally supported with a

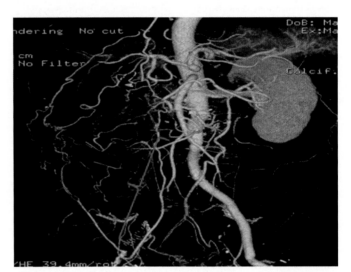

**FIGURE 7-1** Computed tomographic (CT) angiogram illustrating occlusion of the right iliac system indicated by the red bracket.

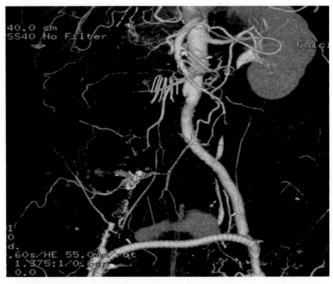

**FIGURE 7-2** Left to right femorofemoral bypass (arrow) redirecting the blood flow from the left iliac system to the right lower extremity.

removable continuous-spiral coil to reduce kinking and compression. Commonly used grafts are ePTFE and Dacron grafts.[1]

## INDICATIONS FOR INTERVENTION

Two primary indications for extra-anatomic bypass are the presence of a contaminated field or hostile abdomen and poor medical condition of the patient. Elderly patients with severe cardiopulmonary disease who are not good candidates for coronary artery revascularization are best managed by extra-anatomic bypass procedures.[2] These patients may not tolerate open abdominal operation and aortic cross-clamping.

## CONTRAINDICATIONS

- Femorofemoral, axillofemoral, and obturator bypass may be contraindicated in patients who are prohibitive medical risks for any surgery or with unusually short life expectancies.

- Thoracofemoral and supraceliac-to-iliofemoral bypass are invasive procedures, and they are inappropriate for patients at high risk for open abdominal or thoracic surgery.

## SURGICAL OPTIONS

### Femorofemoral Bypass

This reconstruction is recommended to patients with symptoms related to unilateral stenosis or occlusion of a common or external iliac artery. Both femoral arteries are exposed through groin incisions and a subcutaneous tunnel is created superior to the pubis (Figure 7-3).

The patency of this bypass depends on the capacity of one iliac artery system to provide adequate blood flow to support both the legs. If the donor artery has a hemodynamically significant lesion the patient may develop "steal syndrome" in that leg. Donor artery with flow-limiting lesions may be amenable to endovascular treatment including angioplasty and stenting. The cumulative patency rates are reported to be 60% to 83% at 5 years.[3]

### Axillofemoral Bypass

The axillary artery is usually a good inflow artery because it is typically spared from atherosclerosis. The axillary artery is exposed through an infraclavicular incision, and a tunnel is created subcutaneously to the ipsilateral femoral artery (Figure 7-4). This is an excellent reconstruction for frail, elderly patients with bilateral iliac artery occlusion and those with other comorbidities such as multiple abdominal surgeries or prior radiation therapy.[1] Advantages include no abdominal incision, faster recovery, shorter hospital stay, no aortic cross-clamping, and no risk of sexual dysfunction. The patency of the graft is determined by the adequacy of inflow, the quality of outflow (runoff vessels), progression of occlusive disease, and technical performance of the procedure. The 5-year patency ranges from 63% to 80%.[4] The most common cause of axillofemoral graft failure is spontaneous thrombosis usually occurring within 1 year. Thrombosis may occur secondary to mechanical factors, including external compression (sleeping on the side of the graft or wearing tight garments). The use of externally ring-supported grafts seems to have offered some protection from thrombosis caused by external compression.[1]

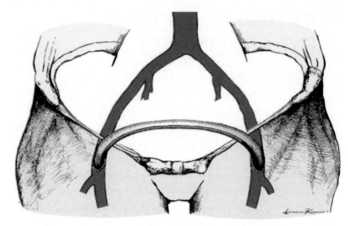

**FIGURE 7-3** Femorofemoral bypass graft connects femoral arteries and redirects flow from normal iliac artery to the leg with occluded iliac artery. (By permission from Extra-anatomic bypass. *Rutherford's Vascular Surgery.* 7th ed. Philadelphia, PA: Elsevier Inc; 2010:1635.)

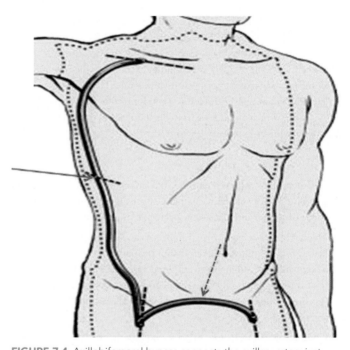

**FIGURE 7-4** Axillobifemoral bypass connects the axillary artery just beyond the clavicle to the femoral artery along the side of the torso (solid arrow) and then a bypass to the contralateral femoral artery if needed (stippled arrow). This bypass avoids entering the thoracic or abdominal cavity. (Reprinted by permission from Extra-anatomic bypass. *Rutherford's Vascular Surgery.* 7th ed. Philadelphia, PA: Elsevier Inc; 2010:1640.)

## Obturator Bypass

Obturator bypass is most commonly employed for femoral arterial reconstruction in patients with groin sepsis, including primary vascular infection; for example, it is used in patients with femoral mycotic aneurysms after puncture for a diagnostic or therapeutic endovascular procedure or recreational drug use, in those requiring removal of an infected arterial prosthesis in the groin, or in patients with otherwise hostile groins (eg, after radiation therapy or previous surgery). A tunnel is created through the obturator foramen, so a graft can be inserted proximal to possible infection and brought into the thigh and distal to the uninvolved artery (Figure 7-5). An obturator bypass may also be performed to restore flow when direct visualization is prohibited. Overall 5-year patency rates range from 66% to 89%.[5]

## Thoracofemoral and Supraceliac
## Aorta-to-Iliofemoral Bypass

Thoracofemoral and supraceliac aorta-to-iliofemoral bypasses are most often employed to avoid reoperation in the infrarenal aorta after failure of aortofemoral bypass or after removal of infected prosthetic aortic grafts. It uses the descending thoracic aorta for inflow source. This is an invasive procedure requiring left thoracotomy and graft positioning, and tunneling might be difficult. The 5-year patency is reported to be 79%.[6]

## COMPLICATIONS OF SURGICAL INTERVENTION

- Extra-anatomic bypasses have complications similar to any arterial operation including graft thrombosis, graft infection, and anastomotic aneurysms.

- Unique complication of femorofemoral bypass includes bladder and viscera injury while tunneling the graft.

- Axillofemoral graft can be complicated by brachial plexus injury, thromboembolic event to the donor arm, and axillary pullout syndrome (disruption of the axillary artery to graft anastomosis).[1]

- The most serious complication of extra-anatomic bypass is persistent or recurrent infection since many of these patients have been treated for failure of other reconstructions or for infected graft.

## FOLLOW-UP AND PATIENT EDUCATION

- Surveillance and patient education are important factors in the success of any vascular reconstruction. However, routine surveillance of extra-anatomic bypass grafts with noninvasive duplex ultrasonography is questionable at this time.[1]

- Although there are some reports of predictors of impending graft thrombosis, there is not uniform consensus or data to support routine surveillance with duplex scanning at the present time.

- Patients should be educated to palpate pulses over their extremities and over the graft routinely. Any changes they appreciate should be communicated with their surgeon.

- Patients should also avoid any external compression on their bypasses such as tight belts, constrictive clothing, or lying on the bypass itself.

- As with all patients with vascular disease, risk factor modifications including smoking cessation, control of hypertension and diabetes, and a low-fat diet should be emphasized.[1,2]

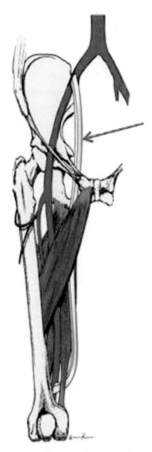

**FIGURE 7-5** The obturator bypass originates from the most proximal portion of the external iliac artery, passes through the obturator foramen, and terminates at the popliteal artery (arrow). This bypass avoids "hostile" groin. (Reprinted by permission from Extra-anatomic bypass. *Rutherford's Vascular Surgery.* 7th ed. Philadelphia, PA: Elsevier Inc; 2010:1648.)

## REFERENCES

1. Schneider JR. Extra-anatomic bypass. In: Cronenwett JL, Johnston KW, eds. *Rutherford's Vascular Surgery*. 7th ed. Philadelphia, PA: Elsevier; 2010:1633-1652.

2. Fahey VA, Milzrek A. Extraanatomic bypass surgery. *J Vasc Nurs*. 1999;17(3):71-75.

3. Ricco J-B, Probst H. Long-term results of a multicenter randomized study on direct versus crossover bypass for unilateral iliac artery occlusive disease. *J Vasc Surg*. 2008;47:45-54.

4. Passman MA, Taylor LM, Moneta GL, et al. Comparison of axillofemoral and aortofemoral bypass for aortoiliac occlusive disease. *J Vasc Surg*. 1996;23:263-271.

5. van Det RJ, Brands LC. The obturator foramen bypass: an alternative procedure in iliofemoral artery revascularization. *Surgery*. 1981;89:543-547.

6. Passman MA, Farber MA, Criado E, et al. Descending thoracic aorta to iliofemoral artery bypass grafting: a role for primary revascularization for aortoiliac occlusive disease? *J Vasc Surg*. 1999;29:249-258.

# 8 BLUE TOE SYNDROME (ATHEROMATOUS EMBOLIZATION)

Irina Shakhnovich, MD

## PATIENT STORY

A 62-year-old woman with a history of smoking presented to the emergency room complaining of acute onset of pain and color change of the left toes. All five of her toes turned purple-blue in color (Figure 8-1). The patient also reported a low-grade fever but denied any precipitating events. Her past medical history was significant for hypertension and coronary artery disease. Her feet were warm, and she had diminished bilateral femoral pulses and absent distal pulses on physical examination. Upon further questioning, the patient admitted to short-distance claudication.

Computed tomographic arteriogram (CTA) showed severely calcified atherosclerotic disease of the abdominal aorta and iliac arteries (Figure 8-2).

The final diagnosis was of blue toe syndrome or atheromatous embolization secondary to severe atherosclerotic disease of abdominal aorta.

## EPIDEMIOLOGY

- Usually affects elderly population with multiple risk factors for atherosclerosis, but it may occur in younger individuals with advanced atherosclerosis.

- The incidence varies, based on population selection and diagnostic criteria. The unselected autopsy studies show that incidence is 0.85% to 2.4%.[1-3] However, autopsy studies performed in selected patients with atherosclerosis and patients who had undergone aortic manipulation showed a prevalence ranging from 12% to 77%.[4,5]

- There is an increased frequency in males. This may be explained by the difference in the prevalence of atherosclerosis between the genders.

- Less likely to occur in blacks than in whites (32:1 ratio).[1] This may represent failure to recognize the pathology because of skin pigmentation.

## ETIOLOGY AND PATHOPHYSIOLOGY

- The most important risk factor is established atherosclerosis.

- This is a process in which emboli from proximal lesions (plaque) produce ischemia in distal arterial beds.

- It may be associated with significant pain and risk of tissue loss such as gangrenous tissue changes (Figure 8-3).

- Emboli may consist of thrombus, platelet-fibrin material, or a combination of both. Macroemboli may arise from thrombus originating in aortic or peripheral aneurysms or atheromatous ulcers, or from the dislodgement of atheromatous plaques. Microemboli are

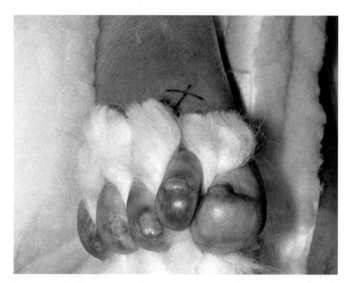

FIGURE 8-1 Cyanotic toes in a 62-year-old female patient diagnostic of blue toe syndrome. (Reprinted by permission from Atheromatous embolization. *Rutherford's Vascular Surgery.* 7th ed. Philadelphia, PA: Elsevier Inc; 2010:2427.)

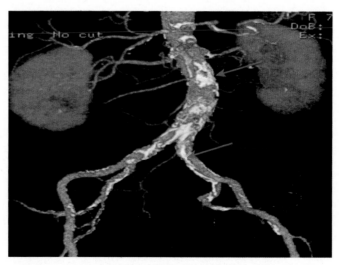

FIGURE 8-2 Severely calcified aorta and bilateral iliac arteries (arrows).

platelet-fibrin emboli or cholesterol crystals. Cholesterol crystals are lightweight and tend to be diffused and lodge in arteries as small as 100 to 200 μm.[6,7]

- Factors that may precipitate lesion (plaque) instability and result in atheroembolization include trauma, vascular surgery, endovascular procedures such as cardiac catheterization, and anticoagulation. Spontaneous embolization was once the most common presentation. With the increase in endovascular interventions, this is now the most frequent underlying cause of distal embolization.[1]

## DIAGNOSIS

- The syndrome is also known as atheromatous embolization, cholesterol embolization, atheroembolism, or "blue toe syndrome."

- It is a poorly recognized and underdiagnosed multisystem disorder that has high morbidity and mortality from associated cardiovascular causes.[1] For this reason a high index of suspicion is needed.

- Any end organ may become affected by distal embolization. Patients may present with cyanotic toes, acute kidney injury, or bowel ischemia if these organs are affected.

- The diagnosis can often be made on clinical grounds alone, based on a history of precipitating events such as recent endovascular procedure and evidence of peripheral embolization on physical examination.

- Definitive diagnosis may require a biopsy of the skin or in the affected organ, such as an amputated extremity in a patient presenting with gangrenous toes, the kidney in a patient with new-onset renal failure, or the gastrointestinal (GI) tract in a patient with abdominal pain and GI bleeding.

- Histologically, cholesterol crystal emboli appear as biconvex, needle shapes that are highly birefringent under polarized light. In addition to mechanical occlusion, cholesterol crystal emboli produce a local inflammatory response, and polymorphonuclear leukocyte infiltrate will be detected in arterioles within 24 hours.

- Atheromatous emboli are insoluble in body fluids and can be detected up to 9 months after an acute event.[1]

## LABORATORY TESTS

- No specific laboratory tests are diagnostic.

- Eosinophilia can be found in up to 80% of cases and is probably related to the generation of complement C5, which has chemotactic properties for eosinophils. The eosinophilia, however, tends to be transient and short lived.

- Laboratory markers of inflammation, including C-reactive protein, fibrinogen, and erythrocyte sedimentation rate, are elevated in many patients.[1]

## DIAGNOSTIC IMAGING MODALITIES

- Invasive vascular procedures requiring aortic instrumentation should be avoided as a diagnostic modality because of high risk of producing recurrent atheroembolism.

- Noninvasive imaging studies such as multidetector CTA, magnetic resonance angiography (MRA), and transesophageal echocardiogram (TEE) can assist in confirming the diagnosis if a markedly irregular and shaggy aorta is demonstrated (Figure 8-4).

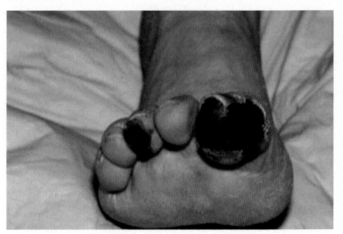

**FIGURE 8-3** Severe case of blue toe syndrome that progressed to gangrene.

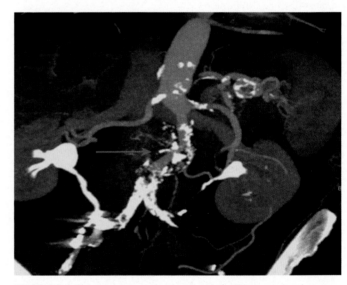

**FIGURE 8-4** Shaggy aorta and severely calcified iliac arteries that can be a source of distal embolization (arrow).

## DIFFERENTIAL DIAGNOSIS

- In the absence of any embolic sources one should consider systemic abnormalities such as necrotizing vasculitis, leukocytoclastic vasculitis, thrombotic thrombocytopenic purpura, antiphospholipid antibody syndrome, and multiple myeloma.[1]
- Cardiac sources of emboli such as atrial myxoma, nonbacterial thrombotic endocarditis, and infective endocarditis need to be excluded.

## MANAGEMENT

The most important aspect of therapy is prevention. Once atheromatous embolization has occurred, therapy is mostly supportive. Good control of hypertension and heart failure, dialysis support, and adequate nutrition are the mainstays of treatment.

### Medical Therapy

- Although the inflammatory process caused by atheromatous embolization may suggest a role for the use of corticosteroids, the data do not support their usage. Based on the available literature, corticosteroid use cannot be recommended on a routine basis for this patient population.[8]
- Statins are reportedly beneficial in the treatment of renal and lower limb cholesterol emboli syndrome.[9]
- In theory, antiplatelet agents such as aspirin and dipyridamole may help stabilize the source of atheroemboli. Unfortunately, no controlled trials have shown that any of these therapies are beneficial.[1]
- Use of anticoagulation with heparin and warfarin is controversial. There is some evidence that anticoagulation agents can promote further plaque instability and embolization.[10]

### Surgical and Endovascular Therapy

- Goal for both therapies is to eliminate the embolic source and improve perfusion to end organs.
- Because of the instability of these lesions, surgical treatment has been perceived as safer than endovascular approaches because the surgeon can clamp the artery proximal and distal to the lesion before manipulating the diseased vessel in an attempt to decrease the risk of recurrent embolization.
- Because of the limited studies available regarding the role of endovascular therapy for atheromatous embolization, its clinical efficacy is difficult to compare with operative treatment.[1]

## FOLLOW-UP

- In general, the prognosis of patients with atheroembolic disease is poor, most likely related to the severe and diffuse atherosclerosis in this patient population. The reported 1-year mortality varies from 64% to 81%. Causes of death are multifactorial and include cardiac, central nervous system, and GI ischemia.[11-13]
- All patients should receive aggressive risk factor modification with an antiplatelet agent (aspirin, clopidogrel, or both), a statin, and an angiotensin-converting enzyme inhibitor, all of which can improve mortality in patients with underlying atherosclerotic disease.

## REFERENCES

1. Rutherford RB, Olin JW, Bartholomew JR. Atheromatous embolization. In: Cronenwett JL, Johnston KW, eds. *Rutherford's Vascular Surgery.* 7th ed. Philadelphia, PA: Elsevier; 2010: 2422-2434.
2. Fine MJ, Kapoor W, Falanga V. Cholesterol crystal embolization: a review of 221 cases in the English literature. *Angiology.* 1987;38:769-784.
3. Blauth CI, Cosgrove DM, Webb BW, et al. Atheroembolism from the ascending aorta. An emerging problem in cardiac surgery. *J Thorac Cardiovasc Surg.* 1992;103:1104-1111.
4. Moolenaar W, Lamers CB. Cholesterol crystal embolization in the Netherlands. *Arch Intern Med.* 1996;156:653-657.
5. Cross SS. How common is cholesterol embolism? *J Clin Pathol.* 1991;44:859-861.
6. Rhodes JM. Cholesterol crystal embolism: an important "new" diagnosis for the general physician. *Lancet.* 1996;347:1641.
7. Ghannem M, Philippe J, Ressam A, et al. Systemic cholesterol embolism. *Ann Cardiol Angeiol (Paris).* 1995;44:422-426.
8. Fabbian F, Catalano C, Lambertini D, et al. A possible role of corticosteroids in cholesterol crystal embolization. *Nephron.* 1999;83:189-190.
9. Woolfson RG, Lachmann H. Improvement in renal cholesterol emboli syndrome after simvastatin. *Lancet.* 1998;351: 1331-1332.
10. Haimovichi H. *Haimovici's Vascular Surgery: Principles and Techniques.* 4th ed. Norwalk, CT: Appleton and Longe; 1996: 466-479.
11. Lye WC, Cheah JS, Sinniah R. Renal cholesterol embolic disease. Case report and review of the literature. *Am J Nephrol.* 1993;13:489-493.
12. Saleem S, Lakkis FG, Martinez-Maldonado M. Atheroembolic renal disease. *Semin Nephrol.* 1996;16:309-318.
13. Dahlberg PJ, Frecentese DF, Cogbill TH. Cholesterol embolism: experience with 22 histologically proven cases. *Surgery.* 1989;105(6):737-746.

# PART 2

# AORTIC AND UPPER EXTREMITY ARTERIAL DISEASE

# 9 ATHEROSCLEROTIC ARCH VESSEL DISEASE

Jean M. Ruddy, MD
Thomas E. Brothers, MD
Nitin Garg, MBBS, MPH

## PATIENT STORY

A 59-year-old Caucasian woman presented for evaluation after a recent right hemispheric stroke. She had residual short-term memory loss but no sensory or motor deficits. She reported previous episodes of dizziness, syncope, and left arm fatigue upon exertion prior to the stroke. Despite a 60 pack-year cigarette smoking history, she had recently quit and was compliant with her statin and antiplatelet therapy. On physical examination she had a right cervical bruit, absent left radial pulse, and her lower extremity vascular examination was unremarkable. There was significant discrepancy in upper extremity pressures.

Computed tomography (CT) and digital subtraction arteriogram (DSA) demonstrated occlusion of the left subclavian and the origin of the left common carotid arteries, but the latter was reconstituted by collaterals at the level of the bifurcation (Figure 9-1A). The right common carotid artery (CCA) had greater than 90% ostial stenosis and the right subclavian artery had significant stenosis, as suggested by the poststenotic dilation (Figure 9-1B). The right vertebral artery was dominant (Figure 9-1C). The innominate artery demonstrated diffuse calcific irregularity with moderate distal stenosis (Figure 9-2). The left vertebral artery was patent with retrograde flow on duplex ultrasonography.

After extensive discussion with the patient regarding the risks and benefits of open versus endovascular management strategies, she proceeded to the operating room for a hybrid procedure. Retrograde open right subclavian artery access was obtained with placement of a balloon expandable stent from the proximal subclavian artery extending into the innominate artery (Figure 9-3A and B). A right subclavian to carotid artery bypass was then constructed with a prosthetic graft, and the proximal common carotid was ligated. She was discharged home on postoperative day 1 (POD1) and had no adverse events. She was doing well with no further neurologic problems at subsequent follow-up.

## EPIDEMIOLOGY

- The incidence, and consequence, of atherosclerosis in the aortic arch vessels has been described in few reports. In an autopsy study of patients who suffered a fatal stroke, approximately 50% of subjects had plaque deposition at the origin of the innominate, left common carotid, or left subclavian arteries.[1]

- Arch multivessel atherosclerotic disease is most common in middle-aged Caucasian females. The majority of them are asymptomatic, even in the presence of flow reversal through the vertebral, and should be managed conservatively. However, more clinically relevant is the 0.6% to 4% incidence of concurrent internal carotid

and proximal arch vessel atherosclerotic disease, raising questions regarding preprocedure imaging and indications for treatment of arch vessel disease.[2]

## ETIOLOGY AND PATHOPHYSIOLOGY

- The well-recognized vascular risk factors associated with atherosclerotic disease, including diabetes mellitus, hypertension, hyperlipidemia, obesity, family history of accelerated atherosclerosis, and cigarette smoking, also contribute to the deposition of plaque in the aortic arch vessels.

- Differential distribution of atherosclerotic disease is likely related to flow dynamics and is an independent risk factor for stroke.[3] In some patients, underlying inflammatory arteritis (eg, Takayasu disease) hastens atherosclerotic degeneration.

## DIAGNOSIS

### Clinical Presentation

- Patients with disease of the supra-aortic trunk vessels may present with symptoms of global cerebral ischemia, upper extremity fatigue upon exertion, subclavian steal syndrome, or coronary-subclavian steal syndrome.[4]

- Transient ischemic attack as well as stroke may result from embolic events from proximal common carotid or innominate artery lesions or acute occlusion.[3]

- Subclavian artery stenosis or occlusion may lead to the sensation of upper extremity cramping or fatigue during heavy activity or repeated use. Alternatively, increased upper extremity workload may precipitate reversal of flow through a patent vertebral artery.[4] These patients report symptoms corresponding to posterior cerebral ischemia such as dizziness, vision changes, and presyncope (subclavian steal syndrome). Similarly, in patients with prior coronary artery bypass grafting utilizing internal thoracic artery conduit, angina pectoris may be elicited by aggressive upper extremity exercise due to reversal of flow through the bypass segment, a phenomenon known as coronary-subclavian steal syndrome.[4]

- Detailed past medical history should be obtained with particular attention to the patient's atherosclerotic risk factors. A personal history of cigarette smoking is almost always associated with multivessel disease[3] and patients should be extensively counseled on cessation. In young patients, a history of fever, malaise, night sweats, weight loss, arthralgias, and fatigue should also be pursued for consideration of large vessel arteritis.

### Physical Examination

- In addition to confirming that the patient's heart has a regular rate and rhythm without evidence of mitral or aortic murmurs (to rule

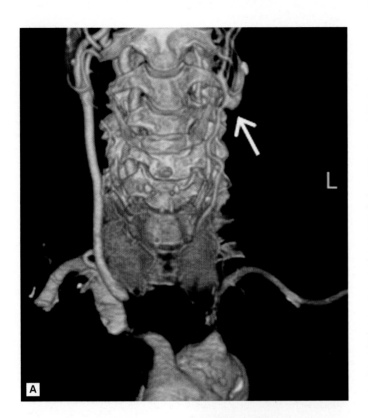

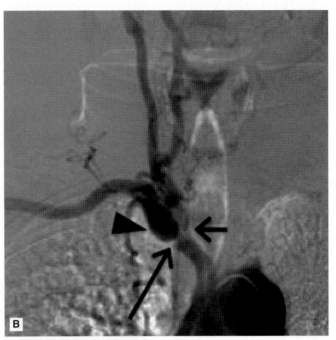

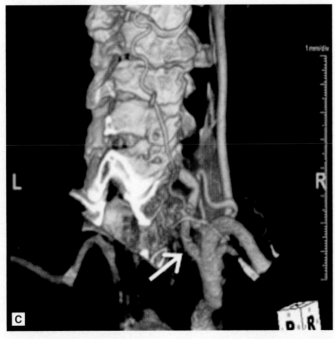

**FIGURE 9-1** Anterior view of a computed tomographic arteriography (CTA) three-dimensional (3D) reconstruction demonstrating occlusion of the left carotid and subclavian arteries with collateralization through the thyroid arteries to reconstitute the left internal carotid artery (ICA) at the level of the bifurcation (arrow) (A). Arch arteriogram of the same patient shows stenosis of the origin of the right subclavian (long arrow) and right carotid arteries (short arrow) with poststenotic dilation in the proximal subclavian (arrowhead) (B). Posterior view of CTA 3D reconstruction exhibiting a large dominant right vertebral artery (arrow) (C).

out secondary cause of embolic event in symptomatic patients), a carotid bruit may be auscultated during evaluation of the neck.

- Palpation of carotid and upper extremity pulsation could provide clues to high-grade proximal disease with associated palpable thrill and diminished pulsation distally. Bilateral brachial blood pressure measurements should be performed.

## Laboratory Evaluation

- Patients with suspected peripheral arterial disease should be evaluated with a complete blood count, a renal function panel, and a fasting lipid panel. In cases where clinical presentation suggests underlying vasculitis, erythrocyte sedimentation rate and C-reactive protein levels should also be obtained.[3]

- Color duplex ultrasonography has been instrumental in the diagnostic evaluation of internal carotid atherosclerotic disease, with the velocity parameters and indications for surgery extensively studied and widely accepted. Its use in CCA lesions, however, has yet to be fully defined. Studies correlating duplex ultrasound to arteriography initially identified delayed systolic upstroke, spectral broadening, and dampening of the peak systolic velocity as indicators of CCA stenosis, but ultrasonographic imaging of the proximal CCA is difficult and dependent on body habitus (Figure 9-4).[5] Alternatively, very low flow velocities in an otherwise disease-free internal carotid artery (ICA) (Figure 9-5A) and diastolic reversal of

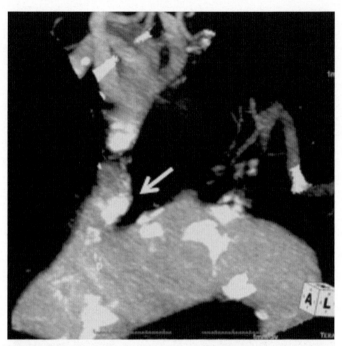

**FIGURE 9-2** Computed tomographic arteriography (CTA) reconstruction of the arch and supra-aortic branch vessels demonstrating scattered atherosclerotic plaque deposition along the arch and heavy disease within the innominate artery (arrow).

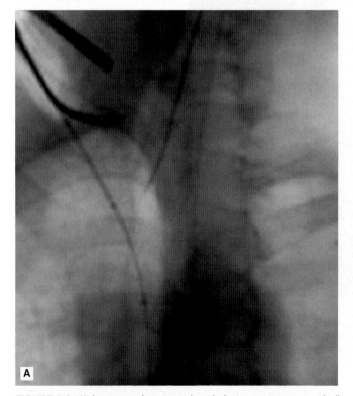

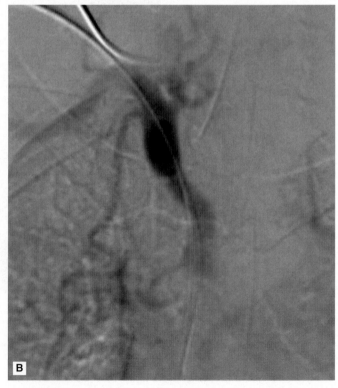

**FIGURE 9-3** With retrograde open right subclavian artery access, a balloon expandable covered stent was placed from the proximal subclavian artery into the innominate artery (A). Completion arteriogram demonstrated hemodynamically insignificant residual stenosis and absence of flow in the right common carotid artery (CCA) (B).

flow in the ipsilateral ICA (Figure 9-5B) represent ultrasonographic findings suggestive of proximal CCA occlusion. In one report using computed tomographic arteriography (CTA) as the gold standard, a CCA peak systolic velocity greater than 182 cm/s had a 64% sensitivity and 88% specificity for indicating a greater than 50% stenosis of the mid or distal CCA (Figure 9-4).[5] In patients undergoing evaluation for cerebrovascular symptoms, the greatest contribution of duplex ultrasound may be identifying those who warrant further vascular anatomic imaging.

- Flow reversal in the ipsilateral vertebral artery (Figure 9-5C), indicating steal physiology, has often been considered diagnostic of significant proximal subclavian stenosis.[6] However, the absence of this sonographic finding does not definitively exclude subclavian disease. Therefore, hemodynamic criteria to describe subclavian atherosclerosis carry considerable clinical relevance. When DSA was used as a comparative standard, duplex ultrasonographic measurement of peak systolic velocity greater than 343 cm/s within the subclavian artery had an 87% sensitivity and 83.2% specificity of identifying a greater than 70% stenosis,[6] whereas slow, monophasic flow may be consistent with ostial occlusion and reconstitution via collaterals (Figure 9-5D). On the right side, occlusive disease of the proximal innominate artery is rare and may result in reversal of flow in both the ipsilateral vertebral and carotid arteries.

## Radiographic Evaluation

- DSA of the aortic arch and branch vessels was once considered as standard preoperative workup for patients with ICA atherosclerotic disease and accurately identified the small subset of patients with tandem carotid or concurrent subclavian artery lesions, but the attendant cost and stroke risk have become prohibitive for routine use.

- CTA of the aortic arch, neck, and circle of Willis has become easily accessible at most major centers, can be achieved with a single contrast bolus, and through manipulation by radiologic software may provide axial, coronal, sagittal, and three-dimensional images ideal for operative planning.[7] The accuracy of CTA measurement of atherosclerotic stenosis when compared to DSA has been extensively studied and confirmed in the carotid arterial system, with regard to both lumen diameter and area, with sensitivity and specificity as high as 97% and 99%, respectively.[7]

- Magnetic resonance arteriography (MRA) has been utilized following an inconclusive duplex ultrasonographic study to investigate atherosclerotic disease of the arch and cerebrovascular system rather than exposing the patient to the risks of arteriography.[8] Specifically within the supra-aortic trunk, MRA had a sensitivity of 93% and specificity of 89% for identifying a significant stenosis, suggesting that it can be a reliable tool in initial diagnosis as well as long-term follow-up of these patients.[8] Although far more limited in the current era, there may still be a role for diagnostic DSA in cases where noninvasive imaging provides disparate results and also when endovascular management is planned (Figure 9-6).

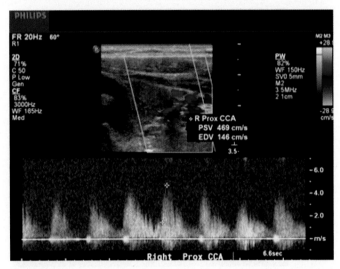

**FIGURE 9-4** When body habitus permits, duplex ultrasonography of the proximal common carotid artery (CCA) may capture turbulent, high-velocity flow.

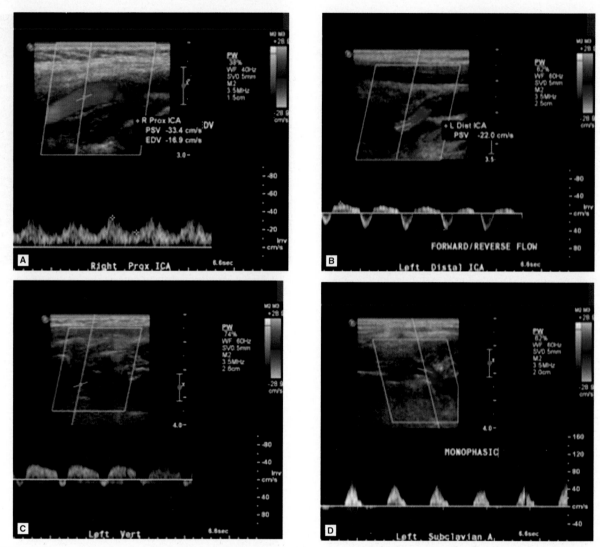

**FIGURE 9-5** Ultrasonographic image of the proximal right internal carotid artery (ICA) showing low flow in the absence of atherosclerotic disease (A) and a rare finding of ICA diastolic reversal of flow (B), suggestive of proximal common carotid artery (CCA) high-grade stenosis or occlusion. Vertebral artery reversal of flow may be diagnostic of subclavian steal syndrome (C). When low velocity, monophasic flow is identified in the subclavian artery (D), ostial occlusion with subsequent reconstitution through collaterals should be considered and cross-sectional imaging pursued.

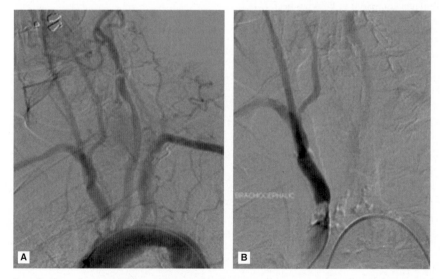

**FIGURE 9-6** Aortic arch and cerebral arteriogram demonstrating tandem lesions with severe occlusive arch disease and occlusion of left internal carotid artery (ICA) (arrow) (A). Selective arteriogram subsequently revealed high-grade densely calcified innominate stenosis with eccentric plaque (B). (Published with permission from *Journal of Vascular and Endovascular Surgery*, originally printed in Garg, et al. Retrograde supra-aortic stent placement combined with open carotid or subclavian artery revascularization. 2011;45(6):527-535.)

## MANAGEMENT

### Medical

- Aggressive medical management is the cornerstone for all patients with atherosclerosis and is imperative to minimize the risk of postintervention complications. The myocardial risk reduction and plaque stabilization realized through angiotensin blockade as well as statin therapy have made these medications standard pharmacotherapy in all patients with atherosclerosis, both perioperatively and in the long term.[9,10]

- Antiplatelet therapy has been recommended in all patients without contraindications and can significantly reduce vascular mortality, nonfatal myocardial infarction, and nonfatal stroke.[11] For patients undergoing operative therapy, perioperative administration of beta-blockade has been shown to decrease the risk of myocardial infarction in appropriately selected patients undergoing a peripheral vascular procedure.[12]

### Surgical

- Surgical reconstruction of the supra-aortic trunk has been performed via either a transthoracic or extra-anatomic cervical approach, depending largely on the distribution of the atherosclerotic disease and the patient's cardiopulmonary risk factors. In a retrospective review of 100 transthoracic reconstructions, 63% of patients had multivessel disease, with the innominate artery being most frequently involved, and most patients underwent reconstruction via a median sternotomy.[13]

- A combined stroke or death rate of 16% was reported along with 3% myocardial infarctions, 7% pulmonary complications, 2% operative re-exploration for hematoma evacuation, and 1% right recurrent laryngeal nerve injury.[13] Overall survival was 52%, and graft patency was 88% at 10 years.[13]

- Alternatively, a review of the extra-anatomic approach for supra-aortic trunk reconstruction reported 61% single vessel disease, allowing for 33% of patients to undergo arterial translocation and the remainder requiring graft placement with either saphenous vein or prosthetic graft.[14] Combined stroke or death rate of 4% was observed, and additional morbidities included 3% myocardial infarctions, 2% wound hematomas, 2% recurrent laryngeal nerve injuries, and 1% graft infections.[14] When necessary to cross the midline, a retropharyngeal tunnel has been favored, although there is a risk of dysphagia with this approach (Figure 9-7). The extra-anatomic approach is associated not only with reduced mortality and morbidity, but also shorter length of stay (6 days vs 11 days).[13,14]

- Long-term patency with either the transthoracic or the extra-anatomic approach has been excellent. Patients suffering from an inflammatory arteritis are eligible for the same surgical interventions, but the procedure should be scheduled during a time of disease quiescence.

### Endovascular

- With the considerable risk of complications following operative revascularization, angioplasty of the arch vessels has emerged as a less morbid therapeutic approach with reportedly excellent technical success but variable patency rates and frequent requirement for repeat intervention.

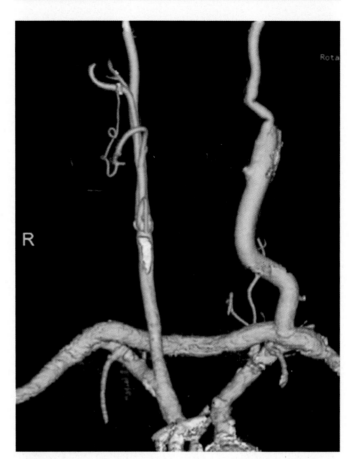

**FIGURE 9-7.** Anterior view of three-dimensional (3D) rendering of a computed tomographic arteriography (CTA) demonstrating an extra-anatomic reconstruction of an aortic arch afflicted with occlusive disease of the innominate, left common carotid, and left internal carotid artery (ICA). A left-to-right retropharyngeal subclavian–subclavian bypass was performed in this patient, with an interposition graft from this bypass to the left carotid bifurcation (with internal carotid endarterectomy).

- The addition of stent placement following supra-aortic trunk angioplasty was subsequently introduced to decrease restenosis, and endovascular therapy has continued to progress with regard to access location, types of stents, methods of cerebral protection, and approach to tandem carotid lesions. Most institutions have reported retrospective reviews of collective stent placement in any arch vessel, making comparative analysis difficult, but technical success rates of 89% to 100% have been described, with the majority of failures attributable to chronic subclavian occlusions.[15]

- Access site hematomas and intimal dissections were more common in the early reports, but alternative access locations, advances in percutaneous closure devices, and the evolution of wire and catheter technology have decreased these considerably. Short segment stenosis or occlusion of the innominate and subclavian arteries has been successfully approached from both the femoral and ipsilateral brachial arteries.[4,15] Additionally, a combined brachial or femoral access approach with one- or two-wire advancement has been described to facilitate stent deployment in occlusive lesions.[4,16] Early studies deployed Palmaz® stents,[15] but self-expanding stents have since gained popularity for nonostial lesions with poststent balloon dilation to optimize expansion, and placement of additional stents to address flow-limiting dissections as needed.[4] Use of cerebral protection devices when addressing lesions of the innominate artery has also been advocated by some centers.[17] Technical success may be assessed by angiography with brisk flow through the stent and less than 10% residual stenosis, or by employing hemodynamic parameters targeting a pressure gradient of less than 5 mm Hg across the stent.[15] A recent large series of transfemoral CCA angioplasty and stenting reported a 99% technical success rate and 2.5% 30-day stroke incidence in a patient population where only 10% were treated with embolic protection devices.[18] On long-term follow-up, 1-, 4-, and 7-year primary patency was 98%, 82%, and 74%, respectively, and secondary patency rates at the same time-points were 100%, 88%, and 88%, respectively.[18] In a contemporary study, embolic stroke was described in less than 1% of patients, and at approximately 5 years of follow-up, primary and secondary patency was reported at 83% and 96%, respectively.[4]

- Angioplasty and stenting of CCA lesions have carried the obvious risk of embolic events, and operative exposure of the distal CCA through a standard neck incision followed by arteriography and retrograde stent placement has been used to reduce this risk.[15,17,19] Technical success rates of 92% to 100% have been reported with no periprocedural strokes documented.[15,17,19] A concerning potential complication of the retrograde technique has been iatrogenic dissection, which may need stent placement to maintain vessel patency or require conversion to subclavian–carotid bypass.[15]

- Tandem lesions of the CCA and bifurcation carry an increased risk of periprocedure stroke compared to CCA lesions alone.[15] The commonly described hybrid approach to these stenoses has involved standard neck incision with distal control of the ICA, retrograde stent placement in the CCA, flushing of embolic debris through the arteriotomy and/or into the external carotid artery (ECA), brief establishment of antegrade flow, and subsequently proceeding with standard carotid endarterectomy of the bifurcation with or without shunt placement.[2,20] Technical success rates of 97% to 100% have been described,[20] and transcranial Doppler confirmed protection from embolic debris in cases with operative distal control via clamping of the ICA. Overall, the concurrent repair of atherosclerotic stenosis of both the CCA and carotid bifurcation by a hybrid open or endovascular procedure has demonstrated safety and efficacy and may be considered as the preferred method.

## CONCLUSION

Arch disease is an uncommon and challenging diagnosis with optimal management achieved by tailoring therapy to each patient's anatomy and comorbidities. Endovascular treatment is applicable to a majority of cases and will continue to evolve, but extra-anatomic surgical options remain safe and effective.

## ACKNOWLEDGMENT

We would like to acknowledge the efforts of Ms Marguerite Cappuccio, RVT, Medical University of South Carolina, Charleston, SC, for her assistance with images used in this manuscript.

## REFERENCES

1. Mazighi M, Labreuche J, Gongora-Rivera F, Duyckaerts C, Hauw JJ, Amarenco P. Autopsy prevalence of proximal extracranial atherosclerosis in patients with fatal stroke. *Stroke*. Mar 2009;40(3):713-718.

2. Garg N, Oderich GS, Duncan AA, et al. Retrograde supra-aortic stent placement combined with open carotid or subclavian artery revascularization. *Vasc Endovascular Surg*. Aug 2011;45(6):527-535.

3. Iribarren C, Sidney S, Sternfeld B, Browner WS. Calcification of the aortic arch: risk factors and association with coronary heart disease, stroke, and peripheral vascular disease. *JAMA*. Jun 7 2000;283(21):2810-2815.

4. Patel SN, White CJ, Collins TJ, et al. Catheter-based treatment of the subclavian and innominate arteries. *Catheter Cardiovasc Interv*. Jun 1 2008;71(7):963-968.

5. Slovut DP, Romero JM, Hannon KM, Dick J, Jaff MR. Detection of common carotid artery stenosis using duplex ultrasonography: a validation study with computed tomographic angiography. *J Vasc Surg*. Jan 2010;51(1):65-70.

6. Hua Y, Jia L, Li L, Ling C, Miao Z, Jiao L. Evaluation of severe subclavian artery stenosis by color Doppler flow imaging. *Ultrasound Med Biol*. Mar 2011;37(3):358-363.

7. Zhang Z, Berg M, Ikonen A, et al. Carotid stenosis degree in CT angiography: assessment based on luminal area versus luminal diameter measurements. *Eur Radiol*. Nov 2005;15(11):2359-2365.

8. Kumar S, Roy S, Radhakrishnan S, Gujral R. Three-dimensional time-of-flight MR angiography of the arch of aorta and its major branches: a comparative study with contrast angiography. *Clin Radiol*. Jan 1996;51(1):18-21.

9. Fukuhara M, Geary RL, Diz DI, et al. Angiotensin-converting enzyme expression in human carotid artery atherosclerosis. *Hypertension*. Jan 2000;35(1 Pt 2):353-359.

10. O'Neil-Callahan K, Katsimaglis G, Tepper MR, et al. Statins decrease perioperative cardiac complications in patients undergoing noncardiac vascular surgery: the Statins for Risk Reduction in Surgery (StaRRS) study. *J Am Coll Cardiol.* Feb 1 2005;45(3): 336-342.

11. Collaboration AT. Collaborative meta-analysis of randomised trials of antiplatelet therapy for prevention of death, myocardial infarction, and stroke in high risk patients. *BMJ.* Jan 12 2002;324(7329):71-86.

12. Bangalore S, Wetterslev J, Pranesh S, Sawhney S, Gluud C, Messerli FH. Perioperative beta blockers in patients having non-cardiac surgery: a meta-analysis. *Lancet.* Dec 6 2008;372(9654):1962-1976.

13. Berguer R, Morasch MD, Kline RA. Transthoracic repair of innominate and common carotid artery disease: immediate and long-term outcome for 100 consecutive surgical reconstructions. *J Vasc Surg.* Jan 1998;27(1):34-41; discussion 42.

14. Berguer R, Morasch MD, Kline RA, Kazmers A, Friedland MS. Cervical reconstruction of the supra-aortic trunks: a 16-year experience. *J Vasc Surg.* Feb 1999;29(2):239-246; discussion 246-248.

15. Sullivan TM, Gray BH, Bacharach JM, et al. Angioplasty and primary stenting of the subclavian, innominate, and common carotid arteries in 83 patients. *J Vasc Surg.* Dec 1998;28(6):1059-1065.

16. Ryer EJ, Oderich GS. Two-wire (0.014 & 0.018-inch) technique to facilitate innominate artery stenting under embolic protection. *J Endovasc Ther.* Oct 2010;17(5):652-656.

17. Peterson BG, Resnick SA, Morasch MD, Hassoun HT, Eskandari MK. Aortic arch vessel stenting: a single-center experience using cerebral protection. *Arch Surg.* Jun 2006;141(6):560-563; discussion 563-564.

18. Paukovits TM, Haasz J, Molnar A, et al. Transfemoral endovascular treatment of proximal common carotid artery lesions: a single-center experience on 153 lesions. *J Vasc Surg.* Jul 2008;48(1):80-87.

19. Queral LA, Criado FJ. The treatment of focal aortic arch branch lesions with Palmaz stents. *J Vasc Surg.* Feb 1996;23(2):368-375.

20. Allie DE, Hebert CJ, Lirtzman MD, et al. Intraoperative innominate and common carotid intervention combined with carotid endarterectomy: a "true" endovascular surgical approach. *J Endovasc Ther.* Jun 2004;11(3):258-262.

# 10 THORACIC AORTIC DISSECTION

Christopher J. Goltz, MD
Daniel J. Reddy, MD

## PATIENT STORY

An otherwise healthy male with a history of systolic arterial hypertension presented to the emergency department (ED) with acute onset of upper back pain, stabbing in nature, with associated shortness of breath. When seen in the ED the patient was noted to be hypotensive and tachycardiac. Physical examination disclosed diminished breath sounds in the left chest, equal pulses in bilateral upper extremities, and diminished bilateral femoral pulses. Initial chest x-ray showed a left hemothorax (Figure 10-1). Vascular surgery was consulted and a thin slice computed tomographic (CT) scan with intravenous contrast and three-dimensional reconstruction indicated an acute Stanford B (DeBakey IIIB) aortic dissection with apparent rupture into the left chest (Figure 10-2). A proximal landing zone just distal to the origin of the left subclavian artery was seen. The dissection was seen to extend to the level of the abdominal aortic bifurcation (Figure 10-3). The celiac, superior and inferior mesenteric, and bilateral renal arteries were seen to be patent, and there was no clinical evidence of malperfusion syndrome of the visceral organs. The patient was taken for compassionate off-label use of a thoracic endovascular stent grafting (TEVAR) as his only option for survival. One day later he returned to the operating room for left thoracotomy and evacuation of the hemothorax. Percutaneous tracheostomy was performed several days later at the bedside. Postoperative imaging showed control of the rupture with resolution of the hemothorax and good position of the thoracic endograft (Figures 10-4 and 10-5). The patient was maintained in the intensive care unit (ICU), and after a prolonged hospital course and weaning from the ventilator, he improved and was subsequently discharged home.

## PATHOLOGY OF AORTIC DISSECTION

Two classification schemes are in common use to define aortic dissections. To define the anatomic landmarks, the takeoff of the left subclavian artery is used as the distal extent of the aortic arch.

The DeBakey classification is as follows:

- Type I dissections involve the ascending aorta and the arch and extend beyond the level of the aortic arch.

- Type II involves the ascending aorta and the arch only.

- Type IIIA involves the descending aorta only, not extending into the abdominal aorta.

- Type IIIB involves the abdominal aorta as well as the descending aorta.

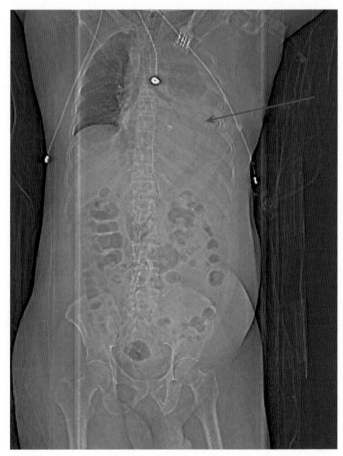

**FIGURE 10-1** A scout film showing a left hemothorax (arrow).

The Stanford classification (Figure 10-6) is as follows:

- Type A involves the ascending aorta and the arch with variable distal involvement.
- Type B involves the descending aorta only.[1]

## EPIDEMIOLOGY

- High mortality is associated with the disease, with 27% in-hospital mortality for all patients presenting with acute dissection.[1]
- Incidence of 0.5 to 2.1 per 100,000 person-years.[2]
- Mean incidence of type A dissection at 61 years.[1]
- Mean incidence of type B dissection at 66 years.[1]
- Acute dissection is defined at 14 days or less from the onset of symptoms as increased mortality and morbidity during this period, as well as stabilization of surviving patients.[1]

## CLINICAL PRESENTATION

- Pain in chest, back, or abdomen, often described as ripping, tearing, sharp, or stabbing, and often acute in onset.[1]
- Syncope may occur, more commonly with type A dissection than type B (12.7% vs 4.1% of patients) with stroke being a less common presentation at 6.1% for type A lesions.[1]
- Spinal cord ischemia.[3]
- Renal or mesenteric involvement causing ischemia, presenting with abdominal pain, tenderness, elevated amylase or liver function tests, diarrhea, or elevation in creatinine.[5]

## DIAGNOSTIC EVALUATION

- Computed tomography (CT) has largely replaced conventional angiography as the initial imaging modality of choice.[4]
- Echocardiography also provides high-quality and real-time evaluation of these lesions, with transthoracic echocardiography allowing imaging of the ascending aorta only.[4]

## TREATMENT

### Medical Therapy

- Control of blood pressure with intravenous (IV) B blockade (eg, esmolol) followed by IV vasodilatory agents (eg, nitroprusside) with invasive hemodynamic monitoring.[4]

### Surgical Therapy

- Stanford A dissections are typically treated operatively as risk of rupture, coronary artery compromise, hemopericardium, and impairment of aortic valve function is significant.[4]
- May be treated with delayed operation if evidence of end-organ malperfusion, limb ischemia, or neurologic involvement is present, and may have intervention to control malperfusion prior to operative repair of ascending portion.[5]
- Asymptomatic Stanford B dissections are treated with medical management alone, as no benefit is seen at 2 years when chronic dissections are treated with thoracic endografts.[6]

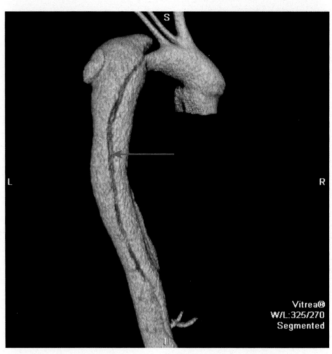

**FIGURE 10-2** Computed tomographic (CT) scan with intravenous contrast and three-dimensional reconstruction indicated an acute Stanford B (DeBakey IIIB) aortic dissection (arrow).

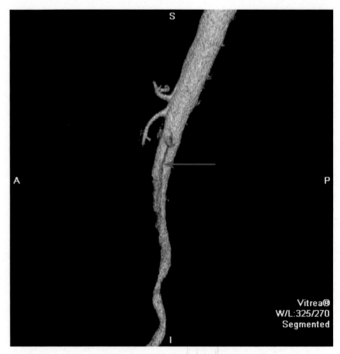

**FIGURE 10-3** The dissection was seen to extend to the level of the abdominal aortic bifurcation (arrow). The celiac and superior mesenteric arteries are also noted to be patent.

- Operative treatment indicated for end-organ malperfusion, progression of dissection, or if actual impending rupture is noted.[4]

- Endovascular options of type B dissections include stent grafting of the proximal tear site, fenestration procedures to widen the opening between true and false lumens, and stenting of impaired arterial branches.[4] No stent graft is approved for this use by the Food and Drug Administration (FDA), making TEVAR an off-label use for dissections. Mortality for the endovascular approach to these problems shows a significant improvement when compared to open surgery or to medical management alone.[2]

- Goals of endovascular therapy include thrombosis of the false lumen, prevention or aneurysmal dilation, and prevention of late rupture. Patency of false lumen is a risk factor for late mortality.[7]

- Open repair has been seen to have a high mortality, prohibiting repair in asymptotic patients except in specific cases where endovascular therapy is contraindicated.[2]

## COMPLICATIONS

Complications can be numerous. A few major ones are listed below.

- Death
- Paralysis or paraplegia
- Stroke
- Postoperative hemorrhage
- Renal failure
- Occlusions of various arteries
- Deep venous thrombosis (DVT)

## PATIENT FOLLOW-UP

- Frequent follow-up visits are necessary considering the major nature of the operation.
- Renal function must be monitored.
- Home rehabilitation is often necessary.
- Signs and symptoms of major organ failure and infection are explained.

## REFERENCES

1. Hagan PG, Nienaber CJ, Isselbacher EM, et al. The international registry of acute aortic dissection (IRAD); new insights into an old disease. *JAMA*. 2000;283(7):897-903.

2. Tang DG, Dake MD. TEVAR for acute uncomplicated aortic dissection: immediate repair versus medical therapy. *Semin Vasc Surg*. 2009;22:145-151.

3. Tsai TT, Fattori R, Trimarchi S, et al. Long-term survival in patients presenting with type B acute aortic dissection: insights from the International Registry of Acute Aortic Dissection. *Circulation*. 2006;114:2226-2231.

4. Ince H, Nienaber C. Diagnosis and management of patients with aortic dissection. *Heart*. 2007;93:266-270.

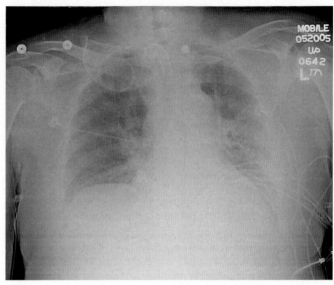

FIGURE 10-4 Postoperative chest x-ray showing resolving hemothorax.

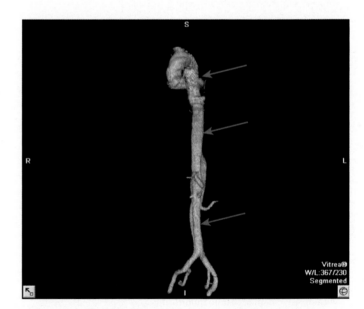

FIGURE 10-5 Postoperative imaging showing obliteration of false lumen and control of rupture, and good position of the thoracic and distal endografts.

5. Patel HJ, Wiliams DM, Dasika NL, Suziki Y, Deeb GM. Operative delay for peripheral malperfusion syndrome in acute type A aortic dissection: a long-term analysis. *J Thorac Cardiovasc Surg.* 2008;135:1288-1296.

6. Nienaber CA, Rosseau H, Eggebrecht H, et al. Randomized comparison of strategies for type B aortic dissection; the investigation of stent grafts in aortic dissection trial. *Circulation.* 2009;120:2519-2528.

7. Conrad MF, Crawford RS, Kwolek CJ, Brewster DC, Brady TJ, Cambria RP. Aortic remodeling after acute complicated type B aortic dissection. *J Vasc Surg.* 2009;50(3):510-517.

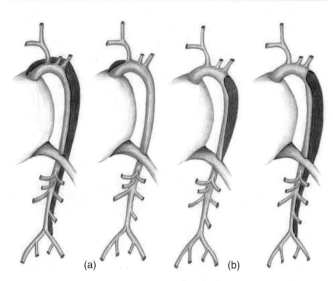

(a)   (b)

**FIGURE 10-6** The Stanford classification consists of type A that involves the ascending aorta and the arch with variable distal involvement; DeBakey type I and II (A and B) and Stanford type B involve the descending aorta only (C and D); and also DeBakey type III.

# 11 INNOMINATE AND SUBCLAVIAN ARTERY PERIPHERAL ARTERIAL DISEASE

Axel Thors, DO

## PATIENT STORY

A 62-year-old woman presented to the emergency department (ED) with worsening digital ecchymosis of her second through fifth fingers of the left hand with progressive pain over the preceding 3 weeks. She denied any history of dizziness, syncope, or symptoms of a stroke in the past. She also denied symptoms of upper extremity claudication. She was examined and found to have weak pulses in the brachial, radial, and ulnar arteries on the left side. The hand did not appear to be acutely threatened.

The patient underwent a computed tomographic angiogram (CTA) with findings of a significant proximal left subclavian artery stenosis (Figure 11-1). She subsequently underwent an angiogram with left subclavian artery stent placement (Figure 11-2). She was maintained on clopidogrel and recovered uneventfully.

## EPIDEMIOLOGY

### Peripheral Arterial Disease

- Progressive narrowing of the arteries due to atherosclerosis.[1]

- Mostly silent in early stages until luminal narrowing exceeds 50% of the vessel diameter.[2]

- Prevalence of peripheral arterial disease (PAD) in adults over 40 years in the United States is approximately 4%.[2]

- Prevalence of PAD in adults over 70 years in the United States is approximately 15%.[2]

- 20% to 25% of patients will require revascularization.[2]

- Approximately 5% of patients will progress to critical limb ischemia.[2]

- Patients with limb loss have 30% to 40% mortality in the first 24 months.[2]

## ETIOLOGY AND PATHOPHYSIOLOGY

### Peripheral Arterial Disease

- Global arterial tree inflammation accounts for atherogenesis and participates in local, myocardial, and systemic complications of atherosclerosis.[3]

- Vascular risk factors including diabetes, hypertension, hyperlipidemia, and tobacco abuse augment cell adhesion molecules, which promote leukocyte binding to the arterial cell wall. This process perpetuates, causing remodeling of the arterial wall and lipid deposition within the tunica media. This process continues and begins to

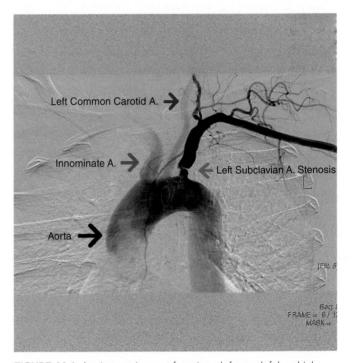

**FIGURE 11-1** Angiogram image of aortic arch from a left brachial artery approach. Red arrow indicates proximal left subclavian artery stenosis. Blue arrow indicates the left common carotid artery. Green arrow indicates the innominate artery. Black arrow indicates proximal ascending aorta.

narrow the vessel lumen, and eventually causes calcification of the arterial wall.[3]

- Disease of the brachiocephalic arteries can manifest in several ways including stroke or transient ischemic attack (TIA), upper extremity ischemia or claudication, and vertebrobasilar insufficiency related to subclavian steal syndrome.[4]

- The brachiocephalic arteries including the innominate and subclavian can be affected by vasculitides like Takayasu arteritis and giant cell arteritis.

- Brachiocephalic atherosclerotic disease can be unifocal or multifocal.

- Aneurysms of the brachiocephalic arteries occur infrequently and can be related to atherosclerotic poststenotic dilatation, trauma, inflammation, or infection.

## DIAGNOSTIC EVALUATION

- Physical examination is the mainstay in evaluating patients for brachiocephalic disease. Careful pulse examination and auscultation for bruits in the subclavian arteries or carotid arteries will narrow the search for any occult disease.

- Duplex ultrasound examination is in general the gold standard for evaluation of the carotid arteries and vertebral arteries. Duplex examination of the subclavian arteries can be performed; however, this examination is more technologist dependent and should be relied on only in accredited vascular laboratories experienced in imaging these arteries.

- CTA or magnetic resonance angiogram (MRA) studies are excellent for evaluating the aortic arch and brachiocephalic arteries. The preference for either study is institution and provider dependent. The ability for three-dimensional (3D) reconstruction is available for both modalities and is very useful for operative planning.

- Angiography is definitive if noninvasive studies are nondiagnostic. There is a similar risk of nephrotoxicity when compared to CT or MR angiography; however, this is dose dependent. There is a small risk of stroke (<1%) when manipulating the aortic arch and brachiocephalic arteries.

## TREATMENT

- The modality of treating brachiocephalic symptomatic lesions varies and can be accomplished with open, endovascular, or hybrid (combination) approaches.

- Initial experience with treatment of the aortic arch arteries was with open repair requiring sternotomy for many of the repairs. Endovascular therapy of symptomatic lesions of the aortic arch has surpassed open repair in frequency and safety.[5]

- Favorable lesions for endovascular repair include nonostial lesions, noncalcified, minimally ulcerated, nonoccluded, and favorable anatomic approaches. These criteria are also individual to the patient and particular circumstances.

- The use of stents in treating brachiocephalic arterial disease has surpassed angioplasty alone.

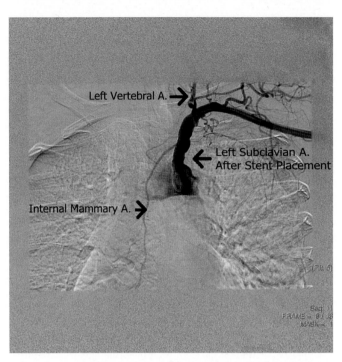

**FIGURE 11-2** Angiogram image of aortic arch from a left brachial artery approach. Arrow marks the left subclavian artery after stent placement. Arrows also demonstrate filling of the internal mammary artery and the left vertebral artery.

## RESULTS

- 1-year and 5-year patency for aortic arch occlusive disease is approximately 80% to 90% and 77% to 89%, respectively.[6]

- In general, the long-term patency rates are better for surgical bypass; however, it carries a higher short-term risk. Endovascular procedures provide excellent patency with lower risk and shorter hospital stay.

- Complication rates ranged from 0% to 20% over a 5-year period and consisted mostly of access-related problems. The incidence of stroke was less than 1%.[6]

## POSTOPERATIVE MANAGEMENT

- Control of PAD risk factors is the mainstay of treatment.

- Patients receiving stents should be maintained initially on dual antiplatelet therapy with aspirin and clopidogrel.

## PATIENT FOLLOW-UP

- Physical examination including bilateral upper extremity blood pressure measurement should be performed every 6 months.

- Duplex evaluation of the stent graft including upper extremity segmental pressures and pulse volume recordings should be performed every 6 months for the first 18 to 24 months and then annually.

- If ultrasound evaluation is not technically feasible, CTA should be performed at the same interval.

## REFERENCES

1. Selvin E, Erlinger TP. Prevalence of and risk factors for peripheral arterial disease in the United States results from the National Health and Nutrition Examination Survey, 1999-2000. *Circulation*. 2004;110:738-743.

2. Garcia LA. Epidemiology and pathophysiology of lower extremity peripheral arterial disease. *J Endovasc Ther*. 2006;13(suppl II): II-3-II-9.

3. Libby P, Theroux P. Pathophysiology of coronary artery disease. *Circulation*. 2005;111:3481-3488.

4. Cronenwett JL, Johnston KW. *Rutherford's Vascular Surgery*. 7th ed. New York, WB Saunders, 2010.

5. Patel SN, White C, Collins T, et al. Catheter-based treatment of the subclavian and innominate arteries. *Catheter Cardiovasc Interv*. 2008;71:969-971.

6. Rodriguez-Lopez JA, Werner A, Martinez R, et al. Stenting for atherosclerotic occlusive disease of the subclavian artery. *Ann Vasc Surg*. 1999;13:254-260.

# 12 UPPER EXTREMITY ISCHEMIA: ACCESS SITE COMPLICATIONS

John Anthony O'Dea, MD
Robert M. Schainfeld, DO, FSVM, FSCAI

## PATIENT STORY

A 63-year-old woman develops progressive pain, tenderness, and discoloration in the right wrist within several days of undergoing a cardiac catheterization using a radial artery approach. Her examination is remarkable for a tender, ecchymotic, and pulsatile protuberance along the distal radial artery. The right hand and fingers are warm and without distal embolic phenomena. Sensorimotor function of the right upper extremity is intact, and the forearm muscle compartments are soft. A duplex arterial ultrasound of the affected area documents a 1.5-cm pseudoaneurysm involving the distal radial artery.

## INTRODUCTION

- Brachial artery access is declining for coronary angiography but still holds an important role for complex endovascular interventions, particularly in cases of concomitant severe peripheral artery disease. The majority of brachial access is achieved percutaneously, with a small minority of cases requiring brachial cutdown.

- Transradial artery access for cardiac catheterization is widely embraced in Europe and increasingly is being adopted in the United States as a potentially safer means of access than the conventional transfemoral approach.

## EPIDEMIOLOGY

- Brachial artery access site complications occur in up to 7% of cases. In a review of 323 cases using brachial artery access, the first and second most common complications were pseudoaneurysm and brachial artery thrombosis, respectively (Figures 12-1 to 12-3).[1]

- This relatively high complication rate is probably a function of low operator volume and declining experience in this access over the transradial approach.

- Radial artery catheterization is typically associated with a complication rate between 0.5% and 15%.[2,3] However, the incidence may be higher than reported due to excellent collateral circulation supplying the hand. For instance, in a 2012 prospective ultrasound-assisted registry, radial access complications developed in 33% of patients when a 6F sheath was utilized.[4]

## ETIOLOGY AND PATHOPHYSIOLOGY

- The majority of brachial and radial artery complications arise in women. This gender difference is attributed to a smaller arterial caliber in females.

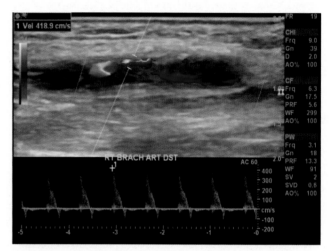

FIGURE 12-1 Duplex ultrasound study illustrating a markedly increased peak systolic velocity (PSV = 419 cm/s) due to subtotal thrombotic brachial artery occlusion following brachial access for an endovascular procedure.

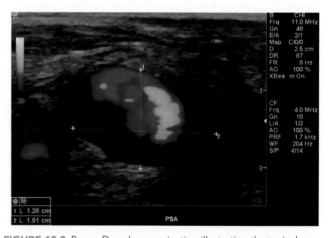

FIGURE 12-2 Power Doppler examination illustrating the typical "Yin and Yang" color findings of a brachial artery pseudoaneurysm.

## Brachial Artery

- Potential complications of brachial artery access include pseudoaneurysm, hematoma, bleeding, thrombotic occlusion, distal emboli, infection, dissection, and arteriovenous fistula.

- Brachial artery pseudoaneurysm is the most commonly encountered complication (Figure 12-2).[1]

- The rate of access site complications increases with sheath diameter at or above 8F and lengths greater than 10 cm, due to the greater strain exerted by these sheaths on a mobile brachial artery.

- Women are anywhere from two to five times more likely than males to develop a complication with brachial artery access.

- Periprocedural aspirin reduces the risk of thrombotic occlusion without increasing the bleeding risk. Conversely, concurrent warfarin use increases the risk of complications.

## Radial Artery

- Reported complications of radial artery access include occlusion, pseudoaneurysm, perforation with bleeding, spasm, compartment syndrome, sterile abscess, cutaneous infection, and even complex regional pain syndrome.

- Radial artery occlusion is the most common access site complication with a variable incidence between 0.5% and 10%.

- When duplex ultrasonography was used to prospectively follow the radial artery, radial artery occlusion occurred in 14% with 5F sheaths compared with 31% with 6F sheaths ($p < .001$).[4]

- Factors influencing radial artery occlusion include sheath size, ratio of the radial artery diameter to the sheath outer diameter, adequacy of anticoagulation, number of cannulation attempts, duration of cannulation and compression, as well as device adopted. Statin use appears to decrease this complication risk.[5]

- Radial artery pseudoaneurysm is extremely rare with an incidence of only 0.1%. It arises in cases of repeated puncture attempts, aggressive anticoagulation, larger sheath size, and inadequate compression postsheath removal (Figure 12-4).

- Radial artery perforation is a rare complication with an incidence between 0.1% and 1% of cases. Perforation is more likely in women of short stature and with difficult to traverse, tortuous arteries. If undetected, a large hematoma, with or without compartment syndrome, may ensue.

- Radial arterial harvesting for coronary artery bypass grafting (CABG) has led to the identification of nonocclusive radial artery injury. The pathophysiology is related to radial artery trauma at the time of sheath insertion, thereby triggering neointimal hyperplasia. Repeated cannulation increases the risk of this phenomenon. Usually nonocclusive radial artery injury is of little clinical significance, having no impact on quality of life or dexterity. However, it does have a potential impact on graft patency when harvested as a conduit for CABG.

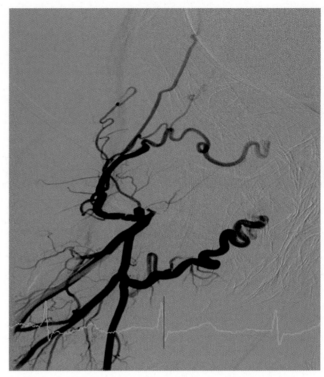

FIGURE 12-3 Digital subtraction arteriogram of a postcatheterization asymptomatic brachial artery occlusion with extensive collaterals.

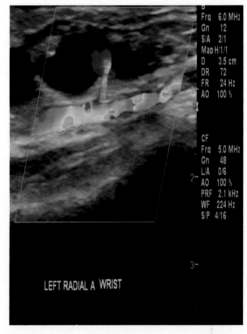

FIGURE 12-4 Color duplex Doppler findings in a case of radial pseudoaneurysm due to catheterization.

## DIAGNOSIS

### Clinical Features

- Brachial and radial pseudoaneurysms present as a pulsatile mass or swelling days to weeks after a procedure, which may be associated with pain, dysesthesias, and/or rarely acral ischemia.

- Brachial artery thrombosis may present with severe distal ischemic thromboembolic manifestations. The brachial, radial, and ulnar pulses are weak to absent.

- Radial artery thrombosis is typically asymptomatic if the ulnar and interosseous arteries as well as the palmar arches are patent. However, a reverse Allen test is abnormal and the distal radial pulse is weak to absent. In the setting of inadequate collateral flow, the hand and fingers may become severely ischemic when the radial artery occludes (Figure 12-5).

- Bertrand et al. have classified bleeding into the forearm into five possible grades. Grades I and II represent local superficial hematomas; grades III and IV indicate intramuscular bleeds; and grade V is consistent with a limb-threatening compartment syndrome.[6]

- The physical examination findings in acute compartment syndrome are notoriously unreliable, and the classic "5 P's of pain, pressure, pulselessness, paralysis, and paresthesia" are more indicative of arterial injury or occlusion. Pain out of proportion to the physical examination in addition to pain with passive muscle compartment stretching is the most sensitive physical examination finding.

### Imaging

- Definitive diagnosis of the majority of the brachial and radial artery access site complications listed earlier is best made with duplex arterial ultrasound (Figures 12-1, 12-2, 12-4, and 12-6).

- If a duplex arterial ultrasound is inconclusive, arteriography may be helpful (Figure 12-3).

- In rare circumstances, a computed tomograph (CT) or magnetic resonance image (MRI) of the antecubital fossa/forearm/wrist will be required for diagnostic purposes.

- If acute compartment syndrome is a possibility, obtaining compartment pressures is essential. When intracompartmental pressures obtained via a Stryker tonometer exceed 15 to 20 mm Hg, surgical decompression may be indicated.

## DIFFERENTIAL DIAGNOSIS

A true aneurysm of the brachial or radial artery can present in a similar fashion as a pseudoaneurysm, yet the duplex arterial ultrasound can distinguish between these two entities (Figure 12-6). The latter diagnosis displays the characteristic turbulent "Yin and Yang" color flow turbulence within the chamber and a "to and fro" spectral Doppler appearance within the pseudoaneurysm neck.

## MANAGEMENT

### Brachial Artery Complications

- Prevention of brachial access site complications is best achieved by using excellent technique with use of a micropuncture system and ensuring that the arteriotomy lies just proximal to the antecubital fossa.

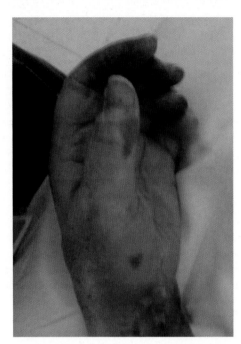

FIGURE 12-5 Rare case of a severe acral ischemia in a patient who underwent radial artery catheterization. The deep and superficial palmar arches were arteriographically incomplete and anomalous.

This is visualized fluoroscopically over the olecranon process that facilitates manual compression upon removal of the sheath on completion of the procedure.

- Most complications (60%) require surgical correction for either a thrombotic occlusion or pseudoaneurysm of the brachial artery. Open surgical correction is required more commonly for women (75%) than for men (25%). Half of the pseudoaneurysm cases require surgical intervention, with the remainder treated with either ultrasound-guided (USG) thrombin injection or USG manual compression.

- Surgical intervention for brachial artery occlusion entails cutdown, thrombectomy, and Fogarty embolectomy, followed by repair of the vessel. Given the frequency of surgical intervention for brachial access site complications, it is imperative to be vigilant for these complications during the postsheath pull period of monitoring. The use of closure devices has been reported but is discouraged due to the absence of an adequate track and brachial-specific devices.

## Radial Artery Complications

- It is imperative to detect radial artery thrombosis early following device removal, as compression of the ulnar artery can facilitate recanalization. With good screening via the (reverse) Allen test and plethysmography, the incidence of *symptomatic* radial artery occlusion is extremely rare.

- Radial artery pseudoaneurysm can be managed with a simple conservative, surgical, or minimally invasive approach. Conservative methods include manual compression or the use of the Terumo TR Band (Terumo Medical Corporation). The neck of the pseudoaneurysm may be injected with thrombin under duplex ultrasound guidance. Surgical interventions such as pseudoaneurysm neck ligation, excision of vessel wall with patch angioplasty, and excision of pseudoaneurysm with or without radial artery ligation have reported technical success.

- Prevention and early detection of radial artery perforation is best achieved by angiography. When resistance to a guidewire or sheath is encountered a decision to abort the procedure may avoid complications.

## PATIENT EDUCATION

Patients should be admonished to immediately notify their caregiver if progressive pain, swelling, bruising, numbness, and/or color and temperature changes develop within the catheterized upper extremity.

## FOLLOW-UP

- A brief outpatient follow-up appointment is typically scheduled in 1 to 2 weeks to assess for any postprocedural problems, to review the findings of the procedure with the patient, as well as to evaluate the patient's response to therapy.

- The physician should remain vigilant for postprocedural complications, especially when the patient is an elderly female.

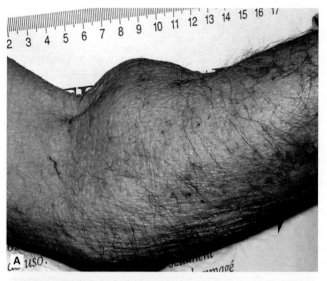

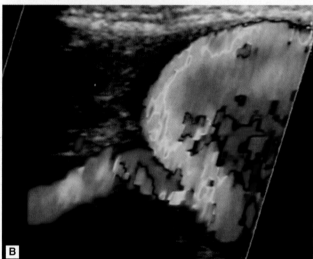

**FIGURE 12-6** Gross (A) and color Doppler (B) findings in a patient with a large true brachial aneurysm that required surgical excision.

## PROVIDER RESOURCES

- http://bmctoday.net/citoday/2010/04/article.asp?f=managing-radial-access-vascular-complications
- http://www.angiosoft.net/img_pwp_case/Gilchrist2008TCT.pdf
- http://www.dicardiology.com/article/patient-satisfaction-and-complications-transradial-catheterization

## PATIENT RESOURCES

- http://www.texasheartinstitute.org/HIC/Topics/Proced/radial_artery_access.cfm
- http://www.youtube.com/watch?v=doB9mqeeryM

## REFERENCES

1. Alvarez-Tostado JA, Moise MA, Bena JF, et al. The brachial artery: a critical access for endovascular procedures. *J Vasc Surg*. 2009;49:378-385.

2. Burzotta F, Trani C, Mazzari MA, et al. Vascular complications and access crossover in 10,676 transradial percutaneous coronary procedures. *Am Heart J*. 2012;163:230-238.

3. Bhat T, Teli S, Bhat H, et al. Access-site complications and their management during transradial cardiac catheterization. *Expert Rev Cardiovasc Ther*. 2012;10(5):627-634.

4. Uhlemann M, Mobius-Winkler S, Mende M, et al. The Leipzig prospective vascular ultrasound registry in radial artery catheterization: impact of sheath size on vascular complications. *J Am Cardiol Interv*. 2012;5(1):36-43.

5. Honda T, Fujimoto K, Miyao Y, et al. Access site-related complications after transradial catheterization can be reduced with smaller sheath size and statins. *Cardiovasc Interv Ther*. 2012;27(3):174-180.

6. Bertrand OF, Larose E, Rodes-Cabau J, et al. Incidence, predictors, and clinical impact of bleeding after transradial coronary stenting and maximal antiplatelet therapy. *Am Heart J*. 2009;157:164-169.

# 13 THORACIC OUTLET SYNDROME AND ARTERIAL ANEURYSM OF UPPER EXTREMITY

Irina Shakhnovich, MD

## PATIENT STORY

A 20-year-old woman presented to the emergency room with sudden onset of cold, pale fingers, and discolored spots in the fingertips of the left hand (Figure 13-1). The patient's medical history was significant for fatigue and weakness of the left hand for about 1 year. She attributed these symptoms to overuse at work as a nursing assistant at the hospital. Her physical examination was significant for discoloration and splinter hemorrhages of the fingers. She had palpable radial and ulnar pulses. With overhead left arm elevation, the patient complained of pain in the entire left upper extremity. The workup included a chest x-ray and left upper extremity angiogram. The chest x-ray showed bilateral cervical ribs (Figure 13-2). Angiogram confirmed the presence of a subclavian artery aneurysm with partial thrombosis (Figure 13-3). Her hand angiogram showed evidence of embolic disease to her digits (Figure 13-4).

The final diagnosis was of thoracic outlet syndrome (TOS) with arterial involvement complicated by subclavian arterial aneurysm and distal microembolization.

### EPIDEMIOLOGY

- Arterial involvement is the least common form of TOS.
- Most patients with symptoms of arterial TOS are young, active adults.
- The mean age in most published series is 37 years, with a similar proportion of men and women reported.[1]
- The condition appears to be related to bony abnormalities or trauma in nearly every circumstance.
- No familial predisposition has been described.[1]

### PATHOPHYSIOLOGY

- The compression of the subclavian artery caused by the cervical rib leads to turbulent blood flow through the narrowed segment of the artery. This type of long-standing stress eventually results in degeneration of the arterial wall, and the poststenotic dilatation then leads to formation of an aneurysm in the location of the artery immediately beyond the stenosis.
- Arterial complications of TOS are associated with bony abnormalities in almost all cases. Cervical ribs that cause subclavian artery damage tend to be short, broad, and complete, and usually articulate with the first rib as a pseudarthrosis.[2] Less common causes include hypertrophic callus from a healed clavicle fracture, anomalous first ribs, and fibrocartilaginous bands associated with the anterior scalene muscle.[3]

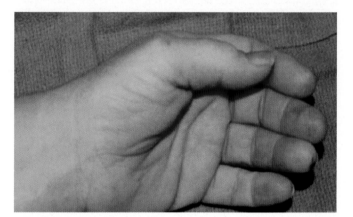

**FIGURE 13-1** Patient's hand with evidence of digital ischemia manifested by splinter hemorrhages at the fingertips.

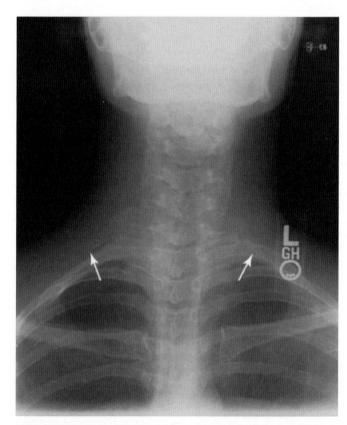

**FIGURE 13-2** Chest radiograph demonstrates bilateral cervical ribs (arrows). (By permission from Upper extremity arterial disease. *Rutherford's Vascular Surgery.* 7th ed. Philadelphia, PA: Elsevier Inc; 2010:1901.)

- The most common manifestation is hand ischemia as a result of microembolization. However, arterial TOS can be associated with less dramatic symptoms and may go unrecognized because it tends to occur in young patients without a history of atherosclerotic risk factors.[1]

## DIAGNOSIS

Arterial TOS is a clinical diagnosis and is made by combining important elements from the history and physical examination. The following studies are important adjuncts that may support the diagnosis and rule out other causes of upper extremity ischemia.

- **Compression maneuvers** can be used to help with the diagnosis of TOS. But none of these techniques are accurate. For example, the Adson test consists of having the patient elevate his or her chin and turn it to the affected side. Disappearance or reduction of the radial pulse with this maneuver is considered a positive test result. This finding has not proved to be diagnostic of TOS. The incidence of false-positive results in normal, healthy volunteers ranges from 9% to 53%.[4] Yet, a negative test result may be helpful in ruling out the diagnosis and prompting evaluation for an alternative cause.

- **Duplex ultrasonographic** examination of the subclavian and axillary arteries may demonstrate aneurysmal changes or elevated flow velocities correlating with a compressive stenosis. This may facilitate rapid diagnoses.

- **Radiographic imaging**

  ○ **Chest radiographs** with cervical spine views can demonstrate bony pathology. Cervical ribs and large clavicle fracture calluses are easily seen on plain films (Figure 13-2). Anomalous first ribs are more difficult to detect and may require other imaging modalities.[3]

  ○ **Catheter-based angiography** of the upper extremity arteriography is the gold standard for evaluation of arterial TOS. This is an important test in operative planning for localization and character of arterial compression. An arteriogram also visualizes the extent of arterial damage and permits evaluation of the distal circulation.

  ○ **Computed tomography** with intravenous contrast-enhanced angiography is an accurate study and an acceptable substitute for invasive angiography. It is gradually replacing catheter-based arteriography in many centers. However, arteriography with magnified views remains the best method for demonstrating embolic occlusion of the small arteries of the hand and fingers (Figure 13-4).[1]

## DIFFERENTIAL DIAGNOSIS

Other causes of upper extremity ischemia may be suspected and need to be ruled out with laboratory studies and imaging studies, as discussed below.

- A history of cardiac arrhythmia such as atrial fibrillation can suggest a cardioembolic etiology. These patients need to be evaluated with surface cardiac echo and bubble study.

- Personal or a family history of venous thromboembolic disease suggests an underlying hypercoagulable state. Further hypercoagulable workup is strongly recommended.

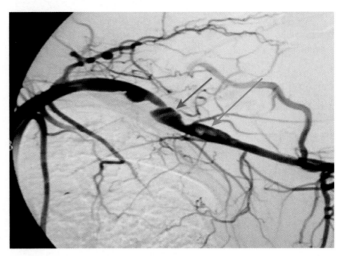

**FIGURE 13-3** Left subclavian arteriogram demonstrating a subclavian artery aneurysm (red arrow) and partial thrombus (blue arrow). Also note the presence of multiple collateral vessels, confirming the presence of chronic disease. (By permission from Upper extremity arterial disease. *Rutherford's Vascular Surgery*. 7th ed. Philadelphia, PA: Elsevier Inc; 2010:1901.)

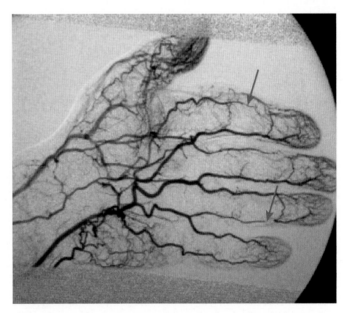

**FIGURE 13-4** Hand angiogram demonstrating distal embolization in the fingers (arrows). (By permission from Upper extremity arterial disease. *Rutherford's Vascular Surgery*. 7th ed. Philadelphia, PA: Elsevier Inc; 2010:1901.)

- Patients with risk factors for atherosclerosis, particularly patients with a history of heavy tobacco use, suggests the possibility of atherosclerotic occlusive disease as the etiology.

- Evaluation for connective tissue disease is suggested for patients with dermatitis and any esophageal dysmotility. Associated symptoms of polymyalgia rheumatica suggest the possibility of vasculitis.[1-3]

- Arterial dissection, radiation injury, and trauma can cause micro-embolization and can be easily detected with imaging studies such as computed tomographic angiography (CTA) or catheter-based angiography.

## MANAGEMENT

### Medical Treatment

There is no role for nonoperative treatment of symptomatic patients with arterial TOS, although it may be appropriate for some asymptomatic patients. Natural history of asymptomatic disease is unknown, and close follow-up is strongly recommended.

### Surgical Treatment

- The three main components of treatment include relieving the arterial compression, removing the source of embolus, and restoring the distal circulation.

- Relieving the arterial compression involves resection of cervical ribs and any other identified anomalies causing impingement in the thoracic outlet. This is performed through a supraclavicular incision, through which the cervical rib and the first rib are identified, divided, and removed. If subclavian reconstruction is planned, the suitable length of the normal artery is identified and adequately mobilized.

- The diseased segment of the artery is removed and an interposition bypass graft is constructed in an end-to-end fashion.

- The best conduit for the subclavian artery is debatable, and both prosthetic bypass graft and autologous vein can be used. The success of arterial reconstruction is usually related to the status of the arterial outflow in the limb. Restoring the distal circulation may involve any combination of thrombolysis, thromboembolectomy, or bypass.[5]

## FOLLOW-UP

- Successful outcome of the surgery is determined by relief of symptoms, patency of arterial bypasses, and limb salvage. Published case series report completes relief of symptoms in more than 90% of patients.[6]

- Long-term results are related to the status of the distal vasculature. Limbs with compromised outflow secondary to embolization have a poor prognosis.

## REFERENCES

1. Smith ST, Valentine RJ. Thoracic outlet syndrome: arterial. In: Cronenwett JL, Johnston, KW, eds. *Rutherford's Vascular Surgery*. 7th ed. Philadelphia, PA: Elsevier; 2010:1899-1906.

2. Green RM. Vascular manifestations of the thoracic outlet syndrome. *Semin Vasc Surg*. 1988;11:67-76.

3. Durham JR, Yao ST, Pearce WH, et al. Arterial injuries in the thoracic outlet syndrome. *J Vasc Surg*. 1995;21:57-70.

4. Plewa MC, Delinger M. The false-positive rate of thoracic outlet syndrome shoulder maneuvers in healthy subjects. *Acad Emerg Med*. 1998;5:337-342.

5. Nehler MR, Taylor LM, Moneta GL, Porter JM. Upper extremity ischemia from subclavian artery aneurysm caused by bony abnormalities of the thoracic outlet. *Arch Surg*. 1997;132:527-532.

6. Cormier JM, Amrane M, Ward A, et al. Arterial complications of the thoracic outlet syndrome: fifty-five operative cases. *J Vasc Surg*. 1989;9:778-787.

# 14 ARTERIAL THORACIC OUTLET SYNDROME

Borzoo Farhang, DO, MS
Nitin Garg, MBBS, MPH

## PATIENT STORY

A 53-year-old woman presented with severe right upper extremity rest pain. She reported a history of bilateral Raynaud phenomenon with cold exposure for many years. She also had progressively worsening right second- and third-digit pallor and pain on arm elevation for 1 year. Physical examination revealed a pale right hand (Figure 14-1A and B) with tender digits, absent radial and ulnar pulses, weakly palpable brachial pulse, and associated hand-grip weakness. No abnormalities were noted on her left upper extremity vascular or neurologic examination.

She had undergone thromboembolectomy and patch angioplasty of the right brachial artery with a normal upper extremity arteriogram 4 months prior for treatment of brachial artery occlusion. She had a negative rheumatology and thrombophilia evaluation at that time, and after initial improvement her symptoms recurred a month later. She underwent a brachioradial bypass, again with temporary resolution of her symptoms.

The patient sought a second opinion and noninvasive vascular studies revealed the absence of right digital laser Doppler signals at baseline and after warming (Figure 14-2). Upper extremity computed tomographic arteriogram (CTA) (Figure 14-3) revealed occlusion of subclavian artery with abduction. Upper extremity arteriogram confirmed occlusion of the mid brachial artery with multiple emboli noted in circumflex humeral and collateral arteries (Figure 14-4A and B; Figure 14-5A and B). The distal radial artery was reconstituted via collaterals through the interosseous artery to provide flow into the palmar arch (Figure 14-5B).

The patient was treated with cervical rib resection, subclavian artery resection and replacement, and brachiointerosseus arterial bypass and was doing well 6 months after the procedure.

## EPIDEMIOLOGY

- Arterial symptoms are present in a minority of patients, encompassing up to 5% of all thoracic outline syndrome (TOS) patients.[1]
- TOS is believed to be the most common cause of acute upper extremity arterial occlusion in adults younger than 40 years; it is more common with occupations or activities that involve prolonged posturing of the neck. However, there is no increased incidence in athletes.[2]

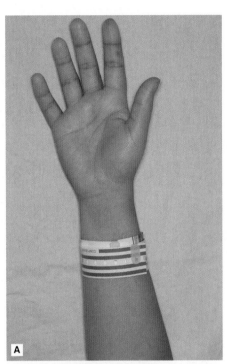

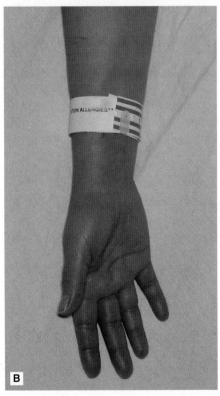

**FIGURE 14-1** Severe pallor noted on arm elevation (A) with dependent rubor on dependency (B) in the right arm.

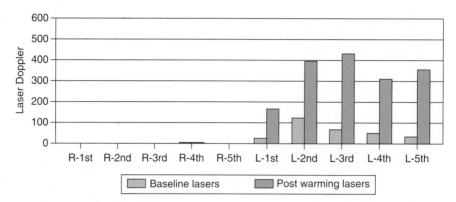

**FIGURE 14-2** Upper extremity noninvasive laser Doppler arterial studies reveal undetectable Doppler signals in the right digits both at rest and postwarming.

- Although strong female preponderance is seen in TOS, arterial TOS affects both genders equally.[3]

- There is a wide variation in age at diagnosis between the second and eighth decades, with a peak in the fourth decade. Younger patients have a greater likelihood of anatomic or structural abnormality (Figure 14-6A).[2]

## CLINICAL FEATURES

Symptoms of arterial TOS include digital ischemia, upper extremity exertional fatigue, pallor, poikilothermia, paresthesia, and pain in the hand. These symptoms are the result of hypoperfusion from arterial thromboemboli or subclavian artery compression during arm abduction. In this situation, the pallor and coldness are due to arterial ischemia and not due to Raynaud disease. Unlike patients with neurogenic TOS, these patients seldom have any symptoms of shoulder or neck pain.[3]

- An absent radial pulse at rest is common, as emboli often lodge near the antecubital space. There is usually no scalene muscle tenderness, commonly observed in neurogenic TOS, and neck rotation or head tilt elicits no symptoms. Varying degrees of ischemic signs are noted on physical examination, depending on chronicity and duration of arterial ischemia.[3]

## ETIOLOGY AND PATHOPHYSIOLOGY

- The subclavian artery courses through the scalene triangle to enter the axillary space and supply the arm. This triangle is bounded by the anterior scalene muscle anteriorly, the middle scalene muscle posteriorly, and the upper border of the first rib inferiorly.[3]

  Arterial TOS results from compression of the subclavian artery at the point where it crosses the first rib (Figure 14-6A and B). Compression or kinking of the subclavian artery as it exits the thoracic cavity results, in effect, from elevation of the floor of the scalene triangle.[3]

- In patients with arterial TOS, cervical rib is present in nearly half, followed by soft tissue anomalies in one-third of patients and scar tissue after clavicle fracture representing 5%,[3] leading to impingement of the artery in this narrow space.

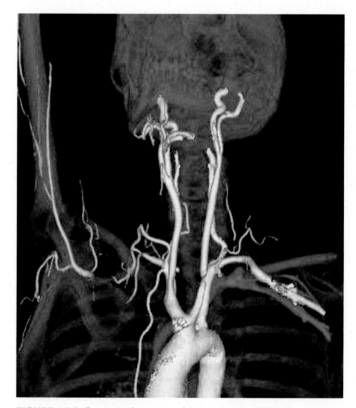

**FIGURE 14-3** Computed tomographic arteriogram (CTA) shows right subclavian artery occlusion with arm in abducted position.

- Chronic compression and trauma to the subclavian artery as it arises out of the thoracic outlet may lead to intimal ulceration (Figure 14-7) or subclavian artery stenosis with poststenotic dilatation or aneurysmal degeneration of the artery just distal to the site of compression. Many of these patients have a subclavian aneurysm at the time of presentation.[4]

- Mural thrombus from the site of damaged intima or within the aneurysm can embolize distally. Patients present with symptoms of pain and transient color changes in the digits that can be difficult to differentiate from Raynaud syndrome or present with ischemic ulceration. Repeated episodes of embolization result in progressive occlusion of the upper extremity arterial tree with progressive symptoms.[5]

## DIAGNOSIS

- Adson test, radial pulse deficit in provocative positions, is of no significant clinical value, but physical examination is important and includes several provocative maneuvers. Upper limb tension test and abducting the arms to 90 degrees in external rotation usually brings on symptoms within 60 seconds.[5]

- Digital occlusion pressure may identify bilateral digital ischemia at rest and help distinguish fixed obstruction from primary Raynaud disease. Multiple imaging studies have been used to demonstrate neurovascular compression.[6]

- Cervical plain radiography should be performed first to assess for bony abnormalities and to narrow the differential diagnosis. CTA or magnetic resonance (MR) imaging performed in association with postural maneuvers is helpful in analyzing dynamic compression. B-mode and color duplex ultrasonography (US) are good supplementary tools for assessment of vessel compression in association with postural maneuvers, especially in cases with clinical features of TOS but negative features of TOS on CT and MR imaging.[5]

- Arteriography is the gold standard, but is not necessary in most cases to make the diagnosis. Primary reason for arteriographic evaluation is to assist with planning arterial reconstruction.[6]

## DIFFERENTIAL DIAGNOSIS

- Adhesive capsulitis
- Carpal tunnel syndrome
- Cervical disk disease
- Cervical myofascial pain
- Cervical spondylosis
- Cervical sprain and strain
- Chronic pain syndrome
- Complex regional pain syndromes
- Fibromyalgia
- Radiation-induced brachial plexopathy
- Rheumatoid arthritis
- Rotator cuff disease
- Traumatic brachial plexopathy
- Workers' compensation claims[2]

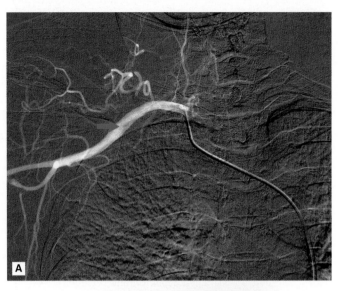

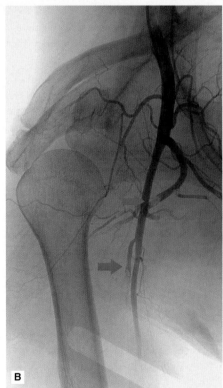

**FIGURE 14-4** Digital subtraction arteriogram showing a patent right subclavian artery with an area of filing defect or lucency (arrow) at level of clavicle and first rib intersection (A). Multiple small filling defects suggestive of thrombus or embolus (arrows) noted in the circumflex and collateral branches (B).

## MANAGEMENT

- Effective treatment of the arterial complications of TOS requires early recognition and prompt correction of the compressive mechanism.

- Management is indicated in most patients with ischemia as well as asymptomatic patients with arterial injury. Goals of treatment include

  ○ Decompression of the structures compressing the artery

  ○ Removal of the source of emboli

  ○ Restoration of distal perfusion[7]

- Thrombolytic therapy has been used effectively in acute management of arterial embolic complications prior to definitive operative decompression of the thoracic outlet with repair of any associated arterial abnormalities; alternatively, operative embolectomy may be employed, either through a subclavian arteriotomy or, if necessary, a separate brachial arteriotomy. Chronic occlusions resulting from emboli may require a bypass if ischemia is severe.[5]

- Anticoagulation following thrombolysis will minimize the risk of rethrombosis and allows adequate evaluation of the thoracic outlet prior to further operative intervention.[5]

- Thrombolysis is a useful adjunct in the management of arterial or venous occlusions, re-establishing early patency and permitting time for further evaluation. A combined approach of thrombolysis and surgical decompression of the thoracic outlet offers a satisfactory outcome in a majority of patients.[5]

## PATIENT EDUCATION

- Educating patients about the causes or perpetuating factors involved in thoracic outlet syndrome is essential. Offering training to minimize the likelihood of recurrence may be considered.

- Proper use of keyboards and adjustment of workstation ergonomics are useful. Specific techniques for exercise and motivation are necessary. Appropriate management of stress and depression also are helpful.[2]

## ACKNOWLEDGMENT

We are sincerely grateful to our patient and Dr. Thomas C. Bower, Mayo Clinic, Rochester, for providing us the pictures used in this chapter.

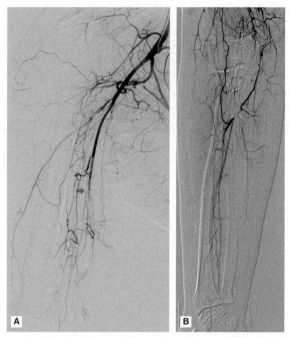

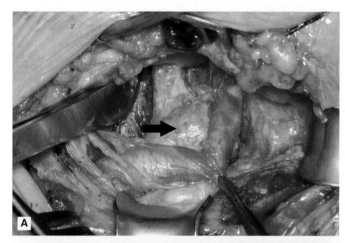

**FIGURE 14-5** Arteriogram of right upper extremity shows occlusion of brachial artery (arrow) with multiple small collaterals (A) and reconstitution of the interosseous artery (arrow) via collateral branches (B).

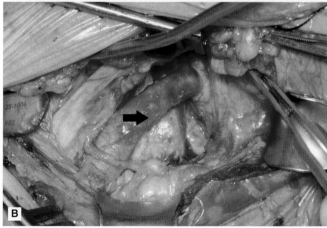

**FIGURE 14-6** Intraoperative images show a broad attachment of the cervical rib (arrow) to the first rib (A) and inflamed proximal subclavian artery overlying this area (arrow) from chronic trauma, with normal-appearing distal subclavian adventitia (B).

## REFERENCES

1. Makhoul RJ. Developmental anomalies at the thoracic outlet: an analysis of 300 consecutive cases. *J Vasc Surg*. 1992;16:534-545.

2. Sucher BM. Physical medicine and rehabilitation for thoracic outlet syndrome. *Differential Diagnoses*. Emedicine: 316715. http://emedicine.medscape.com/article/316715-differential. Accessed May 7, 2013.

3. Davidovic LB. Vascular thoracic outlet syndrome. *World J Surg*. May 2003;27(5):545-550.

4. Cronenwett JL, Johnston W. *Rutherford's vascular surgery* 16th ed. Chapter 124. WB Saunders; 2010.

5. Demondion X. Imaging assessment of thoracic outlet syndrome. *Radiographics*. 2006;26(6):1735-1750.

6. Sanders RJ, Hammond SL. Diagnosis of thoracic outlet syndrome. *J Vasc Surg*. 2007;46(3):601-604.

7. Hood DB. Vascular complications of thoracic outlet syndrome. *Am Surg*. Oct 1997;63(10):913-917.

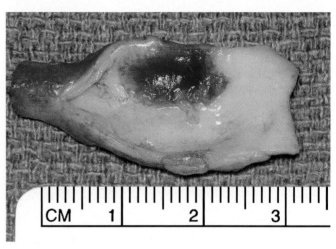

**FIGURE 14-7** Luminal ulcer with overlying thrombus in the subclavian artery in the segment visualized in Figure 14-6B.

# 15 VERTEBROBASILAR INSUFFICIENCY: SUBCLAVIAN STEAL SYNDROME

Mounir J. Haurani, MD

## PATIENT STORY

A 57-year-old left-handed man smoker with hypertension and coronary artery disease presented to the clinic with complaints of left arm pain. He worked predominantly at a desk job but did multiple tasks around the house that required vigorous use of the upper extremity and hand. He stated that when he used his left hand for even short periods of time, he developed cramping and fatigue in his hand and forearm. If he performed a significant amount of work with his left arm he became dizzy and light-headed. He denied any focal neurologic deficits or loss of consciousness.

### HISTORY AND PHYSICAL EXAMINATION

- Symptoms associated with vertebrobasilar ischemia are[1,2]
  - Disequilibrium
  - Vertigo
  - Diplopia
  - Cortical blindness
  - Alternating paresthesia
  - Tinnitus
  - Dysphasia
  - Dysarthria
  - Drop attacks
  - Ataxia
  - Perioral numbness
- The vertebrobasilar system is frequently not symptomatic because it has built-in redundancy via the basilar artery.
- Collaterals from the external carotid artery, the thyrocervical trunk, and multiple small branches of the cervical vertebral artery also supply the vertebrobasilar system.
- In patients with subclavian steal the most frequent symptoms are
  - Arm pain with exercise
  - Dizziness or vertigo
  - Diplopia, bilateral visual blurring
- Motor or sensory symptoms are typically only present with concurrent carotid artery disease.

### EPIDEMIOLOGY

- Vertebrobasilar "spells" that occur in association with subclavian steal syndrome represent a common example of hemodynamically based transient cerebral ischemia. In the presence of subclavian occlusion proximal to the vertebral takeoff (Figure 15-1), exercise of the affected arm may cause flow resistance to drop in the arm because of exercise-induced vasodilation. This drop in resistance may result in retrograde flow down the ipsilateral vertebral artery

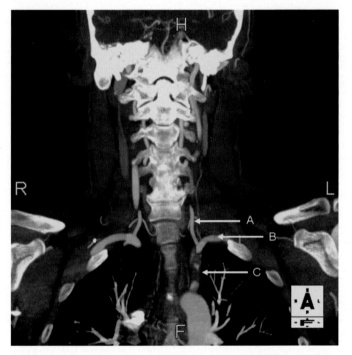

**FIGURE 15-1** Computed tomographic angiography (CTA) is useful in diagnosing the extent of the subclavian lesion or occlusion (C) as well as the patency of the carotid artery, vertebral artery (A), and distal subclavian artery (B). Given the length of the occlusion, extra-anatomic bypass may be preferable in the case depicted in the figure; however, more recently, combined retrograde brachial artery access with simultaneous antegrade access via the femoral artery has been used to revascularize this lesion percutaneously. (H represents the head end and F the foot end of the patient.)

with subsequent steal from the vertebrobasilar distribution and posterior circulation symptoms (diplopia, bilateral visual loss, drop attacks, etc).

- These symptoms subside when the arm is rested.[3] With more severe subclavian disease, steal physiology and symptoms can occur in the absence of ipsilateral arm exercise.

## ETIOLOGY AND PATHOLOGY

- The syndrome exists when a patient has compromised upper extremity blood flow as a result of high-grade stenosis or occlusion in the corresponding subclavian artery proximal to a patent vertebral artery.

- Subclavian steal symptoms occur if vertebrobasilar territory symptoms (eg, syncope or presyncope) develop because of steal of blood from the posterior cerebral circulation down the vertebral artery to supply the arm.

- Disease of the brachiocephalic (innominate) trunk on the right can cause a similar phenomenon secondary to altered vertebral or carotid flow, or both.

- Revascularization of the upper extremity should eliminate the steal. In addition, the presence of anatomic reversed flow in the vertebral artery on angiography or duplex ultrasound imaging at rest or during stress is sometimes referred to as subclavian steal (Figure 15-2).

- There is no evidence that the presence of subclavian steal with or without symptoms is an indicator of a high risk for stroke.[2,4] Again, it may be reasonable to initially consider carotid intervention in patients with global symptoms and severe carotid bifurcation disease.

## DIAGNOSIS

### Physical Examination

- The findings on physical examination may often be diagnostic themselves.

- Imaging is often needed to define the anatomy of the lesions for treatment planning, but the level can be readily ascertained based on physical examination alone.

Findings include the following features:

○ Unequal arm blood pressures
○ Diminished or absent distal pulses in comparison to the contralateral arm
○ Cervical or supraclavicular bruits
○ Evidence of ischemic changes or embolism in the form of ulcers or gangrenous skin changes and nail bed splinter hemorrhages

Of these findings, comparison of the brachial artery pressure difference is the most specific finding. Multiple studies have shown that by using a difference of 15 to 20 mm Hg, the negative predictive value is nearly 100%.

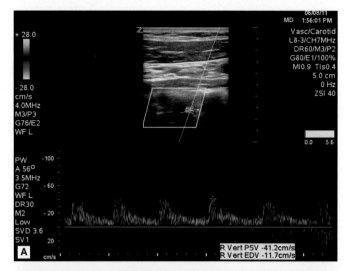

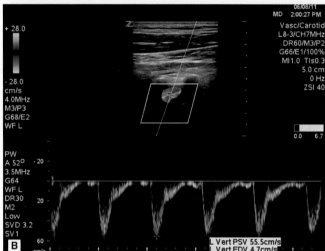

**FIGURE 15-2** Duplex ultrasonography can be useful in detecting the stenosis or occlusion of the subclavian artery directly. Additionally, reversal of flow in the affected vertebral artery may be seen in subclavian steal syndrome as the blood is shunted away from the vertebral artery to supply the upper extremity. In the example depicted in the figure, A the right vertebral artery demonstrates normal antegrade flow, with B being the left side, with a subclavian artery occlusion. Notice that the flow is reversed on the left side.

## Diagnostic Imaging

- Once a significant blood pressure difference is found in a symptomatic patient, diagnostic imaging is indicated.[5]
  - Duplex ultrasound examination is the study of choice.
    - It is noninvasive.
    - It is able to determine whether a significant or hemodynamic obstructive pattern is present.
  - The signs of vertebrobasilar insufficiency on duplex examination of the subclavian artery are
    - Waveform dampening
    - Monophasic changes
    - Color aliasing suggestive of turbulent flow
    - Increased blood flow velocities at the suspected site of stenosis
  - Vertebral arteries may also demonstrate retrograde or altered flow indicative of steal (Figure 15-2).
  - Axial imaging with either computed tomographic angiography (CTA) or magnetic resonance angiography (MRA) is indicated.
    - Both are excellent tools for assessing the anatomy of the subclavian lesion.
    - Can also demonstrate other arterial pathology in the aortic arch as well as the distal head and neck arteries (Figure 15-1).
    - Should be reserved for patients in whom the duplex was not sufficient or an intervention is planned.
    - Angiography via a catheter has the advantage of obtaining diagnostic information as well as the ability to intervene on the lesions at the same time.

## TREATMENT OPTIONS

### Medical Therapy

- The role of medical therapy is for management of risk factors that lead to the atherosclerosis. If a patient is symptomatic from subclavian steal with vertebrobasilar insufficiency, an intervention is usually warranted in the absence of significant systemic risk factors. In the absence of symptoms or steal phenomena, patients should not be intervened based on hemodynamic findings alone.

- Medical therapy should include
  - Antiplatelet therapy
  - Lipid-lowering therapy
  - Blood pressure control
  - Glucose control in diabetics
  - Smoking cessation

### Surgical Repair

- While originally performed via a transthoracic approach and direct revascularization, the current preferred treatment strategy involves extra-anatomic bypasses that is better tolerated with significantly lower morbidity and mortality and excellent long-term patency rates of 91% and 82% at 5 and 10 years.[6]

- Extra-anatomic options include
  - Carotid to subclavian bypass (Figures 15-3 and 15-4).
  - Subclavian transposition.
  - Axillary–axillary bypass.
  - All of these procedures have similar low mortality and stroke rates with excellent long-term patency.

## Endovascular Interventions

- Percutaneous transluminal angioplasty (PTA) was first reported in the literature in the 1970s and 1980s, followed by several reports of PTA of aortic arch vessels.

- Disadvantages of endovascular interventions include
  - Restenosis
  - Lower long-term patency rates compared to surgical correction
  - Potential of embolization into the vertebral artery, although reversal of flow is somewhat protective

- Acute thrombosis is rare given the overall caliber of the subclavian artery.

- Results of endovascular interventions are as follows:
  - Recent studies of endovascular repair of symptomatic subclavian artery stenosis[7-9] showed the following:
    - Stents were placed 58% of the time.
    - Technical and clinical success rate was 93%.
    - There was a low (1%) stroke rate.
    - Primary patency at 5 years was 89% based on duplex scans.
    - Even more modern series have improved on these results and have expanded the application to chronic total occlusions as well.
    - Access site hematomas, distal embolization, and arm arterial thrombosis are also possible but reports of them are low as well.

## FOLLOW-UP

### Postoperative Period

- Early complications related to surgical location:
  - During carotid to subclavian bypass or subclavian artery transposition, the approach involves transection of the anterior scalene and therefore potential injury to the phrenic nerve (Figure 15-3).
  - Scalene fat pad is a source for continued lymph leaks postoperatively. This problem is usually self-limited but may increase the chances of wound complications.
  - Injury to the thoracic duct on the left side may also cause lymph leak and potential wound complications.
  - Injury to the nerves of the brachial plexus (Figure 15-3).

### Long-Term Follow-Up

- Bilateral upper extremity blood pressure monitoring.
  - Thorough history and examination.
  - Any recurrence of symptoms or decrease in pressure should prompt imaging, typically with ultrasound, but CT angiography may also reveal lesions (Figure 15-4).
  - May demonstrate early stenosis or other problems with the graft that can be intervened on prior to thrombosis.

○ Poststenting follow-up should be done at 1-, 6-, and 12-month intervals initially and yearly thereafter.

○ Color Doppler ultrasound with velocity assessment should be performed with any concerning symptoms or a greater than 10 mm Hg change in arm blood pressure difference.

## REFERENCES

1. Delaney CP, Couse NF, Mehigan D, Keaveny TV. Investigation and management of subclavian steal syndrome. *Br J Surg*. Aug 1994;81(8):1093-1095.

2. Savitz SI, Caplan LR. Vertebrobasilar disease. *N Engl J Med*. Jun 23 2005;352(25):2618-2626.

3. Kresowik TF, Harold P, Adams, Jr. *Cerebrovascular Disease: Decision Making and Medical Treatment*. Vol 2. 7th ed. Philadelphia, PA: Saunders Elsevier; 2010.

4. Reivich M, Holling HE, Roberts B, Toole JF. Reversal of blood flow through the vertebral artery and its effect on cerebral circulation. *N Engl J Med*. Nov 2 1961;265:878-885.

5. Berguer R, Higgins R, Nelson R. Noninvasive diagnosis of reversal of vertebral-artery blood flow. *N Engl J Med*. Jun 12 1980;302(24):1349-1351.

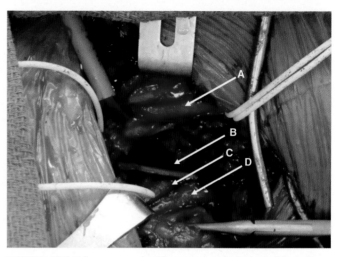

**FIGURE 15-3** When approached from a supraclavicular incision, the common carotid artery (A) and the subclavian artery (C) are in close proximity to each other. In order to gain this exposure, however, the anterior scalene muscle needs to be divided. The phrenic nerve (B), which lies on top of the anterior scalene, needs to be preserved and carefully protected. In addition, the nerve roots of the brachial plexus (D) are closely related to the subclavian artery as it courses under the clavicle.

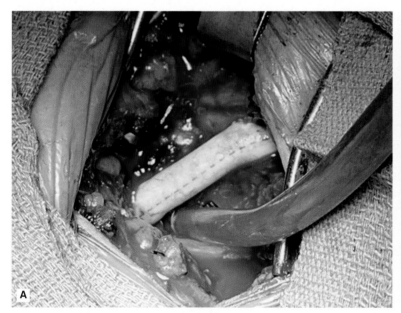

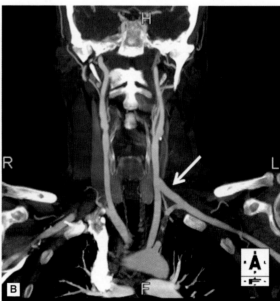

**FIGURE 15-4** A short prosthetic graft is used to fashion an end-to-side anastomosis between the common carotid artery and the subclavian artery (A). On a follow-up examination, the computed tomographic angiography (CTA) demonstrates that the previously occluded subclavian artery is now being supplied via the common carotid artery via the bypass (white arrow, panel B). (H represents the head end and F the foot end of the patient.)

6. AbuRahma AF, Robinson PA, Jennings TG. Carotid-subclavian bypass grafting with polytetrafluoroethylene grafts for symptomatic subclavian artery stenosis or occlusion: a 20-year experience. *J Vasc Surg*. Sep 2000;32(3):411-418; discussion 418-419.

7. Erbstein RA, Wholey MH, Smoot S. Subclavian artery steal syndrome: treatment by percutaneous transluminal angioplasty. *Am J Roentgenol*. Aug 1988;151(2):291-294.

8. Bates MC, Broce M, Lavigne PS, Stone P. Subclavian artery stenting: factors influencing long-term outcome. *Catheter Cardiovasc Interv*. Jan 2004;61(1):5-11.

9. Henry M, Henry I, Polydorou A, Hugel M. Percutaneous transluminal angioplasty of the subclavian arteries. *Int Angiol*. Dec 2007;26(4):324-340.

# 16 SUBCLAVIAN CORONARY STEAL

Bhagwan Satiani, MD, MBA, RPVI, FACS

## PATIENT STORY

A 50-year-old physician presented to his cardiologist with chest pain. He had a remote history of a redo coronary artery bypass graft (CABG) using the left internal mammary artery (LIMA) a few years ago. On physical examination, his left radial pulse was absent. A carotid duplex examination showed no hemodynamically significant lesions in his internal carotid arteries. The left vertebral flow was noted to be reversed (Figure 16-1). His cardiac catheterization showed a patent LIMA graft. However, he was noted to have a tight preocclusive left subclavian artery stenosis (Figure 16-2). He was referred to our Vascular Surgery Division for a surgical opinion.

## PATHOPHYSIOLOGY

- Coronary subclavian steal syndrome (CSSS) is an uncommon cause of angina and occurs due to decreased coronary blood flow in patients with a patent internal mammary to coronary artery graft.[1-4]

- The usual cause of CSSS is ipsilateral subclavian artery stenosis. The term *steal* refers to retrograde flow in the vertebral artery secondary to decreased pressure gradient in the mid-to-distal subclavian

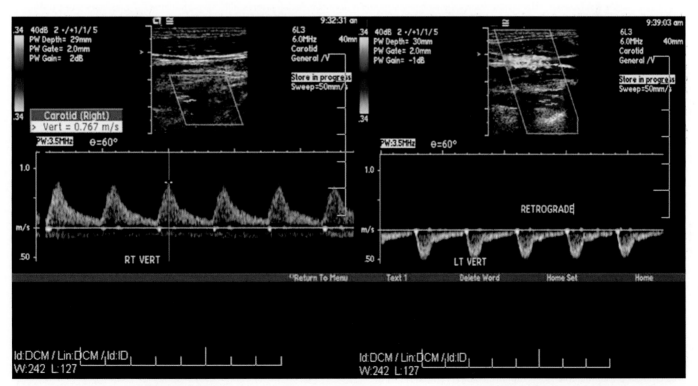

Right Vertebral                    Left Vertebral

**FIGURE 16-1** Duplex ultrasound shows normal antegrade flow in the right vertebral artery and reversed flow in the left vertebral artery.

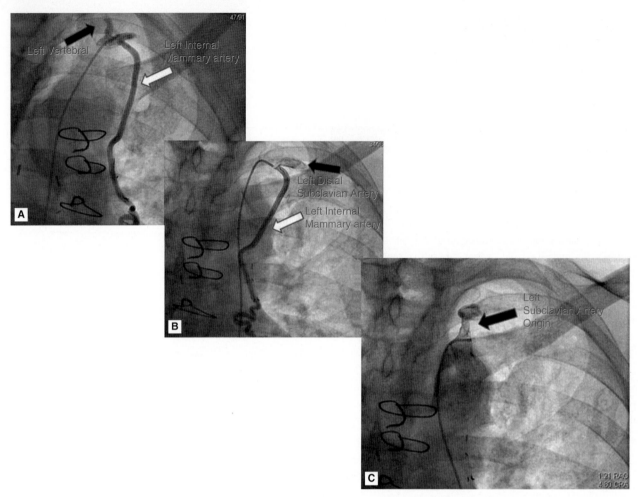

**FIGURE 16-2** **(A)** A subclavian arteriogram shows the catheter entering a tight subclavian artery orifice filling the internal mammary artery (IMA) (white arrow) with a visible left vertebral artery (black arrow). **(B)** The contrast then is visible in the distal subclavian artery (black arrow) and again outlines the IMA (white arrow). **(C)** The final picture shows the origin of the left subclavian artery (black arrow). The sternal wires are visible in all images from the previous coronary artery bypass operation.

artery due to occlusion or high-grade stenosis at its origin. The steal can cause cerebrovascular or ipsilateral arm symptoms.

- In this patient, the angina was due to either a severe decrease in antegrade flow into the coronary artery or because of an obstructive lesion in the proximal subclavian artery. In some cases retrograde flow from the coronary artery into the arm can also cause angina pectoris.

## CLINICAL FEATURES

- Most patients with uncomplicated subclavian steal syndrome are asymptomatic.

- Some patients present with arm claudication on physical exertion and others with vertebrobasilar symptoms due to a relative steal phenomenon occurring from a subclavian stenosis at its origin. This stenosis then results in reversed flow in the ipsilateral vertebral artery causing ischemia of the posterior brain.

- The physical examination shows diminished or absent pulses in the ipsilateral arm and a blood pressure differential between the two arms. A bruit may or may not be heard over the clavicle.

- In CSSS, the physical findings are similar. Neurologic examination is usually normal.

## DIAGNOSIS

- In patients who have previously undergone coronary artery bypass using the LIMA, onset of recurrent angina should prompt a consideration of CSSS as a possible diagnosis. In addition, any upper extremity claudication or vertebral basilar symptoms in association with angina should point to a possible CSSS.

- Duplex ultrasound examination leads to confirmation of a clinical diagnosis of CSSS. The classic findings are those of reversed flow in the left vertebral (Figure 16-1), decreased velocities in the left subclavian artery, and usually normal antegrade flow to the left common carotid artery.

- Once the duplex findings point to a diagnosis of CSSS a contrast angiographic study will show a patent LIMA, high-grade stenosis of the left subclavian artery at its origin, and reverse flow in the left vertebral artery with antegrade flow into the left arm (Figure 16-2).

## DIFFERENTIAL DIAGNOSIS

- The angina can be on the basis of stenosis or occlusion of the LIMA.

- Claudication of the left arm can be due to a lesion in the subclavian or axillary artery beyond the origin of the LIMA.

- Symptoms of vertebral basilar insufficiency can be due to bilateral carotid stenosis or anatomic lesions elsewhere other than the origin of the left subclavian artery.

## MANAGEMENT

- Correction of the subclavian artery lesion leads to relief of the angina.

- The stenosis can be corrected by either percutaneous balloon dilation with or without stenting or a surgical bypass from the ipsilateral common carotid artery into the subclavian artery beyond the origin of the vertebral artery. The surgical option was chosen by the patient with a successful outcome and resolution of his angina pectoris (Figure 16-3).

- The percutaneous option offers a lower immediate risk provided the stenosis is amenable to a guide-wire safely crossing the lesion. There is some risk of restenosis, but repeat intervention can be performed.

- The patient should be offered both options with the risk of a prosthetic bypass and excellent long-term patency versus the less invasive procedure with a higher risk of reintervention.

## PATIENT EDUCATION

- If a surgical option is chosen, the patient should be instructed on care of the incision and signs and symptoms of bleeding or infection.

- The patient should be educated on the physiology of the CSSS and given a diagram showing the direction of flow in the LIMA and how recurrence may cause similar symptoms.

**Coronary Steal**

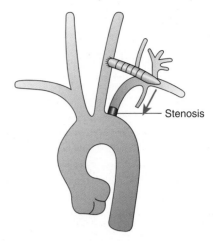

Stenosis

Carotid subclavian
bypass

**FIGURE 16-3** A schematic diagram showing correction of the subclavian coronary steal phenomenon by a carotid subclavian surgical bypass procedure performed in the patient in the case presented.

- Control of the usual risk factors including smoking, diet, and lipid control should be reinforced.

## FOLLOW-UP

- Instruction at discharge should include a return appointment in 2 to 3 weeks to check patency of the procedure.

- If a graft has been placed, physical examination can usually confirm patency.

- If an endovascular procedure has been performed, a palpable axillary, brachial, and radial pulse should be easily detected. If there is some doubt about patency or recurrence of symptoms, a repeat duplex examination of the area can be performed.

### PROVIDER RESOURCES

- http://www.ncbi.nlm.nih.gov/pubmed/7903598

### PATIENT RESOURCES

- http://en.wikipedia.org/wiki/Subclavian_steal_syndrome

## REFERENCES

1. Labropoulos N, Nandivada P, Bekelis K. Prevalence and impact of the subclavian steal syndrome. *Ann Surg*. Jul 2010;252(1):166-170.

2. John A, Hofmann S, Ostowar A, Ferdosi A, Warnecke H. Reversal of flow in the mammary artery to treat subclavian steal syndrome in conjunction with coronary bypass surgery. *Ann Thorac Surg*. 2011;91:283-285.

3. Correia M, Mendes S, Araujo C, et al. Subclavian steal syndrome in a coronary patient. *Rev Port Cardiol*. 2011;30(6):633-635.

4. Carrascal Y, Arroyo J, Fuertes JJ, Echevarría JR. Massive coronary subclavian steal syndrome. *Ann Thorac Surg*. 2010;90:1004-1006.

# 17 CONGENITAL VASCULAR ANOMALIES OF THE UPPER EXTREMITY

Luigi Pascarella, MD
Cynthia K. Shortell, MD, FACS

## PATIENT STORY

A 32-year-old man presents with right lower extremity edema, pain, lipodermatosclerosis, and history of recurrent right ankle ulcers. Physical examination demonstrates port-wine stains overlying his right upper and lower extremity, as well as the right hemithorax and abdomen (Figure 17-1). He states that these lesions have been present since birth. A clear asymmetry of his lower extremity is also noted with the right leg being larger than the left. Some soft tissue masses are also present, mainly in his lower extremity with an overlying cutaneous bluish discoloration. A duplex ultrasound documents a heterogeneous network of hypoechoic vessels with monophasic flow patterns and an incompetent great saphenous vein that is feeding many of the dilated venous structures. The deep venous system is normal and intact.

T2-weighted hyperintense magnetic resonance imaging or magnetic resonance angiography (MRI or MRA) demonstrates low-flow lesions mostly in his upper and right lower extremities (Figure 17-1) with osteomuscular hypertrophy of the right leg. The iliac veins and inferior vena cava are normal and patent.

A diagnosis of the unique vascular malformation, Klippel-Trenaunay syndrome (KTS), is made. The treatment plan is to eliminate the great saphenous vein using thermal ablation, and to treat the remainder of the venous malformations with ultrasound-guided foam sclerotherapy in multiple sessions.

## INTRODUCTION

Congenital vascular anomalies are a unique group of vascular disorders whose treatment remains a significant challenge. The groundbreaking work of Mulliken and Glowacky in characterizing vascular anomalies provides the definition of vascular malformations as "diffuse or localized embryologically developed errors of vascular morphogenesis leading to true structural anomalies."[1] It is critical to understand that with this classification and definition, hemangiomas are considered vascular tumors, as they exhibit a different clinical appearance and biologic behavior. For this reason, vascular malformations and hemangiomas will be discussed separately here.

## HEMANGIOMAS

Hemangiomas are the most common pediatric vascular tumor, and as such represent a proliferative disorder in contrast to vascular malformations, which are nonproliferative.

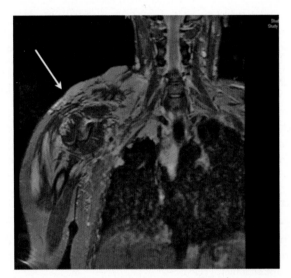

**FIGURE 17-1** Magnetic resonance imaging (MRI) is the imaging modality of choice. The vascular malformation appears as a hyperintense lesion in spin-echo sequences. MRI is also essential in identifying the relationship of the malformation with the normal vasculature.

## Epidemiology

They are congenital and occur in 7% to 10% of children, and 30% are evident at birth, while the remainder appears within the first 4 weeks of life. The female:male ratio is typically 5:1.[2]

## Etiology and Pathophysiology

The etiology is unknown. Recently, overexpression of the notch signaling pathway has been associated with the progression of hemangioma stem cells into hemangioma endothelial cells. Abnormal vascular endothelial growth factor (VEGF) production has also been observed.[2] Increased estrogen levels have been found in children with hemangiomas. In contrast to vascular malformations, hemangioma cells express the *GLUT1* gene, an erythrocyte-type glucose transporter protein.[2,3]

More recently it was hypothesized that hemangiomas may be derived from a stem cell arrested in an early stage of vascular development, as demonstrated by the expression of an immature immunophenotype (Prox-1, SLC, VEGFR-3, CD31, CD34) in tumor cells of infantile hemangioma. This immature immunophenotype tends to fade during the regression of the tumor.[3]

## Histopathology

There are two histologic types of infantile hemangioma. The capillary variant is nonvascular with a spongy appearance, while the cavernous type is characterized by large vessels with thin walls of lined, flat endothelial cells.[2]

## Clinical Presentation and Differential Diagnosis

In contrast to vascular malformations, hemangiomas are benign tumors whose biologic behavior includes a growth phase, a static phase, and then an involutive phase. They commonly affect the head and neck region, while the extremities are less commonly involved (upper extremities are involved in 15% of cases).[2]

Hemangiomas may appear as bright red, raised, or flat patches (Figure 17-2). Deeper lesions may have healthy overlying skin with a bluish discoloration. Hemangiomas are usually warm to touch, firm to palpation, and swell when the child is upset. Ulceration occurs in about 30% of patients.[2,4]

## Diagnosis

- MR is the most common imaging modality.[2,5]
- On MRI, hemangiomas appear as T2 hyperintense, well-circumscribed lesions with some heterogeneity due to feeding and draining vessels.[5]

## Management

As the overwhelming majority of hemangiomas involute spontaneously within the first 7 years of life, the initial approach is observation. It has been reported that 50% of hemangiomas involute by age 5 and 70% by age 7.[2]

Persistent or symptomatic lesions have been treated by oral, systemic, and intralesional steroids with mixed success.[2] Leaute-Labreze et al. initially reported the effectiveness of oral propranolol for treatment of infantile hemangioma.[6] More recently, a large multicenter retrospective study conducted on 71 patients treated with oral propranolol (1 mg/kg/12 h) documented regression of the

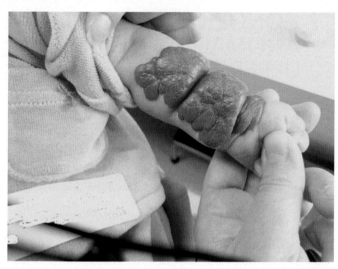

**FIGURE 17-2** Hemangiomas are benign tumors that appear as bright red, raised, or flat patches. (*Adapted from Jacobs BJ, et al.*)

tumor over a 32-week treatment period regardless of gender, age at the initiation of treatment, location, ulceration, and depth.[7,8] Propranol is currently the treatment of choice in patients requiring medical therapy.

Pulsed dye lasers in ulcerated lesions are associated with decreased pain and shorter healing time.[2] Intralesional bleomycin has also been utilized. Common complications are local hyperpigmentation and pulmonary fibrosis.[2]

Surgical treatment is recommended in patients with involvement and impairment of vital structures. In a review of 85 patients over 25 years, surgical excision with clean margins has reduced recurrence rates with the majority of patients reporting excellent function with no impairment.[2]

Kasabach-Merritt syndrome (KMS) was originally described as a life-threatening and localized consumption coagulopathy with thrombocytopenia and microangiopathic anemia, associated with a lesion initially called "capillary hemangioma with extensive purpura."[7] Current opinion indicates that KMS is rarely an epiphenomenon of infantile hemangioma, but is more commonly associated with the kaposiform hemangioendothelioma, an aggressive, rare pediatric vascular tumor.[7]

## VASCULAR MALFORMATIONS

Vascular malformations are congenital nonproliferative vascular disorders, usually evident at birth, although some may present at a later age.

### Epidemiology

• Their incidence has been reported to be 1.5% of the general population with no gender predilection.[4,9]

• Venous malformations are the most common type. In a recent series, the ratio of venous to arteriovenous malformations was 4:1.[4]

• Frequently vascular malformations are mixed and associated with developmental anomalies as in the KTS or the Parkes Weber syndrome, in which case they have shown familiarity and an autosomal pattern of inheritance.[4]

### Classification

Several classification schemes for vascular malformations have been proposed over the years.

In 1996 the International Society for the Study of Vascular Anomalies (ISSVA), based on the initial work of Mulliken and Glowacki, implemented the previous Hamburg classification and approved a classification system in which vascular malformations were divided on the basis of the cellular kinetics, anatomy, and clinical behavior in two major categories: high-flow (HFVMs) and low-flow vascular malformations (LFVMs) (Figure 17-3).[4,9] HFVMs are vascular malformations that involve arterial vessels, often with abnormal connections to the venous system, while LFVMs involve only venous or lymphatic channels. The distinction is critically important to the management of patients as the treatment of LFVM and HFVM differs. LFVMs are further subdivided into venous, capillary, lymphatic, and mixed subtypes.

A further division includes the stage of embryonic developmental arrest. Extratruncular malformations are associated with arrest in

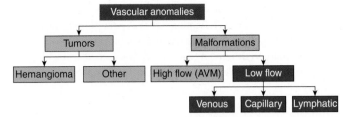

**FIGURE 17-3** Vascular malformations may be divided on the basis of the cellular kinetics, anatomy, and clinical behavior.

the early stages of development, high recurrence rate, and resistance to therapy. Truncular malformations are the result of later stage arrest in development[4] and are associated with improved prognosis and response to therapy. As hemangiomas are vascular tumors, despite being present at birth, they are not considered vascular malformations.

## Etiology and Pathogenesis

Most vascular malformations are present at birth and grow proportionately with the child. Increased lesion growth may be stimulated by puberty and trauma to the lesion. The majority are sporadic.[10] The inherited forms have been recently linked to specific gene mutations.[10]

Recent reports in the literature have documented that the underlying pathogenesis of vascular malformations is a dysfunction of signaling pathways, including receptors for tyrosine kinases, involved in the angiogenesis process.[4,10]

While in the glomuvenous malformation the defect is in the mural smooth muscle cells, developmental disturbances in most lesions are associated with derangements of the vascular endothelial cells.[10]

An endothelial-specific angiopoietin receptor TIE2/TEK on chromosome 9p21 has been identified in the famililal mucocutaneous vascular malformation.[10]

Mutations in *RASA1* have been identified in six families with capillary malformation.[10] The glomulin gene on the short arm of chromosome 1 has been documented in venous malformations with glomus cells. Milroy disease, the hereditary form of primary congenital lymphedema, has been linked to chromosome 5q35.3 within the locus of the *VEGFR3* gene.[4]

## Clinical Presentation

The clinical presentation of congenital vascular malformations (CVMs) varies widely, from the trivial to the life threatening: Cutaneous and/or mucosal birthmarks are often a cosmetic deformity, while HFVMs involving large areas or critical structures represent a serious health risk.

In a Mayo Clinic review of 185 patients, skin discoloration and pain were the most common manifestations (43% and 37%), while 35% had a palpable mass and 34% limb hypertrophy.[4] Additional clues to the diagnosis and indicators of HFVMs are decreased distal pulses and the presence of a thrill or bruit.[4]

In the same review a bruit, which defines an HFVM, was present in 26%, and 20% of patients had skin necrosis and ulcerations (Figure 17-4).

- HFVMs present early in life as warm, often painful masses that do not compress easily, or empty with elevation in contrast with venous lesions.[11] Symptoms of ischemia may occur with increased shunting in more proximal arteriovenous fistula (AVF).[11] In severe cases congestive heart failure may develop.

- HFVMs of the extremities have been subclassified into types A, B, and C.[11] Type A includes single or multiple AVFs, often associated with arterial aneurysms. Type B lesions are anomalies with macro- or microfistulas localized to a single artery of the limb, hand, or digit. These HFVMs have stable flow characteristics with minimal distal steal symptoms. Type C are diffuse vascular malformations with multiple macro- and micro-AVFs. They are associated with severe steal phenomena.[11]

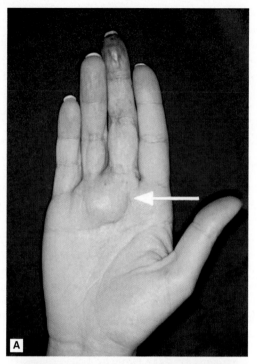

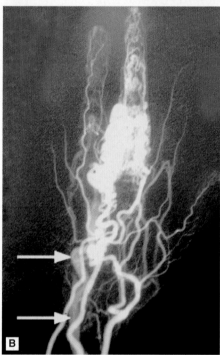

**FIGURE 17-4** Fast-flow vascular malformations may appear as palpable pulsatile masses with the presence of an overlying bruit. Despite magnetic resonance imaging (MRI) being the imaging modality of choice, angiography with selective catheterization is reserved in the case of inconclusive MRI findings and in the case of embolization of the malformation. (*Adapted from Upton J, et al.*)

The truncular form of HFVMs may present with aplasia, obstruction, coarctation, and/or ectasia. Similar malformations include the persistent sciatic artery and the retroesophageal aberrant subclavian artery causing the syndrome of dysphagia lusoria.[4]

- Clinical presentation of LFVM may include varicosities, port-wine stains, limb overgrowth, digital anomalies, edema, pain, or ulceration with bleeding or leaking of lymph fluid.[4] Venous lesions are readily compressible and empty with elevation, while lymphatic lesions are spongy to touch and do not empty with elevation.

- Thrombophlebitis and lymphangitis are not uncommon complications of venous and lymphatic LFVMs, respectively.

- In patients with pelvic involvement, hematuria and hematochezia may be present.[4]

Capillary malformations are usually localized pink or red lesions (Figure 17-5). Darker at birth, they lighten in the first weeks of life.[12]

- In the extremities, LFVMs may be associated with osteomuscular hypertrophy.

- Midline capillary malformations of the posterior neck have been found to have a high degree of association with spinal dysraphism.[13]

- Venous malformations are the most common (Figure 17-1).[14] They appear as bluish, soft, easily compressible nonpulsatile masses that enlarge with activity, dependent posture, and crying. Venous malformations may involve several tissue planes including the central nervous system, abdominal viscera, and muscles.[14] The communicating

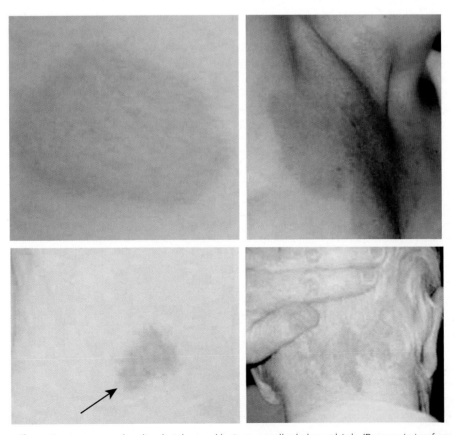

**FIGURE 17-5** Capillary malformations appear as localized pink or red lesions, usually darker at birth. (By permission from Eerola I, Boon LM, Mulliken JB: Capillary malformation-arteriovenous malformation, a new clinical and genetic disorder caused by RASA1 mutations. *Am J Hum Genet* 2003;Dec;73(6):1240-1249.)

variant has connection to the deep venous system and is associated with increased incidence of distal thromboembolic events.[14]

- Lymphatic malformations may be noted at birth. They appear as spongiform lesions with a bluish discoloration of the overlying skin.

- Lymphatic malformations can be macrocystic or microcystic (cysts <2 cc). Bleeding, lymphangitis, lymph leaking, and edema are the most common manifestations. If the malformation involves the head or neck, compression symptoms, including the airway, may arise.[4,9]

Several specific syndromes warrant specific mention and description. The Sturge-Weber syndrome is a neuroectodermal disorder in which capillary malformations are present in the ophthalmic and trigeminal nerves with leptomeningeal involvement.[12]

In KTS, mixed venous, capillary, and lymphatic lesions are associated with osteomuscular dystrophy. Orthostatic hypotension and occult pulmonary embolism from intralesional thrombi may be observed. Deep venous anomalies, including aplasia and hypoplasia, have been described in KTS (Figure 17-6).[15]

## Diagnosis

Evaluation and diagnostic testing should focus on identifying the type (HFVM vs LFVM) and the extent of the malformation. The presence of arterial involvement must be established, which dictates the most appropriate therapeutic approach.

The initial diagnosis is based on clinical findings. A detailed medical history and physical examination are essential. Duplex ultrasound documents hetereogeneous or hypoechoic lesions. Monophasic, low flow is usually present in venous malformations.[16]

While physical examination and duplex scanning are helpful, MRI is the imaging modality of choice and should be performed in all patients in whom intervention and treatment are considered. MRI is highly effective in identifying involvement of deep structures and relationship to normal vasculature, as well as differentiating between high-flow and low-flow lesions. The vascular malformation is hyperintense in T2 spin-echo sequences[5] (Figure 17-1).

Contrast arteriography and venography are reserved for patients who are good candidates for intervention or in the case of inconclusive MRI results[5] in patients requiring treatment. Adjunct tests are a blood count and a coagulation profile to investigate the presence of localized intravascular coagulopathy that manifests with minimally diminished platelet count and increased D-dimer in nonlymphatic vascular malformations.[17]

## Management

The complexity of vascular malformations requires a multidisciplinary approach as emphasized at the ISCVM in 1996.[12] The treatment is dictated by the type of vascular malformation (HFVM vs LFVM). Embolization with selective catheterization has emerged as the main therapeutic approach of high-flow arteriovenous malformations.[4,18] Embolization with polyvinyl alcohol particles, stainless steel coils, absorbable gelatin pledgets, and powder coils has been reported with success.[4] Liquid agents have also been used to occlude at the arteriolar level and capillary bed.[4]

Sclerotherapy has emerged as the main treatment modality for venous malformations, which induces denaturation of the endothelial lining.

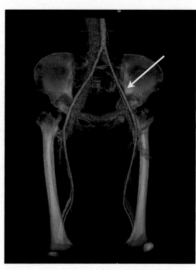

**FIGURE 17-6** Aplasia of the left iliac venous system in a patient with KTS. Note large cross pelvic venous collateral.

Ethanol sclerotherapy yields good results but is associated with significant local and systemic complications such as ulceration and pulmonary hypertension. In addition, ethanol sclerotherapy requires general anesthesia for adequate pain control.[19,20]

Lee et al. reported their experience with 87 patients undergoing ethanol sclerotherapy for LFVMs. They had an initial success rate of 95% in 87 patients undergoing 399 sessions of sclerotherapy. Nerve injury was reported in five patients including one case of permanent peroneal nerve injury. Cutaneous complications were reported in 24 patients (28%).[19]

The efficacy of sodium tetradecyl sulfate (STS) and polidocanol sclerotherapy with foam created using the Tessari[21] technique has been confirmed in several studies.[22,23] A prospective analysis of 135 patients with vascular malformation (77.2% were LFVM), presented at the 2011 Society for Vascular Surgery Meeting, showed improvement of symptoms in 93.5% of patients with no complications following ultrasound-guided STS and polidocanol sclerofoam injection (Figure 17-7). In comparison, a subgroup treated with ethanol achieved symptom improvement in 42.9% of patients, yet 57.1% experienced complications including deep vein thrombosis, ulceration, bradycardia, and/or hypoxia.

- Pulsed dye laser is a frequent modality of treatment of predominantly cutaneous lesions.[2] Reyes et al. reported a good response in 80% of treated patients in capillary malformations.[24] Multiple treatments are usually required every 6 to 8 weeks over several months of therapy.[12]

- Finally, surgical resection, historically associated with high recurrence rates (25%-52%) is currently reserved for encapsulated, localized lesions while generally contraindicated in diffuse and multifocal malformations.[4,25] When high-flow lesions are resected, immediate preoperative embolization may reduce intraoperative blood loss.

## CONCLUSION

Congenital vascular malformations pose a serious diagnostic and therapeutic challenge. Their etiology and pathogenesis is still largely unknown, despite recent advances, and further studies may shed some light on their physiopathology. A multidisciplinary staged diagnostic and therapeutic approach with multiple modalities is recommended, using MRI as the primary means of differentiating between HFVMs and LFVMs.

HFVMs are managed predominantly with transcatheter embolotherapy. Sclerotheraphy with STS or polidocanol foam may be the preferred treatment modality in LFVMs, given the relatively high efficacy and low complication rates compared to ethanol sclerotherapy, although this remains controversial. Pulsed dye lasers are used with success in cutaneous lesions and capillary malformations. Surgical resection is reserved for small, encapsulated lesions and for lesions involving vital structures that cannot be managed with interventional methods.

## PATIENT EDUCATION

Patients should be educated that the primary goal of therapy is symptom control, and that the need for future treatment due to recurrence is likely.

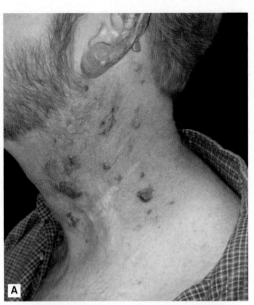
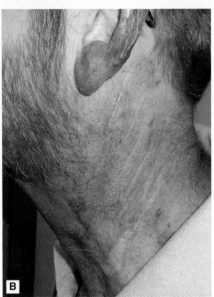

FIGURE 17-7 Venous malformations are the most common vascular anomalies. They appear as bluish, soft, easily compressible nonpulsatile masses that enlarge with activity, posture, and crying. (A). Sclerotherapy with sodium tetradecyl sulfate (STS) or polidocanol foam has recently emerged as the main treatment modality for venous malformations with improvement of symptoms in the majority of patients (B).

**PROVIDER RESOURCES**

- http://vascular.surgery.duke.edu/files/documents/Vasc _Malformations_10-29-09.pdf

- https://www.dcri.org/education-training/meetings/meeting-presentations/venous-disease-2012/Shortell_demystifying%20 venous%20malformations.pdf

**PATIENT RESOURCES**

- http://www.novanews.org/information/vascular-malformations

- http://www.ohsu.edu/xd/health/health-information/topic-by-id.cfm?ContentId=P01841&ContentTypeId=90

## REFERENCES

1. Mulliken JB, Glowacki J. Hemangiomas and vascular malformations in infants and children: a classification based on endothelial characteristics. *Plast Reconstr Surg.* 1982;69(3):412-422.

2. Jacobs BJ, Anzarut A, Guerra S, Gordillo G, Imbriglia JE. Vascular anomalies of the upper extremity. *J Hand Surg Am.* 2010; 35(10):1703-1709; quiz 1709.

3. Dadras SS, North PE, Bertoncini J, Mihm MC, Detmar M. Infantile hemangiomas are arrested in an early developmental vascular differentiation state. *Mod Pathol.* 2004;17(9):1068-1079.

4. Gloviczki P, Duncan A, Kalra M, et al. Vascular malformations: an update. *Perspect Vasc Surg Endovasc Ther.* 2009;21(2):133-148.

5. Ernemann U, Kramer U, Miller S, et al. Current concepts in the classification, diagnosis and treatment of vascular anomalies. *Eur J Radiol.* 2010;75(1):2-11.

6. Leaute-Labreze C, Dumas de la Roque E, Hubiche T, Boralevi F, Thambo JB, Taïeb A. Propranolol for severe hemangiomas of infancy. *N Engl J Med.* 2008;358(24):2649-2651.

7. Enjolras O, Wassef M, Mazoyer E, et al. Infants with Kasabach-Merritt syndrome do not have "true" hemangiomas. *J Pediatr.* 1997;130(4):631-640.

8. Bagazgoitia L, Torrelo A, Gutiérrez JC, et al. Propranolol for infantile hemangiomas. *Pediatr Dermatol.* 2011;28(2):108-114.

9. Marler JJ, Mulliken JB. Vascular anomalies: classification, diagnosis, and natural history. *Facial Plast Surg Clin North Am.* 2001;9(4):495-504.

10. Brouillard P, Vikkula M. Genetic causes of vascular malformations. *Hum Mol Genet.* 2007;16(Spec No. 2):R140-R149.

11. Upton J, Coombs CJ, Mulliken JB, Burrows PE, Pap S. Vascular malformations of the upper limb: a review of 270 patients. *J Hand Surg Am.* 1999;24(5):1019-1035.

12. Lee BB, Bergan J, Gloviczki P, et al. Diagnosis and treatment of venous malformations. Consensus document of the International Union of Phlebology (IUP)-2009. *Int Angiol.* 2009;28(6):434-451.

13. Guggisberg D, Hadj-Rabia S, Viney C, et al. Skin markers of occult spinal dysraphism in children: a review of 54 cases. *Arch Dermatol.* 2004;140(9):1109-1115.

14. Legiehn GM, Heran MK. Venous malformations: classification, development, diagnosis, and interventional radiologic management. *Radiol Clin North Am.* 2008;46(3):545-597, vi.

15. Jacob AG, Driscoll DJ, Shaughnessy WJ, Stanson AW, Clay RP, Gloviczki P. Klippel-Trenaunay syndrome: spectrum and management. *Mayo Clin Proc.* 1998;73(1):28-36.

16. Trop I, Dubois J, Guibaud L, et al. Soft-tissue venous malformations in pediatric and young adult patients: diagnosis with Doppler US. *Radiology.* 1999;212(3):841-845.

17. Mazoyer E, Enjolras O, Bisdorff A, Perdu J, Wassef M, Drouet L. Coagulation disorders in patients with venous malformation of the limbs and trunk: a case series of 118 patients. *Arch Dermatol.* 2008;144(7):861-867.

18. Natali J, Merland JJ. Superselective arteriography and therapeutic embolisation for vascular malformations. (Angiodysplasias). *J Cardiovasc Surg (Torino).* 1976;17(6): 465-472.

19. Lee BB, Do YS, Byun HS, Choo IW, Kim DI, Huh SH. Advanced management of venous malformation with ethanol sclerotherapy: mid-term results. *J Vasc Surg.* 2003;37(3):533-538.

20. Lee BB, Do YS, Yakes W, Kim DI, Mattassi R, Hyon WS. Management of arteriovenous malformations: a multidisciplinary approach. *J Vasc Surg.* 2004;39(3):590-600.

21. Tessari L, Cavezzi A, Frullini A. Preliminary experience with a new sclerosing foam in the treatment of varicose veins. *Dermatol Surg.* 2001;27(1):58-60.

22. Cabrera J, Cabrera J Jr, Garcia-Olmedo MA, Redondo P. Treatment of venous malformations with sclerosant in microfoam form. *Arch Dermatol.* 2003;139(11):1409-1416.

23. Pascarella L, Bergan JJ, Yamada C, Mekenas L. Venous angiomata: treatment with sclerosant foam. *Ann Vasc Surg.* 2005;19(4):457-464.

24. Reyes BA, Geronemus R. Treatment of port-wine stains during childhood with the flashlamp-pumped pulsed dye laser. *J Am Acad Dermatol.* 1990;23(6 pt 1):1142-1148.

25. Tang P, Hornicek FJ, Gebhardt MC, Cates J, Mankin HJ. Surgical treatment of hemangiomas of soft tissue. *Clin Orthop Relat Res.* 2002(399):205-210.

# 18 ALLEN TEST AND EVALUATION OF THE PALMAR ARCH

Bhagwan Satiani, MD, MBA, RPVI, FACS

## PATIENT STORY

A 75-year-old man was sent to the noninvasive vascular laboratory for evaluation of patency of his palmar arch prior to possible harvesting of his radial artery (RA) for use as an autograft in a coronary artery bypass procedure. His saphenous veins and one of his internal mammary arteries had been previously used.

## ANATOMY AND PHYSIOLOGY

- A dual system consisting of the superficial and deep palmar arches formed by the radial and ulnar arteries (UAs) supplies blood flow to the hand in most people.
- Rarely, there is a third artery, the median artery supplying the hand.
- A patent UA and a physiologically complete palmar arch network are necessary for safe harvesting of the RA.
- The UA commonly forms the superficial palmar arch in conjunction with the superficial palmar branch of the RA. This arch is complete in 84.4% of people.[1]
- The deep palmar arch is most often formed by an anastomosis between the deep palmar branch of the UA and the dorsal RA.

## THE ALLEN TEST

- Edgar V. Allen first described the Allen test in1929 when reporting three patients with thromboangiitis obliterans.[2]
- His original description of making a fist with the RA occluded for 1 minute followed by extending the fingers and watching for return of color was later modified and is now called the modified Allen test (MAT).[3]
- The correct technique involves the patient making a fist for 30 seconds while pressure is applied over both the radial and ulnar arteries to occlude them. The patient is then asked to open the fist and the UA is selectively released with the RA still occluded.
- Hyperextension of the hand or wide separation of the digits is avoided to avoid a falsely positive abnormal test. In most normal hands it takes 3 to 12 seconds for the normal color to return if sufficient collateral to the hand is present.[4]
- The MAT is considered positive or abnormal if color does not return in this time interval.

## CLINICAL SIGNIFICANCE

- The RA is the third most common conduit utilized for grafting of coronary artery occlusive disease. Cardiac surgeons need precise information of adequate collateral circulation to the hand to avoid harvesting the RA if this would result in hand ischemia with devastating consequences.
- Furthermore, if prolonged RA catheterization or larger bore lines are inserted with a greater risk of thrombosis, demonstration of a physiologically complete palmar arch is necessary.
- The specificity of the MAT is in the 97% range with a 6-second cutoff.[5]
- The predictive value of a positive (abnormal) MAT is such that it does not necessarily mean hand ischemia will result if the RA is harvested.
- A negative (normal) MAT safely allows RA harvest, although the cutoff point is somewhat controversial and can range between 3 and 12 seconds.
- Because of the lower sensitivity if a MAT is performed and is abnormal, an additional noninvasive test such as a dynamic duplex scan of the palmar arch may be necessary.
- However, it must be remembered that there is not a perfect correlation between the MAT and Doppler or duplex evaluation.
- It is estimated that between 10% and 27.7% of the patients have nonharvestable radial arteries.[5]

## NONINVASIVE TESTING

- There are a variety of noninvasive tests available for determining adequate circulation to the hand. These include digital plethysmography, digital Doppler waveforms and pressures, pulse oximetry, and duplex ultrasonography.
- This patient underwent digital plethysmography, and compression of the RA showed abnormal waveforms in the digits of the left hand (Figure 18-1). The patient then underwent dynamic duplex ultrasonography as described. Baseline RA signals were normal (Figure 18-2). Selective release of the UA and continued compression of the RA resulted in almost no antegrade flow. This pointed to an incomplete palmar arch (Figure 18-3).
- Another advantage of duplex scanning is that the technique allows measurement of the size of the RA as well as identification of any significant atherosclerotic disease, both of which are important to the surgeon in deciding whether to use the RA as a conduit.

## RECOMMENDATION

Based on the physical examination and noninvasive testing the recommendation was to not use the RA from the left arm.

## PATIENT EDUCATION

- Patients must be informed prior to RA harvesting regarding the risks and benefits of RA and reasons for determining patency of a normal palmar arch.

Digit Waveforms

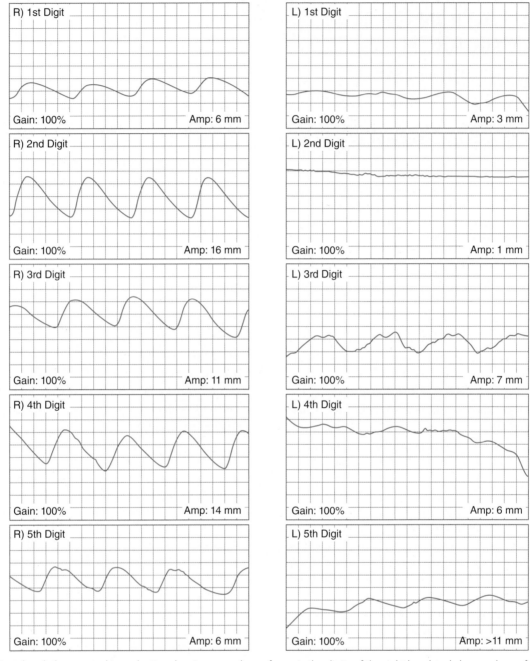

**FIGURE 18-1** Doppler plethysmographic evaluation showing normal waveforms in the digits of the right hand and abnormal waveforms in the left hand.

- Following RA harvest there will be a need to assess postoperative hand function and any evidence of ischemic pain or claudication.

- If there is any hand ischemia, patients must be informed about rehabilitation and any measures to gradually increase the collateral flow.

- Local wound complications resulting in infection at the RA harvest site can also occur. If this occurs, patients are instructed in the care of the wound.

### PROVIDER RESOURCES

- Baetz L, Satiani B. Palmar arch identification during evaluation for radial artery harvest. *Vasc Endovascular Surg*. 2011;45:255-257.

- Habib J, Baetz L, Satiani B. Assessment of collateral circulation to the hand prior to radial artery harvest. *Vasc Med*. 2012;17: 352-361.

### PATIENT RESOURCES

- http://medical-dictionary.thefreedictionary.com/Allen's+test

- http://wiki.answers.com/Q/What_is_the_difference_between_an_Allen's_test_and_a_modified_Allen's_test

### REFERENCES

1. Gellman H, Botte MJ, Shankwiler J, Gelberman, RH. Arterial patterns of the deep and superficial palmar arches. *Clin Orthop Related Res*. 2001;383:41-46.

2. Allen EV. Thromboangiitis obliterans; methods of diagnosis of chronic occlusive arterial lesions distal to the wrist with illustrative cases. *Am J Med Sci*. 1929;178:237-244.

3. Fuhrman TM, Pippin WD, Talmage LA, Reilley TE. Evaluation of collateral circulation of the hand. *J Clin Monit*. 1992;8:28-32.

4. Jarvis MA, Jarvis CL, Jones PM, Spyt TJ. Reliability of Allen's test in selection of patients for radial artery harvest. *Ann Thorac Surg*. 2000;70:1362-1365.

5. Kohonen M, Teerenhovi O, Terho T, Laurikka J, Tarkka M. Non-harvestable radial artery. A bilateral problem? *Interact Cardio-Vasc Thorac Surg*. 2008;7:797-800.

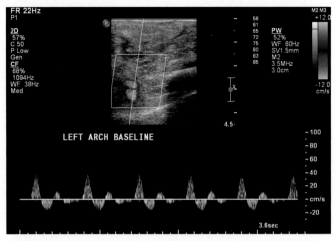

**FIGURE 18-2** Dynamic duplex ultrasound examination showing normal signals in the palmar arch as a baseline.

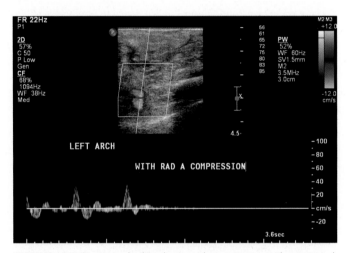

**FIGURE 18-3** Dynamic duplex ultrasound examination with continued compression of the radial artery (RA) and selective release of the ulnar artery (UA) showing almost no antegrade flow in the palmar arch.

# 19 HYPOTHENAR HAMMER SYNDROME

Shankar M. Sundaram, MD, FACS, FCCP

## PATIENT STORY

- A 43-year-old man presented with no relevant past medical, family or social history except for 1 pack-a-day tobacco use.
- Several-week history of right fourth- or fifth-digit coolness, pain, and ulceration of fourth digit.
- No medications.
- Patient's occupation was manual labor.
  His physical examination showed the following:
- There were 2+ carotid, brachial, radial, femoral, popliteal, and pedal pulses. He did not have an ulnar pulse on the right side.
- He had ischemia of his right fourth and fifth fingers, with decreased capillary refill, and there was a dry, and ischemic ulceration over the nail bed laterally on the fourth finger. No signs of infection were present.
- A Doppler signal was present over the palmar arch until the radial artery was manually compressed.

## ETIOLOGY

- Repetitive use of the palm of the hand in activities that include pounding and pushing.
- Anatomic site of injury to the ulnar artery is in the hypothenar eminence (Figure 19-1). The terminal branches of the ulnar artery arise in a groove that is bounded medially by the hamate bone.
- As the distal ulnar artery lies superficially in the palm, it is covered for approximately 2 cm by only the skin, subcutaneous tissue, and the palmaris brevis muscle. Therefore, pounding and pushing of the hand causes the ulnar artery to hit the hamate bone repeatedly.
- When this area is repeatedly traumatized, ulnar or digital spasm, aneurysms, occlusion, or a combination of these can result.

## CLINICAL FINDINGS

- Intimal damage results in thrombotic occlusion. Damage to the media results in palmar aneurysms.
- Fourth digit is most often involved.
- Differentiated from Raynaud phenomenon by the lack of tricolor changes and sometimes absence of thumb involvement.

## DIAGNOSIS

- Suggested by history and physical examination.
- Arteriography defines lesion, rules out other causes, and possibly can be therapeutic (Figures 19-2 to 19-6).

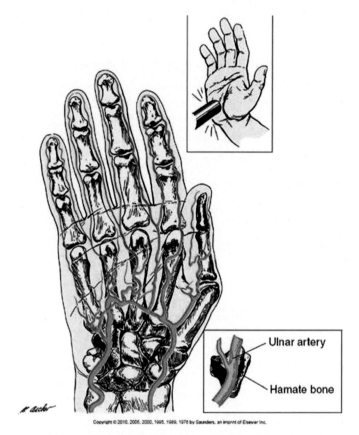

Copyright © 2010, 2006, 2000, 1995, 1989, 1976 by Saunders, an imprint of Elsevier Inc.

**FIGURE 19-1** Schematic showing the mechanism of ulnar artery injury (upper inset) in a patient with hypothenar hammer syndrome. The lower inset shows that the terminus of the ulnar artery is susceptible to injury because of its proximity to the hamate bone. (Modified from Eskandari MK. Occupational vascular problems. In: Cronenwett JL, Johnston KW, eds. *Rutherford's Vascular Surgery*. 7th ed. Philadelphia, PA: Saunders-Elsevier; 2010.)

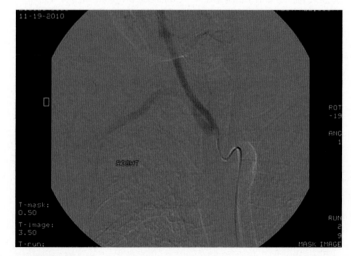

**FIGURE 19-2** Contrast injection into brachiocephalic artery revealing no stenosis in main brachiocephalic artery or proximal right common carotid or proximal right subclavian arteries.

## DIFFERENTIAL DIAGNOSIS

- Atherosclerosis
- Embolic phenomena
- Hypercoagulable states
- Buerger disease (thromboangiitis obliterans)
- Raynaud phenomenon
- Inflammatory vasculitis (systemic lupus erythematosus, rheumatoid arthritis)
- Thoracic outlet syndrome
- Iatrogenic

## TREATMENT

- Supportive
- If acute or semi-acute → intra-arterial thrombolytic therapy
- If aneurysm, can resect and place an interposition vein graft

## PATIENT EDUCATION

- Occupational hazards, the link between their symptoms, and underlying pathology must be explained to patients.
- If thrombolysis is required, the complications of lysis such as hemorrhage must be disclosed.
- The possibility of recurrence, if the underlying causative event is not alleviated, must also be discussed with patients and their families.

### PATIENT RESOURCES

- http://www.nlm.nih.gov/medlineplus/ency/article/000412.htm
- http://www.mayoclinic.com/health/raynauds-disease/DS00433

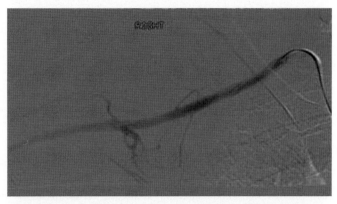

FIGURE 19-3 Normal right subclavian-axillary artery angiogram.

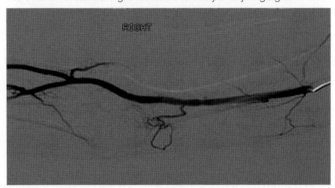

FIGURE 19-4 Normal right brachial artery bifurcating into normal proximal radial and ulnar arteries.

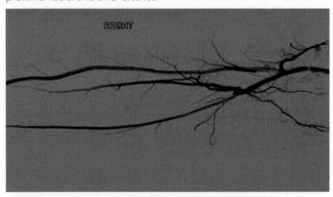

FIGURE 19-5 Normal right mid-radial and ulnar arteries.

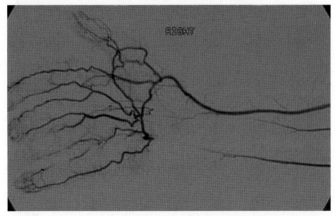

FIGURE 19-6 Distal right ulnar artery is occluded. Also note the small aneurysm at the terminus of the ulnar artery at the palmar arch. A combination of embolization from this aneurysm, spasm, or direct injury is the likely cause of the digital artery occlusion seen in the fourth and fifth digits.

# 20 HAND ISCHEMIA AFTER PLACEMENT OF HEMODIALYSIS ACCESS

Faisal Aziz, MD, RVT, RPVI

## PATIENT STORY

A 78-year-old, right-hand-dominant man was diagnosed with end-stage renal disease. It was deemed that he would require lifetime hemodialysis. Venous mapping with Duplex ultrasound was performed in both upper extremities to locate suitable veins for dialysis access. Left proximal radial artery to cephalic vein arteriovenous fistula was created. Patient had an uneventful postoperative course. He demonstrated an excellent thrill and bruit throughout the course of fistula. He had palpable radial and ulnar pulses. Approximately 8 weeks later, the fistula was used for hemodialysis. The patient started complaining of pain in all the digits of the left hand and noticeable discoloration of the left hand during dialysis. His symptoms resolved completely upon discontinuing dialysis.

## DIAGNOSIS AND TREATMENT COURSE

• Photoplethysmography of the left hand digits showed diminished waveforms in all fingers of the left hand. The waveforms improved upon compression of the fistula (Figures 20-1 and 20-2).

• Duplex ultrasound examination of the fistula showed reversal of flow in the radial artery (Figures 20-3 to 20-5).

• Diagnostic arteriogram of the left upper extremity was performed that showed normal arterial vasculature of left upper extremity. Selective catheterization of the ulnar artery showed antegrade flow

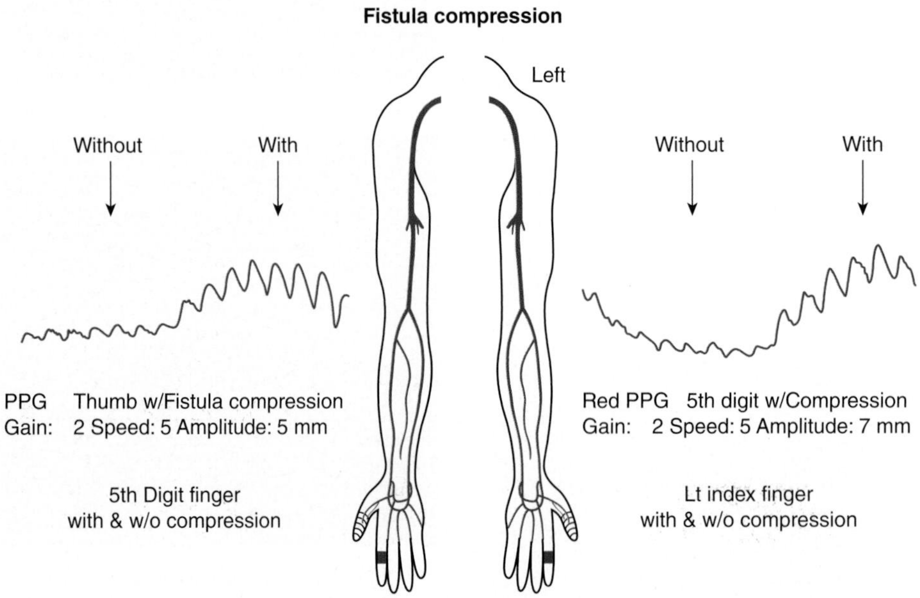

**Fistula compression**

Left

Without        With                         Without        With

PPG     Thumb w/Fistula compression          Red PPG   5th digit w/Compression
Gain:   2 Speed: 5 Amplitude: 5 mm           Gain:   2 Speed: 5 Amplitude: 7 mm

5th Digit finger                              Lt index finger
with & w/o compression                       with & w/o compression

**FIGURE 20-1** Plethysmographic waveforms of left second and fifth digits with and without compression of arteriovenous fistula showing improvement in perfusion with compression of the fistula.

in the ulnar artery, filling of the palmar arch, and retrograde flow
in the radial artery (Figure 20-6).

- The patient was brought to the operating room and under
  local anesthetic, the distal radial artery was ligated. He had dialysis
  after the procedure and had no further symptoms of digit ischemia
  during dialysis.

## EPIDEMIOLOGY

- Ischemic digit pain in a hemodialysis patient with an arteriovenous
  fistula can be a potentially serious complication. In the majority
  of cases, the arterial "steal" causes pain and discomfort, but in
  extreme cases, it can lead to tissue necrosis and eventual loss of
  digits.

- Prevalence of distal hypoperfusion ischemic syndrome varies
  anywhere from 1% to 20%.[1-4] It is more common in patients who
  have arteriovenous fistulae based on inflow from the brachial artery
  as compared to those in whom the radial artery is used for arterial
  inflow.[2]

## CLINICAL PRESENTATION

- Patients with arteriovenous fistulae may present emergently
  with acute ischemia of upper extremity immediately after
  fistula placement. These patients need emergent ligation of
  fistula.

- However, the majority of patients present in a delayed fashion.
  Most of them are symptomatic only during dialysis. According to
  some studies, reversal of flow can be noticed in up to 30% of the
  patients with arteriovenous fistulas; however, intervention is
  indicated in only those patients who are symptomatic.

## TREATMENT OPTIONS

Ischemia due to a post-dialysis access arteriovenous fistula can be
treated in a number of ways:

- Distal revascularization with interval ligation
  In this operation, the artery is ligated distal to the origin of fistula
  and a bypass is done between the proximal and distal portions of
  the artery. The basic principle is to stop the reversal of flow in the
  native artery.

- Banding
  In this operation, the diameter of the anastomosis is narrowed with
  a suture (band), so that the volume of the blood flowing out of
  artery is reduced.

- Distal arterial ligation
  In cases with easily demonstrable reversal of flow on diagnostic
  studies, simple ligation of artery distal to the origin of fistula can
  prevent reversal of flow.

## PATIENT EDUCATION

Patients should be educated about the signs and symptoms of
hand ischemia, so they can make clinicians aware of their
symptoms.

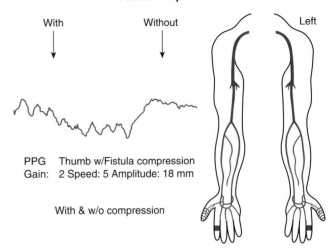

**Fistula compression**

With          Without          Left

PPG     Thumb w/Fistula compression
Gain:   2 Speed: 5 Amplitude: 18 mm

With & w/o compression

**FIGURE 20-2** Plethysmographic waveforms of the right thumb
with and without compression of the arteriovenous fistula showing
improvement in perfusion with compression of the fistula.

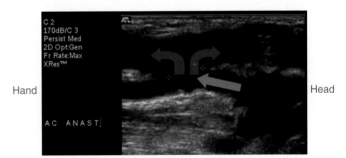

**FIGURE 20-3** Direction of blood flow across the anastomosis into the
proximal and distal cephalic vein (blue arrows). Reversal of blood flow
in the artery distal to the anastomosis is shown by the red arrow.

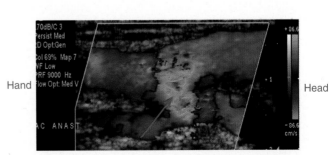

**FIGURE 20-4** Arterial duplex ultrasound study showing the anastomosis (blue arrow).

## REFERENCES

1. Duncan H, Ferguson L, Faris I. Incidence of the radial steal syndrome in patients with Brescia fistula for hemodialysis: its clinical significance. *J Vasc Surg.* 1986;4:144-147.

2. Kwun KB, Schanzer H, Finkler N, Haimov M, Burrows L. Hemodynamic evaluation of angioaccess procedures for hemodialysis. *Vasc Surg.* 1979;13:170-177.

3. DeMasi RJ, Gregory RT, Sorrell KA, et al. Intraoperative noninvasive evaluation of arteriovenous fistulae and grafts. The steal study. *J Vasc Tech.* 1994;18:177-192.

4. Morsy A, Kulbaski M, Chen C, Isiklar H, Lumsden AB. Incidence and characteristics of patients with hand ischemia after a hemodialysis access procedure. *J Surg Res.* 1998;74:8-10.

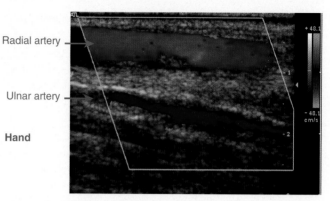

**FIGURE 20-5** Arterial duplex ultrasound study: antegrade flow in radial artery (red color). Retrograde flow in ulnar artery (blue color). The anastomosis is indicated by the blue arrow.

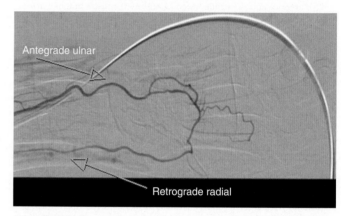

**FIGURE 20-6** Arteriogram showing antegrade flow in the ulnar artery and retrograde flow in the radial artery (arrows).

# PART 3

# CAROTID ARTERY OCCLUSIVE DISEASE

# 21 ARTERIOSCLEROTIC CAROTID OCCLUSIVE: SURGICAL

Michael R. Go, MD

## PATIENT STORY

A 62-year-old Caucasian man presented 1 week after an episode where he spontaneously dropped a cigarette he was holding in his right hand. He immediately noted an inability to grasp objects and numbness in his right hand. These symptoms lasted for 2 minutes and then spontaneously resolved. Currently, his right hand feels completely normal. He denies other symptoms such as amaurosis, paralysis, paresthesias, speech disturbance, or gait disturbance. His past medical history is significant for hypertension, hyper-cholesterolemia, and cramping in his calves when he walks long distances. He has a 30 pack-year history of smoking and denies use of alcohol. A carotid duplex ultrasound shows a left 70% to 99% internal carotid artery (ICA) stenosis. A surgical option was elected by the patient (Figures 21-1 to 21-3).

## EPIDEMIOLOGY

Stroke ranks third among all causes of death in the United States behind heart disease and cancer, with 795,000 strokes occurring per year.[1]

- Annually, 55,000 more women than men are affected, and over 60% of all stroke deaths occur in women. African Americans have twice the stroke risk of Caucasians. Mexican Americans also have an increased incidence of stroke compared to Caucasians.[2]

## ETIOLOGY AND PATHOPHYSIOLOGY

- One-third of all strokes are related to cervical carotid disease.

- Standard risk factors for coronary and systemic atherosclerosis apply to this patient population such as age, male sex, family history, smoking, hypertension, hyperlipidemia, sedentary lifestyle, and high dietary fat.

- The mechanism of cervical carotid stroke is usually emboliza-tion from the carotid bifurcation plaque, but hemodynamic compromise from stenosis may also play a role. The risks of embolization and hemodynamic compromise increase with increasing ICA stenosis.[3]

## DIAGNOSIS

- When carotid territory stroke or transient ischemic attack (TIA) is suspected, carotid duplex in an accredited vascular laboratory to define degree of stenosis is mandatory.

- When carotid duplex is nondiagnostic, computed tomography (CT) or magnetic resonance angiography (MRA) may be used.

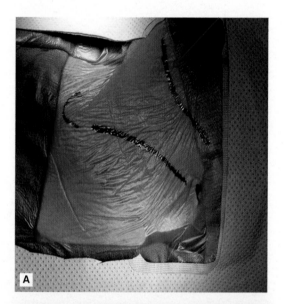

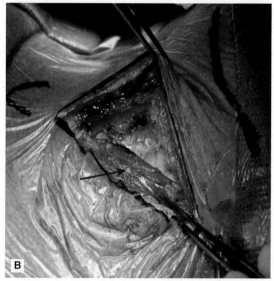

**FIGURE 21-1** (A) Carotid endarterectomy (CEA) can be performed via a neck incision along the anterior border of the sternocleidomastoid muscle (red arrow). The inferior border of the mandible is indicated by the blue arrow. (B) The platysma is divided and the sternocleido-mastoid muscle (blue arrow) and jugular vein are retracted laterally. The head end of the patient is towards the right side of the photos. Procedure is being performed on the left carotid artery.

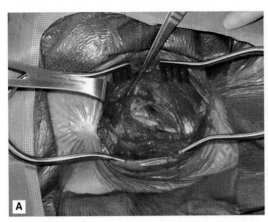
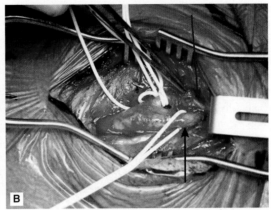

**FIGURE 21-2** (A) The vagus is preserved in the carotid sheath. (B) The hypoglossal nerve is encountered cephalad in the dissection (dark blue arrow). The internal carotid artery (ICA) is shown by the black arrow.

- Catheter angiography is indicated in the setting of conflicting non-invasive studies and when carotid artery stenting (CAS) is planned.[4]

## CLINICAL FEATURES

- Neurologic examination may reveal motor or sensory deficits contralateral to the affected carotid artery. Aphasia, dysphasia, or apraxia may be reported.

- Amaurosis fugax, or sudden complete or partial loss of vision in one eye, is a result of embolization from the cervical carotid artery to the ipsilateral central retinal artery. Up to 70% of stroke survivors can regain functional independence; however, 15% to 30% become permanently disabled and 20% will require long-term care.[5] In patients over 65 years of age, 6 months after a stroke 50% have some residual hemiparesis, 30% require some assistance with walking, 26% cannot perform activities of daily living independently, 19% have aphasia, and 26% are institutionalized.[6]

- Mean lifetime cost of an ischemic stroke in the United States is $140,048. In 2007, the total cost of stroke exceeded 40 billion dollars.[1]

## MANAGEMENT

- Carotid endarterectomy (CEA) has been well established as a treatment for cervical carotid disease. Recently, debate has centered on CEA versus CAS in the management of carotid disease.

- All patients should receive optimal medical therapy. Aspirin is indicated for all patients with atherosclerotic carotid disease.

- Warfarin may be indicated to treat patients who have had stroke from cardiac embolization, but there is no evidence supporting the use of heparin and warfarin or clopidogrel to prevent or treat stroke related to cervical carotid disease.

- Management of hypertension and hypercholesterolemia, smoking cessation, and dietary and activity modification are all mainstays of treatment.

- Patients with asymptomatic carotid stenosis greater than or equal to 60% gain stroke risk reduction with carotid revascularization.

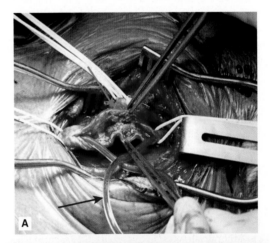

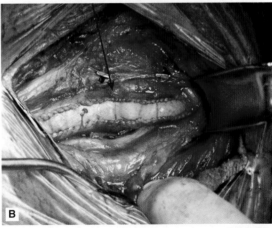

**FIGURE 21-3** (A) The intraoperative carotid clamping is tolerated without neurologic compromise by greater than 85% of patients. The plaque is noted by the green arrow as soon as the carotid bifurcation is opened. Carotid endarterectomy (CEA) may be performed with or without intraoperative shunting (dark blue arrow); if done without shunting, cerebral monitoring of some kind is indicated to detect intolerance of clamping. This can be accomplished by using regional anesthesia with direct monitoring of mental status, or with general anesthesia using electroencephalogram, somatosensory-evoked potential, or internal carotid artery (ICA) stump pressure monitoring. (B) Endarterectomy may be done longitudinally as pictured or using an eversion technique without an effect on outcome, but if longitudinal endarterectomy is performed, patch angioplasty offers better stroke and restenosis rates than primary closure (blue arrow).

However, that risk reduction must be considered in light of the patient's life expectancy, with intervention reserved for patients with at least a 5-year life expectancy.[7,8]

- Current medical therapy may outperform intervention in certain low-risk asymptomatic patients, and there is low absolute risk reduction with intervention for asymptomatic patients. Overall stroke risk in medically managed asymptomatic patients is only 2% per year, thus careful patient selection in asymptomatic carotid disease is paramount.

- Carotid intervention is indicated in patients with symptomatic carotid disease if the stenosis is greater than 50%.[9,10]

- Patients considered high risk for CEA include those with anatomically inaccessible lesions, cervical immobility, prior neck dissection, tracheostomy, contralateral cranial nerve injury, prior radiation therapy, contralateral occlusion, and recurrent stenosis after CEA. Medical comorbidities considered high risk for CEA include presence of chronic obstructive pulmonary disease, New York Heart Association (NYHA) class III or IV heart failure, ejection fraction less than 30%, recent myocardial infarction (MI), and unstable angina.

- Short-term risks in centers of excellence for both CEA and CAS may be equivalent for the composite endpoint of any stroke, death, or MI.

- Age increases risk with CAS. Carotid tortuosity may present problems with stent or embolic protection device deployment.

- Symptomatic patients may be better treated by CEA, especially when older than 70 years or if male.

- In the absence of high risk for CEA criteria, patients aged less than 70 years may be offered CAS or CEA with equivalent composite stroke or MI or death rates. In this group, CAS incurs higher stroke risk in exchange for lower MI risk, and CEA incurs higher MI risk in exchange for lower stroke risk.

- Patients over 70 years may be offered CEA based on a lower periprocedural stroke risk (Figure 21-1).[11-16]

## FOLLOW-UP

- Recurrent stenosis occurs in 6% to 14% of patients undergoing CEA.[17] Surveillance using duplex ultrasound is recommended within 30 days after CEA, and an accepted long-term regimen is duplex ultrasound every 6 months for stenoses over 50% and yearly duplex for stenoses less than 50%.[1]

### PROVIDER RESOURCE

- http://www.jvascsurg.org/article/S0741-5214(11)01635-1/abstract.

### PATIENT RESOURCES

- http://www.vascularweb.org/vascularhealth/Pages/carotid-endarterectomy.aspx
- http://www.ninds.nih.gov/disorders/stroke/carotid_endarterectomy_backgrounder.htm

## REFERENCES

1. Roger V, Go A, Lloyd-Jones D. Heart disease and stroke statistics—2011 update: a report from the American Heart Association Statistics Committee and Stroke Statistics Committee. *Circulation*. 2011;123:e18-e209.

2. *Incidence and Prevalence: 2006 Chart Book on Cardiovascular and Lung Diseases*. Bethesda, MD: National Heart, Lung, and Blood Institute; 2006. Available at http://www.nhlbi.nih.gov/resources/docs/06a_ip_chtbk.pdf. Accessed May 8, 2013.

3. Kleindorfer D, Panagos P, Pancioli A. Incidence and short-term prognosis after transient ischemic attack in a population-based study. *Stroke*. 2005;36:720-723.

4. Ricotta JJ, Aburahma A, Ascher E, Eskandari M, Faries P, Lal BK. Updated Society for Vascular Surgery guidelines for management of extracranial carotid disease: executive summary. *J Vasc Surg*. 2011;54: 832-836.

5. Asplund K, Stegmayr B, Peltonen M. From the twentieth to the twenty-first century: a public health perspective on stroke. In: Ginsberg MD, Bogousslavsky J, eds. *Cerebrovascular Disease Pathophysiology, Diagnosis, and Management*. Malden, MA: Blackwell Science; 1998.

6. Kelly-Hayes M, Beiser A, Kase CS, Scaramucci A, D'Agostino RB, Wolf PA. The influence of gender and age on disability following ischemic stroke: the Framingham study. *J Stroke Cerebrovasc Dis*. 2003;12:119-126.

7. Endarterectomy for asymptomatic carotid artery stenosis. Executive Committee for the Asymptomatic Carotid Atherosclerosis Study. *JAMA*. 1995;273:1421-1428.

8. Halliday A, Mansfield A, Marro J, et al. MRC Asymptomatic Carotid Surgery Trial (ACST) Collaborative Group. Prevention of disabling and fatal strokes by successful carotid endarterectomy in patients without recent neurological symptoms: randomised controlled trial. *Lancet*. 2004;363:1491-1502.

9. Ferguson GG, Eliasziw M, Barr HW. The North American symptomatic carotid endarterectomy trial: surgical results in 1415 patients. *Stroke*. 1999;30:1751-1758.

10. Randomised trial of endarterectomy for recently symptomatic carotid stenosis: final results of the MRC European Carotid Surgery Trial (ECST). *Lancet*. 1998;351:1379-1387.

11. Mantese V, Timaran C, Chiu D. The carotid revascularization endarterectomy versus stenting trial (CREST)—stenting versus carotid endarterectomy for carotid disease. *Stroke*. 2010;41: S31-S34.

12. Yadav JS, Wholey MH, Kuntz RE. Protected carotid-artery stenting versus endarterectomy in high-risk patients. *N Engl J Med*. 2004;351:1493-1501.

13. Eckstein J, Ringleb PA, Allenberg J. Results of the stent-protected angioplasty versus carotid endarterectomy (SPACE) study to treat symptomatic stenoses at 2 years: a multinational, prospective, randomised trial. *Lancet*. 2008;7:893-902.

14. Mas JL, Chatellier G, Beyssen B. Endarterectomy versus stenting in patients with symptomatic severe carotid stenosis. *N Engl J Med*. 2006;355:1660-1671.

15. Mas JL, Chatellier G, Beyssen B. Endarterectomy versus angio-plasty in patients with symptomatic severe carotid stenosis (EVA-3S) trial: results up to 4 years from a randomised, multi-centre trial. *Lancet Neurol*. 2008;7:885-892.

16. Carotid artery stenting compared with endarterectomy in patients with symptomatic carotid stenosis (International Carotid Stenting Study): an interim analysis of a randomised controlled trial. International Carotid-Stenting Study Investigators. *Lancet*. 2010;375:985-997.

17. Roseborough G, Perler B. Carotid artery disease: endarterec-tomy. In: Cronenwett J, Johnston K, eds. *Vascular Surgery*. Philadelphia, PA: Elsevier; 2010.

# 22 ARTERIOSCLEROTIC CAROTID OCCLUSIVE: STENT

Michael R. Go, MD

## PATIENT STORY

A 72-year-old Caucasian man presented 1 week after an episode where he spontaneously dropped a cigarette he was holding in his right hand. He had immediately noted an inability to grasp objects and numbness in his right hand. These symptoms lasted for 2 minutes and then spontaneously resolved. After this episode his right hand felt completely normal. He denied other symptoms such as amaurosis, paralysis, paresthesias, speech disturbance, or gait disturbance. His past medical history was significant for hypertension, hypercholesterolemia, and cramping in his calves when he walked long distances. He had a 40 pack-year history of smoking and denied use of alcohol. A carotid duplex ultrasound examination showed a left 70% to 99% internal carotid artery (ICA) stenosis.

## EPIDEMIOLOGY

- Stroke ranks third among all causes of death in the United States behind heart disease and cancer, with 795,000 strokes occurring per year.[1]

- Annually, 55,000 more women than men are affected, and over 60% of all stroke deaths occur in women. African Americans have twice the stroke risk of Caucasians. Mexican Americans also have an increased incidence of stroke compared to Caucasians.[2]

## ETIOLOGY AND PATHOPHYSIOLOGY

- One-third of all strokes are related to cervical carotid disease.

- Standard risk factors for coronary and systemic atherosclerosis apply to carotid disease such as age, male sex, family history, smoking, hypertension, hyperlipidemia, sedentary lifestyle, and high dietary saturated fatty acids and cholesterol.

- The mechanism of cervical carotid stroke is usually embolization from a carotid bifurcation plaque, but hemodynamic compromise from stenosis may also play a role. The risks of embolization and hemodynamic compromise increase with increasing ICA stenosis.[3]

## DIAGNOSIS

- When carotid territory stroke or transient ischemic attack (TIA) is suspected, carotid duplex in an accredited vascular laboratory to define degree of stenosis is mandatory.

- When carotid duplex is nondiagnostic, computed tomography (CT) or magnetic resonance angiography (MRA) may be used.

- Catheter angiography is indicated in the setting of conflicting non-invasive studies and when carotid artery stenting (CAS) is planned.[4]

## CLINICAL FEATURES

- Neurologic examination may reveal motor or sensory deficits contralateral to the affected carotid artery. Aphasia, dysphasia, or apraxia may also be reported.

- Amaurosis fugax, or sudden complete or partial loss of vision in one eye, is a result of embolization from the cervical carotid artery to the ipsilateral central retinal artery.

- Up to 70% of stroke survivors can regain functional independence; however, 15% to 30% become permanently disabled and 20% will require long-term care.[5] In patients over 65 years old, 6 months after stroke 50% have some residual hemiparesis, 30% require some assistance with walking, 26% cannot perform activities of daily living independently, 19% have aphasia, and 26% are institutionalized.[6]

- Mean lifetime cost of an ischemic stroke in the United States is $140,048. In 2007, the total cost of stroke exceeded $40 billion.[1]

## MANAGEMENT

- Carotid endarterectomy (CEA) has been well established as a treatment for cervical carotid disease. Recently, debate has centered on CEA versus CAS in the management of carotid disease. The decision to revascularize should be relatively independent of the method of revascularization, with case-specific nuances contributing more to the decision of CAS versus CEA.

- All patients should receive optimal medical therapy. Aspirin is indicated for all patients with atherosclerotic carotid disease.

- Warfarin may be indicated to treat patients who have had stroke from cardiac embolization, but there is no evidence supporting the use of heparin and warfarin or clopidogrel to prevent or treat stroke related to cervical carotid disease.

- Management of hypertension and hypercholesterolemia, smoking cessation, and dietary and activity modification are all mainstays of treatment.

- Patients with asymptomatic carotid stenosis greater than and equal to 60% gain stroke risk reduction with carotid revascularization. However, that risk reduction must be considered in light of the patient's life expectancy, with intervention reserved for patients with at least a 5-year life expectancy.[7,8]

- Current medical therapy may outperform intervention in certain low-risk asymptomatic patients, and there is low absolute risk reduction with intervention for asymptomatic patients. Overall stroke risk in medically managed asymptomatic patients is only 2% per year, thus careful patient selection in asymptomatic carotid disease is paramount.

- Carotid intervention is indicated in patients with symptomatic carotid stenosis if greater than 50% diameter reduction is demonstrated.[9,10]

- Patients considered high risk for CEA include those with anatomically inaccessible lesions, cervical immobility, prior neck dissection, tracheostomy, contralateral cranial nerve injury, prior radiation therapy, contralateral occlusion, and recurrent stenosis after CEA. Medical comorbidities considered high risk for CEA include presence of chronic obstructive pulmonary disease, New York Heart Association (NYHA) class III or IV heart failure, ejection fraction less than 30%, recent myocardial infarction (MI), and unstable angina.

- Short-term risks in centers of excellence for both CEA and CAS may be equivalent for the composite endpoint of any stroke, death, or MI.

- Center for Medicare and Medicaid Services (CMS) approval for CAS continues to undergo scrutiny, but currently CAS is reimbursed only for high-risk patients with symptomatic high-grade stenosis. Patients who are at high risk and symptomatic with 50% to 79% stenosis and high-risk asymptomatic patients with over 80% stenosis can be covered in the context of a trial. These criteria were put forth in the formative years of CAS when it was considered more reasonable to attempt CAS in patients with some contraindication to CEA. Evidence that these indications will evolve come in the form of recent FDA approval of several devices for use in nonhigh-risk patients.

- Age alone increases risk with CAS, and this is thought to be related to increased arch calcification and changing arch morphology that can make access difficult (Figure 22-1). Carotid tortuosity

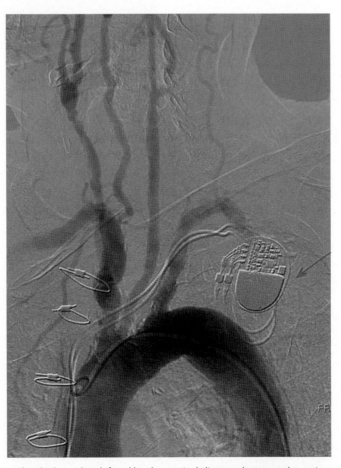

**FIGURE 22-1** Steepness of the aortic arch, which can be defined by the vertical distance between the ostium of the innominate artery and the apex of the greater curve of the aortic arch, adds technical difficulty to carotid artery stenting (CAS). Calcification of the arch and great vessels is thought to increase periprocedural stroke risk during carotid artery stenting. Red arrow indicates a pacemaker in place.

(Figure 22-2) is also associated with age and may present problems with stent or embolic protection device deployment. Symptomatic patients may be better treated by CEA, especially when older than 70 years or if male.

- Patients meeting high risk for CEA criteria with symptomatic high-grade stenosis may be offered CAS as primary treatment (Figures 22-3 and 22-4).

- In the absence of being considered high risk for CEA, patients aged less than 70 years may be offered CAS or CEA with equivalent composite stroke or MI or death rates. In this group, CAS incurs higher stroke risk in exchange for lower MI risk, and CEA incurs higher MI risk in exchange for lower stroke risk.[11-16]

## FOLLOW-UP

- Surveillance after CAS should be done with duplex as after CEA.[17] However, velocity criteria should be altered when interpreting post-CAS degrees of stenosis. Decreased compliance after stenting results in increased flow velocities through the stented area. In this setting, if standard velocity criteria are used, falsely increased estimates of in-stent stenosis will result.[18]

## PATIENT RESOURCE

- http://www.ninds.nih.gov/disorders/stroke/carotid _endarterectomy_backgrounder.htm

## REFERENCES

1. Roger V, Go A, Lloyd-Jones D. Heart disease and stroke statistics—2011 update: a report from the American Heart Association Statistics Committee and Stroke Statistics Committee. *Circulation*. 2011;123:e18-e209.

2. *Incidence and Prevalence: 2006 Chart Book on Cardiovascular and Lung Diseases*. Bethesda, MD: National Heart, Lung, and Blood Institute; 2006. Available at http://www.nhlbi.nih.gov/resources /docs/06a_ip_chtbk.pdf. Accessed May 8, 2013.

3. Kleindorfer D, Panagos P, Pancioli A. Incidence and short-term prognosis after transient ischemic attack in a population-based study. *Stroke*. 2005;36:720-723.

4. Ricotta JJ, Aburahma A, Ascher E, Eskandari M, Faries P, Lal BK. Updated Society for Vascular Surgery guidelines for management of extracranial carotid disease: executive summary. *J Vasc Surg*. 2011;54: 832-836.

5. Asplund K, Stegmayr B, Peltonen M. From the twentieth to the twenty-first century: a public health perspective on stroke. In: Ginsberg MD, Bogousslavsky J, eds. *Cerebrovascular Disease Pathophysiology, Diagnosis, and Management*. Malden, MA: Blackwell Science; 1998.

6. Kelly-Hayes M, Beiser A, Kase CS, Scaramucci A, D'Agostino RB, Wolf PA. The influence of gender and age on disability following ischemic stroke: the Framingham study. *J Stroke Cerebrovasc Dis*. 2003;12:119-126.

7. Endarterectomy for asymptomatic carotid artery stenosis. Executive Committee for the Asymptomatic Carotid Atherosclerosis Study. *JAMA*. 1995;273:1421-1428.

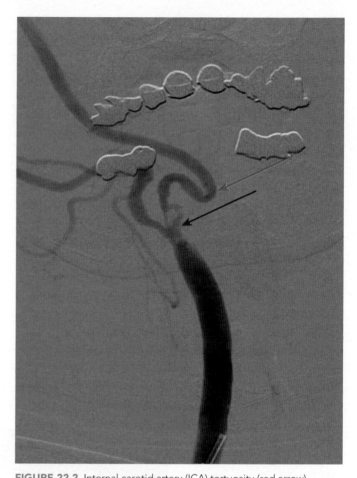

**FIGURE 22-2** Internal carotid artery (ICA) tortuosity (red arrow) increases the technical difficulty of carotid artery stenting (CAS), posing problems with stent or embolic protection device delivery. Stenosis is indicated by the blue arrow. This image is from a different patient to demonstrate the difficulty with tortuous vessels.

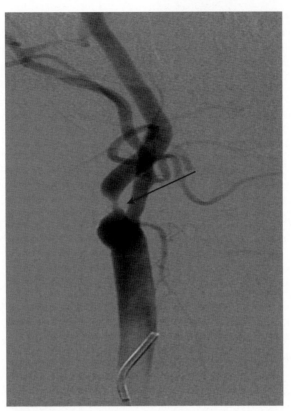

**FIGURE 22-3** A different view of the carotid bifurcation and the origin of the internal carotid artery (ICA) shows the tight stenosis (blue arrow).

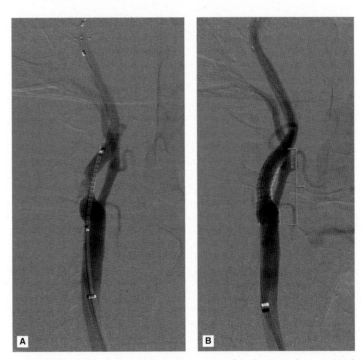

**FIGURE 22-4** (A) Carotid artery stenting (CAS) requires delivery of a percutaneous sheath across the aortic arch and into the ipsilateral common carotid artery. A guide-wire with an embolic protection device is used to cross the lesion; the device is deployed in the distal internal carotid artery (ICA), and then angioplasty and stenting of the ICA lesion is performed. Options for cerebral protection are filters (as depicted in the figure), distal occlusion balloons, and proximal occlusion with flow reversal. Filters are mechanical screens placed distal to the lesion and collect debris that is removed after stent deployment. Lesions must be crossed in order to deliver the filter, but they do offer the advantage of maintaining cerebral blood flow. Distal occlusion devices occlude the distal internal carotid with a balloon. The lesion must be crossed to deliver the balloon, and the ICA is occluded, making this option less attractive to many clinicians. The flow reversal proximal balloon method uses two balloons, one inflated in the common carotid and the other in the external carotid. Reversed flow from the internal carotid is maintained by continuous arteriovenous shunting from the internal carotid to a separate sheath in the femoral vein. This option allows for cerebral protection prior to crossing the lesion, but does require larger sheath access, and not all patients tolerate flow reversal. (B) Completion arteriogram shows the stent in place (red bracket).

8. Halliday A, Mansfield A, Marro J, et al. MRC Asymptomatic Carotid Surgery Trial (ACST) Collaborative Group. Prevention of disabling and fatal strokes by successful carotid endarterectomy in patients without recent neurological symptoms: randomised controlled trial. *Lancet*. 2004;363:1491-1502.

9. Ferguson GG, Eliasziw M, Barr HW. The North American symptomatic carotid endarterectomy trial: surgical results in 1415 patients. *Stroke*. 1999;30:1751-1758.

10. Randomised trial of endarterectomy for recently symptomatic carotid stenosis: final results of the MRC European Carotid Surgery Trial (ECST). *Lancet*. 1998;351:1379-1387.

11. Mantese V, Timaran C, Chiu D. The carotid revascularization endarterectomy versus stenting trial (CREST)—stenting versus carotid endarterectomy for carotid disease. *Stroke*. 2010;41: S31-S34.

12. Yadav JS, Wholey MH, Kuntz RE. Protected carotid-artery stenting versus endarterectomy in high-risk patients. *N Engl J Med*. 2004;351:1493-1501.

13. Eckstein J, Ringleb PA, Allenberg J. Results of the stent-protected angioplasty versus carotid endarterectomy (SPACE) study to treat symptomatic stenoses at 2 years: a multinational, prospective, randomised trial. *Lancet*. 2008;7:893-902.

14. Mas JL, Chatellier G, Beyssen B. Endarterectomy versus stenting in patients with symptomatic severe carotid stenosis. *N Engl J Med*. 2006;355:1660-1671.

15. Mas JL, Chatellier G, Beyssen B. Endarterectomy Versus Angioplasty in Patients With Symptomatic Severe Carotid Stenosis (EVA-3S) trial: results up to 4 years from a randomised, multicentre trial. *Lancet Neurol*. 2008;7:885-892.

16. Carotid artery stenting compared with endarterectomy in patients with symptomatic carotid stenosis (International Carotid Stenting Study): an interim analysis of a randomised controlled trial. International Carotid-Stenting Study Investigators. *Lancet*. 2010;375:985-997.

17. Roseborough G, Perler B. Carotid artery disease: endarterectomy. In: Cronenwett J, Johnston K, eds. *Vascular Surgery*. Philadelphia, PA: Elsevier; 2010.

18. AbuRahma A, Abu-Halimah S, Bensenhaver J, Dean LS, Keiffer T, Emmett M. Optimal carotid duplex velocity criteria for defining the severity of carotid in-stent restenosis. *J Vasc Surg*. 2008;48:589-594.

# 23 ARTERIOSCLEROTIC CAROTID OCCLUSIVE DISEASE: ULCERATIVE

Michael R. Go, MD

## PATIENT STORY

A 58-year-old woman presented 1 week after a single episode of left-eye blindness that lasted 30 seconds. It spontaneously resolved, and she had no further visual disturbances. She denies weakness, numbness, paralysis, paresthesias, speech disturbance, or gait disturbance. A carotid duplex ultrasound suggested a less than 50% left internal carotid artery (ICA) stenosis, but there was a suggestion of a complex plaque. Further imaging with computed tomography (CT) angiography was performed, and showed a left ICA eccentric, ulcerative complex plaque not associated with a significant stenosis.

### ETIOLOGY AND PATHOPHYSIOLOGY

- While degree of carotid stenosis is related to stroke risk, plaque morphology may also play a role.

- Increased risk for neurologic events is seen in patients with less organized, soft, echolucent, complex, or ulcerated plaque, regardless of the degree of stenosis. Plaque that is echolucent, heterogeneous, and ulcerated, and has a high lipid content core may be more unstable and prone to rupture with embolization.[1]

- Intraplaque hemorrhage, or plaque with thin or ruptured fibrous caps, may also present a higher stroke risk (Figure 23-1).

### DIAGNOSIS

- Gross characteristics of plaque morphology, such as presence of ulceration, thrombus, calcification, or eccentricity, can be defined by standard carotid duplex or angiography.

- Duplex imaging has the additional capability of identifying homogeneous or heterogeneous plaque and echogenic or echolucent plaque.

- Intravascular ultrasound performed at the time of carotid angiography can provide even more detail about plaque characteristics.

- Studies on the use of high-resolution computed tomography (CT) and magnetic resonance (MR) imaging, as well as fluorodeoxyglucose positron emission tomography (FDG-PET) imaging, to define what constitutes high- and low-risk carotid plaque are ongoing.

- As these imaging techniques improve at predicting the behavior of carotid plaque, it may become possible to predict which patients are more likely to benefit from intervention for asymptomatic carotid stenosis.[2-4]

### MANAGEMENT

- Diagnosis and clinical features of ulcerative cervical carotid disease are similar to those of nonulcerative disease. However, risk of stroke from these lesions is less well defined.

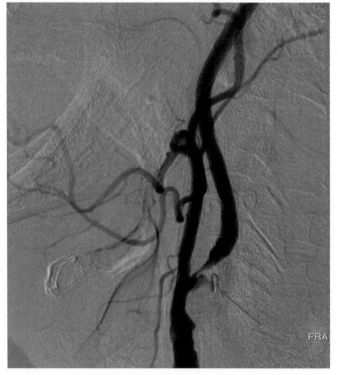

FIGURE 23-1 An ulcerated complex carotid lesion on angiography (red arrow).

- All patients should receive optimal medical therapy. Aspirin is indicated for all patients with atherosclerotic carotid disease.

- Warfarin may be indicated to treat patients who have had stroke from cardiac embolization, but there is no evidence supporting the use of heparin and warfarin or clopidogrel to prevent or treat stroke related to ulcerative (or stenotic) cervical carotid disease.

- Management of hypertension and hypercholesterolemia, smoking cessation, and dietary and activity modification are all mainstays of treatment.

- Some advocate intervention when patients have had stroke or transient ischemic attack (TIA), even when the degree of carotid stenosis is less than 50%.

- Intervention for asymptomatic ulcerative lesions that produce a high-grade stenosis does not differ from nonulcerative lesions.

- Intervention for asymptomatic complex or ulcerative lesions without high-grade stenosis is more controversial but may be appropriate in selected high stroke risk patients.

## PATIENT EDUCATION

- Patients should be informed of the link between atherosclerotic disease in general and carotid disease in particular with controllable risk factors such as hypertension, diabetes, abnormal lipids and high-fat diet, smoking, and sedentary lifestyle.

- Patients with carotid disease should also know the signs and symptoms of TIA or stroke so that they can seek expeditious treatment.

### PATIENT RESOURCES

- http://www.vascularweb.org/vascularhealth/Pages/default .aspx is a website provided by the Society for Vascular Surgery that contains podcasts and online information about carotid disease and other peripheral vascular conditions.

## REFERENCES

1. O'Holleran LW, Kennelly MM, McClurken M, Johnson JM. Natural history of asymptomatic carotid plaque. *Am J Surg*. 1987;154:659-662.

2. Horie N, Morikawa M, Ishizaka S, et al. Assessment of carotid plaque stability based on the dynamic enhancement pattern in plaque components with multidetector CT angiography. *Stroke*. Feb 2012;43(2):393-398.

3. Figueroa AL, Subramanian SS, Cury RC, et al. Distribution of inflammation within carotid atherosclerotic plaques with high risk morphological features: a comparison between PET activity, plaque morphology and histopathology. *Circ Cardiovasc Imaging*. Jan 2012;5(1):69-77.

4. U-King-Im JM, Young V, Gillard JH. Carotid-artery imaging in the diagnosis and management of patients at risk of stroke. *Lancet Neurol*. 2009;8:569-580.

# 24 ARTERIOSCLEROTIC CAROTID OCCLUSIVE DISEASE: OCCLUSION

Michael R. Go, MD

## PATIENT STORY

A 50-year-old man presented with a 1-year history of worsening fatigue and bitemporal headaches. He denied focal neurologic symptoms, but complained of constant dizziness which was exacerbated when he went from a lying to a standing position. Sometimes he experienced syncopal episodes, and a complete syncope workup thus far had been negative. Carotid duplex ultrasound suggested chronic occlusion of his left internal carotid artery (ICA), with a 70% to 99% stenosis of his right ICA. Carotid duplex ultrasound also showed elevated velocities in his external carotid arteries (ECAs) bilaterally indicating significant stenosis.

### EPIDEMIOLOGY

- Symptomatic ICA occlusion has an incidence of 6 per 100,000, though the rate of asymptomatic chronic occlusion is unknown and may be higher.[1]

### ETIOLOGY AND PATHOPHYSIOLOGY

- Total ICA occlusion results from thrombosis of or embolization to the cervical carotid in the setting of chronic stenosis. Cardiogenic embolization to a normal carotid bifurcation or carotid dissection may also cause total occlusion of the ICA.

- Acute occlusion may result in a carotid territory stroke.

- A previously asymptomatic chronic ICA occlusion may become symptomatic related to embolic or hemodynamic issues.

- Embolism may occur from the ipsilateral ECA via collaterals to the cerebral circulation. It may also occur when there is occult patency of the occluded ICA, which then serves as the source of embolic material.

- Hemodynamic insufficiency may occur when any condition that interferes with cerebral perfusion such as orthostasis, hypotension, volume depletion, or cardiac failure is superimposed on the carotid occlusion, especially when contralateral carotid disease is significant (Figure 24-1).[2]

### CLINICAL FEATURES

- The distinction between hemodynamic and embolic stroke in the setting of chronic ICA occlusion is important.

- Embolic symptoms are those of classic stroke or transient ischemic attack (TIA) and typically are focal. They may include contralateral motor or sensory deficits or amaurosis.

- Hemodynamic symptoms may be similar to those of classic stroke or TIA, but may also be less predictable and atypical.

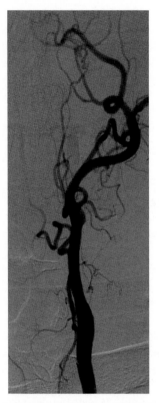

**FIGURE 24-1** Occlusion of the internal carotid artery (ICA) results in collateral formation via the external carotid artery (ECA).

- Symptoms such as limb shaking, retinal claudication, headache from large pulsatile ECA collaterals, syncope, and generalized fatigue have all been reported.[2]

## DIAGNOSIS

- Carotid duplex ultrasound examination typically shows a high-resistant signal in the carotid bulb and the very proximal ICA (Figure 24-2). Distally, there are no Doppler signals audible in the carotid artery.

- Some form of contrast examination such as digital subtraction arteriography, magnetic resonance arteriography (MRA), or computed tomographic (CT) arteriography is generally required to confirm the diagnosis (Figure 24-3).

## MANAGEMENT

- Acute symptomatic carotid occlusion should be treated with urgent revascularization in select cases with immediate presentation. This can be accomplished with carotid endarterectomy (CEA) or interventional techniques including thrombolysis.

- In the setting of chronic total ICA occlusion, medical management is preferred over revascularization.[3]

- However, several special clinical indications exist for procedural intervention.

- Ipsilateral hemodynamic symptoms in the setting of ipsilateral ICA occlusion and contralateral ICA stenosis may benefit from contralateral ICA revascularization to ameliorate hemodynamic insufficiency.

- Ipsilateral embolic symptoms in the setting of ipsilateral ICA occlusion and ipsilateral ECA stenosis may be treated with ipsilateral ECA revascularization to eliminate the source of embolization, which occurs via enlarged ECA collaterals; ligation of the ipsilateral ICA also eliminates that as a source for the embolization.

- Finally, ipsilateral hemodynamic symptoms in the setting of a patent contralateral carotid system, ipsilateral ICA occlusion, and ipsilateral ECA stenosis indicate ipsilateral ECA revascularization to improve ipsilateral hemodynamic flow.

## FOLLOW-UP

- There are no specific criteria for surveillance of patients with chronically occluded ICAs, nor are there criteria to specify the degree of ECA stenosis by duplex ultrasound.

- A reasonable regimen is to follow the patient clinically every 6 months to a year, with or without duplex, to serially follow ECA disease.

- The development of symptoms indicates investigation with imaging of some kind to see if cerebrovascular revascularization is indicated.

## PATIENT EDUCATION

- Patients should be informed of the link between atherosclerotic disease in general and carotid disease in particular with controllable risk factors such as hypertension, diabetes, abnormal lipid levels and high-fat diet, smoking, and sedentary lifestyle.

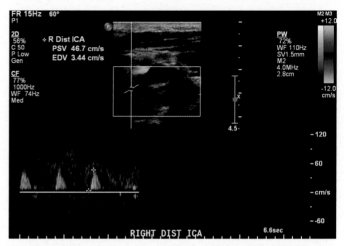

**FIGURE 24-2** Occlusion of the distal internal carotid artery (ICA) results in a high-resistance Doppler waveform when the vessel is interrogated proximally, with no diastolic flow.

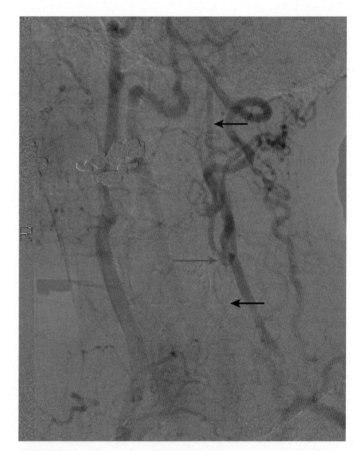

**FIGURE 24-3** An example of collateralization in a patient with left common carotid artery (CCA) occlusion. The left CCA is occluded (black arrow). There is filling of the left external carotid artery (ECA) via collaterals, and the left carotid bifurcation fills via the ECA (red arrow). The distal left internal carotid artery (ICA) then fills antegrade (blue arrow).

- Patients with carotid disease should also know the signs and symptoms of TIA or stroke so that they can seek expeditious treatment.
- Patients with ICA occlusion should also be educated on symptoms of hemodynamic cerebral insufficiency, such as limb shaking, retinal claudication, headache, syncope, and generalized fatigue.

## PATIENT RESOURCES

- http://www.vascularweb.org/vascularhealth/Pages/default .aspx is a website provided by the Society for Vascular Surgery that contains podcasts and online information about carotid disease and other peripheral vascular conditions.

## REFERENCES

1. Flaherty ML, Flemming KD, McClelland R. Population-based study of symptomatic internal carotid artery occlusion. Incidence and long-term follow-up. *Stroke.* 2004;35:e349.

2. Thanvi B, Robinson T. Complete occlusion of extracranial internal carotid artery: clinical features, pathophysiology, diagnosis and management. *Postgrad Med J.* 2007;83:95-99.

3. Powers WJ, Clarke WR, Grubb RL Jr, Videen TO, Adams HP Jr, Derdeyn CP; COSS Investigators. Extracranial-intracranial bypass surgery for stroke prevention in hemodynamic cerebral ischemia: the Carotid Occlusion Surgery Study randomized trial. *JAMA.* 2011;306:1983-1992.

# 25 CAROTID ARTERY FIBROMUSCULAR DYSPLASIA

Jean Starr, MD, FACS, RPVI

## PATIENT STORY

A 57-year-old woman presented to the emergency department (ED) with left arm and leg weakness that resolved after 2 hours. She had a similar episode 1 week previously. She was otherwise healthy and active, although her blood pressure was 160/94 mm Hg, without a previous history of hypertension. She underwent a computed tomogram (CT) of the head that was negative for bleeding or stroke. She then had a carotid duplex ultrasound examination, which showed a focal area of increased velocity in the distal internal carotid artery (ICA) distally without any significant plaque formation at the bifurcation or the proximal ICA. It was felt that she needed a carotid angiogram to better delineate the disease process.

The contrast angiogram revealed fibromuscular dysplasia (FMD) in the mid and distal cervical ICA (Figure 25-1). Further investigation also showed FMD in both common iliac arteries (Figure 25-2) and both renal arteries (Figures 25-3 and 25-4). She denied any claudication symptoms. Renal artery intervention was discussed for her hypertension.

She agreed and a balloon angioplasty of the right renal artery was successfully carried out. Her carotid disease was managed with antiplatelet therapy and she has had no recurrence of her symptoms.

## EPIDEMIOLOGY

- Women are most commonly affected; although it is thought to be a rare disease, it may occur in up to 4% of women.[1]
- In a large carotid duplex imaging study, the overall incidence of FMD was 0.14%.[2]

## ETIOLOGY AND PATHOPHYSIOLOGY

- FMD is a noninflammatory, nonatherosclerotic process that most commonly affects the carotid and renal arteries, although it can occur elsewhere in medium-sized vessels.[1]
- FMD usually occurs in the mid and distal ICA, sometimes extending into the intracranial region.[3] Aneurysms may be a component of the disease process as well.
- There are several pathologic types, with medial fibrodysplasia being the most common.[3] The pathophysiology is mostly unknown.

## CLINICAL FEATURES

- When the carotids are affected, ipsilateral cerebral ischemia, spontaneous dissection, or pseudoaneurysm or true aneurysms may occur, but many times FMD is discovered incidentally on diagnostic studies for workup of other diseases.
- Renal artery FMD typically presents as hypertension, but can be totally asymptomatic.

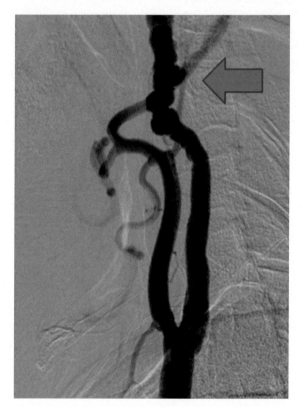

**FIGURE 25-1** Carotid angiogram demonstrating mid and distal internal carotid artery (ICA) fibromuscular dysplastic changes (blue arrow).

- Iliac artery FMD is typically discovered incidentally during angiographic studies for renal or carotid artery disease, although it has been reported to present as acute onset of claudication due to spontaneous dissection.[4]

## DIFFERENTIAL DIAGNOSIS

- When FMD affects multiple arterial beds (carotid, renal, iliac), it may mimic systemic vasculitis.[5]
- Diagnostic imaging studies will help differentiate the two, as may inflammatory markers, as these will typically not be elevated in FMD.

## DIAGNOSTIC STUDIES

- FMD can sometimes be suspected on a routine carotid duplex examination, but is found more commonly on computed tomographic angiography (CTA) or catheter-based angiography. Carotid duplex imaging may have difficulty characterizing FMD due to the more distal location of the disease process in the cervical carotid arteries.[2,6]
- The classic appearance is that of "beads on a string," which represent luminal webs with normal intervening segments of artery.[3] Indirect evidence with elevated velocities suggest that serial stenoses may also aid in the diagnosis when the classic beading is not apparent.[2]

## MANAGEMENT OR INTERVENTION OPTIONS

- Since little is known about the natural history of FMD in any vascular bed, there are no randomized trials and only a few case series reports.
- Treatment is usually reserved for when symptoms occur and can vary from open approaches to endovascular methods[7] or a combination of the two, using covered stents.[8]
- Otherwise, medical management with antiplatelet therapy for carotid FMD is the first-line treatment.
- Balloon angioplasty alone without stenting is often used to treat renal artery FMD when causing hypertension. Intervention for renal artery FMD can have better results than when performed for atherosclerotic disease. Results from renal FMD intervention tend to be worse with advanced age and when hypertension is long standing.[9]

## PATIENT EDUCATION AND FOLLOW-UP

- Patients who present with cervical carotid dissection have a 1% recurrence rate of dissection over time, and most of these patients have FMD. Most recurrences also affect another cervical artery.[10]
- Blood pressure should be controlled to help prevent any recurrence.
- Annual carotid duplex imaging may help monitor for progressive stenosis or aneurysmal formation.

### PROVIDER RESOURCE

- http://www.fmdsa.org/dynamic/files/4Olin4_07.pdf

### PATIENT RESOURCES

- http://my.clevelandclinic.org/heart/disorders/vascular/fibromuscular_dysplasia.aspx
- http://www.fmdsa.org/dynamic/files/4Olin4_07.pdf

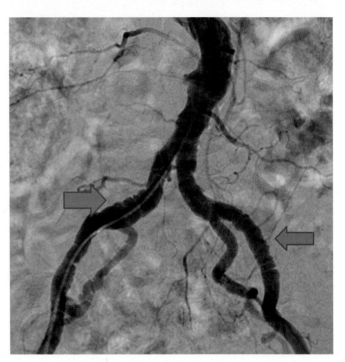

**FIGURE 25-2** Abdominal aortogram showing bilateral iliac artery fibromuscular dysplasia (FMD) (blue arrows).

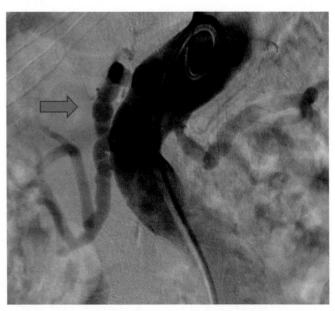

**FIGURE 25-3** Abdominal aortogram showing bilateral renal artery FMD (blue arrow).

## REFERENCES

1. Olin JW, Sealove BA. Diagnosis, management, and future developments of fibromuscular dysplasia. *J Vasc Surg*. Mar 2011;53(3):826-836.

2. Arning C, Grzyska U. Color Doppler imaging of cervicocephalic fibromuscular dysplasia. *Cardiovasc Ultrasound*. Jul 20 2004;2:7.

3. Touzé E, Oppenheim C, Trystram D, et al. Fibromuscular dysplasia of cervical and intracranial arteries. *Int J Stroke*. Aug 2010;5(4):296-305.

4. Akashi H, Nata S, Kanaya K, Shintani Y, Onitsuka S, Aoyagi S. Spontaneous dissection of the iliac artery in a patient with fibromuscular dysplasia. *Ann Vasc Surg*. Oct 2010;24(7):952.

5. Capsoni F, Poletto G, Giorgetti PL. Fibromuscular dysplasia: a rare disease that can mimic vasculitis. *Rheumatol Int*. Dec 2012;32(12):4027-4029.

6. Arning C. Nonatherosclerotic disease of the cervical arteries: role of ultrasonography for diagnosis. *Vasa*. Jul 2001;30(3):160-167.

7. Edgell RC, Abou-Chebl A, Yadav JS. Endovascular management of spontaneous carotid artery dissection. *J Vasc Surg*. Nov 2005;42(5):854-860.

8. Assadian A, Senekowitsch C, Assadian O, Schuster H, Ptakovsky H, Hagmüller GW. Combined open and endovascular stent grafting of internal carotid artery fibromuscular dysplasia: long-term results. *Eur J Vasc Endovasc Surg*. Apr 2005;29(4):345-349.

9. Trinquart L, Mounier-Vehier C, Sapoval M, Gagnon N, Plouin PF. Efficacy of revascularization for renal artery stenosis caused by fibromuscular dysplasia: a systematic review and meta-analysis. *Hypertension*. Sep 2010;56(3):525-532.

10. de Bray JM, Marc G, Pautot V, et al. Fibromuscular dysplasia may herald symptomatic recurrence of cervical artery dissection. *Cerebrovasc Dis*. 2007;23(5-6):448-452.

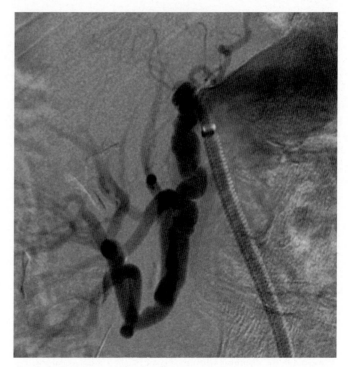

**FIGURE 25-4** Selective right renal angiogram detailing right renal artery FMD changes.

# 26 CAROTID ARTERY DISSECTION

Michael R. Go, MD

## PATIENT STORY

A 30-year-old man was involved in a motor vehicle accident. He had rib fractures, a pulmonary contusion, and mild neck pain, but no other injuries. He denied amaurosis fugax, weakness, numbness, paralysis, paresthesias, speech disturbance, or gait disturbance. On the upper cuts of a chest computed tomography (CT), a dissection of his right internal carotid artery (ICA) was seen, and a focal dissection starting just distal to the right carotid bulb and extending through the cervical ICA was confirmed on a subsequent CT angiogram of the neck.

## EPIDEMIOLOGY

• Dissection causes less than 2% of ischemic strokes, but up to 20% of the ischemic strokes in patients less than 50 years old are related to dissection. It is the second leading cause of cervical carotid disease, behind atherosclerosis.[1-3]

## ETIOLOGY AND PATHOPHYSIOLOGY

• Carotid dissection, as in other vascular beds, starts when a tear in one or more layers of the arterial wall occurs, allowing blood to separate the layers and form a thrombosis or a patent false lumen.

• In the cervical carotid artery, the dissection often occurs after trauma causing a whiplash-type motion.

• Carotid dissections may be spontaneous as well, though often a careful history will reveal a temporally associated trivial trauma such as a cough or neck rotation.

• Predisposing factors such as Marfan disease, Ehlers-Danlos type IV syndrome, or fibromuscular dysplasia may be present in these cases, but these connective tissue disorders are implicated in only 5% of spontaneous dissections.[4]

• The location of the dissection is usually at a mobile point of the artery, such as distal to the carotid bulb.

• Carotid dissection may also present as an extension of aortic dissection (Figure 26-1).

## DIAGNOSIS

• Diagnosis is often made incidentally, perhaps by imaging done at the time of multiple trauma.

• Carotid dissection can be detected with duplex ultrasound (Figure 26-2), CT angiography, magnetic resonance (MR) angiography, or catheter angiography.

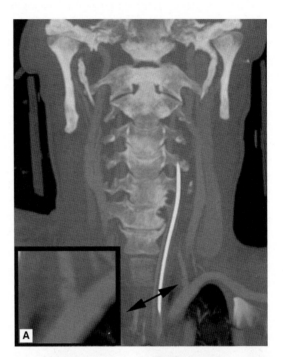

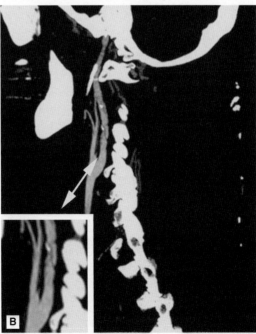

**FIGURE 26-1** Carotid artery dissection may be spontaneous, related to trauma, or result as an extension of aortic dissection. (A) Vertebral artery injury (double-sided black arrow), and (B) carotid artery dissection (double-sided white arrow).

## CLINICAL FEATURES

- When found incidentally, many carotid dissections may be asymptomatic.
- If symptomatic, in addition to cerebral ischemia, carotid dissection can present with unusual or pathognomonic symptoms.
- Headache and neck pain are the most common nonischemic symptoms.
- A Horner syndrome can result from interruption of blood supply to sympathetic fibers at the level of the superior cervical ganglion.
- Rarer symptoms include pulsatile tinnitus and lower cranial nerve palsy from local compression.[5]

## MANAGEMENT

- Many carotid dissections are asymptomatic, with a relatively benign natural history.
- Spontaneous healing of the dissection flap is likely to occur, and even if thrombosis occurs, later recanalization is common.
- If ischemic symptoms do occur, they are typically thromboembolic in nature, thus medical management with antiplatelet agents or anticoagulation is indicated for all dissections.
- There has been no evidence to suggest the superiority of anticoagulation over antiplatelet treatment.
- In cases of persistent ischemia despite medical therapy, intervention with thrombolysis, carotid artery stenting (CAS), or surgical repair if accessible may be indicated, but prognosis is poor.[5]

## PATIENT EDUCATION

1. Although rare, patients with predisposing risk factors mentioned should be educated on the symptoms of dissection.
2. Patients who sustain the type of trauma discussed should warned about the symptoms prior to discharge even if preliminary evaluation seems normal.

## FOLLOW-UP

Clinical follow-up can detect failure of medical therapy, and some advocate serial imaging at weeks to months postdissection to document healing.[6]

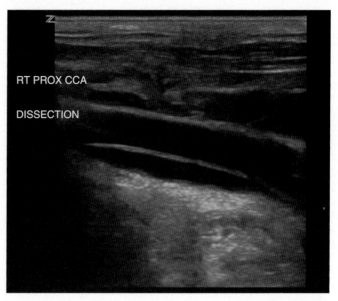

**FIGURE 26-2** Sagittal view of the common carotid artery on duplex ultrasound grayscale imaging showing a large intimal flap in the lumen of the artery.

## REFERENCES

1. Chandra A, Suliman A, Angle N. Spontaneous dissection of the carotid and vertebral arteries: the 10-year UCSD experience. *Ann Vasc Surg*. 2007;21:178-185.

2. Nagumo K, Nakamori A, Kojima S. Spontaneous intracranial internal carotid artery dissection: 6 case reports and a review of 39 cases in the literature. *Rinsho Shinkeigaku*. 2003;43:313-321.

3. Chabrier S, Lasjaunias P, Husson B, Landrieu P, Tardieu M. Ischemic stroke from dissection of the craniocervical arteries in childhood: report of 12 patients. *Eur J Paediatr Neurol*. 2003;7:39-42.

4. Uhlig P, Bruckner P, Dittrich R, Ringelstein EB, Kuhlenbaumer G, Hansen U. Aberrations of dermal connective tissue in patients with cervical artery dissection (sCAD). *J Neurol*. 2008;255: 340-346.

5. Fusco MR, Harrigan MR. Cerebrovascular dissections—a review part I: spontaneous dissections. *Neurosurgery*. 2011;68:242-257.

6. Bromberg WJ, Collier BC, Diebel LN, et al. Blunt cerebrovascular injury practice management guidelines: the Eastern Association for the Surgery of Trauma. *J Trauma*. 2010;68:471-477.

# 27 CAROTID ARTERY ANEURYSM

Jean Starr, MD, FACS, RPVI

## PATIENT STORY

A 70-year-old man with stable coronary artery disease presented to the emergency department (ED) with new onset of right arm and leg weakness, as well as dysphasia.

His workup included a computed tomogram (CT) scan of his head that showed an acute stroke in the distribution of the left middle cerebral artery. A carotid duplex ultrasound examination revealed no significant bilateral carotid artery stenosis but did show a 1.5 cm aneurysm with a small amount of mural thrombus in the proximal left internal carotid artery (ICA) (Figure 27-1). A magnetic resonance angiogram (MRA) of the neck confirmed the presence of the proximal left ICA aneurysm, but there was also a question of stenosis at the proximal and distal extent of the aneurysm (Figure 27-2).

A catheter-directed angiogram was therefore performed to rule out any other intimal defects given the discrepancy between the MRA and the duplex. No significant stenosis was identified, and no other luminal irregularities were seen (Figure 27-3).

After he functionally recovered from his stroke, he was offered left carotid aneurysm repair with a vein interposition graft (Figures 27-4 and 27-5).

This was accomplished and he recovered uneventfully. Further workup revealed no other aneurysmal disease.

### EPIDEMIOLOGY

- Rare pathologic finding. Several series exist that are small and often span decades.[1-5] One study reported the incidence of procedures performed for carotid artery aneurysm to be less than 1% of the total carotid procedures over a 20-year period.[1]

- Men are much more commonly afflicted than women, as would be expected since the most common etiology of carotid aneurysms is a degenerative, atherosclerotic pathology.

- No association with the occurrence of other aneurysms has been shown.

### ETIOLOGY OR PATHOPHYSIOLOGY

- Atherosclerotic degenerative, postoperative or iatrogenic, dissection, post-traumatic, infectious, fibromuscular dysplasia, cystic medial necrosis, and congenital.

- Degenerative aneurysms typically occur at the carotid bifurcation and tend to be more fusiform in nature, while saccular aneurysms tend to be more localized to the mid ICA.[1]

- Aneurysms resulting from dissections often extend to the base of the skull.

- Aneurysms associated with cystic medial necrosis may be a manifestation of Marfan syndrome.

- Postcarotid surgery pseudoaneurysms account for a significant proportion (range 8%-53%) of carotid aneurysms.[1,4,6-8]

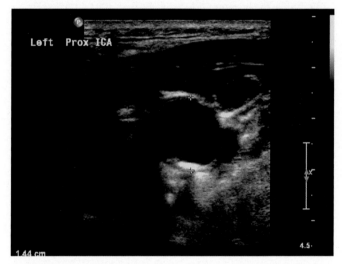

**FIGURE 27-1** Transverse arterial ultrasound image, highlighting the diameter of 1.5 cm (cursor + signs).

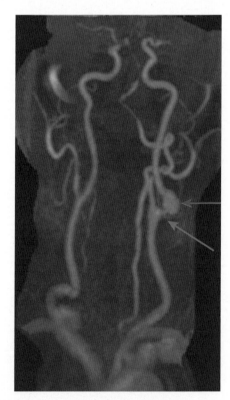

**FIGURE 27-2** Magnetic resonance angiogram (MRA) image showing proximal left internal carotid aneurysm (red arrow) and relatively normal contralateral carotid artery. There is a possible high-grade stenosis at the proximal extent of the aneurysm (blue arrow).

- In one series, fibromuscular dysplasia accounted for 50% of all cervical carotid aneurysms.[4]

## CLINICAL FEATURES

- Patients can present with neurologic symptoms or compressive or mass-effect symptoms, or be totally asymptomatic.

- Patients presenting with either global neurologic symptoms or ipsilateral stroke or transient ischemic symptoms (TIA) vary from 36% to 61%.[1-6,8]

- A pulsatile neck mass was the initial finding in 11% to 33% of patients.[3,5,8] If large enough, the mass effect may cause local compressive symptoms resulting in hoarseness, difficulties swallowing, and pain or pressure.

## DIFFERENTIAL DIAGNOSIS

- Neurologic symptoms may be caused by the more common atherosclerotic process and could be differentiated on duplex imaging or CT or MR studies.

- Cervical mass differential diagnosis may include benign tumors, such as paragangliomas and lymphadenopathy, and malignant processes as well, especially if local nerves are involved.

## RADIOGRAPHIC STUDIES

- The initial evaluation of a pulsatile neck mass may include duplex imaging, CTA examination, or MR imaging.

- Duplex imaging may give information on the size and extent of the aneurysm, but also gives concomitant information on arterial flow disturbances and intra-arterial thrombus formation.

- CT and MR studies help to differentiate an aneurysm presenting as a neck mass from other potential etiologies, such as cancers, paragangliomas and carotid body tumors, lymphadenopathy, and tortuous vessels associated with aging.

- Contrast imaging studies, including catheter-based angiography, may reveal the presence of other aneurysms and associated intimal irregularities, in addition to better delineating the aneurysmal process itself.

## MANAGEMENT OR INTERVENTION OPTIONS

- A consensus on when to recommend intervening on a carotid aneurysm has not yet been reached, most likely due to the rarity and lack of long-term studies examining the natural history of this entity.

- Generally, repair is recommended when the aneurysmal segment measures twice the size of the native vessel in the area or when a patient experiences symptoms that appear to be related to the aneurysm.

- There are several approaches that one could take to repair a carotid artery aneurysm, including resection with vein graft or polytetrafluoroethylene (PTFE) interposition, patch angioplasty, reimplantation into the external carotid artery, primary end-to-end anastomosis, and primary closure.

- Further treatments to be considered include proximal and distal ligation and the recent option of endovascular stent graft repair. Aneurysm resection and interposition graft (prosthetic and autogenous vein graft) was the most commonly performed procedure (range 42%-71%).[1,4,6]

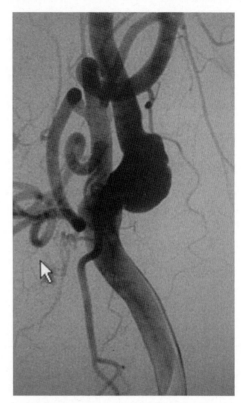

**FIGURE 27-3** Carotid angiogram highlighting the aneurysm.

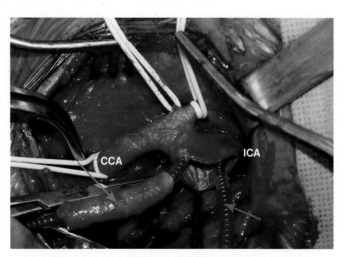

**FIGURE 27-4** Intraoperative photo of carotid shunt in place with reversed saphenous vein graft (blue arrow) assembled over the shunt (green arrow) in preparation for anastomosis.

## COMPLICATIONS

- A large, untreated aneurysm may cause compressive local neurogenic effects as listed earlier.
- Operative complications depend on the extent of repair and may include local nerve injury or neurologic complications such as stroke or TIA. The results vary, but in general, there is a high primary patency rate and fairly low surgical complication rate, with cranial nerve injury being the most common.[3]

## PATIENT EDUCATION AND FOLLOW-UP

- An aneurysm not yet requiring repair should be followed every 6 to 12 months with the same initial imaging study, in order to longitudinally follow the size and the thrombus formation.
- Depending on the type of repair, follow-up after surgery should typically occur every 6 to 12 months with duplex ultrasound imaging to monitor for stenoses.

### PROVIDER RESOURCES

- http://www.ncbi.nlm.nih.gov/pubmed/22341576
- http://www.ncbi.nlm.nih.gov/pubmed/20141956

### PATIENT RESOURCE

- http://my.clevelandclinic.org/disorders/extracranial_carotid _aneurysm/heart_overview.aspx

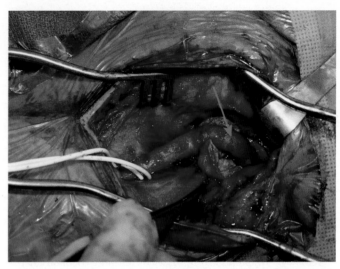

**FIGURE 27-5** Photograph of completed interposition saphenous vein graft (blue arrow) and exclusion of the aneurysm.

## REFERENCES

1. Donas KP, Schulte S, Pitoulias GA, Siebertz S, Horsch S. Surgical outcome of degenerative versus postreconstructive extracranial carotid artery aneurysms. *J Vasc Surg*. Jan 2009;49(1):93-98.

2. Rosset E, Albertini JN, Magnan PE, Ede B, Thomassin JM, Branchereau A. Surgical treatment of extracranial internal carotid artery aneurysms. *J Vasc Surg*. Apr 2000;31(4):713-723.

3. Attigah N, Külkens S, Zausig N, et al. Surgical therapy of extracranial carotid artery aneurysms: long-term results over a 24-year period. *Eur J Vasc Endovasc Surg*. Feb 2009;37(2):127-133.

4. Faggioli GL, Freyrie A, Stella A, et al. Extracranial internal carotid artery aneurysms: results of a surgical series with long-term follow-up. *J Vasc Surg*. Apr 1996;23(4):587-594; discussion 594-595.

5. Zwolak RM, Whitehouse WM Jr, Knake JE, et al. Atherosclerotic extracranial carotid artery aneurysms. *J Vasc Surg*. May 1984;1(3):415-422.

6. Srivastava SD, Eagleton MJ, O'Hara P, Kashyap VS, Sarac T, Clair D. Surgical repair of carotid artery aneurysms: a 10-year, single-center experience. *Ann Vasc Surg*. Jan 2010;24(1):100-105.

7. Szopinski P, Ciostek P, Kielar M, Myrcha P, Pleban E, Noszczyk W. A series of 15 patients with extracranial carotid artery aneurysms: surgical and endovascular treatment. *Eur J Vasc Endovasc Surg*. Mar 2005;29(3):256-261.

8. de Jong KP, Zondervan PE, van Urk H. Extracranial carotid artery aneurysms. *Eur J Vasc Surg*. Dec 1989;3(6):557-562.

# 28 CAROTID ARTERY TRAUMATIC INJURIES

Mounir J. Haurani, MD

## PATIENT STORY

A restrained driver in a high-speed motor vehicle accident was evaluated in the emergency department where he was found to have a Glasgow Coma scale score (GCS) of 6 and significant facial fractures. His injuries were limited to the head, and a computed tomography (CT) scan of the abdomen and pelvis was otherwise negative, and the CT scan of his head showed no intracranial injury. He was admitted and intubated in the intensive care unit (ICU) where he awoke over the next 12 hours. On hospital day 1, he was found to have a new-onset right hemiparesis and aphasia. He was taken for a stat repeat head CT that did not reveal any bleeding but did demonstrate a small left temporal infarct. Angiography showed a left internal carotid artery (ICA) dissection with near-total occlusion in the carotid siphon (Figure 28-1). He was started on antiplatelet therapy (aspirin) and once there was no evidence of bleeding, he was anticoagulated on heparin. Serial head CT scans showed stable infarct size, and he slowly recovered over the next several days.

### EPIDEMIOLOGY

#### Blunt Carotid Artery Injury

- Accounts for 3% to 10% of all carotid injuries.
- Overall incidence of carotid artery injury in blunt trauma is 0.08% to 0.33%.
- Half of the affected patients show no signs of cervical trauma or neurologic deficit at presentation.
- 90% of blunt injuries involve the ICA.
- The most common location is as it enters the siphon.
- Bilateral injury has been reported in 20% to 50% of cases.

  There is an increase in the incidence of reported blunt carotid injuries due in part to better recognition and screening (Figure 28-2).

#### Penetrating Carotid Injury

- The incidence of major vascular trauma following a penetrating injury is 20%.
- The low incidence, anatomic site, and variable presentation have made optimal diagnostic and management strategies difficult.

#### Mechanisms Leading to Blunt Carotid Injury

- The most common mechanism involves hyperextension and rotation of the cervical spine.
- Basilar skull fractures.

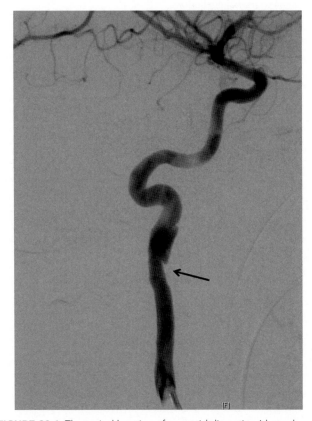

**FIGURE 28-1** The typical location of a carotid dissection (shown by the arrow) is at the relatively fixed point of the internal carotid artery (ICA) near the siphon (S-shaped portion as it enters the skull base). This dissection is focal and is only causing about a 30% stenosis. Management would include anticoagulation or possibly antiplatelet agents for 6 months if the patient can tolerate it.

- Direct blows to the artery.

- Intraoral trauma.

## Sequelae of Injury

- Dissection

- Thrombosis

- Pseudoaneurysm

- Carotid-cavernous sinus fistula

- Complete arterial disruption

The mortality rate of blunt carotid injury varies from 20% to 40% due in part to the extent of concurrent injuries. Permanent neurologic impairment occurs in 25% to 80% of survivors; therefore, the importance of detecting the injury prior to symptoms is crucial in preventing long-term complications.

## DIAGNOSIS

### Screening Criteria (Penetrating Injury)

The management and workup of penetrating neck injuries is dependent on two factors: level of injury and need for emergent operative exploration.

Criteria for emergent exploration are

- Shock

- Refractory hypotension

- Pulsatile bleeding

- Bruit

- Enlarging hematoma

- Neurologic deficit

- Hard signs of a tracheobronchial injury (respiratory distress or air bubbles from the wound)

Clinical features suggestive of injury in hemodynamically stable patients are:

- History of bleeding at the scene

- Stable hematoma

- Nerve injury

- Proximity of the injury track

- Unequal upper extremity blood pressure measurements

- Painful swallowing

- Subcutaneous emphysema

- Hematemesis

- Nerve injury (cranial nerves or brachial plexus injury)

Ninety-seven percent of patients with hard signs have a vascular injury. About 3% of those with soft signs are found to have an injury.[1] A negative physical examination with observation has a negative predictive value of 90% to 100% for vascular injuries.[2]

### Screening Criteria (Blunt Injury)

There are multiple studies that have attempted to develop a consensus as to which signs and symptoms warrant screening for blunt carotid injury.

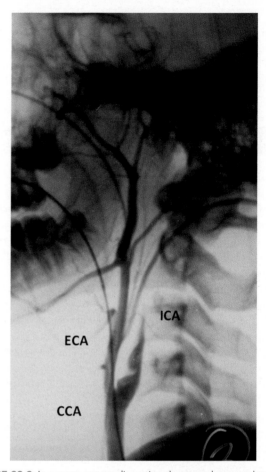

**FIGURE 28-2** In a more severe dissection there can be complete occlusion of the internal carotid artery. The patient above has a normal common carotid artery (CCA) and external carotid artery (ECA). The internal carotid artery (ICA) has a proximal injury that has led to complete occlusion of the distal ICA.

- Denver Health Medical Center[3]
  - This was the first attempt at establishing criteria.
  - 18% of screened patients were found to have an injury.
  - Half of the patients were asymptomatic at presentation.
  - The criteria that prompted screening included
    - Hemorrhage or expanding hematoma
    - Cervical bruit
    - Examination inconsistent with head CT findings
    - Stroke on follow-up head CT
    - Focal neurologic deficit
  - They defined risk factors as below:
    - Le Fort II or III fractures
    - Basilar skull fracture
    - Diffuse axonal injury with GCS less than 6
    - Cervical spine fracture
    - Near-hanging with anoxic brain injury
- The Memphis criteria[4]
  - Had a higher rate of injury using their protocol (29%).
  - This protocol required screening for
    - Neurologic examination not explained by brain imaging
    - Horner syndrome
    - Neck soft tissue injury
    - Le Fort II or III fracture
    - Basilar skull fracture
    - Cervical spine fracture
  - This protocol also had high rates of screening with low positive results.
- Biffl et al. performed a multivariate analysis on a prospectively screened population and found four clinical findings predictive of carotid injury[5]:
  - GCS less than 6
  - Le Fort II or III fractures
  - Petrous fractures
  - Diffuse axonal injury
  - Patients with one finding had a 41% risk of carotid injury, two findings had 56% to 74%, three findings had 80% to 88%, and all four had 93% risk.

## IMAGING MODALITIES

### Duplex Ultrasound

- May be useful for detecting more severe lesions causing greater than 60% stenosis.
- It is limited because it cannot image the carotid artery as it enters the base of the skull, which is where the majority of blunt carotid artery injuries occur.
- Small intimal tears or nonocclusive dissections are hard to detect with ultrasound.

The sensitivity of duplex ultrasound for detecting carotid injury is variable and probably should not be used as a screening tool.[6]

The role in penetrating injuries is limited in that there are often fragments, subcutaneous air, and hematoma that obscure adequate visualization.

### Angiography

Selective angiography is the diagnostic gold standard for screening patients with suspected carotid injury whether by blunt or penetrating mechanisms. It is more sensitive than ultrasound and can detect injuries along the entire course of the internal carotid.

Its limitations are as follows:

- It is an invasive procedure.
- It has the associated risks of arterial access.
- There is a risk of stroke associated with the procedure.
- The resources may not be available at all facilities to perform an angiogram in a timely fashion.[7]

However, the advantage is that it can be not only diagnostic, but also therapeutic in cases of penetrating trauma where the injury is not easily accessible operatively, such as low in the neck near the origin of vessels or high in the neck where the arteries enter the base of the skull.

### CT Angiography

- Helical CT angiography (CTA) is rapid and can be obtained in a matter of minutes.
- Patients who are being screened for blunt carotid artery injury are often being evaluated for other injuries in the abdomen and pelvis, and CT scanning is often performed to evaluate for these.
- The addition of CTA of the head and neck adds minimal increase in time, contrast, or radiation. The benefit is the ability to obtain detailed imaging of the carotid artery with good sensitivity for intimal injuries. With the newer multislice scanners there is also the ability to obtain three-dimensional reconstructions of the head and neck arteries, which increases the ability to manipulate the images to detect subtle injuries.
- Prospective comparative studies have validated 16-slice CTA as a primary screening modality; CTA and digital subtraction angiography (DSA) were 100% concordant for blunt carotid injuries, resulting in sensitivity and specificity of 100% each.[8,9]

Helical CT has become the mainstay of diagnostic evaluation in penetrating injuries as well.[10]

- Initial diagnostic test if no hard signs of injury
- Detects vascular injuries
- Demonstrates location of the tract to the esophagus or trachea
- Shows spinal fractures and cord involvement
- 90% sensitivity and 100% specificity for vascular injuries
- May be limited if there are multiple fragments due to scatter from metallic fragments

### Injury Grades; Blunt Trauma

Depending on the severity of the injury, there is an associated risk of stroke, and therefore a grading scheme has been developed in order to describe this.[7]

- Grade I
  - Luminal irregularity or intramural hematoma with less than 25% luminal narrowing

- Grade II
  - Luminal irregularity or intramural hematoma with less than 25% luminal narrowing
- Grade III
  - Injury with evidence of a pseudoaneurysm
- Grade IV
  - Occlusion of the vessel
- Grade V
  - Transaction of the vessel

Stroke risk increases with the severity of the grade from 3% to 44% (Grade I-IV) with all of Grade IV having strokes.

The mortality also increases with severity of injury from 11% to 22% (Grade I-IV) with all of the Grade V patients dying as well.

## MANAGEMENT

In blunt carotid artery injury, the initial evaluation may be difficult because of the concurrent associated injuries to the head, chest, or abdomen. As in the patient described earlier, there may be no symptoms of cerebral ischemia at initial evaluation.

The presentation of penetrating carotid injuries is far different and less occult than those of blunt injury. The management is largely dictated by the location of the injury. Those patients who have a penetrating injury to the neck that pierces the platysma all warrant further investigation whether it is operative exploration or imaging (Figure 28-3). Direct bleeding, a large hematoma, or any compromise of the airway indicates significant vascular injury and the patient needs operative exploration. Any penetrating injuries in the difficult areas to access surgically (between the cricoid cartilage and clavicles, or between the base of the skull and mandible) would need angiography in a stable patient without the above signs, and management would be based on these findings.

## Medical Treatment; Blunt Trauma

There are no randomized trials comparing the treatment options for blunt carotid artery injuries. The mainstay of treatment is antithrombotic therapy.

- There is improved neurologic outcome associated with the early use of antithrombotic therapy with heparin.[11]
- This should be done in both asymptomatic and symptomatic patients.
- The benefits of anticoagulation need to be weighed in patients with polytrauma especially if there is intracranial hemorrhage.
- Gastrointestinal bleeding, retroperitoneal hemorrhage, blunt solid organ injury with hemorrhage, and rebleeding from surgical wounds are all possibilities in these patients.

Due to these potential complications, an alternative is antiplatelet therapy.[12]

- Initially it was thought to be inferior to full anticoagulation.
- Several studies have failed to show any real difference between heparin or Coumadin and antiplatelet therapy.

Either therapy should be continued for a total of 3 months.

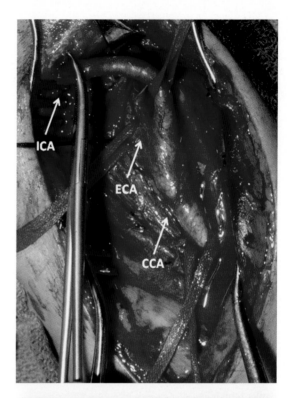

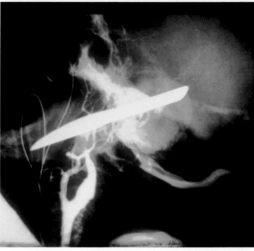

**FIGURE 28-3** In penetrating trauma, the management is dependent on the level of the entry wound and whether there is penetration of the platysma. In the above example on the left, the knife entered just below the angle of the mandible (Zone 2) and there was an expanding hematoma. There was complete transection of the internal carotid artery (ICA) (the end of it is within the hemostat). The patient on the right was managed initially with an angiogram to evaluate for injuries that may not be accessible from the neck, given that the level of penetration was in Zone 3 (above the angle of the jaw). (*Photos courtesy of Dr. Bhagwan Satiani.*)

## Endovascular Treatment

For blunt carotid injuries, invasive procedures are reserved for patients who have failed or are failing medical management with anticoagulation or antiplatelet therapy.

- Intimal flaps or pseudoaneurysms can be repaired without the need for surgical exposure of the vessels.

- Especially useful in vessels difficult or impossible to access.

- Indications for repair are
  - Pseudoaneurysms that fail to resolve
  - Pseudoaneurysms that enlarge
  - Pseudoaneurysms that cause an ischemic injury from embolisms
  - A dissection that is expanding or causes an increased luminal narrowing

Endoluminal therapy with stenting or stent grafting can be employed to tack down the dissection flap or to exclude the pseudoaneurysm. This is true for penetrating injuries as well as in hemodynamically stable patients without hard signs of injury.

## Surgical Treatment

The indications for surgical repair are the same as the indications for endovascular repair in blunt trauma.

- Patients with evolving dissections

- Pseudoaneurysms that persist or enlarge after antithrombotic treatment (Figure 28-4)

- Worsening neurologic symptoms

The decision to proceed with endovascular compared to open repair in large part depends on the associated comorbidities and injuries. Open repair is indicated

- In young patients who are unlikely to comply with antiplatelet therapy.

- In young patients since the long-term effects of stenting or stent grafts is uncertain.

- If the lesion is surgically accessible direct repair or repair with a patch, angioplasty may be advantageous.

The decision to proceed with surgical repair in penetrating injuries is again dictated by the presence of hard signs. Which surgical approach to employ is determined by the location of the injury relative to specific landmarks in the neck.

- Zone I
  - Below the cricoid cartilage and above the clavicles.
  - Proximal control needs to be obtained via the chest via a median sternotomy or high anterolateral thoracotomy.
  - Temporary control with an endoluminal approach is possible but should not delay a sternotomy.

- Zone II
  - Between the cricoid cartilage and the angle of the mandible
  - Approached via a cervical incision
  - Most common injury site and most easily accessed surgically

- Zone III
  - Above the angle of the mandible.
  - Distal control is almost impossible to obtain.

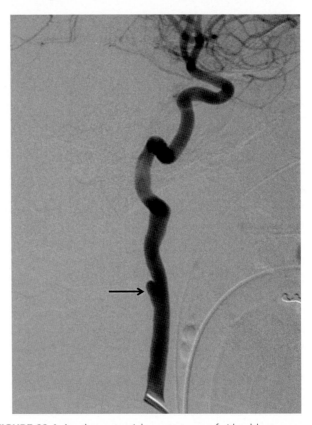

**FIGURE 28-4** Another potential consequence of either blunt or penetrating injury is the formation of a pseudoaneurysm (arrow). The patient above was struck by a car and was found to have a dissection. He was treated nonoperatively, and on follow-up duplex he was found to have a pseudoaneurysm. Angiography confirmed a small pseudoaneurysm. The management could include either open repair or exclusion with a stent graft.

○ Can be obtained by placing a Fogarty balloon (No. 3 or 4) within the vessel lumen.

○ An arteriogram can be performed via a sheath.

○ The artery can be repaired, embolized, stented, or ligated.

## FOLLOW-UP

• For patients who undergo medical management of their blunt carotid injury, follow-up imaging is mandatory in order to assess the intimal flap. Much like the initial evaluation, CTA with a multi-slice detector is recommended.

• Follow-up should occur at 1 week and 3 months.

• Patients with high-grade (Grade IV) injuries do not typically show improvement at follow-up, so they do not require imaging like Grade I to III injuries.

• The follow-up is predominantly to assess for resolution of the intimal injury as well as for development of or resolution of a pseudoaneurysm.

• Pseudoaneurysms will develop in up to one-third of patients and can be a source of embolisms. Pseudoaneurysms are also unlikely to resolve with medical management alone and therefore warrant repair.

## PROVIDER RESOURCES

• http://emedicine.medscape.com/article/757906-overview

• http://www.ncbi.nlm.nih.gov/pubmed/20206804

• http://www.sjtrem.com/content/18/1/61

## REFERENCES

1. Demetriades D, Theodorou D, Cornwell E, et al. Evaluation of penetrating injuries of the neck: prospective study of 223 patients. *World J Surg.* Jan 1997;21(1):41-47; discussion 47-48.

2. Demetriades D, Charalambides D, Lakhoo M. Physical examination and selective conservative management in patients with penetrating injuries of the neck. *Br J Surg.* Dec 1993;80(12):1534-1536.

3. Biffl WL, Moore EE, Ryu RK, et al. The unrecognized epidemic of blunt carotid arterial injuries: early diagnosis improves neurologic outcome. *Ann Surg.* Oct 1998;228(4):462-470.

4. Miller PR, Fabian TC, Croce MA, et al. Prospective screening for blunt cerebrovascular injuries: analysis of diagnostic modalities and outcomes. *Ann Surg.* Sep 2002;236(3):386-393; discussion 393-385.

5. Biffl WL, Moore EE, Offner PJ, et al. Optimizing screening for blunt cerebrovascular injuries. *Am J Surg.* Dec 1999;178(6): 517-522.

6. Mutze S, Rademacher G, Matthes G, Hosten N, Stengel D. Blunt cerebrovascular injury in patients with blunt multiple trauma: diagnostic accuracy of duplex Doppler US and early CT angiography. *Radiology.* Dec 2005;237(3):884-892.

7. Biffl WL, Moore EE, Offner PJ, Brega KE, Franciose RJ, Burch JM. Blunt carotid arterial injuries: implications of a new grading scale. *J Trauma.* Nov 1999;47(5):845-853.

8. Bub LD, Hollingworth W, Jarvik JG, Hallam DK. Screening for blunt cerebrovascular injury: evaluating the accuracy of multi-detector computed tomographic angiography. *J Trauma.* Sep 2005;59(3):691-697.

9. Eastman AL, Chason DP, Perez CL, McAnulty AL, Minei JP. Computed tomographic angiography for the diagnosis of blunt cervical vascular injury: is it ready for primetime? *J Trauma.* May 2006;60(5):925-929; discussion 929.

10. Nunez DB Jr, Torres-Leon M, Munera F. Vascular injuries of the neck and thoracic inlet: helical CT-angiographic correlation. *Radiographics.* Jul-Aug 2004;24(4):1087-1098; discussion 1099-1100.

11. Fabian TC, Patton JH Jr, Croce MA, Minard G, Kudsk KA, Pritchard FE. Blunt carotid injury. Importance of early diagnosis and anticoagulant therapy. *Ann Surg.* May 1996;223(5):513-522; discussion 522-515.

12. Wahl WL, Brandt MM, Thompson BG, Taheri PA, Greenfield LJ. Antiplatelet therapy: an alternative to heparin for blunt carotid injury. *J Trauma.* May 2002;52(5):896-901.

# PART 4

# ANEURYSMAL DISEASE

# 29 ENDOVASCULAR ANEURYSM REPAIR

Joseph Habib, MD

## PATIENT STORY

A 65-year-old man presented to the vascular clinic after his primary care physician felt a pulsatile abdominal mass in his left mid abdomen. The patient was not having any abdominal pain or back pain. His past medical history was significant for hypertension, hyperlipidemia, and tobacco use. An abdominal ultrasound and computed tomographic angiogram (CTA) of the abdomen and pelvis were performed, which showed a 5.7-cm dilation of the infrarenal aorta beginning about 2 cm below the origin of the renal arteries.

This patient had an infrarenal abdominal aortic aneurysm (AAA). Most patients are asymptomatic on presentation. The goal of aneurysm repair is to prevent death from rupture.

## EPIDEMIOLOGY

- The 15th leading cause of death in the United States is ruptured AAA.[1] Abdominal aneurysms are more common in males than in females and generally affect people over age 50. Incidence in the United States is approximately 6.5 per 1000 person-years.[2]
- AAA is defined as a dilation of all three layers of the abdominal aorta greater than $1.5\times$ its native diameter.[3]

## ETIOLOGY AND PATHOPHYSIOLOGY

- There appears to be a familial component to the development of AAA. People with an affected first-degree relative have an 11.6-fold increase in AAA risk.[4]
- The risk factors that have the greatest impact on AAA development appear to be age, male gender, family history, and smoking.[5]
- Most aneurysms are caused by a complex degenerative process.
- Patients with AAAs appear to have increased levels of metalloproteinases.[6]
- Aneurysms may develop in autoimmune inflammatory conditions or as a result of infectious etiology.[7]

## DIAGNOSIS AND CLINICAL FINDINGS

- Nonruptured AAAs are usually asymptomatic and discovered incidentally on imaging obtained for workup of conditions that are unrelated.
- Sometimes a pulsatile mass in the mid abdomen may be felt by an examining physician or the patients themselves.
- Occasionally very large aneurysms may cause early satiety, nausea, vomiting, urinary symptoms, or venous thrombosis secondary to local compression of adjacent structures by the aneurysm.[3]

## LABORATORY

- No specific laboratory tests are diagnostic.
- Blood chemistry including serum creatinine, complete blood count, and coagulation studies should be obtained in preparation for the repair.

## IMAGING

### Ultrasound

- Less expensive, noninvasive
- May underestimate the size of the aneurysm by 2 to 4 mm[8]

### CT

- More expensive, risks associated with contrast and radiation exposure
- More accurate measurement of diameter[8]

### Angiography

- Invasive
- Associated with contrast and radiation exposure
- Can be performed at the time of the repair

## MANAGEMENT

- In general, although somewhat controversial, it may be safe to observe asymptomatic aneurysms less than 5.5 cm in diameter.[2,9]
- Rapidly growing aneurysms (>1.0 cm/year) or symptomatic aneurysms should be referred for repair.[9]
- The ratio of the diameter of the aneurysm to the size of the native aorta may also be considered to determine the rupture risk and the need for subsequent repair, but the validity of this has not been proven.[10]
- After aneurysms reach 5.5 cm they should be referred for elective repair.[2,9]

### Open Versus Endovascular Repair

- The first endovascular repair of an endovascular AAA was performed in 1991.[11]
- Perioperative survival benefit has been demonstrated in randomized trials with endovascular treatment when compared with open repair.[12,13]
- Long-term durability of endovascular repair is unknown.
- EVAR-1 and DREAM trials—the only level-one evidence for comparing open repair with endovascular repair.[14]

- These two clinical trials are reviewed as follows:

## EVAR 1 Trial, 1082 Patients[12]

- 30-day mortality: 1.7% in endovascular group versus 4.7% in open surgical group ($p < .001$)

- Aneurysm-related mortality at 4 years: 4% in endovascular group versus 7% in the open surgical group ($p < 0.04$)

- Post-op complications at 4 years: 41% in endovascular group versus 9% in the open surgical group

- Reinterventions: 20% in endovascular group versus 6% open surgical group

## DREAM Trial, 351 Patients[13]

- Perioperative mortality and severe complications: 4.7% after EVAR versus 9.8% for open surgery

- 2-year survival rates: 89.7% for EVAR and 89.6% for open surgery

## PATIENT SELECTION[15]

- Must have proximal and distal sealing zones (attachment sites or fixation points within the aorta and iliac arteries for the endovascular graft).

- Proximal sealing zone
  - Length of infrarenal aortic neck should be 10 to 15 mm.[15]
  - Angulation of proximal neck should be less than 60 degrees.[15]
  - Calcification and mural thrombus in proximal neck should be less than 90 degrees.[15]

- Distal sealing zone proximal to hypogastric arteries should have a length of 10 to 15 mm.[15]

- Should avoid endovascular repair in patients with small, calcified, and tortuous iliac arteries.[15]

## TECHNIQUE[15]

- Performed in operating room, radiologic angiography suite, or catheterization laboratory.

- General, regional, or local anesthesia may be used.

- Common femoral arteries in the groin are usually used and can be accessed either by direct cut-down or percutaneous measures.

- Large introducer sheaths are inserted through both common femoral arteries.

- Main body of the endograft is delivered through one access sheath over stiff wire into position just distal to the renal arteries.

- Main body is deployed and the stump (gate) of the contralateral limb is cannulated from the opposite groin.

- After cannulation of the contralateral gate, the wire is exchanged out for a stiff wire and the position of the hypogastric arteries is marked.

- The contralateral limb is placed over the stiff wire then deployed with appropriate overlap in the main body device, with the distal end being just proximal to the hypogastric artery.

- Proximal and distal fixation points as well as all overlap points should then be angioplastied (ballooned).

- Final angiogram should then be performed to detect the presence of endoleaks (extravasation of contrast) (Figure 29-1).

- Proximal and distal extensions may be added to resolve endoleaks.

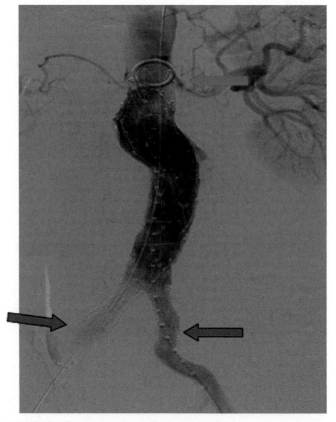

**FIGURE 29-1** Completion angiogram after endovascular aneurysm repair of an infrarenal abdominal aortic aneurysm (AAA) with modular bifurcated prosthesis. Red arrow shows proximal fixation point at the infrarenal aorta and blue arrows show distal fixation points in the common iliac arteries.

## SELECTION OF DEVICES

- Modular devices: for example, Medtronic Endurant (Figure 29-2), Gore Excluder, Cook Zenith
- Unibody devices: for example, Endologix (Figure 29-3)
- Graft materials: for example, PTFE, polyester
- Fixation stents: for example, stainless steel, nitinol

## COMPLICATIONS

- Access-site complications: hematomas, pseudoaneurysm, wound infections, lymphoceles, artery ruptures, or dissections.[15]
- Device-related complications: stent migration or erosion, limb occlusion, persistent endoleaks (see below), stent graft infection, late rupture.[15]
- Systemic complications: stroke, renal insufficiency, pulmonary embolism, deep venous thrombosis, bowel ischemia, spinal cord ischemia, erectile dysfunction, myocardial infarction.[15]
- Endoleak is the presence of persistent blood flow within the aneurysm sac outside the lumen of the stent graft[16] (Figure 29-4).

    Type I: leakage of blood flow around the proximal or distal attachment points of the stent graft resulting from inadequate seal[16] (Figure 29-4).

    Type II: retrograde blood flow into the aneurysm sac from lumbar arteries or the inferior mesenteric artery.[16]

    Type III: leakage of blood into the aneurysm sac from inadequate seal between the components of the stent graft.[16]

    Type IV: leakage of blood through the fabric of the graft secondary to its inherent porosity.[16]

## FOLLOW-UP

- Indefinite follow-up required.
- CTA at 1, 6, 12, and 18 months and then annually is usually recommended.[15]
- Grafts surveyed for endoleaks, migration, patency, sac enlargement.
- Ultrasound, magnetic resonance angiography, plain abdominal x-ray may be used in select cases.

### PROVIDER RESOURCES

- Small aneurysms. http://jama.jamanetwork.com/article.aspx?articleID=1656254&utm_source=Silverchair%20Information%20Systems&utm_medium=email&utm_campaign=MASTER%3AJAMALatestIssueTOCNotification02%2F26%2F2013
- http://www.ncbi.nlm.nih.gov/pubmed/14718853
- http://www.ncbi.nlm.nih.gov/pubmed/19786250

### PATIENT RESOURCES

- http://en.wikipedia.org/wiki/Abdominal_aortic_aneurysm
- http://www.mayoclinic.com/health/abdominal-aortic-aneurysm/ds01194

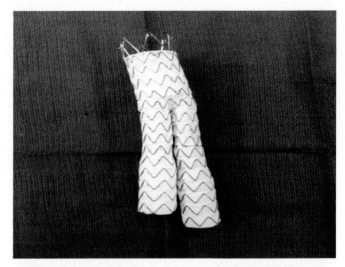

**FIGURE 29-2** Medtronic Endurant graft—modular bifurcated prosthesis with suprarenal fixation.

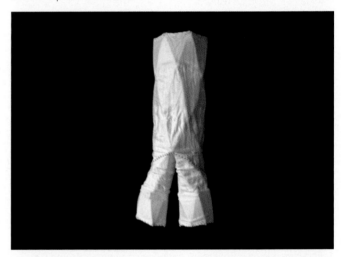

**FIGURE 29-3** Endologix Powerlink—unibody graft.

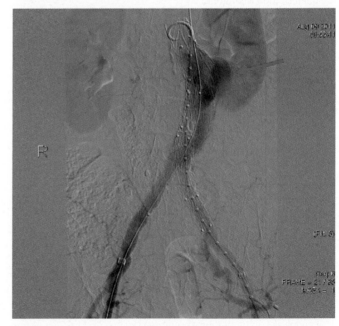

**FIGURE 29-4** Angiogram after endovascular aneurysm repair in an infrarenal abdominal aortic aneurysm. Red arrow shows type IA endoleak.

## REFERENCES

1. Chuter TAM, Schneider D. Abdominal aortic aneurysms: endovascular treatment. In: Cronenwett J, Johnston K, eds. *Rutherford's Vascular Surgery*. 7th ed. Philadelphia, PA: Elsevier; 2010:1972-1993.

2. Parodi JC, Palmaz JC, Barone HD. Transfemoral intraluminal graft implantation for abdominal aortic aneurysm. *Ann Vasc Surg*. 1991;5:491-499.

3. Greenhalgh RM, Brown LC, Kwong GP, et al. Comparison of endovascular aneurysm repair with open repair in patients with abdominal aortic aneurysm (EVAR trial 1), 30-day operative mortality results: randomized controlled trial. *Lancet*. 2004;364:843-848.

4. Lederle FA, Johnson GR, Wilson SE, et al. Yield of repeated screening for abdominal aortic aneurysm after a 4-year interval. Aneurysm Detection and Management Veterans Affairs Cooperative Study Investigators. *Arch Intern Med*. 2000;160:1117-1121.

5. Aortic Aneurysm Fact Sheet. Available at http://www.cdc.gov/dhdsp/data_statistics/fact_sheets/fs_aortic_aneurysm.htm. Accessed April 20, 2013.

6. Johansen K, Koepsell T. Familial tendency for abdominal aortic aneurysms. *JAMA*. 1986;256:1934-1936.

7. Wilmink AB, Quick CR. Epidemiology and potential for prevention of abdominal aortic aneurysm. *Br J Surg*. 1998;85:155-162.

8. Brophy CM, Marks WH, Reilly JM, Tilson MD. Decreased tissue inhibitor of metalloproteinases (TIMP) in abdominal aortic aneurysm tissue: a preliminary report. *J Surg Res*. 1991;50:653-657.

9. Brown SL, Busuttil RW, Baker JD, Machleder HI, et al. Bacteriologic and surgical determinants of survival in patients with mycotic aneurysms. *J Vasc Surg*. 1984;1:541-547.

10. Fillinger MF. Abdominal aortic aneurysms: evaluation and decision making. In: Cronenwett J, Johnston K, eds. *Rutherford's Vascular Surgery*. 7th ed. Philadelphia, PA: Elsevier; 2010:1928-1948.

11. Jaakkola P, Hippelainen M, Farin P, et al. Interobserver variability in measuring the dimensions of the abdominal aorta: comparison of ultrasound and computed tomography. *Eur J Vasc Endovasc Surg*. 1996;12:230-237.

12. The UK Small Aneurysm Trial Participants. Mortality results for randomised controlled trial of early elective surgery or ultrasonographic surveillance for small abdominal aortic aneurysms. *Lancet*. 1998;352:1649-1655.

13. Blankensteijn JD, de Jong S, Prinssen M, van der Ham A. Two-year outcomes after conventional or endovascular repair of abdominal aortic aneurysms. *N Engl J Med*. 2005;352:2398-2405.

14. White GH, Yu W, May J, et al. Endoleaks as a complication of endoluminal grafting of abdominal aortic aneurysms: classification, incidence, diagnosis, and management. *J Endovasc Surg*. 1997;4:152-168.

15. Sambeek MRHM, Cuypers P, Hendriks JM, Buth J. Abdominal aneurysms: endovascular aneurysm repair. In: Hallett J, Mills J, Earnshaw J, Rooke, Reekers J, eds. *Comprehensive Vascular and Endovascular Surgery*. 2nd ed. Philadelphia, PA: Mosby Elsevier; 2009:480-494.

16. Brewster DC, Cronenwett JL, Hallett JW Jr, et al. Guidelines for the treatment of abdominal aortic aneurysms. *J Vasc Surg*. 2003;37(5):1106-1117.

# 30 ENDOVASCULAR ABDOMINAL AORTIC ANEURYSM REPAIR FOR RUPTURED ABDOMINAL AORTIC ANEURYSM

Faisal Aziz, MD

## PATIENT STORY

A 65-year-old man presented to the emergency room with complaints of abdominal pain. He described the pain to be stabbing in nature, radiating to his back and very severe (10 on a scale of 0-10). His past medical history was significant for smoking, hypertension, diabetes, and coronary artery heart disease. On physical examination, he was found to be tachycardic and hypotensive. On abdominal examination, there was a large pulsatile mass in his abdomen. Both femoral pulses were palpable but weak. A computed tomographic (CT) scan of his abdomen showed that there was loss of the fat plane between the aorta and the surrounding tissues and a large retroperitoneal hematoma (Figures 30-1 and 30-2).

## TREATMENT COURSE FOR THE PATIENT

- The patient was brought to the operating room, and under local anesthetic, bilateral groin cut-downs were performed, exposing both common femoral arteries. An occluding balloon was passed via right femoral artery and was inflated proximal to the aneurysm sac, thus temporarily occluding blood flow to the aneurysm.

- A diagnostic catheter was passed via left femoral artery, and an aortogram was performed, identifying the location of both renal and internal iliac arteries.

- Main body of endovascular graft was then deployed via the left femoral artery. Occluding balloon was then placed proximally via the left common femoral artery (Figure 30-3). Then, via the right common femoral artery, the right limb of the endograft was deployed, and then via the left common femoral artery, the left limb of the endograft was deployed (Figure 30-4).

- Balloon insufflation was performed at proximal and distal ends of the endograft and a completion aortogram was performed, which showed that the aneurysm cavity was effectively excluded (Figure 30-5).

- The patient's postoperative course was uneventful, and he was discharged home on the fourth postoperative day.

## EPIDEMIOLOGY

- Rupture of an abdominal aortic aneurysm (AAA) is a catastrophic event. It has been among the 15 most frequent causes of death in the United States and remained steady until 1990, but has gradually declined in the past 15 years.[1,2]

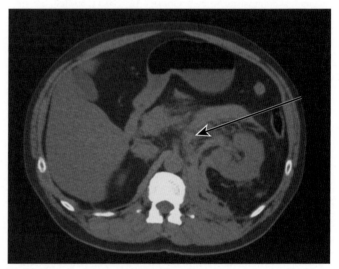

Retroperitoneal Hematoma

**FIGURE 30-1** Computed tomographic (CT) scan of abdomen showing a left retroperitoneal hematoma.

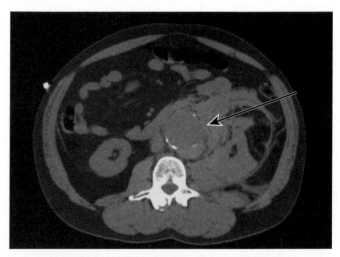

Loss of fat plane between aorta and retroperitoneum.

**FIGURE 30-2** Computed tomographic (CT) scan of abdomen showing loss of fat plane between the aorta and the surrounding tissues. A retroperitoneal hematoma is also visible.

- 30% to 50% of all patients with ruptured AAA die before they reach the hospital.[3]

- About 40% of patients reach the hospital but die before they get operated on.[4,5]

- Bleeding from rupture can occur in the retroperitoneum, peritoneal cavity, gastrointestinal tract, or inferior vena cava.

- Large clinical trials have demonstrated the safety of nonoperative management for AAAs with maximal diameter less than 5.5 cm,[6,7,8] making overall mortality 80% to 90% because of ruptured AAA.[9,10]

- Generally, patients with AAAs larger than 5.5 cm should be offered operative treatment.

## CLINICAL PRESENTATION

- Classically, patients with a ruptured AAA present with a triad of palpable abdominal mass, severe abdominal pain, and hypotension.

- Flank (Grey Turner sign) and periumbilical (Cullen sign) ecchymosis may be seen in patients with more sub-acute or chronic ruptures.

- Hypotension is a sign of active bleeding from rupture of an aneurysm and is an indication for emergent repair of aneurysm.

## TREATMENT OPTIONS

Ruptured AAA can be managed by two surgical techniques.

### Open Surgical Repair

Aneurysm can be accessed either by transperitoneal approach or retroperitoneal approach. Proximal and distal control is achieved, aneurysm cavity is opened, and a Dacron graft (tube or bifurcated) is sutured proximally and distally, effectively excluding the aneurysm sac.

### Endovascular Repair of AAA

Bilateral groin cut-downs are performed, and both common femoral arteries are exposed. Wires are then passed into aorta via common femoral arteries. An endograft is then deployed across the aneurysm cavity. The aneurysm itself remains in its place, but endograft effectively excludes any blood flow in the aneurysm sac.

## FOLLOW-UP AFTER ENDOVASCULAR REPAIR

- Patients who receive endovascular treatment for AAA should be followed with serial CT angiograms to look for any increase in diameter of the aneurysm and to detect any endoleak.

- Any of these findings may warrant further diagnostic studies. Patients with AAA should also be followed for any development of new aneurysms in iliac, femoral, or popliteal arteries, because of high association between these aneurysms.

## PATIENT EDUCATION

- AAAs have a strong genetic component and family members of patients with AAA should be screened for the presence of AAA.

- Men older than 65 years of age who have a strong family history of AAA and are smokers should be offered screening for AAAs.

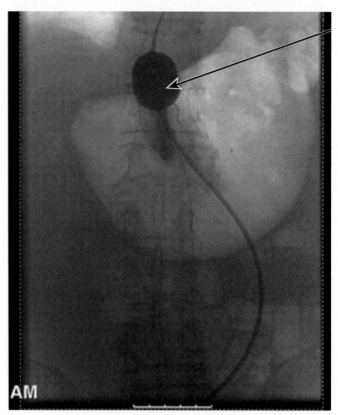

Coda balloon, used to gain proximal control of aorta

**FIGURE 30-3** Occluding balloon, inserted via left common femoral artery and occluding blood flow into the aneurysm sac.

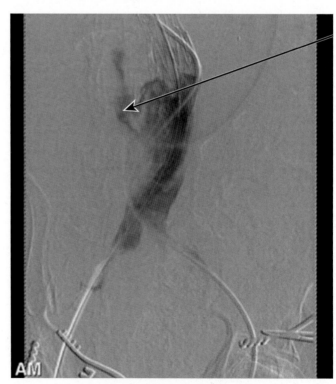

Active extravasation of contrast, consistent with leakage of blood from ruptured aorta

**FIGURE 30-4** Main body of endograft has been deployed and retrograde aortogram shows a leak from the ruptured aneurysm sac.

• Patients with abdominal aortic diameter more than 5.5 cm should be offered intervention.
• Patients with suitable anatomy for endografts should be offered endovascular operation.

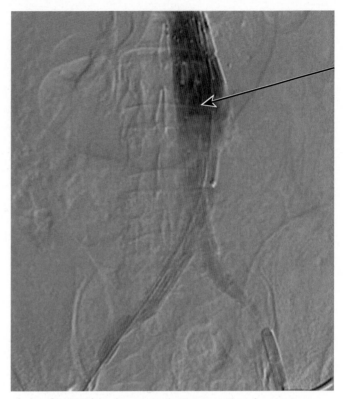

Stent graft in place, no active extravasation of contrast

**FIGURE 30-5** Endograft has been deployed and completion angiogram shows that the aneurysm sac has been completely excluded and there is no leakage of blood flow.

## REFERENCES

1. Silverberg E, Boring CC, Squires TS. Cancer statistics, 1990. *CA Cancer J Clin.* 1990;40:9-26.

2. Aortic Aneurysm Fact Sheet. http://www.cdc.gov/dhdsp/ data_statistics/fact_sheets/fs_aortic_aneurysm.htm

3. Bengtsson H, Bergqvist D. Ruptured abdominal aortic aneurysm: a population-based study. *J Vasc Surg.* 1993;18:74-80.

4. Heller JA, Weinberg A, Arons R, et al. Two decades of abdominal aortic aneurysm repair: have we made any progress? *J Vasc Surg.* 2000;32:1091-1100.

5. Adam DJ, Mohan IV, Stuart WP, et al. Community and hospital outcome from ruptured abdominal aortic aneurysm within the catchment area of a regional vascular surgical service. *J Vasc Surg.* 1999;30:922-928.

6. Brown PM, Pattenden R, Vernooy C, et al. Selective management of abdominal aortic aneurysms in a prospective measurement program. *J Vasc Surg.* 1996;23:213-220.

7. Lederle FA, Wilson SE, Johnson GR, et al. Immediate repair compared with surveillance of small abdominal aortic aneurysms. *N Engl J Med.* 2002;346:1437-1444.

8. Mortality results for randomised controlled trial of early elective surgery or ultrasonographic surveillance for small abdominal aortic aneurysms. The UK Small Aneurysm Trial Participants. *Lancet.* 1998;352:1649-1655.

9. Kantonen I, Lepantalo M, Brommels M, et al. Mortality in ruptured abdominal aortic aneurysms. The Finnvasc Study Group. *Eur J Vasc Endovasc Surg.* 1999;17:208-212.

10. Heikkinen M, Salenius JP, Auvinen O. Ruptured abdominal aortic aneurysm in a well-defined geographic area. *J Vasc Surg.* 2002;36:291-296.

# 31 THORACIC AND THORACOABDOMINAL ANEURYSMS: OPEN REPAIR

Mounir J. Haurani, MD

## PATIENT STORY

A 68-year-old man with hypertension and a history of smoking was 1 week post-op from a right total knee replacement. He presented to the emergency room with acute onset of shortness of breath and right leg swelling. A helical computed tomography (CT) scan of his chest showed a small subsegmental pulmonary embolus (PE) and deep venous thrombosis (DVT) of the right femoral vein. He was incidentally noted to have a 6.7-cm aneurysm of his thoracic aorta that involved the visceral segment (Figure 31-1). Given its size and the involvement of the visceral segment, an open repair was recommended.

### HISTORY AND PHYSICAL EXAMINATION

- Most thoracoabdominal aortic aneurysms (TAAA) are asymptomatic at the time of diagnosis; however, most will become symptomatic before rupture.
- Much like abdominal aneurysms, they are diagnosed incidentally.
- The most common initial symptom is vague pain in the back, flank, chest, or even abdomen.
- The differential diagnosis is extensive in patients who present with these vague symptoms, and they may often be dismissed.
- Compressive symptoms may also occur.
  - Left recurrent laryngeal nerve causing hoarseness.
  - The aneurysm may compress the trachea or esophagus causing cough, dysphagia, or other associated symptoms.
  - Like abdominal aortic aneurysms, embolization to the visceral, renal, and lower extremity arteries has been reported.
- Unless there is an abdominal component to the TAAA there are no specific physical examination findings. If there is an abdominal portion, then a pulsatile mass may be present.

### DIAGNOSTIC EVALUATION

- CT angiography is the mainstay of imaging modalities for evaluation of TAAAs.
  - Depending on the size and rate of growth, imaging for follow-up purposes is typically done at 6- to 12- month intervals.
  - While catheter-directed aortography historically was the modality of choice, helical CT angiography is the current modality of choice.
  - Currently angiography is used for special situations such as mapping the spinal cord circulation or concurrent occlusive disease in the head and neck vessels.

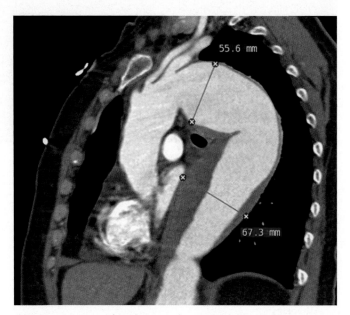

**FIGURE 31-1** As is often the case, thoracic and thoracoabdominal aneurysms are often found incidentally. When the aneurysm is in close proximity to the visceral segment or arch vessels, an open repair is indicated. In cases where this is not an option due to comorbidities, either a hybrid procedure (debranching or extra-anatomic bypass) or non–FDA-approved custom branched or fenestrated endografts are potential options. CT angiography shows the thoracic aorta with diameter measurements indicated in two places.

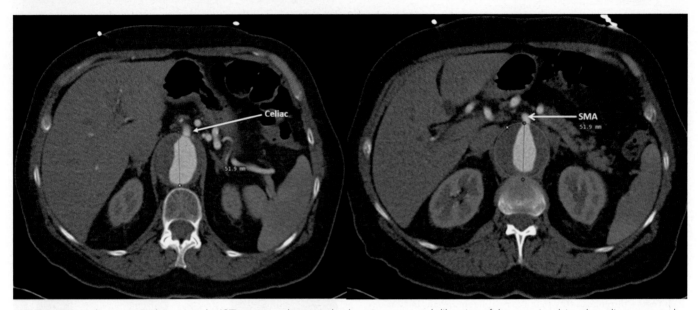

**FIGURE 31-2** In this computed tomography (CT) angiography example, there is aneurysmal dilatation of the aorta involving the celiac artery and the superior mesenteric artery (SMA). Measurements of diameter are also indicated. This is another indication to perform an open repair. In this case if the SMA and celiac artery are in close proximity, they may be included in a single anastomosis. CT angiography such as this is crucial for planning the repair. Consideration of clamp sites, visceral segment revascularization options, and location of the intercostals can be determined with the aid of CT angiography.

- ○ CT angiography allows for reconstructed views of the aorta (Figure 31-1) as well as examination of other organs in the chest, abdomen, and pelvis, which occasionally will reveal incidental pathology.
- ○ CT angiography, like conventional angiography, can also aid in operative planning by identifying large intercostal arteries as well as mural thrombus, inflammatory changes, and other anatomic features that would affect operative planning (Figures 31-1 and 31-2).

## EPIDEMIOLOGY

### Definition

- TAAAs are dilatations in the thoracic and abdominal aortas.
- Once the thoracic aorta is at least 1.5 times its normal size it is considered an aneurysm.
- TAAAs account for 10% of thoracic aneurysms, with ascending thoracic aortic aneurysms being the most common (40%).
- TAAAs have been categorized based on their extent in four types:
  - ○ Type I starts just distal to the left subclavian artery and includes the entire descending thoracic aorta up to the renal arteries.
  - ○ Type II starts at the left subclavian artery and ends at the aortic bifurcation.
  - ○ Type III begins in the distal thoracic aorta and ends at the aortic bifurcation or lower.
  - ○ Type IV starts at the level of the diaphragm (T12) and continues to the aortic bifurcation.
- Most TAAAs are fusiform aneurysms, which are diffuse dilatations involving the entire circumference of the aorta.

## Natural History

- The mean aortic diameter of ruptured TAAAs is 6.1, and the mean growth rate is 0.4 cm yearly.[1,2]
- The growth rates of TAAAs are not predictable or linear; however, larger aneurysms tend to grow faster.[1]

## Population Affected

- Average age is 65 years.
- Male-female ratio of 1.7:1.[3]
- 20% of patients will have a first-degree relative affected by aneurysmal disease.[4]

## Risk Factors for Disease and Rupture

- Hypertension
  - Diastolic pressure greater than 100 mm Hg has been associated with enlargement and rupture.[1]
- Smoking
- Atherosclerosis
- Usually degenerative, but in 20% of patients result of chronic aortic dissection
- Risks associated with rupture
  - Chronic obstructive pulmonary disease.
  - Renal failure.
  - Increased age.
  - Size of TAAA.
  - Rate of growth.
  - Patients with a TAAA diameter of 8 cm have an 80% risk for rupture within 1 year of diagnosis.
  - Expansion by more than 1 cm/y also signals impending rupture.[5]

## Incidence or Prevalence

- The incidence of thoracic aortic disease is 16.3 per 100,000 per year in men, and 9.1 per 100,000 per year in women.
- The prevalence and incidence of thoracic aortic disease is increasing.[6]
- This has been attributed to improved imaging techniques, an aging population, and increased patient and physician awareness.

## PATHOGENESIS

The pathogenesis of TAAA development involves multiple factors.

- These range from genetic factors to hemodynamic factors.
- The processes involved include cellular processes as well as extracellular factors.
- Inflammation and pathologic remodeling occurs and degradation exceeds matrix production and repair.
- Histologically, degeneration of the media is seen, and this is accelerated by hypertension and atherosclerosis.
- Genetic abnormalities such as Marfan syndrome also accelerate aortic medial degeneration.

## MANAGEMENT

### Medical Management

- Once a TAAA has been diagnosed, the evidence is not as clear as it is with abdominal aortic aneurysms in regard to size criteria for intervention.
- In general, once the aneurysm has reached twice the size of normal contiguous aorta, a repair or intervention is indicated.
- Several studies have suggested that 6.5 cm ought to be the point at which intervention in TAAAs should be considered.
- If a patient is symptomatic or there is rapid enlargement of the aneurysm, then size criteria are not as critical, and intervention is indicated.
- Medical management consists of
  - Antihypertensive medication
    - Beta-blockers for decreasing the force of myocardial contraction.
    - Angiotensin-converting enzyme inhibitors reduce oxidative stress.
  - Statins
    - Inhibit inflammation via the suppression of nicotinamide adenine dinucleotide phosphate oxidase
  - Smoking cessation

## OPERATIVE REPAIR

- With the advent of thoracic stent grafting, isolated descending thoracic aneurysms are increasingly being repaired in this fashion.
- When the aneurysm involves the arch or visceral segments, off-label use of stent grafts with fenestrations are needed, or the standard open repair (Figures 31-1 and 31-2).
- In the modern era, open repair consists of[7]
  - Cardiopulmonary bypass.
  - Sequential clamping of the aorta in order to minimize the ischemic complication to the spinal cord and visceral segment.
  - Cerebrospinal fluid drainage.
  - Monitoring of evoked motor potentials allows for spinal cord protection.
  - By utilizing retrograde perfusion of the visceral segment, lumbar arteries, and intercostals during creation of the proximal anastomosis, the mortality and paralysis rates at centers of excellence have been greatly reduced.
    - Mortality rate of 4.8% was attained compared to 20% seen in administrative databases.[8]
    - Paralysis and stroke was as low as 3.4% and 2.7%, respectively.
    - 5- and 10-year survival rates were 60% and 38%, respectively.
  - Often there is a need for concurrent revascularization of either the arch vessels or the visceral and renal vessels, which is a contraindication to endovascular repair.
  - If the left subclavian artery is involved, a left carotid to subclavian bypass may be performed followed by ligation of the subclavian artery during the repair.

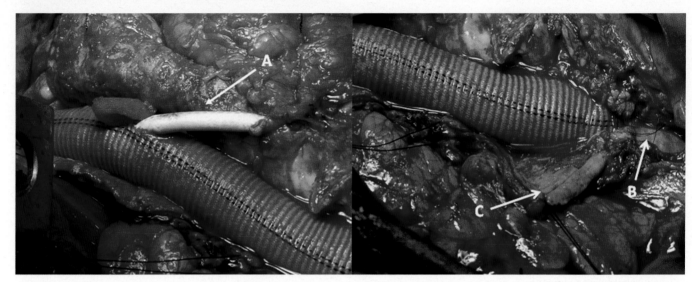

**FIGURE 31-3** During open repair, sequential clamping allows for continued perfusion of the visceral segment and the intercostals as the proximal anastomosis is fashioned (right panel). The native descending aorta (B) is repaired first and the native aneurysmal aorta (C) is reapproximated over the graft. The left renal artery is often revascularized via a retrograde branch sewn onto the main graft (A).

- ○ If the TAAA involves the visceral segment and renal arteries, a small patch of the visceral vessels can be reimplanted into the prosthetic graft. Typically, if the left renal artery is involved then a separate bypass graft is fashioned in a retrograde fashion to revascularize the kidney (Figure 31-3).
- ○ Large intercostals, especially in the T9-12 region, can also be similarly reimplanted as a patch onto the graft in order to prevent spinal cord ischemia.

## FOLLOW-UP

### Postoperative Management

During the first 48 hours postoperatively we can observe the following:

- Cerebrospinal fluid continues to be drained.
- Spinal cord pressures are measured in order to prevent increased pressures and potential spinal cord ischemia.
- Hypotension must be strictly avoided in order to prevent delayed paralysis.
- Neurovascular checks need to be frequently performed.

### Long-Term Follow Up

- Surveillance is necessary because subsequent aneurysm formation is possible.
- These can be either in native tissues or anastomotic aneurysms.
- Once a year, in uncomplicated cases, with magnetic resonance imaging (MRI) or CT angiography is recommended by some.

## REFERENCES

1. Dapunt OE, Galla JD, Sadeghi AM, et al. The natural history of thoracic aortic aneurysms. *J Thorac Cardiovasc Surg.* May 1994;107(5):1323-1333.

2. Elefteriades JA. Natural history of thoracic aortic aneurysms: indications for surgery, and surgical versus nonsurgical risks. *Ann Thorac Surg*. Nov 2002;74(5):S1877-S1880.

3. Bickerstaff LK, Pairolero PC, Hollier LH, et al. Thoracic aortic aneurysms: a population-based study. *Surgery*. Dec 1982;92(6):1103-1108.

4. Biddinger A, Rocklin M, Coselli J, Milewicz DM. Familial thoracic aortic dilatations and dissections: a case control study. *J Vasc Surg*. Mar 1997;25(3):506-511.

5. Coady MA, Rizzo JA, Hammond GL, et al. What is the appropriate size criterion for resection of thoracic aortic aneurysms? *J Thorac Cardiovasc Surg*. Mar 1997;113(3):476-491; discussion 489-491.

6. Olsson C, Thelin S, Stahle E, Ekbom A, Granath F. Thoracic aortic aneurysm and dissection: increasing prevalence and improved outcomes reported in a nationwide population-based study of more than 14,000 cases from 1987 to 2002. *Circulation*. Dec 12 2006;114(24):2611-2618.

7. Safi HJ, Miller CC 3rd, Subramaniam MH, et al. Thoracic and thoracoabdominal aortic aneurysm repair using cardiopulmonary bypass, profound hypothermia, and circulatory arrest via left side of the chest incision. *J Vasc Surg*. Oct 1998;28(4):591-598.

8. Cowan JA Jr, Dimick JB, Henke PK, Huber TS, Stanley JC, Upchurch GR Jr. Surgical treatment of intact thoracoabdominal aortic aneurysms in the United States: hospital and surgeon volume-related outcomes. *J Vasc Surg*. Jun 2003;37(6):1169-1174.

# 32 THORACIC ENDOVASCULAR ANEURYSM REPAIR

Joseph Habib, MD

## PATIENT STORY

A 72-year-old white man underwent a computed tomographic (CT) scan of the chest to evaluate a pulmonary nodule and incidentally found to have a 6-cm descending aortic aneurysm beginning distal to the subclavian artery and ending proximal to the celiac axis. The patient denied any chest or back pain. His past medical history was significant for hypertension, hyperlipidemia, and chronic obstructive pulmonary disease. He also relayed that his father died as a result of a ruptured aneurysm. Auscultation of the chest revealed distant lung sounds but otherwise his physical examination was unremarkable. Risks and benefits of open and endovascular repair of the aneurysm were discussed with the patient, and he elected to undergo endovascular repair.

This patient has a descending thoracic aortic aneurysm (TAA). Most patients are asymptomatic on presentation. The goal of aneurysm repair is to prevent death from rupture.

## EPIDEMIOLOGY

- Aortic disease is the 12th leading cause of death in the United States.[1]
- A descending aortic aneurysm is defined as a dilatation of the thoracic aorta to at least 1.5 times its normal diameter.[1]
- Descending thoracic aneurysms are less common than abdominal aortic aneurysms (AAAs).[1]
- Incidence is approximately 5.9 cases per 100,000 person-years.[1]
- Found mostly in the elderly with a male predominance.[1]

## ETIOLOGY AND PATHOPHYSIOLOGY

- Genetics, cellular imbalance, and altered hemodynamics are all factors involved in the development of a TAA.
- The loss and fragmentation of elastic fibers and smooth muscle cells within the aortic wall is referred to as medial degeneration. It is responsible for approximately 80% of thoracic aneurysms.[1]
- As people age, medial degeneration occurs, but it is accelerated by hypertension and atherosclerosis.[2] Patients with Marfan syndrome have accelerated medial degeneration.[3]
- Dissections, connective tissue disorders, autoimmune disorders, and infections are also responsible for the development of thoracic aneurysms.[1]

## DIAGNOSIS

Thoracic aneurysms are usually asymptomatic and often discovered incidentally during the workup for unrelated conditions.[1]

## LABORATORY TESTING

No laboratory test is currently available to detect the presence of a TAA. Serum chemistry including serum creatinine, complete blood count, and coagulation studies should be obtained in preparation for repair.

## IMAGING

- Computed tomography angiogram (CTA)—Chest or abdomen or pelvis is the primary modality utilized for preoperative planning; 64-slice CT provides excellent detailed imaging and can also be reconstructed for three-dimensional viewing.[4]
- Arteriography—used in conjunction with the CTA to help provide additional anatomic information; invasive; usually performed at time of repair[4] (Figure 32-1).
- Magnetic resonance angiogram (MRA)—may be used in place of the CTA in patients with severe allergies; no radiation risk[4] but contraindicated in those with renal failure secondary to nephrogenic systemic fibrosis.

## MANAGEMENT OR TREATMENT

- Medical management includes maintaining strict blood pressure control usually with beta-blockade, smoking cessation, and periodic imaging of the aneurysm to assess for growth.[1]
- Surgical repair is indicated for thoracic aneurysms greater than 6 cm in diameter and may be performed with either open or endovascular techniques—thoracic endovascular aneurysm repair (TEVAR).[1]

The first TEVAR was performed in 1994.[5] Three industry-supported trials comparing TEVAR to open surgical repair exist. These include the Gore TAG trial, the Cook TX2 trial, and the Medtronic VALOR trial. All three trials are nonrandomized but report lower mortality with TEVAR when compared with open repair. Cardiovascular and pulmonary complications and spinal cord injury were found to be less in the TEVAR group when compared to the open group.[4]

## PATIENT SELECTION

- Indications: Aneurysm should be greater than 6 cm in diameter or symptomatic.[4]
- Need at least 2-cm proximal and distal landing zones (attachment or fixation points within the aorta for the endovascular graft).[4]
- Usually need minimum iliac artery diameter of 8 mm.[4]
- Five landing zones of the thoracic aorta are[6]
  ○ Zone 0: origin of the innominate
  ○ Zone 1: origin of the left common carotid artery (CCA)

- Zone 2: origin of the left subclavian artery
- Zone 3: proximal descending thoracic aorta down to T4 vertebral body
- Zone 4: rest of the descending thoracic aorta

## DEVICE SELECTION

- Three devices currently exist:
  - GORE TAG: ePTFE/nitinol self-expanding stent that deploys from the middle of the graft toward each end[4] (Figure 32-2)
  - Medtronic Talent: Woven polyester fabric or self-expanding nitinol wire frame[4]
  - Cook Zenith TX2: Dacron or self-expanding stainless steel Z-stents[4] (Figure 32-3)
- Diameter is oversized by 10% to 20%.[4]
  - If the graft diameter is too small, it leads to endoleak and migration.
  - If the graft diameter is too large, it leads to folding of the graft.

## TECHNIQUE

- Access to the femoral vessels is obtained either percutaneously or by direct cut down.[4]
- Stiff wire and pigtail catheter are stationed in ascending aorta.[4]
- Angiogram is performed; left subclavian and celiac arteries are identified.[4]
- Proximal and distal landing zones are identified.[4]
  - Proximal graft should be landed in Zone 3 or 4.
  - Distal graft usually lands proximal to celiac.
- Selected graft is placed over stiff wire and into position and deployed.[4]
- Completion angiogram (Figure 32-3) is performed to assess for endoleaks (see later).
- Left subclavian may be covered to achieve adequate proximal landing zone.
- If covered, left subclavian should be revascularized either with carotid subclavian bypass or left subclavian transposition to minimize risk of stroke and spinal cord ischemia.[7]
- Celiac artery may be covered to extend distal landing zone if adequate collateral circulation exists through the superior mesenteric artery or gastroduodenal artery.[8]

## COMPLICATIONS

- Systemic complications—cardiopulmonary complications (15.6%),[4] renal failure or insufficiency
- Vascular complications—pseudoaneurysms, dissections, artery rupture, and hematomas (5%-10%) usually occur in the access vessels that are atherosclerotic and calcified[4]
- Neurologic complications—stroke (3%-5%) and spinal cord injury, paraplegia, or paraparesis (3%-6%)[4]
- Endoleaks—persistent blood flow within the aneurysm sac outside the lumen of the stent graft (4%-12%) at 1 year[4]
- Sac enlargement—persistent endoleaks may lead to sac enlargement (7%-14%) at 1 year[4]

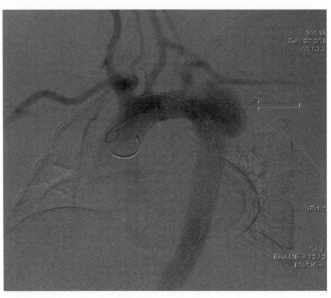

FIGURE 32-1 Arch angiogram in a patient with a descending thoracic aortic aneurysm (TAA). Red arrow indicates the descending TAA.

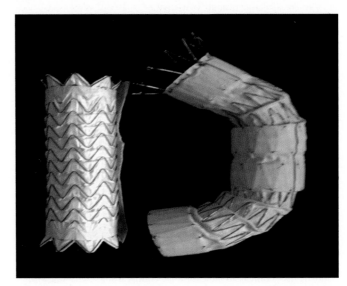

FIGURE 32-2 GORE TAG thoracic endograft (left) and Cook Zenith TX2 (right).

- Migration—stent graft may migrate proximally or distally (0%-30%)[4]

- Reinterventions—2.1% to 10.7%[4]

## FOLLOW-UP

- Scheduled follow-up with CT scans of the chest with and without intravenous (IV) contrast should be obtained at 1, 6, and 12 months during the first year.

- Annual CT scans should then be obtained for life to detect endoleaks and assess the graft.[4]

### PROVIDER RESOURCES

- http://www.uptodate.com/contents/thoracic-endovascular -aneurysm-repair
- http://www.ncbi.nlm.nih.gov/pubmed/20888533
- http://www.ncbi.nlm.nih.gov/pubmed/20888533

### PATIENT RESOURCES

- http://en.wikipedia.org/wiki/Endovascular_aneurysm_repair
- http://my.clevelandclinic.org/heart/disorders/aorta_marfan /endovascularaorticaneurysm.aspx

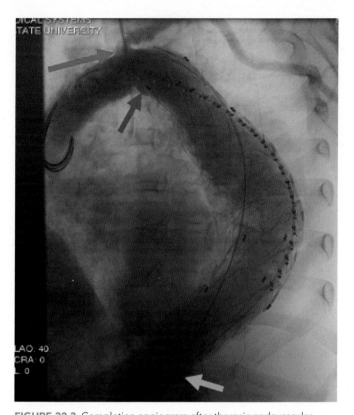

**FIGURE 32-3** Completion angiogram after thoracic endovascular aneurysm repair (TEVAR) of descending thoracic aortic aneurysm (TAA). Red arrow indicates the left subclavian artery. Blue arrow indicates the proximal fixation in descending thoracic aorta. Green arrow indicates the distal fixation point in the descending thoracic aorta.

## REFERENCES

1. Cho JS, Makaroun M. Thoracic and thoracoabdominal aneurysms: endovascular treatment. In: Cronenwett J, Johnston K, eds. *Rutherford's Vascular Surgery*. 7th ed. Philadelphia, PA: Elsevier; 2010:2054-2074.

2. Schlatmann TJ, Becker AE. Histologic changes in the normal aging aorta: implications for dissecting aortic aneurysm. *Am J Cardiol*. 1977;39:13-20.

3. Carlson RG, Lillehei CW, Edwards JE. Cystic medial necrosis of the ascending aorta in relation to age and hypertension. *Am J Cardiol*. 1970;25:411-415.

4. Mitchell RS, Ishimaru S, Ehrlich MP, et al. First International Summit on Thoracic Aortic Endografting: roundtable on thoracic aortic dissection as an indication for endografting. *J Endovasc Ther*. 2002;9(suppl 2):II98-II105.

5. Fairman RM, Farber M, Kwolek CJ, et al. Pivotal results of the Medtronic Vascular Talent Thoracic Stent Graft System for patients with thoracic aortic disease: the VALOR trial. *J Vasc Surg*. 2008;48:546-554.

6. Peterson BG, Eskandari MK, Gleason TG, Morasch MD. Utility of left subclavian artery revascularization in association with endoluminal repair of acute and chronic thoracic aortic pathology. *J Vasc Surg*. 2006;43:433-439.

7. Sunder-Plassmann L, Orend KH. Stent-grafting of the thoracic aorta—complications. *J Cardiovasc Surg (Torino)*. 2005;46: 121-130.

8. Dake MD, Miller DC, Semba CP, et al. Transluminal placement of endovascular stent-grafts for the treatment of descending thoracic aortic aneurysms. *N Engl J Med*. 1994;331:1729-1734.

# 33 FEMOROPOPLITEAL ANEURYSMS

NavYash Gupta, MD, FACS

## PATIENT STORY

A 76-year-old man presented to the emergency room (ER) with acute onset of coolness, pain, and pallor of the left lower extremity. The patient had a history of hypertension and hypercholesterolemia as well as tobacco use in the past. He denied a history of claudication and had no symptoms related to the right leg. Motor and sensory functions of the left foot were mildly diminished. Femoral pulses were palpable bilaterally, but there were no palpable or Doppler signals distally on the left side, and a prominent right popliteal pulse was noted. The patient was suspected to have an acutely thrombosed left popliteal artery aneurysm.

### EPIDEMIOLOGY

- Femoral and popliteal artery aneurysms are second only to aortic aneurysms in occurrence. Popliteal aneurysms account for over 70% of all peripheral aneurysms.

- Incidence increases with advancing age and is higher in males.

- Associated with arteriomegaly.

- Up to 50% of patients will be found to have an abdominal aortic aneurysm (AAA).

- Bilateral aneurysmal degeneration is common (Figure 33-1).

### ETIOLOGY

- Pathogenesis of these aneurysms is believed to be primarily atherosclerotic.

- Genetics and inflammation with enzymatic degradation of the elastin and collagen in the vessel wall are also believed to play a role.

- Rarely popliteal artery entrapment syndrome can result in repetitive trauma and subsequent development of a popliteal artery aneurysm.

### CLINICAL MANIFESTATIONS

- In an elderly patient, especially male, presenting to the ER with a sudden ischemic lower extremity, the diagnosis should be entertained; however, if the aneurysm is thrombosed a prominent popliteal pulse may not be appreciated on examination.

- Aneurysms of the femoral artery usually affect the common femoral artery but can rarely be isolated to the superficial femoral or profunda femoral arteries. Typically, femoral artery aneurysms are asymptomatic. Large femoral artery aneurysms can result in femoral vein compression and leg edema and pain or paresthesias caused by nerve compression. Although rupture is rare, thrombus within the aneurysm can result in distal embolization or thrombosis.

- With popliteal artery aneurysms, symptoms resulting from local compression and rupture are rare. Over 50% of patients with these aneurysms present with acute limb ischemia (Figure 33-2).[1,2]

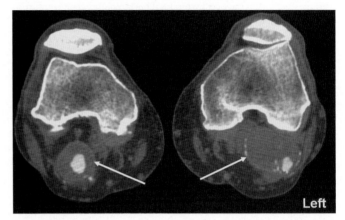

**FIGURE 33-1** Bilateral popliteal artery aneurysms (arrows), left larger than right.

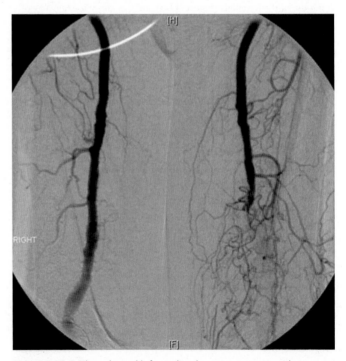

**FIGURE 33-2** Thrombosed left popliteal artery aneurysm with no outflow vessels identified.

- Occurrence of symptoms is correlated with size (>2 cm in diameter) and the presence of thrombus.

- Asymptomatic patients may have already had distal emboli that can progressively occlude the outflow tibial vessels but not necessarily result in acute ischemia.

- Symptoms of chronic ischemia include claudication and atheroemboli to the digits. Pain can occur from local nerve compression, rupture, or acute venous thrombosis, all of which are relatively rare.[2]

## DIAGNOSIS

- Diagnosis of these aneurysms can be made on physical examination, especially when the index of suspicion is high.

- Femoral aneurysms are more easily detected on physical examination, but can be missed.

- Small popliteal artery aneurysms are difficult to detect on physical examination alone.

- Duplex ultrasound is excellent for diagnosis of femoral and popliteal aneurysms, as well as for detecting thrombus and the status of the outflow vessels.[3]

- Computed tomography (CT) and magnetic resonance imaging (MRI) are useful in providing additional information to plan treatment; arteriography gives the most accurate information regarding the outflow vessels (Figure 33-3) and can allow for delivery of thrombolytic agents.

## DIFFERENTIAL DIAGNOSIS

- Acutely ischemic limb from atheroembolism—The most likely source of an arterial embolus to the extremity is cardiac. Often these patients will have no prior arterial insufficiency symptoms, and pulses in the contralateral extremity may be completely normal.

- Chronic peripheral arterial disease with stenosis and acute thrombosis of a chronically diseased and stenotic vessel—Usually, these patients will describe claudication symptoms prior to the acute event. Also, signs of chronic ischemia of the foot such as hypertrophied nails, loss of hair on the dorsum of the foot, and dry, scaly skin may be present.

- Acute thrombosis of a popliteal artery aneurysm—The patient may describe vague symptoms of knee discomfort or leg swelling, but usually has no chronic claudication symptoms. A prominent contralateral popliteal pulse should lead one to suspect a popliteal artery aneurysm. Atheroemboli to the digits of the feet can also occur from the thrombus inside the aneurysm cavity.

## TREATMENT OR MANAGEMENT

- Indications for repair include aneurysms over 2 cm in size in good-risk patients and smaller aneurysms containing a significant amount of thrombus.[4]

- Traditional repair of femoral artery aneurysms is based on the extent of the aneurysm, but typically involves either resection of the aneurysm and placement of a prosthetic interposition graft, or the "inlay" technique of placing the prosthetic graft on the inside of the aneurysm and then closing the sac over the graft.

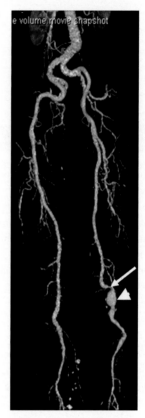

**FIGURE 33-3** Computed tomography (CT) angiogram showing large left popliteal artery aneurysm (arrow head); note stenosis of proximal popliteal artery and angulation of vessel (arrow).

- When the femoral bifurcation is involved, all attempts should be made to include preservation of flow to the profunda femoris artery.

- Popliteal artery aneurysms can be repaired via a medial approach with exclusion of the popliteal artery and bypass with saphenous vein conduit. A posterior approach provides adequate exposure when the popliteal aneurysm is limited to the popliteal space[5] (Figures 33-4 and 33-5). If the small saphenous vein is of adequate caliber, it can be harvested at the same time with the patient prone; however, if the conduit is the great saphenous vein, it is most easily harvested through a separate incision, either with the patient prone, or with the patient supine to start with. Prosthetic interposition grafting has also been used with this approach with almost equivalent patency.

- Endovascular repair of popliteal aneurysms is feasible using polytetrafluoroethylene (PTFE)-lined nitinol stent grafts; however, several early series reported an inferior patency rate compared to open repair. Some of this may be related to crossing the knee joint and movement with walking.

- Use of clopidogrel in the postoperative period may improve the success rate of endovascular treatment.[6]

- Patients presenting with thrombosed popliteal aneurysms usually undergo arteriography, and if a distal target vessel is identified then bypass is performed. If no tibial vessels are noted to be patent, thrombolysis to open up the tibial vessels followed by revascularization is the treatment of choice[7] (Figure 33-6). If the aneurysm is chronically thrombosed and the patient is asymptomatic, no urgent surgical treatment may be required.

## PATIENT EDUCATION

- Once the diagnosis has been established, the patient should be informed about the risks and benefits of various treatment modalities.

- In addition, the patient needs to understand the association with AAAs and the high likelihood of contralateral disease.

## FOLLOW-UP

- Follow-up is done with duplex imaging to assess the patency of the reconstruction. Imaging is generally done at regular intervals, more so in the first year after a bypass.

- Long-term follow-up is recommended to evaluate for aneurysmal degeneration of the native vessels or a vein bypass graft more than 5 years after the initial procedure.

### PATIENT AND PROVIDER RESOURCES

- http://www.vascularweb.org/vascularhealth/pages/peripheral-aneurysms.aspx
- http://emedicine.medscape.com/article/461910-overview#

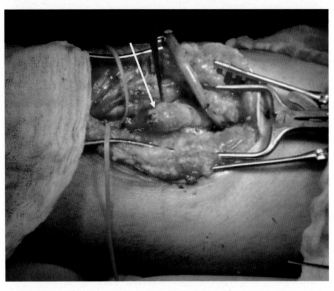

**FIGURE 33-4** Posterior approach to repair of popliteal artery aneurysm. Here the aneurysm (arrow) is being resected in preparation for a vein graft.

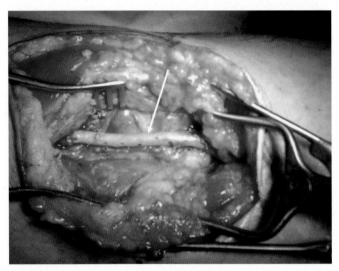

**FIGURE 33-5** Interposition vein graft (arrow) sewn in place via the posterior approach.

## REFERENCES

1. Shortell CK, DeWeese JA, Ouriel K, Green RM. Popliteal artery aneurysms: a 25-year experience. *J Vasc Surg*. 1991;14:771-776.

2. Dawson I, Sie RB, van Bockel JH. Atherosclerotic popliteal aneurysm. *Br J Surg*. 1997;84:293-299.

3. Diwan A, Sarkar R, Stanley JC, Zelenock GB, Wakefield TW. Incidence of femoral and popliteal aneurysms in patients with abdominal aortic aneurysms. *J Vasc Surg*. 2000;31:863-869.

4. Ascher E, Markevich N, Schutzer RW, Kallikuri S, Jacob T, Hingorani AP. Small popliteal artery aneurysms: are they clinically significant? *J Vasc Surg*. 2003;37:755-760.

5. Beseth BD, Moore WS. The posterior approach for repair of popliteal artery aneurysms. *J Vasc Surg*. 2006;43:940-945.

6. Tielliu IF, Verhoeven ELG, Zeebregts CJ, Prins TR, Span MM, van den Dungen JJ. Endovascular treatment of popliteal artery aneurysms: results of a prospective cohort study. *J Vasc Surg*. 2005;41:561-567.

7. Carpenter JP, Barker CF, Roberts B, Berkowitz HD, Lusk EJ, Perloff LJ. Popliteal artery aneurysms: current management and outcome. *J Vasc Surg*. 1994;19:65-72.

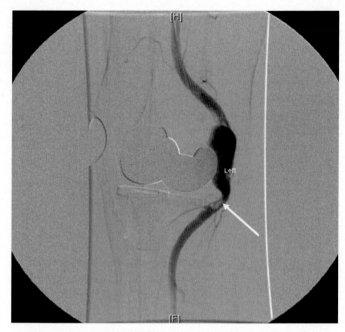

**FIGURE 33-6** Angiogram post-thrombolysis of left popliteal artery aneurysm; note the small amount of residual thrombus in the below-knee popliteal artery (arrow).

# 34 ARTERIAL PSEUDOANEURYSMS

Benjamin J. Aumiller, MS, MD
Raghu L. Motaganahalli, MD, FRCS, FACS

## PATIENT STORY

A 70-year-old obese man underwent cardiac catheterization for coronary stenting. He received dual antiplatelet therapy with the use of glycoprotein inhibitors during the intervention. He presented a week later to his cardiologist with increasing painful groin swelling. He underwent a duplex examination of the groin that demonstrated a pseudoaneurysm (PSA) measuring approximately 4 cm with a long narrow neck and a "Yin-Yang" or "to-and-fro" sign (Figure 34-1A). Doppler evaluation of the neck of the aneurysm demonstrated arterial waveforms (Figure 34-1B).

He was treated with percutaneous ultrasound-guided thrombin injection (UGTI) into PSA sac that led to resolution of his symptoms with occlusion of flow into aneurysm sac (Figure 34-1C).

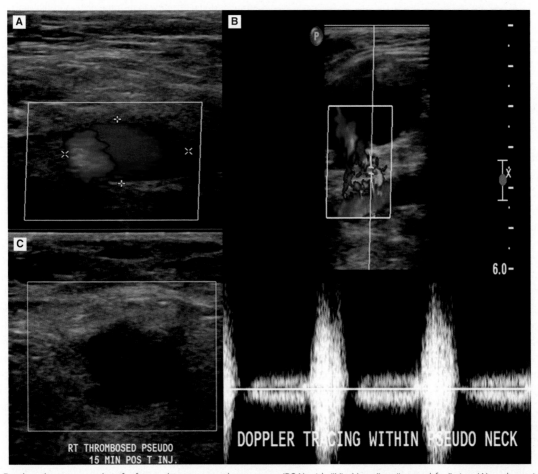

**FIGURE 34-1** Duplex ultrasonography of a femoral artery pseudoaneurysm (PSA) with "Yin-Yang" or "to-and-fro" sign (A) and arterial waveforms on Doppler interrogation of the neck of the PSA (B). Thrombosed aneurysm sac after injection of thrombin (C).

## PATHOPHYSIOLOGY

A true aneurysm of the arterial system involves all the three layers of an artery while PSAs do not involve all the three layers. It is simply a pulsatile hematoma with active extravasation of blood around the arterial wall. The hematoma may tamponade the bleeding artery allowing a spontaneous closure of the PSA sac. Alternatively, it may form a well-organized fibrous capsule with persistent flow maintained at the center of the sac via a neck communicating with the arterial lumen.[1] A PSA may expand, rupture, lead to distal embolization, or cause arterial compression with resultant ischemia.

## EPIDEMIOLOGY

- Femoral artery PSAs are the most common complication resulting after percutaneous procedures.
- The incidence has been reported between 0.5% and 9% of all interventional procedures.[2]
- Other causes include various surgical interventions as well as blunt and penetrating trauma.[3-5]

## RISK FACTORS OR ETIOLOGY

There is a steadily increasing frequency of PSAs due to increased number of percutaneous interventions.[1]

Factors that increase the likelihood for a PSA include

- Large sheath size
- Interventional procedures compared to diagnostic evaluation that require large caliber sheath access
- Poor technique (low or high femoral artery puncture)
- Obesity and significantly calcific arteries
- Need for anticoagulation
- Female gender
- Chronic renal failure requiring hemodialysis[6-8]

## CLINICAL FEATURES

- Symptoms: Painful pulsatile mass is the common presentation. Continued expansion may lead to ecchymosis, cutaneous ischemia, and skin necrosis. Expansion may lead to compression of surrounding femoral nerve, weakness of hip flexion, swelling due to femoral vein compression. Distal embolization and acute limb ischemia are rare but not uncommon. Rupture can lead to cardiovascular collapse and death. Patients can have a large retroperitoneal bleed without any swelling in the groin due to high femoral arterial puncture.
- Signs: Physical examination may elicit tenderness, a thrill or a pulsatile mass. Additionally, a bruit may also be auscultated if there is a coexistent arteriovenous fistula. Peripheral pulses should be assessed and ankle-brachial indices (ABIs) obtained to ensure that there is no distal embolization.

## NATURAL HISTORY

- More than 50% of PSAs will regress spontaneously with reports up to 89% spontaneous closure rate in PSAs less than 3 cm. Thus, it may be advisable to treat small, nonenlarging PSAs in hemodynamically stable patients with no laboratory evidence of hemorrhage with observation.

- Observation requires strict compliance and frequent follow-up testing places a financial burden on the patient.[1,2]
- Patients who have ongoing blood loss, continued expansion, patients who are on anticoagulation, aneurysms that do not regress with 2 months of expectant treatment will benefit from either surgical or percutaneous intervention to occlude flow into aneurysm sac.[9]

## PREVENTION

- Routine use of duplex ultrasonography or fluoroscopic guidance should be encouraged while obtaining arterial access.
- Femoral arterial access should be obtained in the segment of artery that overlies the femoral head. This will ensure the ability to compress the artery against the head of the femur to obtain adequate hemostasis. A high puncture will likely result in a large retroperitoneal bleed without any groin hematoma. A low puncture usually results in injury to the profunda femoris artery, superficial femoral artery, and leads to PSA that cannot be well compressed.
- A large sheath access (beyond 6 F) in upper extremities should be done with planned surgical exposure of the artery so that the arteriotomy can be repaired under direct vision.

## DIAGNOSIS

Imaging modalities for PSAs include duplex ultrasonography (DUS) with a sensitivity of 94% to 97%. Duplex ultrasound will demonstrate a to-and-fro flow (Yin-Yang or to-and-fro sign) between the aneurysm sac and the femoral artery. An adequate examination will include the dimensions, description of sac and the neck as this will guide further treatment. The proximal and distal arteries should also be evaluated for thrombus extruding from the aneurysm sac. Large hematomas or difficult anatomy may necessitate further imaging such as computed tomographic (CT) angiography.[1,2]

## TREATMENT

- Options include
  - Open surgical repair
  - Ultrasound-guided compression (UGC)
  - Ultrasound-guided thrombin injection (UGTI)
  - Coil embolization
  - Covered stent placement
- Surgical repair of PSA is an option when PSA cannot be repaired with a minimally invasive approach such as when there is extensive skin necrosis requiring inguinal decompression and debridement or due to an associated arteriovenous fistula. Surgical repair should also be considered when there is ongoing hemodynamic instability or limb-threatening ischemia and involves obtaining arterial control both proximal and distal to the aneurysm with evacuation of the hematoma and primary repair of the arterial defect. Patients with hemorrhagic shock should have exploration of hematoma with direct digital compression of the bleeding site followed by with vascular control.[1,2]
- A retroperitoneal incision maybe required for obtaining external iliac artery exposure in large PSAs of the groin. If the femoral artery cannot be repaired primarily then a vein graft should be used

to reconstruct the arterial system. Complications of surgical repair include infection, seroma formation, and delayed discharge from the hospital. Death is unusual except in circumstances of shock.

- UGC utilizes the ultrasound transducer to visualize the neck of the PSA and apply pressure until it is occluded. Studies have shown procedural success ranging between 74% and 90% as well as demonstrating its cost-effectiveness.[10] Care is taken to avoid compression of the femoral artery. UGC is successful when PSAs are less than 2 cm. Anticoagulation has also been negatively linked to success of the procedure. If flow is demonstrated in the sac beyond 1 hour of compression then alternate mode of therapy should be considered. Complications of compression include rupture, especially above the inguinal ligament. PSAs located above the inguinal ligament are contraindicated due to the risk of uncontrollable bleeding. Other contraindications include anastomotic PSA, thrombosis resulting in distal ischemia or ischemia of the overlying skin, and infection. Long procedure times, patient and technician fatigue, patient discomfort, and availability of more successful treatment modalities have led to this technique falling out of favor.

- UGTI is a minimally invasive procedure that involves injecting thrombin into the PSA sac with ultrasound guidance.[10] Ideally patients considered for UGTI should have a well-visualized neck that should be fairly long, and narrow. However, patients who have a wide neck, short neck, nonvisualized neck are at a risk for complications of thrombin injection[11] and should be carefully selected for this procedure. Using B-mode imaging, a spinal needle (22-25 gauges) is inserted into the PSA sac. While visualizing the needle throughout the procedure (to avoid accidental thrombin injection into the arterial system) approximately 100 to 1000 U/mL of thrombin is injected into the sac at approximately 0.1 mL increments until thrombosis is achieved. Color-flow imaging is used while injecting thrombin to demonstrate successful closure of the sac. Several series have reported success rates between 93% and 100%. UGTI is the procedure of choice in patients who are on anticoagulation.[12,13] Meta-analysis has suggested superiority of UGTI over UGC.[14]

Complications include the risk of skin necrosis, femoral vein thrombosis or, embolization into the arterial system in up to 2% cases. A postinjection duplex scan should demonstrate no flow in the sac.

- Additional modes of minimally invasive treatments include endovascular techniques such as coil embolization [15] (Figure 34-2A and B) and covered stent deployment[16] (Figure 34-3A and B). Indications differ depending on the anatomy. Risks of endovascular approaches include failure of treatment as well as additional PSA formation.

## PATIENT EDUCATION

- If no intervention is planned for a small PSA, the patient and family must be informed of the activity level permissible, travel restrictions and symptoms and signs of expansion. A proper plan for follow-up ultrasound and examination must be outlined.

## REFERENCES

1. Ahmad F, Turner SA, Torrie P, Gibson M. Iatrogenic femoral artery pseudoaneurysms—a review of current methods of diagnosis and treatment. *Clin Radiol.* Dec 2008;63(12):1310-1316.

2. Patrick AS, Ali FA, Sarah KF, et al. Femoral pseudoaneurysms. *Vasc Endovascular Surg.* 2006;40(2):109-116.

3. Megalopoulos A, Siminas S, Trelopoulos G. Traumatic pseudoaneurysm of the popliteal artery after blunt trauma: case report and a review of the literature. *Vasc Endovascular Surg.* Dec 2006-Jan 2007;40(6):499-504.

4. Sloan K, Mofidi R, Nagy J, Flett MM, Chakraverty S. Endovascular treatment for traumatic popliteal artery pseudoaneurysms after knee arthroplasty. *Vasc Endovascular Surg.* Jun-Jul 2009;43(3):286-290.

5. Barman P, Farber A. Traumatic pseudoaneurysm of the visceral aortic segment managed using both open surgery and endovascular therapy. *Ann Vasc Surg.* Aug 2011;25(6):840.

6. Lumsden AB, Miller JM, Kosinski AS, et al. A prospective evaluation of surgically treated groin complications following percutaneous cardiac procedures. *Am Surg.* 1994;60:132-137.

7. Katzenschlager R, Ugurluoglu A, Ahmadi A, et al. Incidence of pseudoaneurysm after diagnostic and therapeutic angiography. *Radiology.* 1995;195:463-466.

8. McCann RL, Schwartz LB, Pieper KS. Vascular complications of cardiac catheterization. *J Vasc Surg.* 1991;14:375-381.

9. Kent KC, McArdle CR, Kennedy B, et al. A prospective study of the clinical outcome of femoral pseudoaneurysms and arteriovenous fistulas induced by arterial puncture. *J Vasc Surg.* 1993;17:125-131.

10. Fellmeth BD, Roberts AC, Bookstein JJ, et al. Postangiographic femoral artery injuries: nonsurgical repair with ultrasound guided compression. *Radiology.* 1991;178:671-675.

11. Cope C, Zeit R. Coagulation of aneurysms by direct percutaneous thrombin injection. *AJR Am J Roentgenol.* 1986;147:383-387.

12. Morrison SL, Obrand DA, Steinmetz OK, Montreuil B. Treatment of femoral artery pseudoaneurysms with percutaneous thrombin injection. *Ann Vasc Surg.* 2000;14:634-639.

13. Sheiman RG, Brophy DP. Treatment of iatrogenic femoral pseudoaneurysms with percutaneous thrombin injection: experience in 54 patients. *Radiology.* 2001;219:123-127.

14. Tisi PV, Callam MJ. Surgery versus non-surgical treatment for femoral pseudoaneurysms. *Cochrane Database Syst Rev.* 2006;1:CD004981.

15. Abisi S, Chick C, Williams I, Hill S, Gordon A. Endovascular coil embolization for large femoral false aneurysms: two case reports. *Vasc Endovascular Surg.* Oct-Nov 2006;40(5):414-417.

16. Criado E, Marston WA, Ligush J, et al. Endovascular repair of peripheral aneurysms, pseudoaneurysms, and arteriovenous fistulas. *Ann Vasc Surg.* May 1997;11(3):256-263.

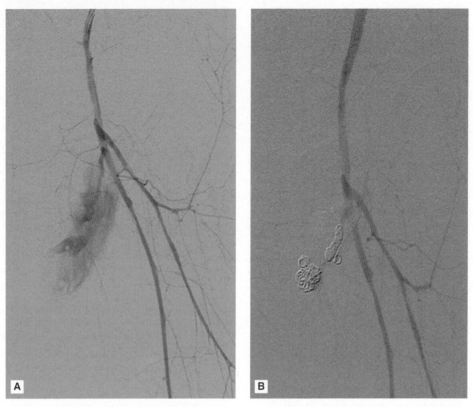

**FIGURE 34-2** A large pseudoaneurysm arising from superficial femoral artery (A) that was treated with coil embolization (B).

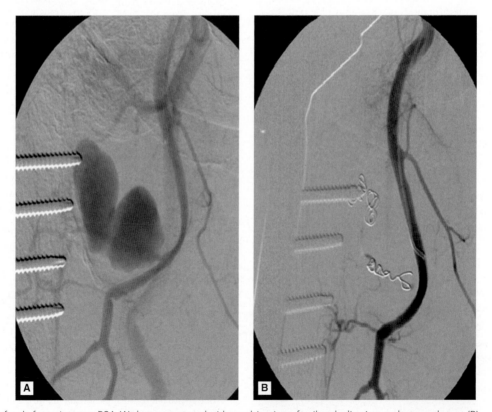

**FIGURE 34-3** A Profunda femoris artery PSA (A) that was treated with combination of coil embolization and covered stent (B).

# 35 MYCOTIC ANEURYSMAL DISEASE

Jean Starr, MD, FACS, RPVI

## PATIENT STORY

A 36-year-old man was admitted to the hospital with signs and symptoms of sepsis. He had a history of intravenous drug abuse as well as hepatitis B and C. He was discovered to have a left forearm abscess at an intravenous drug access site, as well as septic arthritis of the left hip with methicillin-resistant *Staphylococcus aureus* (MRSA) bacteremia.

He underwent incision and drainage of the left hip and conservative management of the left forearm. A computed tomographic arteriogram (CTA) of the abdomen for abdominal pain showed inflammation around the distal abdominal aorta consistent with aortitis (Figure 35-1). Although his clinical course improved, his abdominal pain persisted and a repeat CTA 1 week later showed a large false aneurysm of the distal aorta (Figure 35-2).

Options were discussed and he underwent successful endovascular repair of the aorta (Figures 35-3 and 35-4) and was discharged eventually on long-term antibiotics.

### EPIDEMIOLOGY

- Infectious aortitis represents a rare etiology of aortic aneurysm with one of the largest reviews revealing that 2.8% of 673 consecutive abdominal aortic aneurysm (AAA) patients presented with infectious aortitis as the etiology, including locations in the thoracic and abdominal aortas.[1]

- The disease is significantly more devastating than traditional aneurysmal disease with a large proportion of patients with a mycotic aneurysm (19%-48%) presenting for the first time with rupture.[1-3]

### ETIOLOGY OR PATHOPHYSIOLOGY

- The term *mycotic* is actually a misnomer for infectious aortitis since most aortic infections are not secondary to a fungal pathogen. Many organisms have been implicated with *S aureus* being the most common.

- Others include *Streptococcus pneumoniae*, *Listeria monocytogenes*, *Pseudomonas aeruginosa*, *Morganella morganii*, *Pasteurella multocida*, and *Salmonella* species.[4-9]

- Infections in native vessels are most commonly the result of seeding from a remote source or infections in an immunocompromised host. Infections also occur in previously placed prosthetic grafts, but this is a different disease entity and not the subject of this chapter.

### DIAGNOSIS

#### Clinical Features

- The diagnosis of infectious aortitis is often made late, adding to the complexities and hazards of treating the disease.

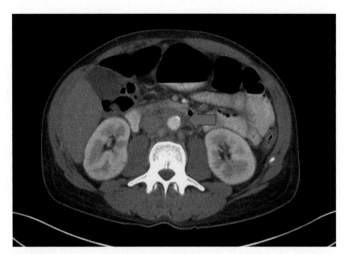

**FIGURE 35-1** Computed tomographic (CT) scan with periaortic inflammation consistent with aortitis (blue arrow).

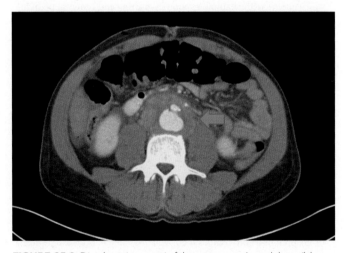

**FIGURE 35-2** Distal aortic mycotic false aneurysm 1 week later (blue arrow).

- Patients may be younger and have evidence of remote infection or even a systemic infectious process.

- The hosts may be immunocompromised from various causes, including cancer.

- Initial signs and symptoms may be cryptogenic and include vague abdominal or back pain, nonspecific fevers, elevated white count, and sepsis of unknown etiology. A high index of suspicion is necessary so that treatment can be rendered as early as is feasible.[5]

## RADIOGRAPHIC STUDIES

- Typically, the most common radiographic study obtained to evaluate a source of abdominal infection is a contrasted CT scan.

- Early in the disease process, inflammation around a normal sized aorta may be the only evidence of aortitis.

- As the disease progresses, one may see development of an aortic aneurysm and subsequent rapid enlargement (within days to weeks). The aneurysm may have an unusual configuration if a pseudoaneurysm (PSA) has developed.

## MANAGEMENT OR INTERVENTION OPTIONS

- Conservative management of this disease process typically results in death.

- No standard operative treatment option for patients with infectious aortitis exists. More traditional approaches include in situ graft replacement with rifampicin-bonded grafting and omental pedicle closure,[3] extra-anatomic bypass with aortic debridement,[4] and in situ graft replacement with cryopreserved arterial homograft.[2]

- More modern approaches to complex vascular diseases include endovascular management. Endovascular aneurysm repair for mycotic aneurysmal disease has been reported more frequently as an alternative strategy to open methods with reasonable early (5%) and late (11%) mortality.[10,11]

- The infectious process may involve the visceral segment of the abdominal aorta, usually resulting in worse outcomes. New techniques and experience with visceral debranching may offer better options to patients with a more extensive aortic disease process.[12]

## COMPLICATIONS

- In-hospital mortality ranges from 9% to 23%.[1,2,4] Still, a significant number (23%) are reported to die soon after discharge.[1] Reinfection rates during follow-up range from 0% to 8%.[1,2,4]

## PATIENT EDUCATION AND FOLLOW-UP

- Patients may be advised to remain on long-term suppressive antibiotic therapy, although recommended length of time has not been established. They should be educated as to the warning signs for recurrent infection.

- Imaging studies every 6 to 12 months may help to monitor for recurrent infection, PSAs, or other complications, depending on the type of repair.

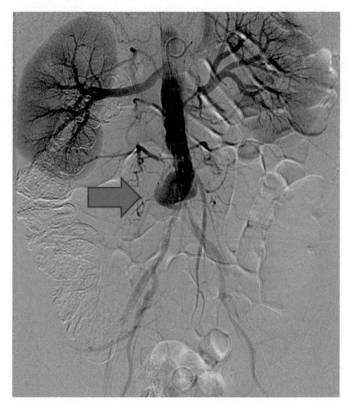

FIGURE 35-3 Aortogram demonstrating distal aortic false aneurysm (blue arrow) and involvement of the iliac vessels.

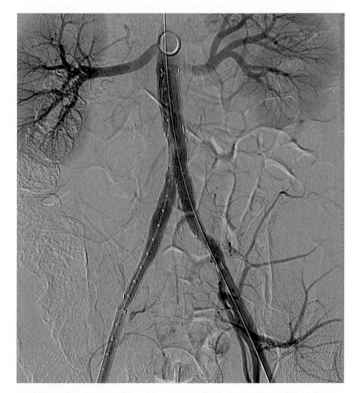

FIGURE 35-4 Successful aortic endograft placement, resolving the false aneurysm.

## REFERENCES

1. Dubois M, Daenens K, Houthoofd S, Peetermans WE, Fourneau I. Treatment of mycotic aneurysms with involvement of the abdominal aorta: single-centre experience in 44 consecutive cases. *Eur J Vasc Endovasc Surg.* Oct 2010;40(4):450-456.

2. Bisdas T, Bredt M, Pichlmaier M, et al. Eight-year experience with cryopreserved arterial homografts for the in situ reconstruction of abdominal aortic infections. *J Vasc Surg.* Aug 2010;52(2):323-330.

3. Uchida N, Katayama A, Tamura K, Miwa S, Masatsugu K, Sueda T. In situ replacement for mycotic aneurysms on the thoracic and abdominal aorta using rifampicin-bonded grafting and omental pedicle grafting. *Ann Thorac Surg.* Feb 2012;93(2):438-442.

4. Yu SY, Hsieh HC, Ko PJ, Huang YK, Chu JJ, Lee CH. Surgical outcome for mycotic aortic and iliac anuerysm. *World J Surg.* Jul 2011;35(7):1671-1678.

5. Cartery C, Astudillo L, Deelchand A, et al. Abdominal infectious aortitis caused by *Streptococcus pneumoniae*: a case report and literature review. *Ann Vasc Surg.* Feb 2011; 25(2):266.e9-e16.

6. Bal A, Schönleben F, Agaimy A, Gessner A, Lang W. *Listeria monocytogenes* as a rare cause of mycotic aortic aneurysm. *J Vasc Surg.* Aug 2010;52(2):456-459.

7. Kwon OY, Lee JS, Choi HS, Hong HP, Ko YG. Infected abdominal aortic aneurysm due to *Morganella morganii*: CT findings. *Abdom Imaging.* Feb 2011;36(1):83-85.

8. Koelemay MJ. *Pasteurella multocida* infection, a rare cause of mycotic abdominal aortic aneurysm. *J Vasc Surg.* Dec 2009;50(6): 1496-1498.

9. Dick J, Tiwari A, Menon J, Hamilton G. Abdominal aortic aneurysm secondary to infection with *Pseudomonas aeruginosa*: a rare cause of mycotic aneurysm. *Ann Vasc Surg.* Jul 2010;24(5): 692.e1-e4.

10. Kan CD, Lee HL, Luo CY, Yang YJ. The efficacy of aortic stent grafts in the management of mycotic abdominal aortic aneurysm— institute case management with systemic literature comparison. *Ann Vasc Surg.* May 2010;24(4):433-440.

11. Clough RE, Black SA, Lyons OT, et al. Is endovascular repair of mycotic aortic aneurysms a durable treatment option? *Eur J Vasc Endovasc Surg.* Apr 2009;37(4):407-412.

12. Soule M, Javerliat I, Rouanet A, Long A, Lermusiaux P. Visceral debranching and aortic endoprosthesis for a suspected mycotic pseudoaneurysm of the abdominal aorta involving visceral arteries. *Ann Vasc Surg.* Aug 2010;24(6):825.e13-e16.

# 36 VASCULAR EHLERS-DANLOS SYNDROME

Angela H. Martin, MD
Raghu Motaganahalli, MD, FRCS, FACS

## PATIENT STORY

A 23-year-old woman was seen in a vascular surgery clinic for a pulsatile mass over the calf for a few weeks' duration. She recollected sustaining a minor injury while she was horse riding. She also had a history of easy bruisability. Her brother also has similar history of skin bruising with hypermobile joints and thin skin.

Further investigation suggested a pseudoaneurysm arising from the anterior tibial artery (Figure 36-1A). She was treated with retrograde coil embolization of the anterior tibial artery (Figure 36-1B) via a direct exposure of the artery at the ankle. The arteriotomy site was closed with pledgeted sutures. She did well in the postoperative period without any complications. Additional investigation with skin biopsy and collagen electrophoresis analysis that suggested a vascular Ehlers-Danlos syndrome (EDS). She was treated with vitamin C supplements and advised to avoid contact sports and of the need for continued follow-up.

## EPIDEMIOLOGY

- Heterogeneous group of inherited connective tissue disorders.

- Six main forms of EDS identified with several rare variants.[1]

- Majority are autosomal dominant inheritance; some less common forms are autosomal recessive or sex linked.[2]

- Prevalence of 1/10,000 to 1/25,000.[3]

- The vascular (AKA type IV or ecchymotic variant) accounts for 5% to 10% of all cases of EDS with a prevalence of less than 1/100,000 overall.[3,4]

- The vascular form has the worst prognosis of all forms of EDS with median age of death at 48 years.[2]

## PATHOPHYSIOLOGY

- Genetic defects cause mutations in collagen synthesis.[2]

- Vascular EDS is associated with type III procollagen deficiencies due to mutations in the COL3A1 gene, resulting in structural defects in the proalpha 1 (proα1) chain of type III collagen[5,6] that leads to extreme vascular fragility.

- The abnormal collagen III molecule cannot fold stably into a triple helix, and is degraded slowly in the rough endoplasmic reticulum of the fibroblast and is never secreted extracellularly. This instability or nonsecretion of mutant protein has been referred to as protein suicide.[7]

- Incomplete penetrance and varying expressivity lead to variations in clinical presentation and symptoms.[5]

- There is a diffuse thinning of the media with reduced elastin and fragmented internal elastic membranes in vessels.[3]

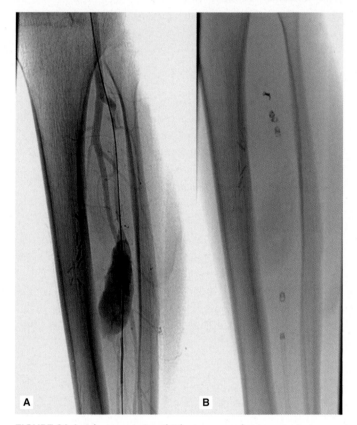

A B

**FIGURE 36-1** A large anterior tibial artery pseudoaneurysm in a 23-year-old patient with minimal trauma (A) that was treated with retrograde coil embolization. (*Courtesy of Dr. Gary Lemmon and Michael C Dalsing, Indiana University School of Medicine, Indianapolis, IN*).

- Patients with EDS have only a quarter of normal skin thickness so it appears translucent and reveals a network of subcutaneous veins, which is one of the major criterion of affected individuals.

- Vessels have reduced collagen fibril cross-sectional area in the media of the vessel wall as well as reduced collagen content.

## FORMS OF EDS

- Classical type associated with skin hyperextensibility, joint hypermobility, and skin scarring.[2,6]

- Hypermobility type is the most common form and is associated with smooth, velvety skin; joint hypermobility; easy bruising; and frequent inguinal hernias.[2,6]

- Vascular type is associated with acrogeria, lobeless ears, and thin, translucent skin in addition to spontaneous arterial and uterine or hollow viscus ruptures.[2,6]

- Less common variants include kyphoscoliosis (associated with scleral fragility, joint laxity, and marfanoid habitus), arthrochalasia (congenital bilateral hip dislocation and joint hyper mobility), dermatosparaxis (doughy redundant skin with large umbilical hernias, blue sclera, dwarfism, and severe skin fragility), and several rarer forms.[2,3,6]

## CLINICAL MANIFESTATIONS OF VASCULAR EDS

- A newborn may present with lobeless ears, bulging eyes with telangiectasia on the eyelids, or spontaneous pneumothorax.[2]

- In pregnancy, uncontrolled uterine hemorrhage necessitating hysterectomy is common. There is a 12% peripartum mortality due to arterial or uterine rupture.[2] Maternal mortality is approximately 25% with each pregnancy.[5]

- Skin changes include easy and extensive bruising with translucent skin and prominent superficial veins. Joint hypermobility and skin elasticity are not always present.

- Spontaneous colon rupture can occur and is usually of the sigmoid colon.[4] Only 16% have a diagnosis of EDS prior to a major vascular catastrophe[4]; 80% have a major complication of EDS by the age 40[8] (Figure 36-2).

- Spontaneous arterial rupture is most common in the abdomen from the splenic or renal arteries rather than the aorta[6] (Figure 36-2).

- Average age of arterial rupture is 23 years.[2]

- In addition to spontaneous arterial rupture, individuals can develop multiple aneurysms, arteriovenous (AV) fistulae, and aortic dissection[6] (Figure 36-3A and B).

- Aneurysm formation is most commonly seen in the visceral, carotid, and aortic arteries.

- AV fistulae are most common at the carotid-cavernous site.

## DIAGNOSTIC CRITERIA FOR VASCULAR EDS

Presence of two or more major criteria is diagnostic of vascular EDS.

- Major criteria: (1) thin and translucent skin; (2) arterial, uterine, or intestine fragility or rupture; (3) easy bruising; (4) characteristic facial appearance—thin nose, thin lips, hollow cheeks

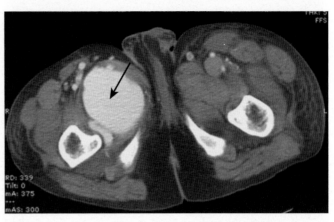

**FIGURE 36-2** A large obturator artery aneurysm (black arrow) in a 40-year-old man with vascular Ehlers-Danlos syndrome (EDS).

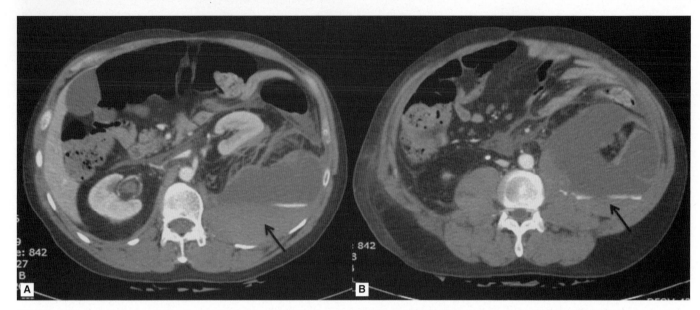

**FIGURE 36-3** Spontaneous retroperitoneal hematoma (arrows) in a patient with vascular Ehlers-Danlos syndrome (EDS) with abdominal compartment syndrome required decompression laparotomy and retroperitoneal packing.

- Minor criteria: acrogeria (taut, thin skin), joint hypermobility, tendon or muscle rupture, club foot, early onset of varicose veins, AV fistula, pneumothorax, gingival recession, family history of sudden death

## DIAGNOSIS OF VASCULAR EDS

- Skin biopsy for collagen analysis revealing abnormal electrophoretic mobility.[2]

- Sodium dodecyl sulphate–polyacrylamide gel electrophoresis (SDS–PAGE) of fibroblast cultures from skin identifies nearly all individuals with a defect in type III collagen. It can detect quantitative and qualitative defects[6]. (Figure 36-4).

- Sequence analysis testing of mutations for genetic counseling.[2]

- Family history of sudden death of a close relative in an individual with suspicion for EDS warrants further investigation.

- Coagulation studies, clotting factors, platelet counts, and bleeding times are typically normal.[6]

## DIFFERENTIAL DIAGNOSIS OF VASCULAR EDS

- Marfan syndrome—defect in fibrillin-1, presents with marfanoid body habitus, lens dislocation, aortic dilatation or dissection, mitral valve prolapsed without increased fragility of smaller arteries and veins.[6]

- Loeys-Dietz syndrome is an autosomal dominant syndrome similar to Marfan syndrome with widely spaced eyes, cleft palate or a bifid uvula, and arterial aneurysms and dissections.[9,10]

- Severe bruising in children often leads to a thorough evaluation for hematologic disorders and child abuse.

## MEDICAL THERAPY

- Avoid contact sports and weight lifting, and wear protective pads to avoid excessive bruising.

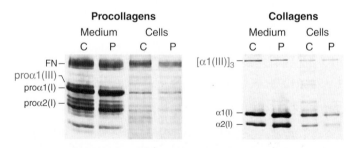

**FIGURE 36-4** Sodium dodecyl sulphate–polyacrylamide gel electrophoresis (SDS–PAGE) collagen screening gel showing diminished amount of proalpha 1 (proα1) chain of type III collagen and relative increase in type III collagen in the cell layer. C, control; P, patient with vascular EDS. (*Courtesy of Dr. Peter Byers, University of Washington, Seattle, WA.*)

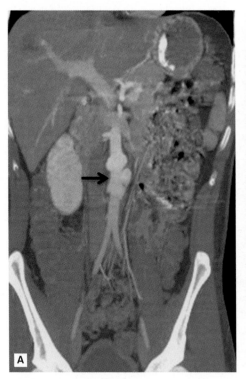 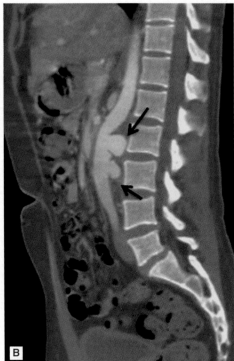 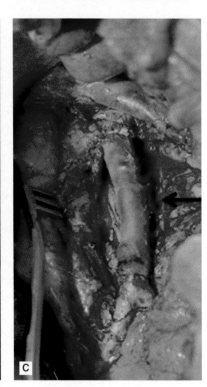

**FIGURE 36-5** Infrarenal aortic aneurysm (A, B—black arrows) in a 29-year-old patient treated with open repair using femoral vein graft (C).

- Vasopressin (DDAVP) can be given to normalize bleeding time via stimulation of von Willebrand factor release if having epistaxis or uncontrolled bruising, or prior to procedures.[4,6]

- Ascorbic acid supplementation can help collagen fibril cross-linking, leading to decreased bruising.[6]

- Avoid medications that inhibit platelet function (NSAIDs, aspirin, clopidogrel, penicillins, cephalosporins).[6]

- Prophylactic management of blood pressure to keep systolic less than 120 mm Hg and atherosclerotic disease at a minimum is advised.[10]

- The beta-blocker celiprolol in a randomized controlled trial was shown to decrease the rate of spontaneous arterial rupture three fold over a period of 47 months independent of any change in blood pressure or heart rate.[10]

- Initial imaging includes echocardiogram, carotid ultrasound, and noninvasive imaging of the chest and abdomen.[8]

- Suggested follow-up for asymptomatic patients includes annual physical examination, carotid ultrasound, and noninvasive imaging of the chest and abdomen. If a patient has developed symptoms he or she needs closer follow-up every 3 to 6 months with imaging.[8]

- Genetic counseling is mandatory. Vascular-type EDS is inherited in an autosomal dominant fashion, so the child of an affected parent has a 50% likelihood of inheriting EDS.

## SURGICAL CONSIDERATIONS

- Avoid diagnostic angiography or other invasive testing as lethal hemorrhage can occur. Arteriography is associated with a 22% to 67% complication rate and 5% to 16% mortality.[4,10,12] Recent reports suggest access site complications of less than 2% for endovascular procedures (combined diagnostic or interventions in both arterial and venous systems).[13]

- If angiography is required then it should be performed with vessel exposure so as to repair the vessel directly.

- Anesthetic considerations should include avoiding central venous lines, placing arterial lines, intramuscular injections, cross-matching adequate blood, and gentle intubation.

- Surgical intervention should be avoided unless absolutely warranted. When intervention is necessary for ruptured pseudoaneurysms, visceral artery aneurysms, and carotid-cavernous fistulas, endovascular coil embolization should be the initial treatment of choice. Successful embolization of aortic branch vessels has been reported.[10]

- When feasible a transvenous access approach is associated with fewer complications. Open closure of approach sites should be performed to lessen the risks from the access site.

- Stent grafting is contraindicated in connective tissue disorders[10] due to long-term durability concerns as well as threat to fixation zones in the setting of chronic outward radial force as this may increase the frequency of secondary interventions.

- Uncontrollable hemorrhage can occur with gentle placement of vascular clamps. Vascular occlusion, when possible, should be accomplished with tourniquets.[4] When not possible, shodded or soft-jawed vascular clamps should be used.[12]

- The surgical treatment of choice for vascular lesions is ligation with reconstruction offered only when essential and when the risks are carefully explained to the patient (Figure 36-5A, B and C). Ligation should be performed even when sacrifice of a limb or nonessential organ will result.[4]

- Reinforcement of sutures and ligation sites is essential. A cuff of polytetrafluoroethylene or comparable material should be placed over all anastomoses.[4]

- Mortality from a vascular rupture is 44% prior to surgical intervention, and another 19% do not survive the operation and immediate postoperative course. Mortality from a hollow viscus rupture is 20%.[4]

## PROVIDER RESOURCES

- http://www.ncbi.nlm.nih.gov/pubmed/19879095
- http://www.jvascsurg.org/article/S0741-5214(07)00522-8 /abstract

## PATIENT RESOURCES

- www.ednf.org
- www.ehlersdanlosnetwork.org

## REFERENCES

1. Beighton P, De Paepe A, Steinmann B, Tsipouras P, Wenstrup RJ. Ehlers-Danlos syndromes: revised nosology, Villafranche, 1997. Ehlers-Danlos National Foundation (USA) and Ehlers-Danlos Support Group (UK). *Am J Med Genet*. 1998;77:31-37.

2. Lawrence E. The clinical presentation of Ehlers-Danlos syndrome. *Adv Neonatal Care*. 2005;5(6):301-314.

3. Germain DP. Ehlers-Danlos syndrome type IV. *Orphanet J Rare Dis*. 2007;2:32.

4. Maltz SB, Fantus RJ, Mellett MM, Kirby JP. Surgical complications of Ehlers-Danlos syndrome type IV: case report and review of the literature. *J Trauma*. 2001;51:387-390.

5. Badauy CM, Gomes SS, Sant'Ana Filho M, Chies JA. Ehlers-Danlos syndrome (EDS) type IV. Review of the literature. *Clin Oral Investig*. 2007;11(3):183-187.

6. De Paepe A, Malfait F. Bleeding and bruising in patients with Ehlers-Danlos syndrome and other collagen vascular disorders. *Br J Haematol*. 2004;127(5):491-500.

7. Prockop DJ. Osteogenesis imperfecta: phenotypic heterogeneity, protein suicide, short and long collagen. *Am J Hum Genet*. May 1984;36(3):499-505.

8. Oderich GS, Panneton JM, Bower TC, et al. The spectrum, management and clinical outcome of Ehlers-Danlos syndrome type IV: a 30-year experience. *J Vasc Surg*. 2005;42(1):98-106.

9. Loeys, BL, Chen J, Neptune ER, et al. A syndrome of altered cardiovascular, craniofacial, neurocognitive and skeletal development caused by mutations in TGFBR1 or TGFBR2. *Nat Genet*. 2005;37(3):275-281.

10. Lum YW, Brooke BS, Black JH. Contemporary management of vascular Ehlers-Danlos syndrome. *Curr Opin Cardiol*. 2011;26(6):494-501.

11. Ong KT, Perdu J, De Backer J, et al. Effect of celiprolol on prevention of cardiovascular events in vascular Ehlers-Danlos syndrome: a prospective randomised, open, blinded-endpoints trial. *Lancet*. 2010;376:1476-1484.

12. Parfitt J, Chalmers RT, Wolfe JH. Visceral aneurysms in Ehlers-Danlos syndrome: case report and review of the literature. *J Vasc Surg*. 2000;31(6):1248-1251.

13. Lum YW, Brooke BS, Arnaoutakis GJ, Williams TK, Black JH. Endovascular procedures in patients with Ehlers-Danlos syndrome: a review of clinical outcomes and iatrogenic complications. *Ann Vasc Surg*. 2012;26(1):25-33.

# 37 MARFAN SYNDROME

Jovan N. Markovic, MD

## PATIENT STORY

On a routine medical examination, a 19-year-old man is found to have a mid systolic click followed by a heart murmur. His height is 78 in, and weight is 157 lb. Physical examination shows arms that are disproportionately long compared with his trunk (arm span of 81 in), thumbs that can be extended to the wrist, pectus excavatum, and laxity of ligaments. Ocular examination demonstrates dislocation of one lens. Family history is positive for sudden death of his father at the age of 41 due to heart problems.

## EPIDEMIOLOGY

- With an estimated prevalence of 1 in 3000 to1 in 5000 individuals, Marfan syndrome (MFS) represents the most common autosomal dominant multisystem disorder of the connective tissue with primary predilection of the skeletal, cardiovascular, and ocular system with consequent bone overgrowth, aortic root dilation, and/or aortic dissection and ectopia lentis, respectively.

## ETIOLOGY AND PATHOPHYSIOLOGY

- The underlying pathophysiology responsible for the development and progression of MFS is the mutation of the fibrillin-1 (FBN1) gene located on chromosome 15q12. FBN1 regulates expression of the protein fibrillin-1 (composed of 2871 amino acids).[1] There have been more than 1200 identified mutations that affect the FBN1 gene, the majority of which are missense mutations with high affinity for highly conserved cysteine residues. Other mutation types include nonsense small deletions and duplications, splice-site alterations, and mutations involving calcium-binding residues.

- Fibrillin is the major protein component of the 10 nm microfibrils of the extracellular matrix that forms the scaffold for the deposition of elastin in tissues of the heart valves, aorta, lens suspensory ligaments, and other ligamentous structures.[2] In addition, data from numerous genetic studies show that fibrillin has an important function in nonelastic tissues, such as ciliary zonules of the eye, tendons, and periosteum of the bone.

## DIAGNOSIS

### Clinical Features

- The clinical features of MFS, including tall stature and slender digits, were first described by the French pediatrician Dr. Antoine Marfan in 1896 in a 5-year-old female patient. Today, initial diagnosis is usually made clinically utilizing the Ghent criteria, an international diagnostic algorithm based largely on clinical findings in the various earlier-mentioned organ systems, as well as on family history. Given that MFS demonstrates a wide phenotypic variety, in which mildly affected patients may be overlooked, the Ghent criteria underwent a revision in 2010 to decrease the risk of misdiagnosis[3] (Table 37-1). The authors of the 2010 revision placed more emphasis on aortic root aneurysm and/or dissection and ectopia lentis and removed some of the less specific manifestations from the diagnostic algorithm. The Ghent criteria are best applied by a geneticist.

- A high index of suspicion for MFS should be raised in patients with the presence of the following clinical features: characteristic tall and thin body habitus with long extremities, long fingers (arachnodactyly), pectus excavatum, protuberant frontal eminence, laxity of joints, and/or scoliosis (and other degenerative changes of the spine). Cardiovascular and ocular manifestations include proximal aortic dilatation resulting in aortic insufficiency, mitral valve prolapse (hence, the mid systolic click), and aortic dissection, as well as ectopia lentis (Figures 37-1 and 37-2). Other less specific clinical findings include pes planus, camptodactyly, high-arched palate, skin striae, protrusion of the medial wall of the acetabulum into the pelvic cavity, and recurrent hernias and/or pneumothorax.

- Disproportionate overgrowth can be assessed by an arm span length greater than 1.05 times height or a reduced upper-to-lower body segment ratio. On physical examination arachnodactyly is assessed with testing for wrist and thumb signs: The wrist sign is positive when the thumb of one hand overlaps the distal phalanx of the small finger when grasping the contralateral wrist (Figure 37-3). The thumb sign is positive when the entire thumb nail protrudes beyond the ulnar border of the hand when the thumb is clenched without assistance (Figure 37-4).

- Scoliosis is present in approximately 60% of MFS patients. Compared to idiopathic scoliosis, MFS scoliosis is characterized by higher prevalence of double thoracic and triple major curves. Up to 40% of patients have kyphosis greater than 50. Another common clinical finding in patients with MFS is dural ectasia (an enlargement of the outer layer of the dural sac and nerve root sleeves), which most commonly affects the L5-S2 lumbosacral spine region. Data from several magnetic resonance imaging (MRI) studies demonstrate that dural ectasia is present in as many as 95% of MFS patients. Most frequently dural ectasia causes lower back pain, followed by leg, abdominal, and/or perineal pain.

- Degenerative changes occasionally affect the cervical spine of patients with MFS. In a review of 104 consecutive MFS patients, Hobbs et al. documented that 16% and 54% of patients had focal cervical kyphosis and increased atlantoaxial translation, respectively.[4] Data from this study also showed that patients with MFS have an increased radiographic prevalence of basilar impression (36%) and increased odontoid height.

- The protrusion of the medial wall of the acetabulum into the pelvic cavity is seen in 27% of MFS patients. Pectus excavatum is found in approximately two-thirds of pediatric patients with MFS, which

**TABLE 37-1** Revised Ghent Criteria for the Diagnosis of Marfan Syndrome and Related Disorders[3]

In the absence of a family history

    (1) Ao (Z ≥ 2) and EL = MFS[a]
    (2) Ao (Z ≥ 2) and *FBN1* = MFS
    (3) Ao (Z ≥ 2) and Syst (≥ 7 points) = MFS[a]
    (4) EL and *FBN1* with known Ao = MFS

EL with or without Syst and with an *FBN1* not known with Ao or no *FBN1* = ELS
Ao (Z < 2) and Syst (≥ 5) with at least one skeletal feature without EL = MASS
MVP and Ao (Z < 2) and Syst (> 5) without EL = MVPS

In the presence of a family history

    (5) EL and FH of MFS (as defined above) = MFS
    (6) Syst (≥ 7 points) and FH of MFS (as defined above) = MFS[a]
    (7) Ao (Z ≥ 2 above 20 years old, ≥ 3 below 20 years) + FH of MFS (as defined above) = MFS[a]

Scoring of systemic features

    Wrist and thumb sign–3 (wrist or thumb sign–1)
    Pectus carinatum deformity–2 (pectus excavatum or chest asymmetry–1)
    Hindfoot deformity–2 (plain pes planus–1)
    Pneumothorax–2
    Dural ectasia–2
    Protrusio acetabuli–2
    Reduced US/LS and increased arm/height and no severe scoliosis–1
    Scoliosis or thoracolumbar kyphosis–1
    Reduced elbow extension–1
    Facial features (3/5)–1 (dolichocephaly, enophthalmos, downslanting palpebral fissures, malar hypoplasia, retrognathia)
    Skin striae–1
    Myopia > 3 diopters–1
    Mitral valve prolapse (all types)–1

Maximum total: 20 points; score ≥ 7 indicates systemic involvement

Ao, aortic diameter at the sinuses of Valsalva above indicated Z-score or aortic root dissection; EL, ectopia lentis; ELS, ectopia lentis syndrome; *FBN1*, fibrillin-1 mutation; *FBN1* with known Ao, *FBN1* mutation that has been identified in an individual with aortic aneurysm; FH, family history; MASS, myopia, mitral valve prolapse, aortic root dilation, skeletal findings, striae syndrome; MVPS, mitral valve prolapse syndrome; Syst, systemic score; US/LS, upper segment/lower segment ratio; Z, Z-score.
[a]Caveat: without discriminating features of Shprintzen-Goldberg syndrome, Loeys-Dietz syndrome or vascular Ehlers-Danlos syndrome.

can negatively affect respiratory function in the most severe cases. Spontaneous pneumothorax occurs in approximately 4.4% of patients with MFS. Recurrence rates of pneumothorax are high.

- Aortic dissection is the most severe, and potentially life threatening, cardiovascular complication of MFS. The underlying pathology that can lead to this potentially catastrophic complication is related to cystic medial degeneration of the aortic wall, which is characterized by fragmented elastic fibers, a decrease in the amount of smooth muscle cells, and the deposition of collagen and mucopolysaccharides between cells of the aortic tunica media. Elastic fiber fragmentation leads to decreased aortic compliance, which results in aortic root dilatation and, in the most severe cases, aortic dissection. Diameter of the sinus of Valsalva greater than 5 cm, dilatation rate of more than 1.5 mm/y, and a positive family history are the most common risk factors for aortic dissection. These patients require lifelong monitoring of the progression of the aortic dilatation (Figure 37-5). In a significant number of patients, pathology of the aortic wall results in aortic valve insufficiency. Laxity of the mitral valve is frequently seen in MFS, resulting in mitral valve prolapse in approximately 50% to 80% of cases. Other cardiovascular manifestations associated with MFS include left ventricular dilatation and dilatation of the pulmonary and iliac arteries (Figure 37-6).

- Ectopia lentis (Figures 37-1 and 37-2) is the most common ocular abnormality associated with MFS. It develops in utero and can be clinically apparent at the first ophthalmologic visit. Pathophysiologically, ectopia lentis is characterized by the displacement of the lens(es). Most frequently there is a bilateral displacement of the lenses upward. It is estimated that ectopia lentis is present in approximately 60% of MFS patients. On transmission electron microscopy the ciliary zonular filaments appear stretched or interpositioned by disrupted microfibril bundles. It has to be emphasized that ectopia lentis is not pathognomonic for MFS since it is associated with other disorders, which include Ehlers-Danlos syndrome, Weill-Marchesani syndrome, congenital contractural arachnodactyly, sulfite oxidase deficiency, and homocystinuria. Other less specific ocular disorders associated with MFS include myopia, glaucoma, cataracts, and retinal detachment.

- Lastly, patients with MFS have a high incidence of pain: Grahame et al. demonstrated that as many as 70% to 96% of patients report pain in at least one location in the body. The underlying etiology of the pain is idiopathic and remains to be elucidated.

## Laboratory Studies

- In addition to a detailed history and physical examination, other diagnostic modalities including ECG, echocardiography, x-ray, and MRI are utilized to detect major and minor criteria conditions. Which imaging modality is used depends on the presenting symptoms. For example, a pelvis x-ray can identify protrusio acetabuli, while an MRI scan of the lumbar spine is an imaging modality of choice to detect dural ectasia. Since the management of MFS exceeds the level of expertise of any single medical specialty, consultations with ophthalmology and cardiology specialists is critical for the proper assessment of the respective ocular and cardiovascular manifestations.

- It has to be emphasized that family history is not always positive, and approximately one out of four MFS cases are the result of new mutations. Thus, genetic testing for *FBN1* mutations are used to confirm the diagnosis, save that *FBN1* mutations may also cause other Marfan-like disorders and that as many as 9% to 34% of MFS patients have no detectible *FBN1* mutations. The inability to detect a genetic mutation in *FBN1* does not absolutely exclude the diagnosis. Currently, molecular diagnosis modalities are characterized with low sensitivity and specificity.

## Differential Diagnosis

- Despite distinct clinical, genetic, and pathophysiologic findings, MFS can be confused with other disorders that involve skeletal, cardiac, or ophthalmologic manifestations, especially in patients without a family history positive for MFS. In these patients clinical follow-up may be the only way to differentiate MFS from some of the other disorders. The differential diagnosis of MFS includes

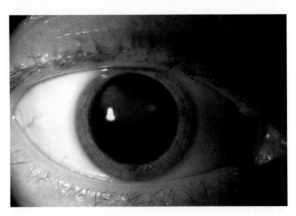

FIGURE 37-1 Ectopia lentis or lens dislocation in Marfan syndrome (MFS). (*Photograph courtesy of Robin Vann, MD, and Brian Lutman, CRA.*)

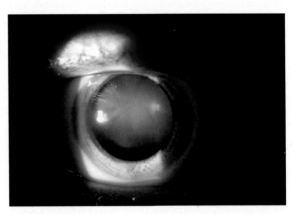

FIGURE 37-2 This figure demonstrates unilateral (right eye) ectopic lens that is displaced supero-laterally (most common displacement location) in a 57 years old female patient with Marfan syndrome. The genetic mutations responsible for Marfan syndrome presumably cause more severe derangements in composition of the microfibrils than those found in ectopia lentis that is not associated with Marfan syndrome which consequently leads to more profound lens displacement. (*Photograph courtesy of Robin Vann, MD and Brian Lutman, CRA.*)

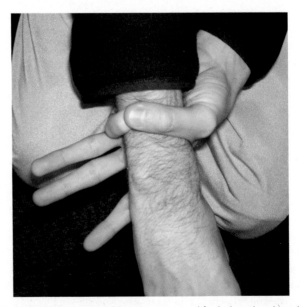

FIGURE 37-3 A positive wrist sign is exemplified when thumb and fingers overlap when encircling the contralateral wrist. (*Photograph courtesy of Rocio Moran, MD.*)

○ Homocystinuria is characterized by several overlapping skeletal and ocular features with MFS, and mitral valve prolapse. However, the aortic enlargement is typically not seen in them. It is an autosomal recessive disorder and is characterized by elevated urinary homocysteine, mental retardation, a predisposition to thromboembolic events, and high prevalence of coronary artery disease.

○ Ehlers-Danlos syndrome type IV (the vascular type) includes skin laxity, scarring, easy bruising, as well as arterial dilatation and dissection.

○ MASS phenotype (an acronym for mitral valve prolapse, aortic root diameter at upper limits of normal for body size, striae of the skin, and skeletal disorders) is a familial disorder that includes features similar to MFS with the aortic enlargement that is usually milder and nonprogressive.

○ Beals syndrome (congenital contractural arachnodactyly) is an autosomal dominant disorder characterized by multiple joint contractures, significant scoliosis, abnormal pinnae, and muscular hypoplasia in addition to a marfanoid appearance.

○ Familial thoracic aortic aneurysm and dissection is inherited as an autosomal dominant trait and is characterized by progression at a faster rate than other aortic disorders, and frequently it does not show typical systemic manifestations of MFS.

○ Congenital bicuspid aortic valve disease and associated aortopathy is a cardiovascular disorder with similar histopathologic findings to MFS yet differs as the dilatation of the ascending aorta is often seen at the mid ascending aortic section rather than at the aortic sinuses. The bicuspid aortic valve may function normally.

○ Loeys-Dietz syndrome is another autosomal dominant connective tissue disorder characterized by arterial tortuosity and aneurysms, craniofacial malformations, and skeletal abnormalities, with an increased risk of dissection throughout the arterial tree including small-size arteries. Additional features include hypertelorism without ectopia lentis and a broad or bifid uvula.

## MANAGEMENT

• In addition to genetic counseling and evaluation, patient care in MFS should focus on the treatment of presenting symptoms and prophylactic measures to maintain and improve cardiovascular health. Serial echocardiograms performed yearly or more frequently and regular computed tomography (CT) surveillance are necessary for detecting and monitoring dilatation of the aorta. Beta-blockers are indicated in all MFS patients (including pediatric patients) to decrease the risk of aortic dissection by reducing ejection fraction and controlling heart rate. In a randomized prospective trial that involved 70 MFS patients, Shores et al. demonstrated that prophylactic treatment with beta-blockers was effective in slowing the rate of aortic dilatation and reducing the risk of aortic dissection.[5] In the same study, data from the Kaplan-Meier survival analysis showed that prophylactic beta-blocker treatment was associated with improved survival of MFS patients. The beta-blocker dose should be adjusted for age and weight with a goal to maintain a heart rate at 60 to 70 and 100 beats/min in patients at rest and after submaximal exercise, respectively. Calcium antagonists and angiotensin-converting enzyme inhibitor drugs are an alternative in patients with beta-blocker intolerance.

• Early prophylactic surgical repair of aortic root dilatation is recommended when the diameter at the aortic sinuses of the ascending

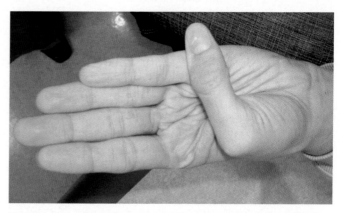

FIGURE 37-4 A positive thumb sign is present if the phalanx of the thumb extends beyond the ulnar border. (*Photograph courtesy of Rocio Moran, MD.*)

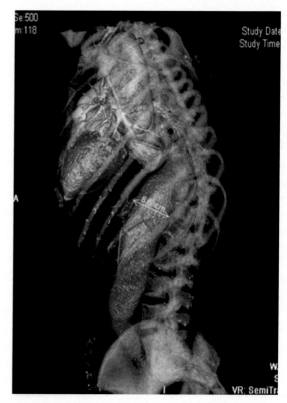

FIGURE 37-5 CT-3D scan demonstrating a massive thoracoabdominal aortic aneurysm (diameter = 8.6 cm) in a patient with Marfan syndrome (MFS).

aorta reaches 5 cm.[6] In patients with a diameter of the ascending aorta less than 5 cm, surgical repair is recommended based on other indications such as family history of aortic dissection, rapid progression of aortic dilatation (defined as aortic root growth of >2 mm per year or 5% per year), symptomatic aortic valve regurgitation and progressive left ventricular dilatation or dysfunction, and the feasibility of a valve-sparing operation. The rationale for surgical intervention is based on data showing that the outcomes of prophylactic aortic root surgery are superior to those of emergent surgery. Impact of the preservation of the aortic valve during aortic root surgery on indications for the surgical intervention is controversial and is a matter of debate.

- The incidence of aneurysmal dilatation and dissection of the descending thoracic and abdominal aorta is significantly lower when compared to the ascending aorta and aortic root in MFS, and the majority of surgical procedures on the descending thoracic aorta are performed for expansion of a chronic dissection. The initial management of dissection of the descending thoracic aorta is pharmacologic therapy. Hagan et al. demonstrated that surgical mortality exceeds that for medical management by a factor of 3.[7] Moreover, connective tissue disease, such as MFS, is considered a contraindication for stent-graft insertion in acute dissection by most surgeons. In nonacute settings a maximum descending aortic diameter greater than 6.5 cm or rate of growth 0.5 cm/6 mo is considered as an indication for intervention (Figure 37-7). The risk of dissection in pregnant patients increases with an aortic diameter greater than 4 cm. Thus, frequent cardiovascular monitoring is necessary for such patients.

- Progressive mitral valve regurgitation that requires mitral valve repair or replacement occurs in up to 50% of MFS patients. Symptomatic mitral valve prolapse and regurgitation or progressive left ventricular dilatation and/or dysfunction are an indication for surgical intervention.[8] However, most patients with MFS will not require mitral valve surgery. When feasible, the mitral valve should be repaired rather than replaced in patients undergoing concomitant aortic valve-sparing root replacement. In patients where the aortic valve is being replaced with a mechanical valve, mitral valve replacement rather than repair should be considered.

- Surgical interventions for spinal deformities in MFS patients (ie, spinal fusion) are associated with high complication rates. Data from a retrospective study showed that the rate of fixation failure was 21% in MFS and that dural tear, infection, and pseudarthrosis complications found in 8%, 10%, and 10% of MFS patients, respectively.[9] Failure of fixation is a common complication in MFS patients because of the thin laminae, thin pedicles, and osteopenia. Because of these properties, some authors suggested that the number of fixation points should be maximized.

- When the protrusion of the medial wall of the acetabulum into the pelvic cavity results in symptomatic osteoarthritis in older patients, total hip arthroplasty is recommended. Nonstructural bone grafting of the medial wall cavity is frequently performed.[10] Younger patients (<40 years of age) with minimal symptoms are treated with valgus intertrochanteric osteotomy. Valgus intertrochanteric osteotomy relieves pain by reducing the transverse vector of forces that drive the head into the acetabulum.

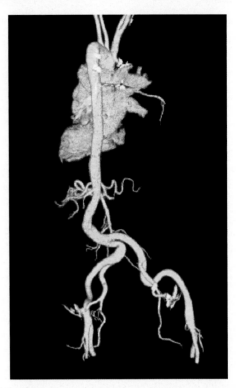

**FIGURE 37-6** Mild dilation of the infrarenal abdominal aorta, an aneurysm of the left common iliac artery (2 cm in diameter), and mild dilatation of the right common iliac artery in a patient with Marfan syndrome (MFS) who underwent St. Jude aortic valve replacement with an ascending aortic graft.

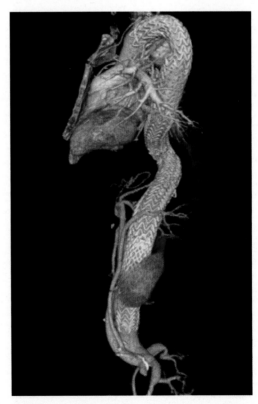

**FIGURE 37-7** Postoperative CT-3D scan illustrating a Marfan syndrome (MFS)-associated thoracoabdominal aorta after staged aneurysm repair with total abdominal visceral debranching procedure followed by concomitant endovascular repair of thoracic and abdominal aortic aneurysm.

## PATIENT EDUCATION

- Counseling on lifestyle modification regarding moderate restriction of physical activity and reduction of emotional stress is very important, especially to protect the cardiovascular system in MFS patients. Established guidelines for adult patients recommend isotonic, low-intensity dynamic activity (eg, swimming, biking, jogging) with aerobic level of work (50% of capacity) and a pulse rate target less than 110 beats/min (<100 beats/min if patient is on beta-blockers). Recommendations can be stricter and are determined on an individual basis based on the patient's echocardiogram findings and earlier-mentioned diagnostic assessment. Contact sports (eg, martial arts), high-intensity activities such as static exercise (eg, weight lifting), and physical activity that require rapid acceleration or deceleration (eg, football, basketball, soccer, skiing, sprinting, etc) need to be avoided.

- Genetic counseling should be offered to patients who plan to start a family. Prospective parents should be informed that approximately 50% of all offspring will inherit the genetic mutation for MFS due to the autosomal dominant pattern of inheritance. Ultrasonographic diagnosis in utero is not sensitive, and newborns should be followed for the development of earlier-mentioned clinical signs.

- Patients should be educated to recognize warning symptoms of acute, possible life-threatening complications including any acute chest, back, or abdominal pain; syncope; sudden change in vision or sense of impending doom, and to seek urgent medical evaluation for any of the earlier-mentioned symptoms. Patients should also be counseled that the treatment with beta-blockers is beneficial in most but not all MFS patients, and beta-blockers do not absolutely prevent aortic dissection.

## FOLLOW-UP

- All patients with MFS require lifelong medical treatment and monitoring for the development of symptoms, especially those related to cardiovascular pathology and aortic dissection. Annual cardiovascular examination that includes transthoracic two-dimensional echocardiography, computerized tomographic angiography, magnetic resonance imaging angiography, or standard aortography of the entire aorta is recommended for all MFS patients (especially in patients after aortic surgery). Biannual evaluation is recommended in some MFS patients with more complex comorbidities.

- Annual ophthalmologic examination, including screening for detachment of retina, glaucoma, myopia, and cataracts, is recommended for all MFS patients regardless of presenting symptoms.

## REFERENCES

1. Dietz HC, Cutting GR, Pyeritz RE, et al. Marfan syndrome caused by a recurrent de novo missense mutation in the fibrillin gene. *Nature*. 1991;352:337-339.

2. Hollister DW, Godfrey M, Sakai LY, Pyeritz RE. Immunohistologic abnormalities of the microfibrillar-fiber system in Marfan syndrome. *N Engl J Med*. 1990;323:152-159.

3. Loeys BL, Dietz HC, Braverman AC, et al. The revised Ghent nosology for the Marfan syndrome. *J Med Genet*. 2010;47:476-485.

4. Hobbs WR, Sponseller PD, Weiss AP, Pyeritz RE. The cervical spine in Marfan syndrome. *Spine*. 1997;22:983-989.

5. Shores J, Berger KR, Murphy EA, Pyeritz RE. Progression of aortic dilatation and the benefit of long-term beta-adrenergic blockade in Marfan's syndrome. *N Engl J Med*. 1994;330:1335-1341.

6. Elefteriades JA. Natural history of thoracic aortic aneurysms: indications for surgery and surgical versus nonsurgical risks. *Ann Thorac Surg*. 2002;74:S1877-S1880.

7. Hagan P, Nienaber CA, Isselbacher EM, et al. The International Registry of Acute Aortic Dissection (IRAD): new insights into an old disease. *JAMA*. 2000;283:897-903.

8. Bhudia S, Troughton R, Lam B, et al. Mitral valve surgery in the adult Marfan syndrome patient. *Ann Thorac Surg*. 2006;81:843-848.

9. Jones KB, Erkula G, Sponseller PD, Dormans JP. Spine deformity correction in Marfan syndrome. *Spine*. 2002;27:2003-2012.

10. Van de Velde S, Fillman R, Yandow S. Protrusio acetabuli in Marfan syndrome: history, diagnosis, and treatment. *J Bone Joint Surg Am*. 2006;88:639-646.

# 38 LOEYS DIETZ SYNDROME AND RELATED DISORDERS

Rocio Moran, MD, FACMG
Christina Rigelsky, MS, CGC

## PATIENT STORY

A 26-year-old woman was referred for evaluation of a possible connective tissue disorder. She first came to medical attention in early childhood when she was diagnosed with a pectus excavatum and joint hypermobility. Additional history included mitral valve prolapse, inguinal and umbilical hernias, as well as scoliosis. She carried the diagnosis of hypermobile Ehlers-Danlos syndrome (EDS) for many years yet had normal collagen studies for EDS type IV. At the age of 19 years, mitral valve repair for severe mitral valve regurgitation was performed. Six years later, she presented to the emergency room for evaluation of sudden-onset tachycardia and chest pain. Echocardiogram revealed a dilated aorta, and computed tomographic (CT) scan showed bilateral subclavian artery aneurysms. The physical examination was notable for normal height, weight, and body mass index (BMI). Marfan syndrome assessment revealed a systemic score of 6 with points for increased arm span to height ratio, pectus excavatum, positive wrist sign, mitral valve prolapse, and hindfoot deformity. Additional physical examination findings were notable for a bifid uvula and normal palate. A transforming growth factor beta (TGF-β) spectrum disorder was suspected and a c.1363T>A mutation in the *TGFβR2* gene consistent with the diagnosis of Loeys Dietz syndrome (LDS) was confirmed on sequencing.

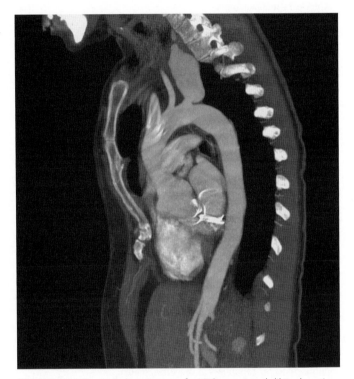

**FIGURE 38-1** Sagittal plane image of a LDS associated dilated aortic root and large left subclavian artery aneurysm.

## EPIDEMIOLOGY

- The prevalence of LDS is unknown. There is no enrichment in any particular ethnic or racial group or gender.

## ETIOLOGY AND PATHOPHYSIOLOGY

- Due to point mutations and (rarely) deletions in the *TGFβR1*, *TGFβR2*, *TGFβ2*, or *SMAD3* genes.

- Autosomal dominant disorder.

- Highly variable disorder even within families with incomplete penetrance.

- Mutations in other genes involved in the TGF-β signaling pathway are likely to emerge as disease contributing.

## CLINICAL FEATURES

LDS is a disorder of connective tissue characterized by:[1]

### Vascular

- Dilatation or dissection of the aorta most commonly thoracic (Figure 38-1)

- Other arterial aneurysms and dissections (Figure 38-1)

- Arterial tortuosity

## Skeletal

- Pectus excavatum or pectus carinatum
- Scoliosis
- Joint laxity
- Arachnodactyly
- Talipes equinovarus or hindfoot deformity
- Osteoarthritis (*SMAD3*)
- Cervical spine instability

## Craniofacial

- Ocular hypertelorism
- Bifid uvula or cleft palate (Figure 38-2)
- Craniosynostosis

## Cutaneous

- Translucent skin (Figure 38-3)
- Easy bruising
- Dystrophic

## IMAGING

- If diagnosis is confirmed or highly suspected, patients should undergo imaging from head to pelvis to investigate for additional arterial disease.
- Cervical spine films should be obtained to evaluate for instability.

## HISTOPATHOLOGY

- Histologic examination of aortic tissue reveals fragmentation of elastic fibers, loss of elastin content, and accumulation of amorphous matrix components in the aortic media.
- Findings of cystic medial necrosis do not distinguish LDS from other causes of aortic aneurysm.

## DIFFERENTIAL DIAGNOSIS

- EDS type IV has many overlapping features with LDS. The diagnosis of EDS type IV is confirmed by abnormal type III collagen biosynthesis and/or identification of a disease-causing mutation in *COL3A1*. Inheritance is autosomal dominant.
- Marfan syndrome also shares many overlapping features with LDS. Cardinal manifestations involve the ocular, skeletal, and cardiovascular systems with new revised clinical criteria to help aid in the diagnosis. Ocular findings play a more prominent role in Marfan syndrome than LDS. Molecular testing of *FBN1* can help aid the clinical diagnosis.[2]
- Arterial tortuosity syndrome is a rare autosomal recessive connective tissue disorder characterized by severe tortuosity, stenosis, and aneurysms of the aorta and middle-sized arteries. Skeletal and skin involvement is common. The underlying genetic defect is loss-of-function mutations in *SLC2A10*.[3]
- Familial aneurysms and dissections should be considered in patients with aneurysms and/or dissections of the thoracic aorta involving either the ascending or descending aorta. While isolated aortic

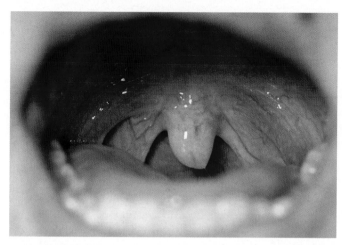

**FIGURE 38-2** Wide, bifid uvula characteristic of Loeys Dietz syndrome (LDS).

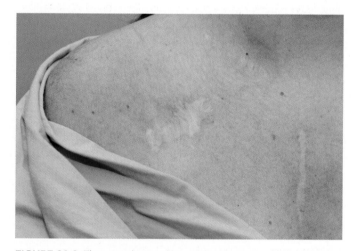

**FIGURE 38-3** Thin, translucent skin with large scars in a patient with Loeys Dietz syndrome (LDS).

disease does occur, additional findings include abdominal aortic aneurysms, cerebral and peripheral artery aneurysms, patent ductus arteriosus, bicuspid aortic valve, livedo reticularis (a purplish skin discoloration in a lacey pattern typically on the extremities), iris flocculi (asymptomatic, ruptured papillary epithelial cysts), and early-onset occlusive vascular diseases. Mutations in the following genes have been associated with this diagnosis: *TGFBR2, TGFBR1, MYH11, ACTA2, MYLK, SMAD3*.[4]

## MANAGEMENT

Evaluation and treatment for patients with LDS is aimed at establishing the extent of disease and treatment of manifestations.[5] Recommendations include

- Echocardiography with attention to absolute aortic size and Z-scores. Magnetic resonance angiography (MRA) or CT scan from head to pelvis to identify arterial aneurysms and arterial tortuosity distal to the thoracic aorta.
  - The interval of follow-up imaging will depend on the clinical findings but usually requires monitoring at frequent intervals to assess for progression of disease.
- Radiographs to assess for skeletal manifestations (eg, scoliosis, cervical spine instability).
  - A referral to orthopedics may be necessary for surgical correction.
- Ophthalmology evaluation.
- The approach for surgical intervention should proceed with the caveat that vascular disease is not limited to the aorta and that aortic dissection occurs at smaller aortic diameters than observed in other connective tissue disorders such as Marfan syndrome.
- Beta-adrenergic blockers are used to reduce hemodynamic stress. Angiotensin receptor blockade is also used due to its inhibition of TGF-β signaling.

- Activity and other restrictions should include the avoidance of contact sports, competitive sports, and isometric exercise.

## PATIENT EDUCATION

Patients suspected of LDS should undergo genetic counseling. Genetic counseling provides patients and their families information on the nature of the disorder and inheritance to help them make informed medical and personal decisions.

### PATIENT AND PROVIDER RESOURCES

- Loeys Dietz Syndrome Foundation: http://www.loeysdietz.org/
- National Marfan Foundation: http://www.marfan.org/marfan/

## REFERENCES

1. Loeys BL, Dietz HC. Loeys-dietz syndrome. In: Pagon RA, Bird TD, Dolan CR, Stephens K, Adam MP, eds. *Genereviews*. Seattle, WA; 1993.

2. Loeys BL, Dietz HC, Braverman AC, et al. The revised ghent nosology for the marfan syndrome. *J Med Genet*. 2010;47:476-485.

3. Callewaert BL, Willaert A, Kerstjens-Frederikse WS, et al. Arterial tortuosity syndrome: clinical and molecular findings in 12 newly identified families. *Hum Mutat*. 2008;29:150-158.

4. Milewicz DM, Regalado E. Thoracic aortic aneurysms and aortic dissections. In: Pagon RA, Bird TD, Dolan CR, Stephens K, Adam MP, eds. *Genereviews*. Seattle, WA; 1993.

5. Williams JA, Loeys BL, Nwakanma LU, et al. Early surgical experience with loeys-dietz: a new syndrome of aggressive thoracic aortic aneurysm disease. *Ann Thorac Surg*. 2007;83:S757-763; discussion S785-790.

# PART 5

# NON-ATHEROSCLEROTIC DISORDERS

# 39 POPLITEAL ARTERY ENTRAPMENT SYNDROME

Bhagwan Satiani, MD, MBA, RPVI, FACS

## PATIENT STORY

A 28-year-old male athlete presented with increasing difficulty running, resulting in severe bilateral calf cramping. He consulted with orthopedics and neurosurgery with no definite etiology identified. Vascular surgery was consulted with a provisional diagnosis of a compartment syndrome. On physical examination he had normal pulses at rest. Diminution of dorsalis pedis and posterior tibial pulses was appreciated on both plantar flexion and dorsiflexion. Duplex ultrasound examination showed normal signals at rest, obliteration of arterial signals on plantar flexion, and reactive hyperemia on a neutral foot position.

## PATHOPHYSIOLOGY

Popliteal entrapment syndrome consists of a group of conditions where vascular and/or neurologic compression symptoms result due to compression of the popliteal artery, vein, or nerve. The compression is due to a congenital anomaly where the popliteal artery becomes functionally occluded by passing medial to and under the medial head of the gastrocnemius muscle or a slip of that muscle, with consequent compression of the artery.

- Relationship of muscle and artery in the popliteal fossa resulting in extrinsic arterial compression.

- Repetitive insult to the popliteal artery can cause arterial damage and lead to aneurysm, thromboembolism, and arterial thrombosis.

   Although there are several classifications, the four types of embryologic entrapment in a commonly used classification system are shown in Figure 39-1.[1,2]

## CLINICAL FEATURES

- The mean age of patients is 32 years.[3]
- Patients are more commonly male.
- About one-third of patients have bilateral entrapment.[4]
- History of leg pain or aching and tiredness; cramping on walking or exercise (intermittent claudication), which is relieved by rest, is the most common presenting symptom. Some swelling may also be described.
- A number of patients may remain completely asymptomatic until the artery is either severely narrowed or completely thrombosed.
- Occasionally patients may present with acute arterial ischemia due to thrombosis of the popliteal artery from long-standing entrapment, intimal damage, and eventual thrombosis. The tip-off is the young age of the patient, no evidence of arteriosclerosis elsewhere, and the prior history of claudication as described above.

- Examination can show arterial compression elicited by maneuvers such as plantar flexion and dorsiflexion of the feet.

## DIAGNOSIS

- The diagnosis is made by history and physical examination and confirmed by noninvasive studies.
- Duplex ultrasound can be diagnostic, although some authors have reported false-positive studies in athletes.[5]
- A baseline duplex ultrasound examination is performed with the foot in the neutral position. Normal triphasic Doppler signals are documented (Figure 39-2). While the Doppler probe is insonating the popliteal artery, the foot is dorsiflexed and plantar flexed to assess Doppler signals in the distal popliteal artery. Typically, the arterial signals are severely attenuated or absent during one of these maneuvers (Figure 39-3). After documenting occlusion of the artery, once the provocative maneuver is released the arterial signals resume, often with reactive hyperemia (Figure 39-4).
- A contrast arteriogram shows deviation of the popliteal artery from the middle of the popliteal fossa (Figure 39-5). The artery often appears narrowed, although this is due to extrinsic compression not intrinsic pathology. Long-standing compression can result in post-stenotic dilatation, aneurysm formation, or even occlusion of the artery.
- Computed tomography (CT) or computed angiography and magnetic resonance angiography (MRA) can be diagnostic and may replace contrast arteriography.

## DIFFERENTIAL DIAGNOSIS

- Arterial occlusive disease.
- Unstable plaque or thrombosis.
- Cystic adventitial disease.
- Compartment syndrome.
- Arterial embolism: acute limb ischemia due to thrombosis of the popliteal entrapment.
- Sometimes there is a functional popliteal entrapment syndrome where there is no anatomic abnormality but a functional entrapment due to gastrocnemius hypertrophy and resulting arterial compression. Those with functional entrapment are younger, more commonly females, highly trained athletes, and have normal noninvasive tests.
- Another problem is that up to 56% of asymptomatic individuals can exhibit evidence of popliteal artery occlusion by duplex scanning with provocative maneuvers.[3]

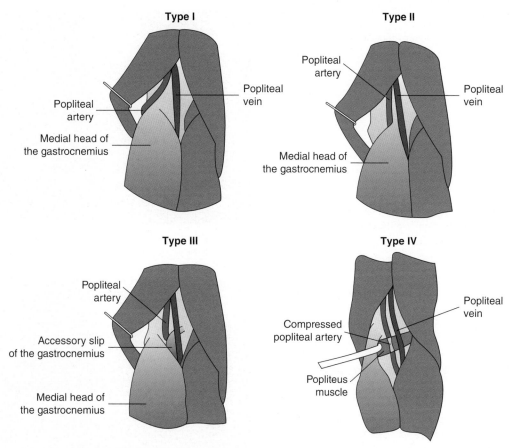

**FIGURE 39-1** Types of popliteal artery entrapment.
Type 1 shows location of the medial head of gastrocnemius muscle, which is attached more laterally than is normal, with resulting popliteal artery entrapment. Type 2 shows an abnormal course of the popliteal artery, with entrapment. Type 3 shows location of an anomalous muscle band with abnormal attachment, with resulting popliteal artery entrapment. Type 4 shows primitive position of the distal popliteal artery posterior to the popliteus muscle. (Reprinted from Pillai J. A current interpretation of popliteal vascular entrapment. *J Vasc Surg*, 2008;48:S61-S65, with permission from Elsevier.)

## MANAGEMENT

- A definitive diagnosis can be established by arteriography, magnetic resonance arteriography, or sometimes a computed tomographic angiography. These studies typically show medial deviation of the popliteal artery, occlusion, or a post-stenotic dilatation. If the artery is normal, plantar or dorsiflexion is performed with stress positional contrast study repeated to demonstrate the abnormalities. In severe cases, the artery may be occluded.

- The surgical approach is either a medial or posterior calf incision in order to access the artery and resect the musculotendinous abnormality in addition to either repairing or replacing the artery when necessary. Results are excellent when the condition is treated early before progression to thrombosis or loss of collaterals.

- Endovascular stenting of the popliteal artery has occasionally been performed for relief of the entrapment. However, recurrence has been the norm, and surgical intervention is the preferred treatment option.[6]

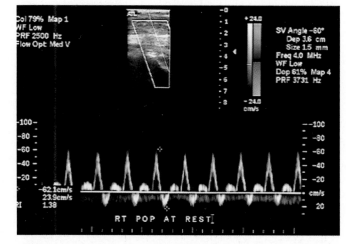

**FIGURE 39-2** Duplex ultrasound examination at rest showing normal Doppler signals.

## PATIENT EDUCATION

Complications after surgical release with or without arterial repair (besides the usual surgical complications such as wound problems) include

- Compartment syndrome
- Lymph leaks
- Arterial thrombosis of the repair
- Venous thrombosis
- Neurologic side effects: superficial or deep nerve injury
- Late recurrence

Patients must be advised on the possibility of these complications as well as immediate and late follow-up and the chance of the contralateral limb being symptomatic later on.

## FOLLOW-UP

Although recurrence of this condition is rare, clinical follow-up is recommended. Athletic activity can be resumed once wound healing has occurred and physical therapy has returned muscle strength and tone back to normal.

### PATIENT RESOURCES

- http://en.wikipedia.org/wiki/Popliteal_artery_entrapment_syndrome
- http://www.livestrong.com/article/183579-popliteal-artery-entrapment-symptoms/

## REFERENCES

1. Pillai J. A current interpretation of popliteal vascular entrapment. *J Vasc Surg.* 2008;48:S61-S65.

2. Delaney TA, Gonzalez LL. Occlusion of popliteal artery due to muscle entrapment. *Surgery.* 1971;69:97-101.

3. Sinha S, Houghton J, Holt PJ, Thompson MM, Loftus IM, Hinchliffe RJ. Popliteal entrapment syndrome. *J Vasc Surg.* 2012;55:252-262.

4. Gourgiotis S, Aggelakas J, Salemis N, Elias C, Georgiou C. Diagnosis and surgical approach of popliteal artery entrapment syndrome: a retrospective study. *Vasc Health Risk Manag.* 2008;4:83-88.

5. Turnipseed WD. Popliteal entrapment syndrome. *J Vasc Surg.* 2001;35:910-915.

6. Di Marzo L, Cavallaro A, O'Donnell SD, Shigematsu H, Levien LJ, Rich N. Endovascular stenting for popliteal vascular entrapment is not recommended. *Ann Vasc Surg.* 2010;24(8): 1135.e1-3.

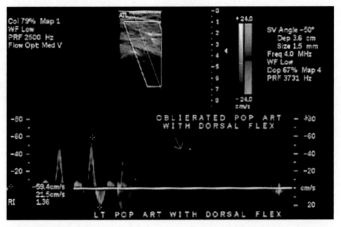

**FIGURE 39-3** Duplex ultrasound examination indicating cessation of arterial signals on dorsiflexion of the foot, confirming popliteal artery entrapment.

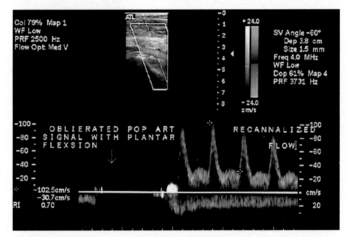

**FIGURE 39-4** Duplex ultrasound examination showing cessation of arterial signals with plantar flexion and resumption of normal arterial signals in the popliteal artery on releasing the foot from plantar flexion.

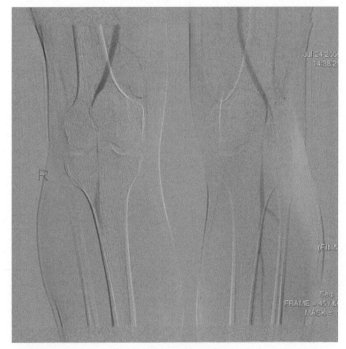

**FIGURE 39-5** Arteriogram showing bilateral popliteal artery deviation from the midline in the popliteal fossa with narrowing due to entrapment.

# 40 ILIAC ARTERY ENDOFIBROSIS

Jean Starr, MD, FACS, RPVI

## PATIENT HISTORY

A 47-year-old woman presented to the outpatient vascular clinic with a 1-year history of left leg pain that began with cramping in the left calf area, progressed up to the thigh, and now is in the buttock and hip region. Even walking a short distance had become significantly uncomfortable, and the pain had progressively gotten worse. She denied any rest pain or nonhealing ulcers. She was an avid runner and was training for a marathon when her symptoms began and now had stopped exercising. She was initially told she had a muscular strain and to limit activities, but she found the discomfort unbearable, even with walking. She was a lifelong nonsmoker and had no significant past medical history.

Physical examination showed a 5-ft, 1-in, 105-lb female with a diminished left femoral pulse with no palpable left pedal pulses and normal contralateral pulses.

Noninvasive Doppler testing showed an ankle-brachial index (ABI) on the right of 1.2, which did not change with exercise. The ABI on the left at rest was 0.7, which indicated moderate disease, and this further dropped to 0.45 with exercise (Figure 40-1). The left femoral waveform was monophasic (Figure 40-2). Duplex ultrasound imaging confirmed a left external iliac occlusion (Figure 40-3).

The options were discussed with her, including conservative management, open surgery, and endovascular methods.

She opted to undergo angiography (Figures 40-4 and 40-5) with concomitant left external iliac stenting. The occlusion required antegrade and retrograde approaches in order to successfully cross the lesion (Figure 40-6) and place a stent (Figure 40-7).

Her postprocedural ABI returned to normal (Figure 40-8).

## EPIDEMIOLOGY

- Iliac endofibrosis was first described in cyclists in 1986 by Chevalier.[1] The true incidence of iliac artery endofibrosis is not known, and few cases have been reported.

- It has been described in young, high-performance athletes, typically runners and cyclists, with few, if any, other risk factors for vascular disease.

## ETIOLOGY AND PATHOPHYSIOLOGY

- The external iliac artery lies distally and posteriorly in the pelvis. Endofibrosis has been postulated to arise from repeated trauma from a hypertrophied psoas muscle where it apposes the external iliac artery during hip flexion.[1] Proximally, the external iliac artery is fixed by the common iliac bifurcation, and distally it adheres to the inguinal ligament structures. It is in this relatively fixed segment

**Exercise pressures**

| | Rest | 1 | 2 | 3 | 4 | 5 | 6 | 7 | 8 | 9 | 10 |
|---|---|---|---|---|---|---|---|---|---|---|---|
| R Ankle (DP): | 158 | 174 | | | | | | | | | |
| L Ankle (DP): | 102 | 62 | | | | | | | | | |
| L Brachial: | 131 | 138 | | | | | | | | | |
| R ABI: | 1.21 | 1.26 | | | | | | | | | |
| L ABI: | 0.78 | 0.45 | | | | | | | | | |

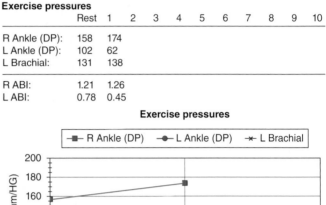
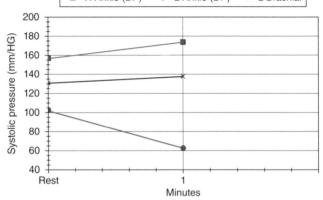

**FIGURE 40-1** Noninvasive exercise test demonstrating drop in left ankle-brachial index (ABI) after exercise.

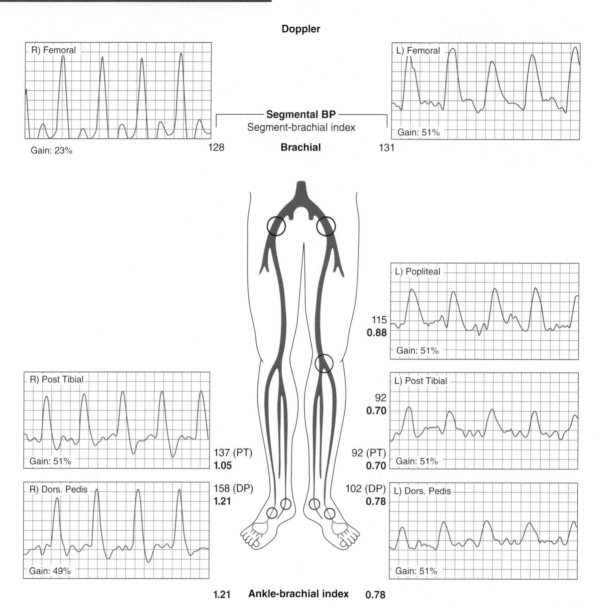

**FIGURE 40-2** Diminished left femoral and distal waveforms.

that external forces may cause vessel mechanical stress and elongation, as well as compression, resulting in luminal stenosis.[2]

- Other theories involve high flow rates through this segment of artery, resulting in endothelial damage, as well as kinking due to arterial side branches tethering the artery in place.[3]

- There tends to be distinct morphologic characteristics of endofibrosis to differentiate it from atherosclerotic lesions, including a lower incidence of calcification[4] and intimal fibrosis.[3]

## CLINICAL FEATURES

- Claudication is classically characterized as the onset of muscle fatigue, cramp, or discomfort, which is reproducible and predictable, usually occurring one level distal to an arterial occlusive process.

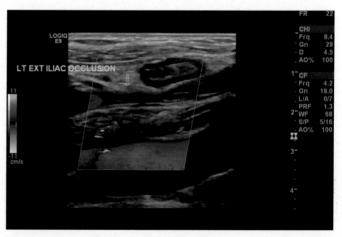

**FIGURE 40-3** Duplex imaging of left iliac artery occlusion (yellow arrow).

- When claudication is secondary to iliac artery endofibrosis, patients often do not possess other stigmata of vascular disease and often present with proximal thigh muscle fatigue or weakness.

- Initially, these high-performance athletes may be told they have muscular strains or sprains or even compartment syndrome. Physical therapy may be prescribed, which will obviously not remedy the underlying pathology or symptomatology.

## DIFFERENTIAL DIAGNOSIS

- Claudication secondary to the more common atherosclerosis process and pseudoclaudication due to spinal stenosis should be considered, although unusual in this unique athletic patient group.

- Claudication is typically worked up by first obtaining noninvasive studies in the vascular laboratory. This may include physiologic studies to assess quantitative blood flow, ABI measurement,[5] arterial duplex imaging, or any combination of these.

- Exercise testing may help unmask underlying occlusive disease in the patient who presents with a normal resting ABI, which may especially occur in patients with iliac artery endofibrosis who do not yet have an occlusion.[6,7]

- Color duplex imaging may help to characterize kinks and intravascular lesions in the external iliac artery, especially with the use of provocative maneuvers.[8]

- Contrast studies are usually next in line. This may involve computed tomographic (CT) angiography, magnetic resonance (MR) angiography, or catheter-based angiography. Each has its own inherent advantages and disadvantages.

- Although CT and MR are noninvasive, catheter-based angiography offers the advantage of potentially treating the disease at the same time by minimally invasive means. Angiographic findings may range from subtle stenosis to complete occlusion, with possible intraluminal thrombosis.[9] Typically, there may be no other signs of vascular occlusive disease, although there may be evidence of contralateral disease in the same location.

## MANAGEMENT OR INTERVENTION OPTIONS

- The ideal treatment for iliac artery endofibrosis would include alleviating the obstruction, as well as eliminating the inciting cause. Most likely, the latter is not feasible unless the same activities that caused the vessel injury (running, cycling) were avoided.

- Treatment aimed at relieving the obstruction includes iliofemoral bypass (for longer segment of disease), iliac endarterectomy with patching, shortening of the arterial segment (for hemodynamic kinking), and endovascular approaches with balloon angioplasty and stenting.[3,10,11]

- Open surgical approaches typically require a retroperitoneal and possible groin incision, which may not be desirable in endurance athletes.

- Endovascular procedures offer a minimally invasive means to improve arterial flow, thereby returning an athlete to endurance activities more expediently. Good results have been obtained from

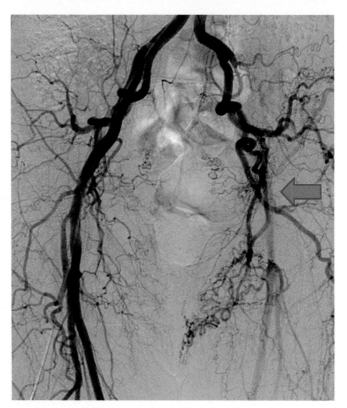

FIGURE 40-4 Angiogram revealing left iliac occlusion, reconstitution of left femoral, and large left pelvic collateral bed (blue arrow).

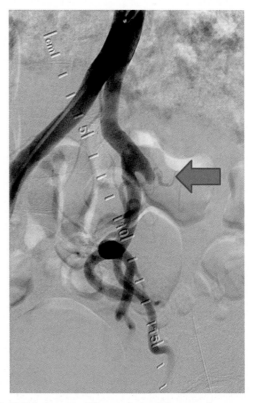

FIGURE 40-5 Left external iliac occlusion (blue arrow).

the surgical approaches; however, few long-term results exist after endovascular management.

## COMPLICATIONS

- Nontreatment results in continued symptoms and is typically not tolerated by this high-performance group of patients. The natural history of untreated iliac artery endofibrosis is unknown.
- Surgical and endovascular intervention can result in typical revascularization complications of graft stenosis or occlusion, infection, nerve injury, and pseudoaneurysm formation, among others.

## PATIENT EDUCATION AND FOLLOW-UP

- Patients should be advised to avoid the activities that caused the initial arterial injury, but this may not be palatable to most athletes.
- Follow-up should be advised every 6 to 12 months to assess for recurrence of symptoms and graft patency.

### PATIENT RESOURCES

- http://www.livestrong.com/article/183579-popliteal-artery -entrapment-symptoms/
- http://cyclingtips.com.au/2011/11/exercise-induced-arterial -endofibrosis/

## REFERENCES

1. Chevalier JM, Enon B, Walder J, et al. Endofibrosis of the external iliac artery in bicycle racers: an unrecognized pathological state. *Ann Vasc Surg.* Nov 1986;1(3):297-303.

2. Scavèe V, Stainier L, Deltombe T, et al. External iliac artery endofibrosis: a new possible predisposing factor. *J Vasc Surg.* Jul 2003;38(1):180-182.

3. Ford SJ, Rehman A, Bradbury AW. External iliac endofibrosis in endurance athletes: a novel case in an endurance runner and a review of the literature. *Eur J Vasc Endovasc Surg.* Dec 2003;26(6):629-634.

4. Vink A, Bender MH, Schep G, et al. Histopathological comparison between endofibrosis of the high-performance cyclist and atherosclerosis in the external iliac artery. *J Vasc Surg.* Dec 2008;48(6):1458-1463.

5. Taylor AJ, George KP. Ankle to brachial pressure index in normal subjects and trained cyclists with exercise-induced leg pain. *Med Sci Sports Exerc.* Nov 2001;33(11):1862-1867.

6. Fernández-García B, Alvarez Fernández J, Vega García F, et al. Diagnosing external iliac endofibrosis by postexercise ankle to arm index in cyclists. *Med Sci Sports Exerc.* Feb 2002;34(2):222-227.

7. Abraham P, Bickert S, Vielle B, Chevalier JM, Saumet JL. Pressure measurements at rest and after heavy exercise to detect moderate arterial lesions in athletes. *J Vasc Surg.* Apr 2001;33(4):721-727.

8. Schep G, Bender MH, Schmikli SL, Wijn PF. Color Doppler used to detect kinking and intravascular lesions in the iliac arteries in endurance athletes with claudication. *Eur J Ultrasound.* Dec 2001;14(2-3):129-140.

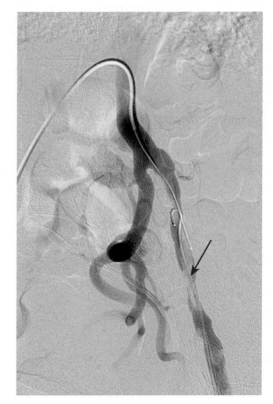

**FIGURE 40-6** Lesion crossing (blue arrow).

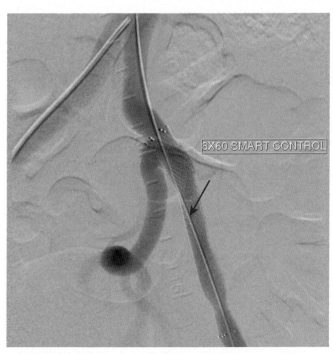

**FIGURE 40-7** Post-stent placement (blue arrow at proximal stent).

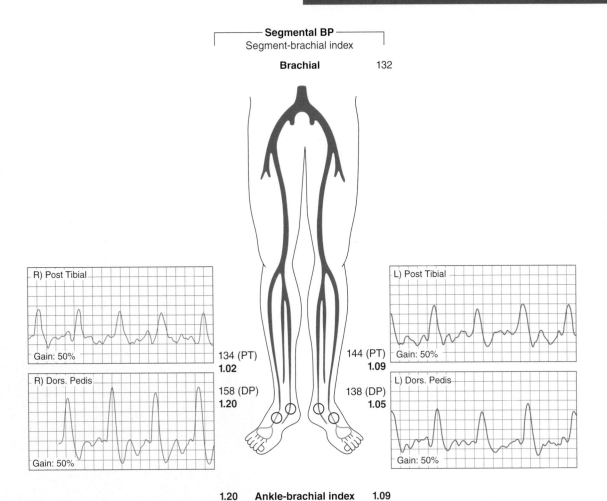

**FIGURE 40-8** Postprocedure ankle-brachial index (ABI).

9. Kral CA, Han DC, Edwards WD, Spittell PC, Tazelaar HD, Cherry KJ Jr. Obstructive external iliac arteriopathy in avid bicyclists: new and variable histopathologic features in four women. *J Vasc Surg.* Sep 2002;36(3):565-570.

10. Bucci F, Ottaviani N, Plagnol P. Acute thrombosis of external iliac artery secondary to endofibrosis. *Ann Vasc Surg.* Jul 2011;25(5):698.e5-7.

11. Maree AO, Ashequl Islam M, Snuderl M, et al. External iliac artery endofibrosis in an amateur runner: hemodynamic, angiographic, histopathological evaluation and percutaneous revascularization. *Vasc Med.* Aug 2007;12(3):203-206.

# 41 KLIPPEL-TRENAUNAY SYNDROME

Maria E. Litzendorf, MD

## PATIENT STORY

A 16-year-old girl presented with painful right-leg varicosities. She was actively involved in several sports, and noticed increasingly painful varicosities in her posterior-lateral thigh and extending distally down to her foot. Shortly after her birth purple-red superficial discoloration along her right leg extending up to her flank that abruptly terminated prior to crossing midline was identified. Several right limb-shortening procedures were required. Initial management included gradient compression hose with improvement in her pain. She presented several years later with worsening symptoms and underwent resection of her symptomatic vein clusters followed by targeted sclerotherapy several months postoperatively. Figure 41-1 illustrates a typical case of Klippel-Trenaunay syndrome (KTS). While generally benign, KTS can have unusual presentations that benefit from surgery, sclerotherapy, and/or thermal ablation treatment.

## EPIDEMIOLOGY

- Rare condition, sporadic in nature, no clear genetic inheritance pattern, but may have multifactorial inheritance pattern

- Occurs in all ethnic groups equally[1]

- Affects males and females equally

- Lack of large studies, but incidence postulated at 1 in 100,000 live births[2]

- Most commonly diagnosed in childhood

## ETIOLOGY AND PATHOPHYSIOLOGY

- Unclear and controversial etiology. Competing theories include the partial persistence of an embryologic vascular system, meso-dermal developmental abnormalities, and venous hypertension as a result of vascular agenesis, atresia, or hypoplasia possibly related to compression of the deep venous system by abnormal muscles or fibrovascular cords.[3-5]

- May be associated with increased maternal age, increased paternal age, and increased number of pregnancies. Vascular malformations are found at increased rates in family members of patients with KTS.[2]

## DIAGNOSIS

- Classic triad described by Klippel and Trenaunay in 1900 consists of capillary malformations, varicose veins or venous malformations, and osseomuscular limb hypertrophy.

- Cutaneous appearance of capillary malformations (previously referred to as a port-wine stain) that are usually present at or soon after birth.

- Limb hypertrophy involves both bone and soft tissue, and in rare circumstances involves a truncal location.[6] Although it may

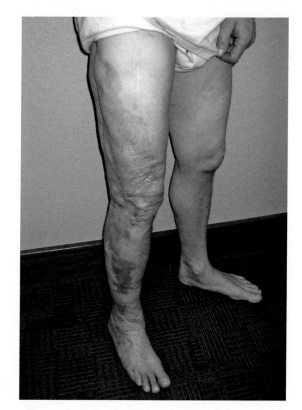

**FIGURE 41-1** Characteristic KTS appearance of unilateral capillary malformations (formerly known as port-wine stain) with varicose veins and associated limb hypertrophy. (*Photograph courtesy of Steven M. Dean, DO, FACP, RPVI.*)

be evident early, limb hypertrophy is often recognized after the affected individual begins walking.

- Lymphatic abnormalities can often be present and range from hypoplasia to aplasia. Lymphedema can exacerbate limb hypertrophy and venous congestion.

- A related syndrome, Parkes-Weber syndrome (PWS), is often confused with KTS, and is characterized by the presence of arteriovenous fistulae or arteriovenous malformations in addition to the constellation of clinical findings classically described with KTS.

- Diagnosis is made clinically, with the presence of at least two of the three main features.

## CLINICAL FEATURES

- Capillary malformations—The most common clinical findings are typically present at birth and have a flat, patchy appearance with a red to purple color. When found in the truncal location, there is generally a sharp border that fails to cross the midline (Figure 41-2). They may or may not blanch with pressure, and are most frequently seen on the same extremity affected with hypertrophy. Moreover, although most commonly at the superficial level, these malformations can also be seen in the subcutaneous tissues.[7] While some of these lesions do progress, and are especially aggravated during puberty and pregnancy, others may fade with capillary thrombosis.[6]

- Limb hypertrophy, the least common clinical finding, occurs in approximately 67% of patients with KTS. The lower extremities are predominantly affected, with the upper extremities accounting for only about 5% of cases[6] (Figures 41-3 and 41-4). Although hypertrophy of the affected limb is the classic finding with KTS, there are reports of both equal or shorter limb size on the affected side. In addition, the bony overgrowth can involve one or more bones on the affected extremity, and can be seen in conjunction with syndactyly and polydactyly.[8] The limb discrepancy is usually greater than 2 cm and accompanied by soft tissue and muscle hypertrophy as well as increased skin thickness that may be due in part to lymphatic involvement. Although growth rate is unpredictable, parents can be reassured that the syndrome is not characterized by progressive involvement of additional limbs.

- Venous malformations—Patients characteristically present with painful, large, and extensive varicosities. There are variable manifestations of venous involvement including complete agenesis of the deep venous system, hypoplasia, aneurysmal dilatation, venous reflux, and persistence of embryonic structures. Up to 80% of patients will have a persistent lateral marginal vein, also known as the "vein of Servelle."[6] This vein originates in the lateral foot and courses proximally along the lateral leg for a variable distance, draining most commonly into either the internal iliac vein or a branch of the profunda femoris vein. It is usually thick walled, superficial, and incompetent along its entire length. Persistent sciatic veins can provide a main source of outflow in patients with a hypoplastic deep system. The venous component of KTS can also involve the intra-abdominal organs. Manifestations vary and include rectal bleeding, hematuria, and esophageal variceal bleeding. Cerebrospinal involvement, though extremely rare, can also occur.

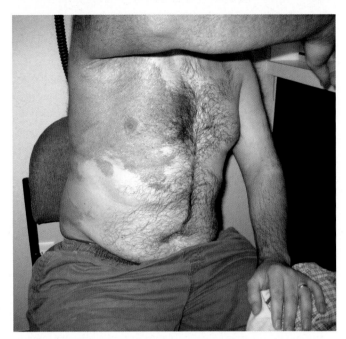

**FIGURE 41-2** Truncal capillary malformations with typical red-purple, flat appearance that fail to cross midline. (*Photograph courtesy of Steven M. Dean, DO, FACP, RPVI.*)

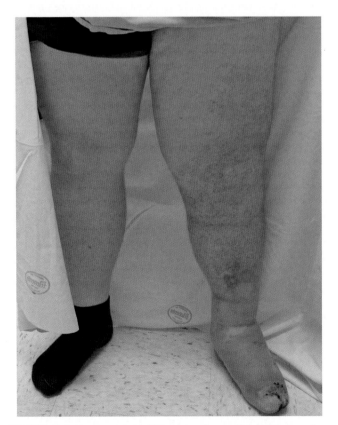

**FIGURE 41-3** Lower extremity KTS with capillary malformation, as well as underlying pedal lymphovenous malformation via magnetic resonance imaging (MRI). (*Photograph courtesy of Steven M. Dean, DO, FACP, RPVI.*)

## DIFFERENTIAL DIAGNOSIS

• Most commonly confused with PWS.

• The presence of a high-flow arteriovenous fistula in addition to a capillary malformation with limb hypertrophy characterizes PWS.

• Although low-flow arteriovenous malformations have recently been described in patients with KTS using advanced imaging techniques, the presence of an easily palpable thrill or prominent pulsation portends a more serious clinical course associated with PWS.

• While KTS is often managed nonoperatively, with control of symptoms using gradient compression and management of associated lymphedema, patients with PWS can require frequent interventions due to the high-flow nature of their malformations.

## MANAGEMENT

• Capillary malformations—Generally, do not require any specific treatment as they rarely become symptomatic. If bleeding or ulceration occurs and surgical excision is undertaken, wound complications occur at higher rates.[6] Pulse dye lasers can be used to decrease the appearance of capillary malformations but may require multiple treatments for optimal results.

• Limb hypertrophy—If the limb discrepancy is less than 2 cm, treatment consists of a contralateral shoe insert. Discrepancies of greater than 2 cm can result in significant gait disturbances that merit surgery. Epiphysiodesis is undertaken to prevent the irreversible sequelae of limb discrepancy including permanent gait disturbance and scoliosis.

• Venous malformations—The initial treatment of varicosities associated with KTS is leg elevation and gradient compression stockings. If symptoms cannot be alleviated with these measures, then both sclerotherapy and operative resection or ablation of the affected veins can be safely undertaken. Prior to any intervention, imaging to delineate the presence or absence of the deep system in conjunction with the presence of any persistent or anomalous embryonic structures is paramount. Duplex ultrasound, magnetic resonance imaging (MRI), and venography aid in planning any intervention. Surgery is reserved for highly symptomatic patients. Only after confirmation of adequate outflow veins should ligation be considered. Stripping of the lateral marginal vein as well as selective ligation of varicosities can be performed with good results.[8] Most authors advocate use of a tourniquet during surgery. Endovenous ablation including radiofrequency and laser has been reported in selected cases. Sclerotherapy is a low-risk treatment that can be used either alone or in conjunction with these other modalities to treat symptomatic varicosities in patients with KTS.

• Lymphedema—The goal of lymphedema management with KTS mimics lymphedema management in general, and is centered on control of local manifestations and prevention of infections. Manual lymphatic massage, graduated compression stockings, intermittent pneumatic compression, leg elevation, and attention to skin hygiene all play a role in the management of lymphedema. Operative debulking procedures can be undertaken in severe cases, and lymphatic reconstructions have been reported in some centers.

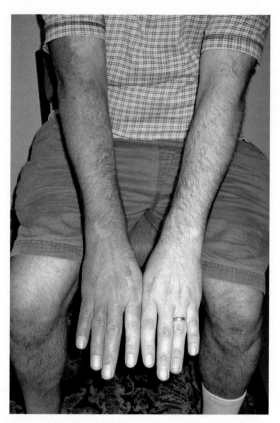

**FIGURE 41-4** KTS affecting the upper extremity with capillary malformation extending distally to involve the hand and digits. (*Photograph courtesy of Steven M. Dean, DO, FACP, RPVI.*)

## FOLLOW-UP

- Patient follow-up is dictated by the severity of symptoms and interventions that are planned. Patients whose symptoms are controlled with compression alone are reassured, as most patients with KTS have a benign course.

### PATIENT RESOURCES

- http://k-t.org/
- http://www.ninds.nih.gov/disorders/klippel_trenaunay /klippel_trenaunay.htm
- http://ghr.nlm.nih.gov/condition/klippel-trenaunay -syndrome

## REFERENCES

1. Berry SA, Peterson C, Mize W, et al. Klippel-Trenaunay syndrome. *Am J Med Genet*. 1998;79(4):319-326.

2. Lorda-Sanchez I, Prieto L, Rodriguez-Pinilla E, Martinez-Frias ML. Increased parental age and number of pregnancies in Klippel-Trenaunay-Weber syndrome. *Ann Hum Genet*. 1998;62(pt 3):235-239.

3. Servelle M. Klippel and Trenaunay syndrome: 768 operated cases. *Ann Surg*. Mar 1985;201(3):365-373.

4. Bourde C. Classification des syndromes de Klippel-Trenaunay de Parkes-Weber d'apres les donees angiographiques. *Ann Radiol (Paris)*. 1974;17(2):153-160.

5. Baskerville PA, Ackroyd JS, Browse NL. The etiology of the Klippel-Trenaunay syndrome. *Ann Surg*. Nov 1985;202(5): 624-627.

6. Capraro P, Fisher J, Hammond DC, Grossman JA. Klippel-Trenaunay syndrome. *Plast Reconstr Surg*. May 2002;109(6): 2052-2060.

7. Gloviczki P, Hollier L, Telander R, et al. Surgical implications of Klippel and Trenaunay syndrome. *Ann Surg*. Mar 1983;197(3): 353-362.

8. Gloviczki P, Driscoll DJ. Klippel-Trenaunay syndrome: current management. *Phlebology*. 2007;22(6):291-298.

# 42 CONGENITAL ARTERIOVENOUS MALFORMATIONS

James Laredo, MD, PhD
Byung Boong Lee, MD, PhD

## PATIENT STORY

A 35-year-old Caucasian man with a pulsating painful flank mass was referred for further evaluation and treatment. The mass had been present for over 15 years and had enlarged over the past year along the right lower back and flank in an area underlying a birth mark (Figure 42-1). Examination confirmed a 15-cm tender mass with overlying erythematous skin changes. A thrill was palpable over the mass, and a continuous bruit was present on auscultation.

The lesion was confirmed to be a localized arteriovenous malformation (AVM) with minimal involvement of the surrounding tissues, as demonstrated on abdominal computed tomography (CT) scanning with angiography including three-dimensional (3D) reconstruction (Figure 42-2).

Conventional angiography (Figure 42-3) confirmed the presence of an extensive AVM lesion with multiple feeding arteries. The massively dilated venous outflow due to the fistulous lesion producing a hemodynamically advanced condition.

Direct puncture, transvenous embolization utilizing 0.035 Bentsen wires was performed preoperatively for subsequent open resection of the lesion to reduce intraoperative bleeding. Complete excision of the lesion filled with the coils was performed safely (Figure 42-4), leaving a minor residual lesion that was treated with conventional sclerotherapy (Figure 42-5). Follow-up CT angiography and 3D reconstruction demonstrated an excellent result (Figure 42-6).

### EPIDEMIOLOGY

#### Congenital Vascular Malformation (Arteriovenous Malformation Subtype)

- Congenital vascular malformations (CVMs) are inborn vascular defects that present at birth and may become clinically evident later in life.

- The AVM is the least common CVM, representing 10% to 15% of all clinically significant CVMs.

- The majority of CVMs (85%-90%) are either a venous malformation (VM)[1] or a lymphatic malformation (LM).[2]

#### Hemangioma

- The neonatal or infantile hemangioma is not a vascular malformation but a vascular tumor.

- Hemangioma is a vascular tumor that originates from endothelial cells and is present in the early neonatal period.

- Hemangiomas occur in approximately 1% to 2% and 10% of white infants at birth and at age 1 year, respectively.

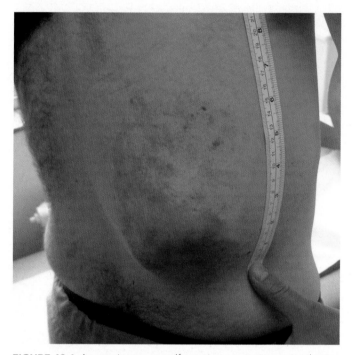

**FIGURE 42-1** An arteriovenous malformation presenting as a pulsating back or flank mass. A 35-year-old Caucasian man shown with a pulsating mass on his back and right flank. The mass had been present for over 15 years and had enlarged over the past year. The mass was associated with pain and developed in an area underlying a birth mark.

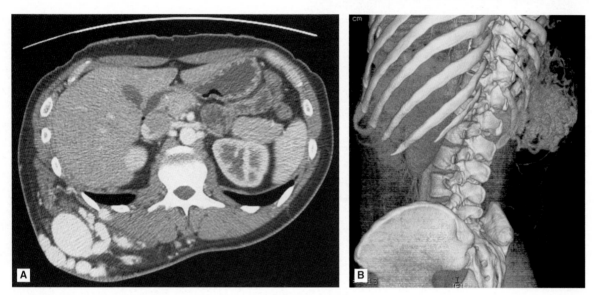

**FIGURE 42-2** Abdominal computed tomography (CT) demonstrating an arteriovenous malformation (AVM) of the right back and flank. The AVM lesion was confined to the superficial tissues. Conventional CT scanning with intravenous contrast (A) with three-dimensional (3D) reconstruction (B) was performed.

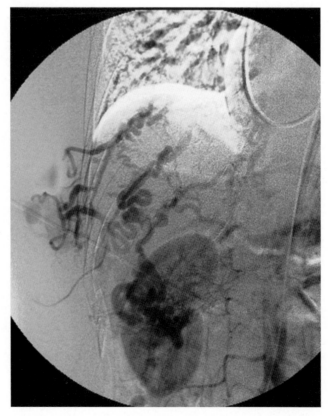

**FIGURE 42-3** Angiography of an arteriovenous malformation (AVM) of the right back and flank. Note the extensive AVM lesion with multiple feeding arteries and massively dilated venous outflow.

- Hemangiomas occur most commonly in white infants, with an incidence rate 10 to 12 times that of black and Asian infants.
- Females are affected more often than males by a ratio of 3:1.

## ETIOLOGY AND PATHOPHYSIOLOGY

### Congenital Vascular Malformation (Arteriovenous Malformation Subtype)

- CVMs are inborn vascular defects that present at birth and continue to grow at a rate proportional to the growth rate of the body.
- The AVM is a congenital anomaly of the vascular system where the anatomic defect produces shunting of arterial blood into the venous system.
- The vast majority of the AVMs exist alone as independent lesions, but occasionally occur with other CVM lesions.
- AVM itself is further subgrouped into two different types, based on the embryological stage where developmental arrest has occurred: extratruncular and truncular lesions.[3]

The AVM type most often associated with unpredictable biological behavior is the extratruncular lesion that has unique, pathologic, embryological characteristics. Its proliferative potential is derived from the mesenchymal cells of origin where developmental arrest has occurred at an earlier stage of in utero organogenesis.

In contrast, the other type of AVM, the truncular form, does not have a mesenchymal cell origin or characteristics. Both forms are classified based on the Hamburg classification (Table 42-1).

In addition to its unique embryological characteristics, AVM exhibits complicated hemodynamics. Both truncular and extratruncular AVM lesions are associated with altered cardiovascular hemodynamics occurring centrally, peripherally, and locally, involving the arterial, venous, and lymphatic systems. These characteristics make the AVM the most hemodynamically complex type of CVM. The AVM also carries a high rate of progression and significant destructive potential of the primary lesion and its secondary effects.[4]

The AVM, especially the infiltrating extratruncular-type lesion, is the most dangerous, primitive CVM that is associated with high rates of recurrence and potentially life-threatening and limb-threatening complications.

Proper treatment of AVMs requires accurate diagnosis and precise classification of its embryological subtype (as either truncular or extratruncular), and determination of its hemodynamic status.

### Extratruncular AVM Lesion

This type of AVM develops during an early stage of embryogenesis. It persists as an embryonic tissue remnant following developmental arrest that occurs during the reticular stage of embryogenesis, prior to maturation of the vascular system into vascular trunks. Extratruncular lesions maintain the original reticular network, resulting in AV shunting with no capillary check valve system. The nidus of the lesion retains its nonfistulous condition (in contrast to the truncular lesion and the fistulous condition). The extratruncular lesion produces a significant hemodynamic alteration to both the arterial and venous systems, resulting in shunting of arterial blood into the venous system that also has a mechanical impact on the surrounding tissues and organs.

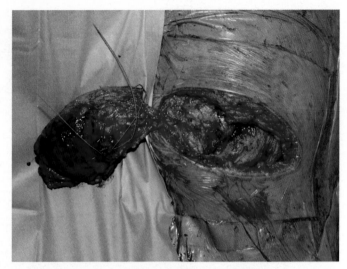

**FIGURE 42-4** Surgical resection of an arteriovenous malformation (AVM) of the right back and flank. Direct puncture, transvenous embolization utilizing 0.035 Bentsen wires was performed prior to open resection of the lesion to reduce intraoperative bleeding. The Bentsen wires are seen protruding from the lesion.

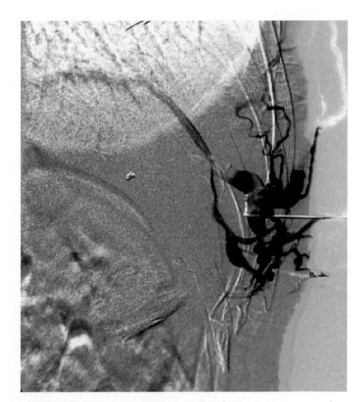

**FIGURE 42-5** Postoperative angiography after surgical resection of an arteriovenous malformation (AVM) of the right back and flank. Note the minor residual lesion, which was treated with conventional sclerotherapy.

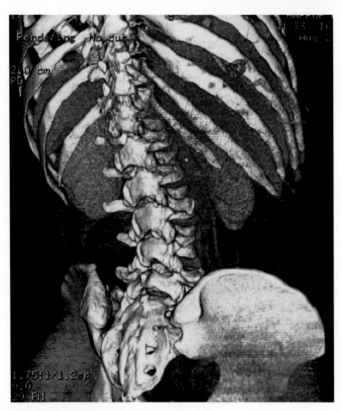

**FIGURE 42-6** Follow-up abdominal computed tomography (CT) with three-dimensional (3D) reconstruction after combined endovascular and open surgical treatment of an arteriovenous malformation (AVM) of the right back and flank. Note the excellent result with no significant residual lesion.

**TABLE 42-1** Hamburg Classification of Congenital Vascular Malformations[a,b]

Main classification based on its predominant vascular component
- Predominantly arterial defects
- Predominantly venous defects
- Predominantly arteriovenous (AV) shunting defects
- Predominantly lymphatic defects
- Predominantly capillary malformation
- Combined vascular defects

Subclassification based on the embryological stage of the defect
- Extratruncular forms—developmental arrest at the earlier stages of embryonal life
  - Diffuse, infiltrating
  - Limited, localized
- Truncular forms—developmental arrest at the later stages of embryonal life
  - Aplasia or obstruction
    - Hypoplasia, aplasia, hyperplasia
    - Stenosis, membrane, congenital spur
  - Dilatation
    - Localized (aneurysm)
    - Diffuse (ectasia)

[a]Both extratruncular and truncular forms may exist together in the same vascular malformation; may be combined with other various malformations (eg, capillary, arterial, AV shunting, venous, hemolymphatic, and/or lymphatic); and/or may exist with hemangioma.
[b]Based on the consensus on the congenital vascular malformation (CVM) classification through the international workshop in Hamburg, Germany, 1988, which was upheld by subsequently founded International Society for Vascular Anomaly (ISSVA).

Furthermore, the lesion retains its ability to proliferate and its mesenchymal cell characteristics derived from mesodermal cells (angioblasts). Lesions proliferate in response to stimulation (eg, trauma, surgery, hormone, menarche, pregnancy), resulting in an increase in their size, extent, and severity. Suboptimal treatment of extratruncular AVMs often results in lesion recurrence.

## Truncular AVM Lesion

This type of AVM develops during a later stage of embryogenesis compared with the extratruncular form. It is the result of a defective arterial system that develops during arterial trunk formation (truncal stage). The truncal stage of fetal development occurs after the reticular stage of vascular development and results in the formation of a mature lesion. Truncular AVMs no longer possesses mesenchymal cell (angioblast) characteristics and carry no risk of recurrence. However, these lesions often have more serious hemodynamic consequences to the vascular system compared with the extratruncular form. Truncular AVMs persist as fistulous lesions with a direct connection between an artery and vein, with no defined nidus. This fistulous lesion produces significantly more serious hemodynamic problems: cardiac failure, arterial insufficiency (eg, gangrene), and/or chronic venous insufficiency.

## Hemangioma

- The hemangioma is a self-limited vascular tumor.
- The growth cycle of a hemangioma is characterized by a proliferation phase of early rapid growth, followed by an involutional phase of slow regression that usually occurs before the age of 5 to 10 years in the majority of cases.
- Most hemangiomas are small and pose only minor clinical problems before they involute and become clinically silent.
- Up to 20% of hemangiomas require treatment. Indications for treatment include aggressive growth, proximity to vital structures, or complications such as ulceration, bleeding, or high-output cardiac failure.[5]

## DIAGNOSIS

CVMs commonly occur as mixed lesions presenting with AVM, VM, LM, and/or congenital malformation components. Therefore, the evaluation of any suspected AVM should proceed in a logical, step-wise manner, bearing in mind that the proposed AVM lesion may actually prove to be a mixed CVM lesion. Diagnosis of a suspected AVM requires specific evaluation and confirmation as AVM.

As a general rule, the extent and severity of any CVM affecting the vascular system (anatomically and hemodynamically) usually determines the type of clinical manifestations observed. The history and physical examination should be followed by diagnostic imaging in order to distinguish the AVM from the various CVMs (eg, duplex ultrasonography and magnetic resonance imaging [MRI]). Most AVMs occur as single lesions.

When AVMs present with additional elements derived from other CVMs (eg, VM, LM), they are classified as hemolymphatic malformation (HLMs). These mixed lesions are considered to be an extended form of Klippel-Trenaunay syndrome (KTS), which is also known as

Parkes-Weber syndrome (PWS). In this situation, the initial priority of investigation should be to confirm the presence of an AVM.

## IMAGING

Initial diagnostic imaging should be performed with a combination of baseline noninvasive to less-invasive tests. More specific diagnostic procedures then follow for precise and detailed assessment of the AVM as a whole in order to define its embryological subtype as either extratruncular or truncular.

The most common initial studies include

- Duplex ultrasonography (arterial and venous)
- MRI with T1- and T2-weighted imaging
- CT angiography with contrast enhancement, with 3D CT reconstruction
- Whole body blood pool scintigraphy (WBBPS)
- Transarterial lung perfusion scintigraphy (TLPS)

The final diagnosis should be confirmed with an invasive study to further define the lesion and plan proper treatment. These studies include

- Selective and superselective angiography
- Percutaneous direct puncture arteriography
- Percutaneous direct puncture phlebography

In addition to the assessment of the primary AVM lesion, assessment of the secondary impact on the nonvascular organ systems, especially to the musculoskeletal system, is warranted. Early detection of vascular-bone syndrome with long bone length discrepancy is essential for appropriate management.

Duplex ultrasonographic evaluation allows hemodynamic assessment of the arterial and venous components involved with the AVM directly and indirectly. Duplex ultrasound is extremely valuable for the clinical follow-up and remains the first-choice study among the various noninvasive tests available for CVM evaluation in addition to MRI.

MRI remains the major diagnostic study for the entire group of CVMs. MRI allows assessment of lesion extent, severity, and anatomic relationship to the surrounding tissues or structures or organs. MRI of the AVM lesion is usually followed up with CT angiography as confirmatory study.

Among the many newly developed noninvasive to less-invasive tests for the evaluation of CVMs, TLPS has a unique role in determining the degree of arteriovenous shunting that occurs within an extremity AVM lesion. TLPS is able to detect and assess a micro-AV shunting lesion. These types of lesions are notoriously difficult to diagnose and detect with conventional arteriography and can be easily missed. Micro-AVMs frequently occur in the combined form of CVM, the HLM (eg, PWS). Misdiagnosis of this potentially limb-threatening lesion can be avoided with TLPS alone. TLPS also provides quantitative measurement of the shunting status during therapy. TLPS may replace the substantial role of traditional arteriography as a follow-up assessment tool for extremity AVMs.

## MANAGEMENT

### New Concept of Multidisciplinary Approach

The AVM remains the most challenging malformation among the various CVMs due to its effects on the cardiovascular system and its hemodynamic consequences. The clinical manifestations associated with the AVM are dependent on lesion location, where centrally and peripherally located lesions may produce cardiac failure and arterial or venous insufficiency, respectively. In addition, local effects of AVMs may include ulceration and gangrene. Indications for treatment are listed in Table 42-2.

Because of the virulent nature of the AVM, all AVM lesions will eventually progress to the point of anatomic, physiologic, and hemodynamic deterioration, resulting in a potentially life-threatening or limb-threatening lesion. Therefore, ideally, an early aggressive approach to all AVM lesions, with either macro- or micro-AV shunting, is favored.

AVM lesion recurrence rates following currently available conventional (surgical or nonsurgical) treatment are much higher than those associated with other CVMs, making recurrence a hallmark of this CVM subtype. One of the major reasons for such dismal results over the last several decades was a flawed approach to the AVM, combined with a lack of a thorough understanding of the fundamental embryological characteristics among extratruncular lesions. The old strategy where the goal was to shut off the feeding artery, while leaving the nidus of the lesion intact, resulted in stimulating a more aggressive neovascular response by the surviving primitive lesion, ultimately making the condition worse.

This often ill planned and improper treatment strategy (eg, incomplete resection, ligation of the feeding arteries) only stimulates the AVM lesion to transform from a dormant state to a proliferative state, resulting in massive growth with uncontrollable complications. Aggressive control of the lesion nidus is therefore essential in order to prevent recurrence and eventual deterioration of the AVM lesion.

A controlled, aggressive approach must be exercised in the management of AVMs where the benefit of treatment must always exceed the risk of the associated morbidity. Only in situations where treatment morbidity and mortality are exceedingly high should a palliative approach be considered. In reality, not every AVM can be treated or should be treated by virtue of its simple existence. Although AVMs can be far more serious than any other CVMs and associated with dismal long-term outcomes, careful assessment of the treatment strategy and an accurate assessment of the risk-to-benefit ratio prior to initiating treatment are essential for success, along with clearly defined treatment goals and realistic expectations.

A relatively new multidisciplinary team approach to the treatment of AVMs resulted in significant improvements in the workup, diagnosis, and treatment of these lesions.[6] Reductions in morbidity, mortality, and recurrence rates associated with the treatment of AVMs have been reported with the multidisciplinary approach. A fully integrated specialty team for advanced diagnosis and treatment of AVMs will provide the full spectrum of endovascular and surgical therapy. The multidisciplinary team approach will allow maximum coordination among the various CVM-related specialists (Table 42-3).

**TABLE 42-2** Indications for Treatment of Arteriovenous Malformations

- Hemorrhage
- High-output heart failure
- Secondary arterial ischemic complications
- Secondary complications of chronic venous hypertension
- Lesions located at life-threatening region (eg, proximity to the airway), or located at the region threatening vital functions (eg, seeing, eating, hearing, or breathing)
- Disabling pain
- Functional impairment
- Cosmetically severe deformity
- Vascular-bone syndrome
- Lesions located at the region with potentially high risk of complication (eg, hemarthrosis)

**TABLE 42-3** Multidisciplinary Team for the Contemporary Management of the Arteriovenous Malformation

- Vascular Surgery
- Pediatric Surgery
- Plastic and Reconstructive
- Surgery
- Orthopedic Surgery
- Neurosurgery
- Oral-Maxillary-Head and Neck Surgery
- Anesthesiology
- Pathology
- Physical Medicine and Rehabilitation
- Cardiovascular Medicine
- General Medicine
- Pediatrics
- Interventional Radiology
- Diagnostic Radiology
- Nuclear Medicine
- Dermatology
- Neurology
- Psychiatry

## Vascular and Endovascular Therapy

Surgical resection has long been the gold standard for the treatment of AVMs despite high rates of complication, morbidity, and recurrence. Complete eradication of the nidus of AVM is required to achieve an effective cure. Surgical resection has long been the only means of eradicating the AVM nidus. Incomplete resection in many cases is unavoidable due to the prohibitively high morbidity associated with radical surgical therapy.

The role of surgical resection changed with the development of endovascular therapy over the last several years. Open surgical resection outcomes have significantly improved with the use of adjunctive endovascular therapy. Preoperative embolo/sclerotherapy has been shown to improve the safety and efficacy of subsequent surgical resection, resulting in significantly reduced morbidity and mortality (eg, intraoperative bleeding). Postoperative supplemental endovascular therapy has also been shown to be of benefit in the surgical treatment of AVMs.

Endovascular therapy with various embolization and sclerotherapy modalities is a fully accepted therapeutic option in the treatment of AVM lesions. Endovascular therapy alone has been shown to be beneficial in patients with prohibitively high surgical risks and in patients with surgically inaccessible lesions. It remains the treatment of choice for AVM lesions that extend beyond the deep fascia and involve muscle, tendon, and bone—the diffuse infiltrating type of extratruncular form of AVMs.

Precise delivery of the embolosclerosants directly into the nidus of the AVM lesion (extratruncular form) is required for successful endovascular therapy. The outdated approach where the goal of treatment was embolization of the AVM feeding arteries is no longer viable and should be condemned. A combination-type therapy approach where all three routes of delivery (transarterial, transvenous, and direct puncture) are utilized in order to obliterate the AVM lesion nidus is most efficacious.

Multisession endovascular therapy is preferred and allows administration of the minimally effective volume of embolization and sclerotherapy agents during each session in order to reduce the risk of associated acute and chronic morbidity. The most commonly utilized treatment agents include absolute ethanol, onyx, N-butyl cyanoacrylate (NBCA), coils, and contour particles (eg, Ivalon).

## Ethanol Sclerotherapy

Absolute ethanol is associated with significant morbidity. To minimize injury to surrounding tissues, ethanol may be effectively diluted to 60% when used to treat superficial AVMs that carry a high risk of skin necrosis and AVM lesions in close proximity to nerves. Administration of smaller volumes in divided doses also minimizes the risk of surrounding tissue injury. The residual ethanol may be drained before removal of needles. If localized swelling and tissue reaction is severe, light compression may be applied for 5 to 10 minutes after treatment. Direct compression of the vein draining the AVM during treatment may prevent early drainage during ethanol injection.

Appropriate precautions for the potential risk of cardiopulmonary complications during ethanol sclerotherapy should be made with the minimal possible amount of ethanol allowed (1 mg/kg of body weight in maximum per session).

The importance of close monitoring of the cardiopulmonary-vascular system during the ethanol sclerotherapy cannot be overemphasized; appropriate or immediate handling of the increased pulmonary pressure when the ethanol should reach to the pulmonary bed is absolutely mandatory.

Pulmonary hypertension is a potentially fatal morbidity by chemical toxicity of the ethanol, and pulmonary spasm, can lead to cardiopulmonary arrest.

Special precaution to the increased risk of skin necrosis should be exercised via arterial puncture; do not allow the ethanol to reflux to the arterial side.

## Coil and Glue Embolotherapy

A major liability of coil embolotherapy is it only exerts mechanical effects to block flow to induce thrombosis and does not have any direct effect on the endothelium to induce permanent damage; therefore, recanalization of the nidus will ultimately recur.

Therefore, it is desirable to have further control of the nidus with additional permanent therapy via absolute ethanol. Although the fistulous AVM, which often requires coils, is a mostly truncular lesion with lack of evolutional potential.

Before injecting ethanol into a high-flow draining vein, coil embolization should be undertaken with one or more of the following modalities: platinum spiral coil, tornado coil, and/or detachable coil(s).

Glue (NBCA) embolization also should be considered with 30% to 50% concentration to minimize foreign body reaction, and its use should be limited to surgical candidates, if possible; try to puncture as close as possible to the AV-connection nidus to make a glue cast from the nidus to proximal draining vein.

## PATIENT EDUCATION

Patients with AVM and other CVMs can experience recurrence of their lesion. The likelihood of a recurrence is directly related to the lesion type and extent of treatment. Patients are instructed to report any new lesions and symptoms to the doctor with regular follow-up and ongoing monitoring and imaging as indicated.

## FOLLOW-UP

After treatment, patients should be reassessed at 3-month intervals or more frequently, if needed for the first year, and then at yearly intervals as appropriate, to monitor for symptoms associated with lesion recurrence.

## CONCLUSION

Arteriovenous malformation is a potentially life- and limb-threatening lesion. This is especially true with the fistulous truncular form, due to its unique embryologic and hemodynamic characteristics.

A multidisciplinary team and early, aggressive approach to the treatment of AVMs utilizing fully integrated endovascular and surgical therapy can achieve effective control of AVM lesions. As with the treatment of any CVM, careful assessment of the risks and benefits associated with the AVM and proposed treatment should serve to guide subsequent therapy.

**PROVIDER RESOURCES**

- http://emedicine.medscape.com/article/1160167-overview
- http://www.phlebolymphology.org/2011/11/congenital-arteriovenous-malformations-what-are-the-perspectives/

**PATIENT RESOURCES**

- http://children.webmd.com/arteriovenous-malformation
- http://www.sickkids.ca/PlasticSurgery/What-we-do/Vascular-Anomalies-Clinic/Vascular-Malformations/Arteriovenous-Malformations/index.html

## REFERENCES

1. Lee BB. Current concept of venous malformation (VM). *Phlebolymphology*. 2003;43:197-203.

2. Lee BB, Laredo J, Seo JM, Nevilles R. Hemangiomas and vascular malformations. In: Mattassi R, Loose DA, Vaghi M, eds. *Treatment of Lymphatic Malformations.* Milan, Italy: Springer-Verlag; 2009:231-250.

3. Belov St. Classification of congenital vascular defects. *Int Angiol*. 1990;9:141-146.

4. Sumner D. Hemodynamics and pathophysiology of arteriovenous fistulas. In: Rutherford RB, ed. *Vascular Surgery*. Vol 8. 3rd ed. Philadelphia, PA: WB Saunders Company; 1989.

5. Lee BB, Mattassi R, Loose D, Yakes W, Tasnadi G, Kim HH. Consensus on controversial issues in contemporary diagnosis and management of congenital vascular malformation—Seoul Communication. *Int J Angiol*. 2004;13(4):182-192.

6. Lee BB, Bergan JJ. Advanced management of congenital vascular malformations: a multidisciplinary approach. *Cardiovasc Surg*. Dec 2002;10(6):523-533.

# PART 6

# ARTERIOVENOUS VISCERAL DISEASE

# 43 ATHEROSCLEROTIC RENAL ARTERY STENOSIS

Ido Weinberg, MD
Michael R. Jaff, DO

## PATIENT STORY

A 67-year-old man treated for hypertension (HTN) for the past 25 years is now having difficulty with his blood pressure control. His medical history is notable for long-standing hypercholesterolemia and former tobacco abuse (25 pack-years) until 1 month ago when he was hospitalized for chest pain. At that time his blood pressure was 195/110 mm Hg. He has noted that blood pressure control has been gradually worsening over the past several years. Most recently, his blood pressure measurements have not been below 160/95 mm Hg. He has eliminated salt from his diet, has been watching his weight, and has been compliant with his three antihypertensive medications, all of which have been prescribed at maximal doses (hydrochlorothiazide 25 mg/d, lisinopril 40 mg/d, and amlodipine 10 mg/d). On physical examination he has a midline systolic bruit just above the umbilicus radiating to his right flank. Figures 43-1 to 43-3 demonstrate the typical appearance of atherosclerotic renal artery stenosis (ARAS) by duplex ultrasonography, computed tomography (CT), and contrast angiography.

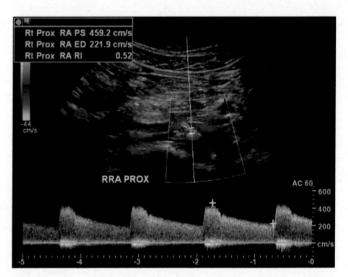

FIGURE 43-1 Duplex ultrasound of right renal artery ostial stenosis.

## EPIDEMIOLOGY

- ARAS is prevalent with advancing age and has been found to affect 6.8% of patients in a population-based study of elderly people.

- ARAS is most prevalent in at-risk populations, including patients with systemic atherosclerosis, patients with coronary artery disease (18%-20%), or patients with peripheral artery disease, where it was found in up to 59% of patients.[1]

## PATHOPHYSIOLOGY

- ARAS is anatomically in the artery ostium as a continuation of plaque from the abdominal aorta.[2]

- HTN in ARAS results from activation of the renin-angiotensin-aldosterone pathway. The kidney ipsilateral to the stenosis responds by secreting renin, which promotes sodium retention and vasoconstriction via the renin-angiotensin-aldosterone pathway. The nonstenotic contralateral kidney responds by natriuresis that promotes intravascular volume depletion. The stenotic kidney excretes more renin as its perfusion pressure has been reduced. At some point natriuresis is overpowered by the renin-angiotensin-aldosterone pathway, resulting in HTN.

- Renal failure in patients with ARAS results from multiple potential etiologies: long-standing systemic HTN, renal ischemia, recurrent atheromatous embolization from an atherosclerotic aorta, and contrast nephropathy following multiple imaging studies.

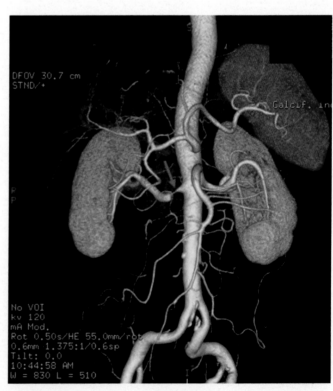

FIGURE 43-2 Three-dimensional reconstructed computed tomography angiography (CTA) image of right renal artery stenosis (arrow).

- While ARAS is more prevalent in patients with end-stage renal failure than those without it, there is no linear relationship between the degree of ARAS and HTN or renal dysfunction.

## DIAGNOSIS

### Clinical Features

- ARAS has been implicated as a cause for HTN, deteriorating renal function, and cardiac disturbance syndromes (recurrent unexplained congestive heart failure, refractory angina, and flash pulmonary edema).

- HTN related to underlying ARAS should be suspected in the following patients: patients older than 55 years at the time of onset, persons with resistant HTN (the inability to achieve goal blood pressure of 140/90 mm Hg or lower despite the use of three antihypertensive medications at maximum tolerable doses used in appropriate combinations), or in patients who experience exacerbation of previously well-controlled HTN.

- ARAS should be suspected when there is deterioration in renal function following initiation of angiotensin-converting enzyme inhibitors or angiotensin receptor antagonists, unexplained azotemia, and an unexplained discrepancy in renal size.

### Noninvasive Imaging Studies

- Renal artery duplex ultrasonography is accurate, inexpensive, and painless, and thus is an ideal noninvasive option for confirming or refuting the diagnosis of renal artery stenosis.[3]

- Duplex ultrasound criteria for the diagnosis of renal artery stenosis combines peak systolic velocities within the renal artery as well as the ratio of the peak systolic velocity as measured in the aorta at the level of the superior mesenteric artery and the peak systolic velocity at the level of the renal artery origin, known as the renal-to-aortic ratio.

- Acceptable duplex criteria for the diagnosis of renal artery stenosis are presented in Table 43-1.

- Computed tomography angiography (CTA) and magnetic resonance angiography (MRA) accurately assess ARAS, while providing excellent three-dimensional images of the renal arteries. Advantages include the ability to visualize accessory (polar) renal arteries and the abdominal aorta and kidneys, as well as other important pathologies such as aneurysms. Disadvantages of CTA include exposure to radiation, the need for iodinated contrast agents, and the inability to differentiate completely between calcification and the renal artery lumen. Disadvantages of MRA include the need for contrast agents (ie, gadolinium), a tendency to overestimate the severity of arterial stenosis, inability to visualize within metallic stents, and the rare occurrence of nephrogenic systemic fibrosis.

- Other than the degree of stenosis, other noninvasive measurements and laboratory findings have been proposed to suggest which patients will respond to renal artery revascularization: cortical thinning, resistive index,[4] and preprocedural proteinuria. The utility of resistive index has not been reproduced by all.

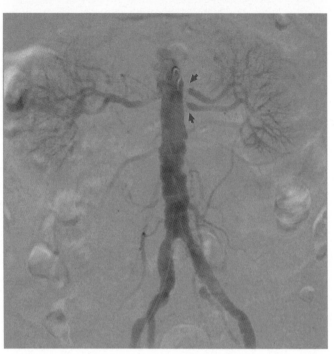

**FIGURE 4-3** Angiography of left renal artery ostial stenosis in a renal artery and an accessory renal artery (arrowheads).

**TABLE 43-1** Duplex Ultrasound Criteria for Native Renal Artery Stenosis

| Degree of Stenosis | PSV[a] | RAR (Renal/ Aortic Ratio)[b] |
|---|---|---|
| Normal | <200 cm/s | <3.5 |
| 1% to 59% stenosis | <200 cm/s | <3.5 |
| 60% to 99% | >200 cm/s + poststenotic turbulence | >3.5 |
| Occlusion | No flow can be detected in the renal artery | |

[a]PSV, peak systolic velocity.
[b]The RAR cannot be used if the aortic PSV is greater than 100 cm/s or less than 40 cm/s.

## Angiographic Features

- Catheter-based contrast angiography is the gold standard for the diagnosis of ARAS (Figure 43-4).

- Intravascular ultrasound and translesional pressure gradients may aid in the assessment of the hemodynamic significance of a renal artery stenosis.

- Some measurements acquired during angiography may assist in predicting the clinical benefit of renal artery revascularization including baseline translesional pressure gradient, hyperemic systolic gradient of the stenosis of greater than or equal to 21 mm Hg, fractional-flow reserve, and renal frame count.[5]

## DIFFERENTIAL DIAGNOSIS

- Fibromuscular dysplasia (FMD) is a noninflammatory, nonatherosclerotic arterial disease that most commonly occurs in women aged 20 to 60 years. The renal arteries are affected in 75% of patients.[6] Differentiating features from ARAS are younger age at presentation and imaging characteristics including a more distal involvement and a typical, often beaded appearance of the renal artery (Figure 43-5A). When indicated, percutaneous transluminal angioplasty has proven to be successful in patients with FMD (Figure 43-5B).

- Takayasu arteritis is a large vessel arteritis. Diagnostic criteria include young age, intermittent claudication of more than one extremity (classically the upper extremity), a decreased brachial pulse, an interbrachial systolic blood pressure difference greater than 10 mm Hg, a bruit over a subclavian artery, and imaging evidence of narrowing of the aorta or one of its large branches. Inflammatory markers are elevated in the active stages of disease. While typically affecting the aortic arch and the great vessels, Takayasu arteritis may also result in a mid-aortic variant that can manifest with renovascular HTN.

- Segmental arterial mediolysis (SAM) is a noninflammatory, nonatherosclerotic condition with a predilection to visceral arteries. Lesions appear as strands of arterial narrowing on imaging (often CTA or MRA). SAM may be asymptomatic and thus incidentally discovered or manifest with abdominal or flank pain.

## MANAGEMENT

- Optimal pharmacologic management of atherosclerotic risk factors is the backbone of the treatment of ARAS. This includes lipid-lowering therapy, tobacco cessation, glycemic control in diabetes mellitus, antiplatelet medications (despite a lack of direct evidence of benefit in patients with ARAS), and blood pressure control as per Joint National Committee VII goals.[7]

- Current guidelines assigned a class IIa recommendation for renal artery revascularization for patients with hemodynamically significant RAS and accelerated, resistant, or malignant hypertension, HTN with an unexplained unilateral small kidney, and HTN with intolerance to medication. Other indications included progressive chronic kidney disease over the past 3 to 6 months with bilateral renal artery stenosis or a renal artery stenosis to a solitary functioning kidney, unstable angina, recurrent unexplained congestive heart failure, or sudden unexplained pulmonary edema.[1]

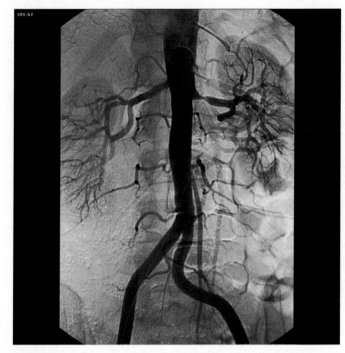

**FIGURE 43-4** Arteriographic image of atherosclerotic renal artery stenosis (ARAS) involving left aorto-ostial segment.

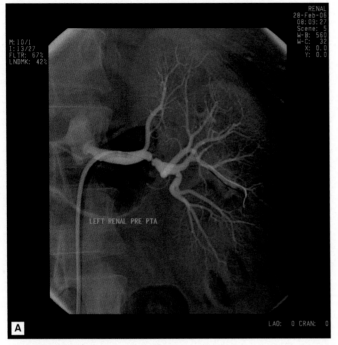 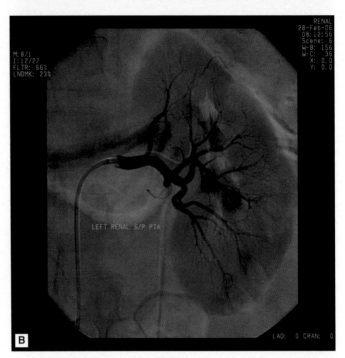

**FIGURES 43-5** Arteriographic images of intimal fibroplasia variant of fibromuscular dysplasia (FMD) in the mid/distal renal artery before (A)/after (B) percutaneous transluminal angioplasty.

- The mechanism underlying ARAS is often bulky atheromatous aortorenal plaque, thus percutaneous transluminal angioplasty does not provide durable patency.[8] Endovascular renal artery stent placement, on the other hand, offers an acute procedural success rate of up to 98%.

- Patient selection for endovascular renal artery stent placement is problematic, as all patients do not respond favorably to intervention.[9,10]

## PATIENT EDUCATION

ARAS can often be managed medically; however, some patients may benefit from intervention. Patients with clear indications as outlined earlier should be offered endovascular renal artery stent placement. However, other patients should be informed of the therapeutic options and about current gaps in the ability to predict response to treatment of ARAS, and a joint decision should be made regarding the method of treatment.

## FOLLOW-UP

- Follow-up of patients with ARAS should incorporate both clinical assessments and imaging studies.

- Renal artery duplex ultrasound is often the most useful tool for surveillance of ARAS, whether revascularization has been performed or not.

- The natural history of ARAS is incompletely understood; therefore, surveillance protocols are often dictated by local practice.[2] If stenosis is 60% in a renal artery supplying a normal-sized kidney and the contralateral renal artery is widely patent, a repeat examination is performed in 6 months, and if unchanged, annual renal artery duplex ultrasonography is reasonable. Factors that may prompt more frequent testing include deterioration in blood pressure control, progression of renal dysfunction, or renal atrophy.

- There are currently no prospective studies evaluating the surveillance of stented renal arteries. The criteria for in-stent restenosis have been proposed (Table 43-2). A reasonable protocol for poststent duplex ultrasonography is within 30 days of the procedure, after 6 and 12 months, and then annually if there is no suspicion of restenosis.

**PROVIDER RESOURCE**
- http://emedicine.medscape.com/article/245023-overview

**PATIENT RESOURCES**
- http://kidney.niddk.nih.gov/kudiseases/pubs/RenalArtery Stenosis/
- http://www.effectivehealthcare.ahrq.gov/repFiles/RAS _Consumer.pdf

**TABLE 43-2** Proposed Criteria for Stented Renal Arteries

| Degree of Stenosis | PSV[a] | RAR (Renal/ Aortic Ratio)[b] |
|---|---|---|
| 0% to 59% | <240 cm/s without PST | |
| 60% to 99% | >300 cm/s | >4.3 |
| Occlusion | No flow can be detected in the renal artery | |

[a]PSV, peak systolic velocity.
[b]The RAR cannot be used if the aortic PSV is greater than 100 cm/s or less than 40 cm/s.

## REFERENCES

1. Hirsch AT, Haskal ZJ, Hertzer NR, et al. ACC/AHA 2005 Practice Guidelines for the management of patients with peripheral arterial disease (lower extremity, renal, mesenteric, and abdominal aortic): a collaborative report from the American Association for Vascular Surgery/Society for Vascular Surgery, Society for Cardiovascular Angiography and Interventions, Society for Vascular Medicine and Biology, Society of Interventional Radiology, and the ACC/AHA Task Force on Practice Guidelines (Writing Committee to Develop Guidelines for the Management of Patients With Peripheral Arterial Disease): endorsed by the American Association of Cardiovascular and Pulmonary Rehabilitation; National Heart, Lung, and Blood Institute; Society for Vascular Nursing; TransAtlantic Inter-Society Consensus; and Vascular Disease Foundation. *Circulation.* 2006;113(11):e463-e654.

2. Dworkin LD, Cooper CJ. Clinical practice. Renal-artery stenosis. *N Engl J Med.* 2009;361(20):1972-1978.

3. Olin JW, Piedmonte MR, Young JR, DeAnna S, Grubb M, Childs MB. The utility of duplex ultrasound scanning of the renal arteries for diagnosing significant renal artery stenosis. *Ann Intern Med.* 1995;122(11):833-838.

4. Radermacher J, Chavan A, Bleck J, et al. Use of Doppler ultrasonography to predict the outcome of therapy for renal-artery stenosis. *N Engl J Med.* 2001;344(6):410-417.

5. White CJ. Optimizing outcomes for renal artery intervention. *Circ Cardiovasc Interv.* 2010;3(2):184-192.

6. Slovut DP, Olin JW. Fibromuscular dysplasia. *N Engl J Med.* 2004;350(18):1862-1871.

7. Chobanian AV, Bakris GL, Black HR, et al. The seventh report of the Joint National Committee on Prevention, Detection, Evaluation, and Treatment of High Blood Pressure: the JNC 7 report. *JAMA.* 2003;289(19):2560-2572.

8. van de Ven PJ, Kaatee R, Beutler JJ, et al. Arterial stenting and balloon angioplasty in ostial atherosclerotic renovascular disease: a randomised trial. *Lancet.* 1999;353(9149):282-286.

9. Bax L, Woittiez AJ, Kouwenberg HJ, et al. Stent placement in patients with atherosclerotic renal artery stenosis and impaired renal function: a randomized trial. *Ann Intern Med.* 2009;150(12):840-848, W150-151.

10. ASTRAL Investigators, Wheatley K, Ives N, et al. Revascularization versus medical therapy for renal-artery stenosis. *N Engl J Med.* 2009;361(20):1953-1962.

# 44 FIBROMUSCULAR DYSPLASIA–ASSOCIATED RENAL ARTERY STENOSIS

Sachin Sheth, MD
Robert Lookstein, MD, FSIR, FAHA

## PATIENT STORY

A 48-year-old woman is evaluated for newly diagnosed hypertension in the absence of atherosclerotic risk factors. A systolic abdominal bruit is discovered on clinical examination. Neither carotid nor femoral bruits are auscultated, and her remaining examination is otherwise unremarkable.

Laboratory investigation for secondary causes of hypertension is unrevealing. However, a duplex arterial ultrasound of her mid renal arteries illustrates 60% to 99% bilateral renal artery stenosis in the absence of plaque. A peculiar beaded appearance exists along the arterial walls. A diagnosis of fibromuscular dysplasia (FMD) is subsequently made.

## OVERVIEW

FMD is a noninflammatory, nonatherosclerotic arterial disease that most commonly affects the renal and internal carotid arteries (ICAs) but has been observed in almost every artery in the body. It is characterized by smooth muscle cell and fibrous tissue overgrowth in one or more layers of the renal arterial wall.

The renal arteries compromise 65% to 75% of cases of FMD, occurring bilaterally in 35% of cases. The carotid and vertebral arteries are involved in 25% to 30% of cases. Multivessel involvement is common.

FMD occurs most frequently in women aged between 20 and 60 years, but may also be seen in men, older individuals, and in the pediatric population.[1,2] It is estimated to affect anywhere between 5.8 and 8.6 million women in the United States.

Hypertension, headache, and pulsatile tinnitus are the most common presenting manifestations. Other signs and symptoms include dizziness, cervical and abdominal bruits, neck pain, flank or abdominal pain, nonpulsatile tinnitus, transient ischemic attack (TIA), and stroke. The clinical presentation is dictated by the affected arteries.

FMD can be asymptomatic and incidentally identified on an imaging study performed for a different clinical indication. In addition to arterial stenosis, patients with FMD can present with aneurysms and dissections. A history of FMD in first- or second-degree relatives is rare and occurs in around 7% of patients.

## TYPES

FMD is classified into three categories related to the pathologic layer of the arterial wall that is affected—intima, media, and adventitia (perimedial).

## Medial FMD

It is by far the most common type and is further subdivided into medial fibroplasia, perimedial fibroplasia, and medial hyperplasia.

*Medial fibroplasia* accounts for 80% to 90% of all types of FMD. This subtype is defined histologically by alternating areas of thinned media and thickened collagen-containing medial ridges. Multiple stenotic webs cause arterial stenosis and poststenotic dilation, often displaying the typical "string of beads" appearance on angiography (Figures 44-1 and 44-2). The bead component is often larger and weaker than the normal arterial lumen, and in a subset of patients with FMD, aneurysms are present that may require treatment.

*Perimedial fibroplasia* (less numerous and smaller beads than medial fibroplasia) is quite uncommon and usually occurs in young females aged between 5 and 15 years who present with hypertension and renal impairment.

*Medial hyperplasia* is extremely rare and requires a pathologic specimen for diagnosis.

## Intimal FMD

This category accounts for approximately 10% of all FMDs. Intimal fibroplasia is due to a collagen deposition within the intima complicated by an often fragmented or duplicated internal elastic lamina. Angiography shows it is distinct from medial disease because the intima causes a focal fibrotic band-like constriction that results in a concentric stenosis (Figure 44-3) and/or long tubular narrowing.

## Adventitial FMD

This has an unknown frequency. The angiographic appearance looks similar to intimal disease (tubular narrowing).

## DIAGNOSIS

Noninvasive imaging studies include duplex ultrasonography, computed tomographic angiography (CTA), and magnetic resonance angiography (MRA).[3-5]

Duplex ultrasound of the renal arteries typically reveals evidence of arterial stenosis including elevated velocity in the main renal artery or a delayed systolic upstroke (tardus parvus waveform) in arterial branches distal to the stenosis. Turbulence or spectral broadening on color Doppler as well as the presence of beading on power and color Doppler distal to the proximal main renal artery should lead to the diagnosis of FMD (Figure 44-4). Intravascular ultrasound (IVUS) may show endoluminal filling defects.

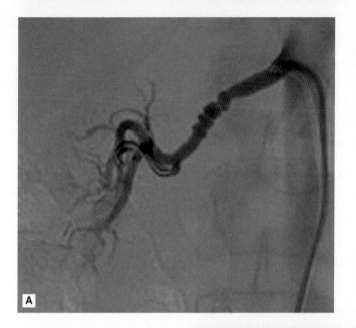

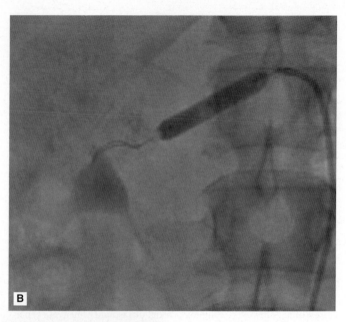

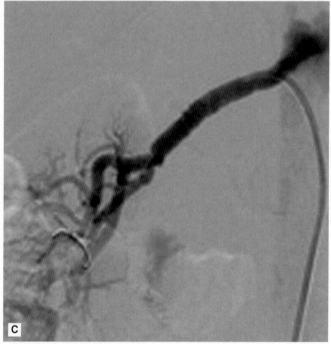

**FIGURE 44-1** (A) Medial fibromuscular dysplasia (FMD) in a 48-year-old woman with stenosis and poststenotic dilatation, giving the appearance of beads on a string. (B) Balloon angioplasty and (C) postangioplasty image.

CTA findings include the classic "string of beads" of the renal artery in patients with medial fibroplasia (Figure 44-5) and a focal concentric stenosis in those with intimal or nonmedial disease. Wedge-shaped renal infarcts can be seen in patients with FMD complicated by dissection. Hypertrophied ureteral arteries can be seen in cases with long-standing hemodynamically significant stenoses. Renal artery macroaneurysms are readily visible.

MRA is a good modality in the diagnosis of renal FMD involvement, particularly in patients who cannot receive IV contrast for CT angiography. MR angiography features of FMD are similar to those seen on CTA (Figure 44-6).

Conventional angiography remains the gold standard imaging modality for renal artery FMD due to its unsurpassed spatial resolution (<0.1 mm). Catheter-based renal angiography is a minimally invasive procedure and can be performed on an outpatient basis. The normal renal artery is smooth in contour and gently tapers from its origin as it courses to the renal hilum. In the setting of medial FMD, the renal artery is irregular in contour and typically displays a classic "beads on string" appearance with multifocal stenoses accompanied by small foci of poststenotic dilatation (accounting for the beads). Alternatively, a focal stenosis or long tubular stenosis can be seen in the less common, nonmedial form of the disease. Secondary signs include ureteral notching due to hypertrophied ureteral arteries. Atrophy of the kidney may also be seen in the setting of long-standing hypoperfusion. Rare manifestations such as macroaneurysms and renal artery dissection may also be observed.

Selective angiography allows for the optimal visualization of the main renal artery, all renal artery branches, and the parenchyma to assess for any primary or secondary signs of FMD. It also offers the advantage of assessing pressure gradients to gauge severity of the stenoses (a gradient of less than 10 mm Hg is considered normal). Lastly, conventional angiography allows for the additional use of IVUS to characterize the renal artery.

## DIFFERENTIAL DIAGNOSIS

### Atherosclerosis

FMD can be distinguished from atherosclerotic disease due to the younger age and lack of traditional atherosclerotic risk factors in some patients. In addition, atherosclerosis occurs at the ostium or proximal portion of the renal and carotid arteries, whereas FMD occurs in the middle or distal portion of these arteries. Because FMD has been observed in elderly persons, it is not uncommon to encounter patients with both FMD and atherosclerosis.

### Vasculitis

FMD is a noninflammatory process, whereas there is marked inflammation of the blood vessel in vasculitis. Therefore, clinical laboratory measurements such as erythrocyte sedimentation rate and C-reactive protein are usually within normal reference ranges in FMD unless there is end-organ ischemia or infarction. FMD may also be confused with a vasculitis because it may occur in multiple vascular territories and cause accelerated hypertension, kidney impairment, TIA, stroke, and complications such as dissection, aneurysm, or stenosis.

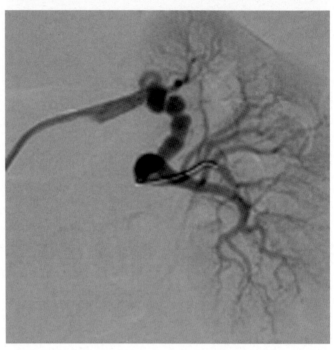

**FIGURE 44-2** Medial fibromuscular dysplasia (FMD) in a 57-year-old woman with hypertension.

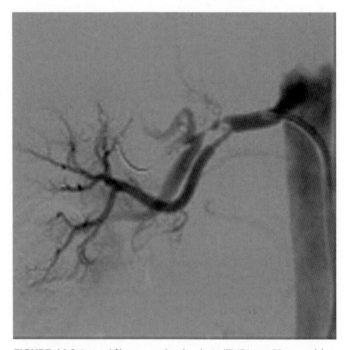

**FIGURE 44-3** Intimal fibromuscular dysplasia (FMD) in a 53-year-old woman demonstrating characteristic concentric stenosis and long tubular narrowing.

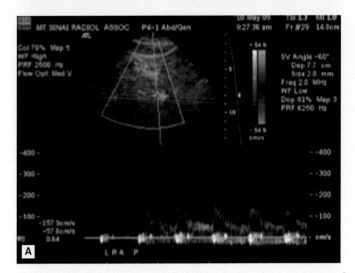

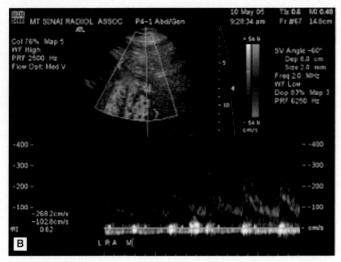

**FIGURE 44-4** Duplex images of the left renal artery show a step up in flow velocity from the proximal artery (A) to the mid artery (B) suggesting an FMD mediated arterial stenosis.

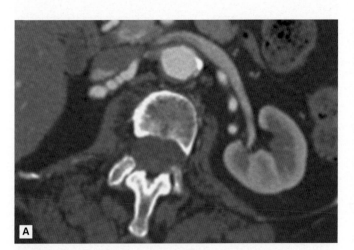

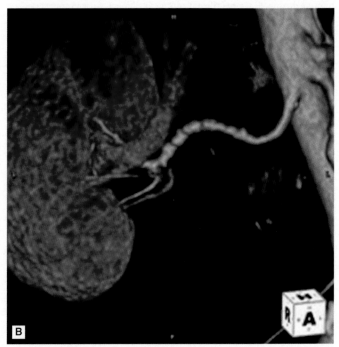

**FIGURE 44-5** (A) Computed tomographic angiogram (CTA) and (B) CTA three-dimensional (3D) volume-rendered images showing the typical "beads on a string" appearance of the right main renal artery.

## Segmental Arterial Mediolysis

Segmental arterial mediolysis (SAM) is a poorly understood condition, and it is unclear whether it is a distinct abnormality or a subtype of FMD. It is characterized by spontaneous dissection(s), occlusion, and/or aneurysm formation. It is often difficult to differentiate from FMD; however, SAM is typically limited to one arterial bed, whereas FMD is more often multifocal. The angiographic appearance may also be indistinguishable from FMD. In contrast to FMD, segmental arterial mediolysis responds poorly to angioplasty.

## TREATMENT OR MANAGEMENT

The primary goal in treating patients with renal artery FMD is the control of blood pressure to prevent the sequelae of long-standing, poorly controlled hypertension.

In patients in whom hypertension is newly diagnosed and secondary to renal artery FMD, the initial treatment may be percutaneous transluminal balloon angioplasty (PTA). The chance of cure (normal blood pressure on no antihypertensive medications) is the highest when the patient is young, the duration of hypertension is short, and the gradient is completely obliterated at the time of angioplasty.

Patients in whom FMD was not diagnosed at the onset of high blood pressure and the hypertension was present for more than several years, antihypertensive medications should be continued as long as the hypertension is well controlled.

Balloon angioplasty alone is a very effective treatment for renal artery FMD; therefore, there is no need for stent implantation under most circumstances.

The two indications for stenting in renal artery FMD are (1) if the gradient cannot be obliterated with angioplasty alone and (2) to treat a dissection.

The primary role for surgical revascularization is to treat aneurysms in patients in whom endovascular therapy is not an option or if PTA fails. PTA has replaced surgery as the preferred treatment of renal artery FMD.

Angioplasty has a number of advantages over open surgical revascularization. It may be performed with a high degree of technical and clinical success with minimal complications; it is less invasive; it has a markedly shorter recovery time; it is less expensive; and it may be performed on an outpatient basis.

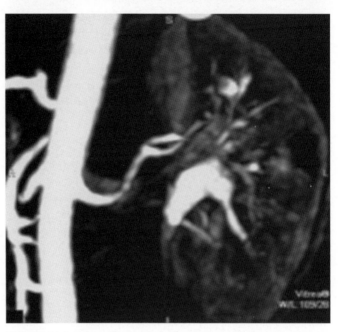

**FIGURE 44-6** Magnetic resonance angiography (MRA) in the same patient as Figure 44-4 reveals beading of the mid-left renal artery typical of fibromuscular dysplasia (FMD).

### PATIENT AND PROVIDER RESOURCES

• Fibromuscular Dysplasia Society of America: http://www.fmdsa.org/

• Fibromuscular Dysplasia on Medscape: http://emedicine.medscape.com/article/1161248-overview

## REFERENCES

1. Slovut DP, Olin JW. Fibromuscular dysplasia. *N Engl J Med.* 2004; 350:1862-1871.

2. Olin JW, Sealove BA. Diagnosis, management, and future developments of fibromuscular dysplasia. *J Vasc Surg.* Mar 2011; 53(3):826-836.e1. Epub 2011 Jan 13. Review.

3. Prasad A, Zafar N, Mahmud E. Assessment of renal artery fibromuscular dysplasia: angiography, intravascular ultrasound (with virtual histology), and pressure wire measurements. *Catheter Cardiovasc Interv*. Aug 1 2009;74(2):260-264.

4. Rountas C, Vlychou M, Vassiou K, et al. Imaging modalities for renal artery stenosis in suspected renovascular hypertension: prospective intraindividual comparison of color Doppler US, CT angiography, GD-enhanced MR angiography, and digital substraction angiography. *Ren Fail*. 2007;29(3):295-302.

5. Sabharwal R, Vladica P, Coleman P. Multidetector spiral CT renal angiography in the diagnosis of renal artery fibromuscular dysplasia. *Eur J Radiol*. Mar 2007;61(3):520-527.

# 45 ACUTE MESENTERIC ISCHEMIA

John C. Wang, MD, MSc
Vikram S. Kashyap, MD

## PATIENT STORY

A 74-year-old hypertensive male presents with a four-hour history of acute-onset severe diffuse abdominal pain. Two weeks prior he was hospitalized with a large anterior wall MI complicated by intermittent atrial fibrillation. Due to a history of frequent falls, he was not anticoagulated. Physical examination is remarkable for an uncomfortable individual with an irregularly irregular heart rhythm and a minimally tender abdomen without peritoneal signs. Laboratory assessment is remarkable for a leukocytosis of 14,000 and mild metabolic acidosis. Electrocardiography indicates atrial fibrillation with a rapid ventricular response between 120 and 140 beats/minute. CT scan of the abdomen illustrates a distended small bowel and a questionable filling defect within the superior mesenteric artery (SMA). Mesenteric arteriography displays a "mercury meniscus sign" within the SMA 4 cm from the aorta. A diagnosis of cardioembolic acute mesenteric ischemia is made and the patient is immediately taken to the operating suite.

## EPIDEMIOLOGY

- Incidence: 3 to 5 per 100,000.

- Sixth to seventh decade of life; more often women.

- Etiology: thromboembolism 50%, thrombosis 20%, nonocclusive mesenteric ischemia (NOMI) 20%, others 10%.[1]

- Clinical presentation depends on adequacy of visceral perfusion by the three mesenteric arteries: celiac artery (CA), superior mesenteric artery (SMA), and inferior mesenteric artery (IMA) (Figure 45-1). There are usually collateralizations among the mesenteric arteries that compensate for flow if there are stenoses or occlusions, hence the common adage; two of the three mesenteric arteries need to be involved before symptoms arise. However, single mesenteric artery occlusion can be symptomatic in the absence of adequate collateralization, such as in acute thromboembolism.

## PATHOPHYSIOLOGY

### Thromboembolism

- Thromboembolism to the SMA is common due to its obtuse angle and path, diverging gently away from the aorta and its flow.

- Embolus source: cardiac arrhythmias (atrial or ventricular), atherosclerotic aorta, proximal thoracic aneurysms. Proximal small intestines may be uninvolved if embolus occludes the SMA a few centimeters beyond its origin, sparing proximal jejunal branches. Transverse colon may be spared if occlusion is beyond the middle colic branch of the SMA.

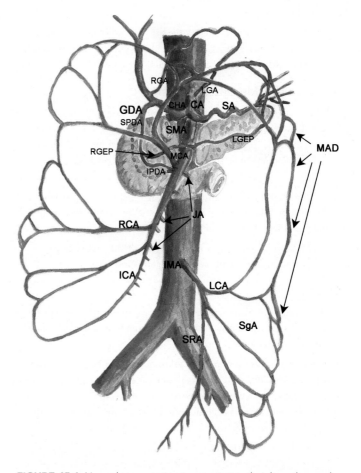

FIGURE 45-1 Normal mesenteric artery anatomy, their branches and natural collateralization. Celiac artery (CA), superior mesenteric artery (SMA), inferior mesenteric artery (IMA), common hepatic artery (CHA), splenic artery (SA), gastroduodenal artery (GDA), superior pancreaticoduodenal artery (SPDA), inferior pancreaticoduodenal artery (IPDA), left gastric artery (LGA), right gastric artery (RGA), right gastroepiploic artery (RGEP), left gastroepiploic artery (LGEP), jejunal arteries (JAs), middle colic artery (MCA), right colic artery (RCA), ileocolic artery (ICA), marginal artery of Drummond (MAD)—between left branch of MCA and ascending branch of left colic artery (LCA), sigmoidal artery (SgA), superior rectal artery (SRA).

## Thrombosis

- Patients are generally older and usually women.

- Evidence of atherosclerotic disease in other vascular beds (coronary, lower extremities) is usually present.

- More than half have chronic mesenteric ischemia (CMI) symptoms (postprandial pain, food fear, weight loss).[2] Thus, patients develop acute mesenteric ischemia (AMI) in the setting of CMI secondary to occlusive disease.

- AMI can also be precipitated in the background of hemodynamic compromise during other cardiovascular events (acute myocardial infarction [MI], coronary artery bypass, sepsis, shock).

## Nonocclusive Mesenteric Ischemia

- Vasospasm of the mesenteric arteries in the absence of critically stenotic lesions can be incited by digitalis, alpha-adrenergic agents, low-flow states (cardiac failure, shock, etc), and less commonly early enteral feeding after revascularization for CMI.

- Diagnosis is angiographic, and features include narrowing at origins of SMA branches, "string of sausage" sign—alternate narrowing and dilations of SMA intestinal branches—mesenteric arcades spasm, and nonfilling of the intestinal intramural branches.[3]

- NOMI has a high mortality rate as patients tend to have more severe underlying conditions and diagnosis is often delayed.

## Others

- Other causes of AMI include mesenteric vein thrombosis (MVT), aortic dissections, Takayasu arteritis, fibromuscular dysplasia, and polyarteritis nodosa.

- Superior mesenteric vein (SMV) thrombosis is associated with hypercoagulability, visceral malignancies (eg, pancreatic mass causing extrinsic compression of the SMV or portal vein), pancreatitis, and cirrhosis. Venous occlusion and hypertension lead to intestinal edema and infarction.

- Aortic dissection intimal flaps can exclude, compress, or extend into the mesenteric arteries resulting in thrombosis (Figure 45-2A and B).

## CLINICAL PRESENTATION

### Symptoms

- Acute-onset abdominal pain (90%); nausea, vomiting, diarrhea—30% to 40%, blood per rectum, 10% to 15%[2]

### Signs

- Abdominal pain out of proportion to examination, initially

- Peritoneal signs (diffuse abdominal tenderness, guarding, rebound tenderness, abdominal rigidity, absent bowel sounds); if intestinal necrosis ensues, sepsis, and shock

## DIAGNOSIS

### Laboratory Testing

- Nonspecific

- Leukocytosis, base deficit, lactic acidosis, hyperphosphatemia

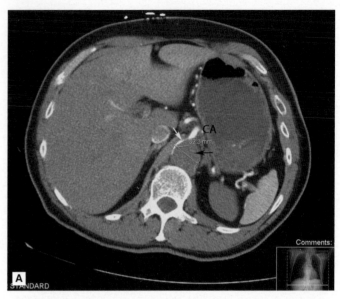

**FIGURE 45-2A** Type-B aortic dissection with significantly narrowed true lumen (small white arrow) due to compression from thrombosed false lumen (small black arrow), and patent celiac artery (CA) origin.

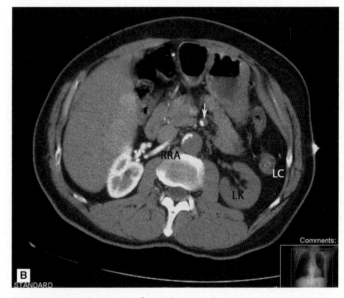

**FIGURE 45-2B** Extension of type-B aortic dissection into superior mesenteric artery (SMA) (small white arrow), patent and perfused right renal artery (RRA), and malperfusion or ischemia to the left kidney (LK) without contrast enhancement, ischemia to the left colon (LC) with mural thickening. (*Image courtesy of Henry Baele, MD.*)

## Imaging Studies

### Duplex Ultrasound Scan

- Absence of flow or thrombus within mesenteric arteries can be visualized.
- Imaging is limited by intestinal gas from paralytic ileus associated with ischemia.
- Reversal of flow in the hepatic artery is pathognomonic of CA occlusion.

### CT Scan of Abdomen and Pelvis

- Bowel distension and wall thickening, pneumatosis intestinalis (Figure 45-3), portal venous gas

### Mesenteric Angiogram (or CT Angiogram)

- Oblique or lateral angiographic projections visualize the mesenteric vessels best as they come off the aorta ventrally.
- Filling defects in proximal SMA, meniscus sign at the site of embolic occlusion (Figure 45-4). Distal branches of SMA may reconstitute on delayed images. Other mesenteric arteries may be stenotic; typically at least two of three mesenteric arteries are involved.
- Prominent collaterals may be present: marginal artery of Drummond, arc of Riolan (meandering mesenteric of Moskowitz), arc of Bühler, arc of Barkow (Figures 45-5 and 45-6).

## TREATMENT

### Preoperative Optimization

- Nothing by mouth (NPO), nasogastric tube (NGT), intravenous fluid (IVF) resuscitation, repletion of serum electrolytes, systemic anticoagulation (heparin), and urine output monitoring.
- Patients with signs of peritonitis require immediate exploratory laparotomy, resection of gangrenous bowel, and on-table mesenteric angiogram.
- Definitive treatment for revascularization is dependent on the etiology of ischemia.
- Patients with symptoms suggestive of AMI without evidence of peritonitis or shock should undergo mesenteric angiography prior to surgery as select patients may be candidates for catheter-directed thrombolytic therapy followed by endovascular revascularization.[4]

### Operative Surgery

#### Thromboembolism

- Peritonitis from AMI is a surgical emergency that requires immediate exploration. Goals of treatment are restoration of mesenteric flow and resection of gangrenous bowel.
- Embolism to the SMA can have a palpable proximal "water-hammer" pulse at the base of the mesentery but absent distal mesenteric pulses.
- Other signs of extensive emboli may manifest as patchy cyanosis or necrosis at other sites along the small and large intestines, or solid organ infarcts (Figure 45-7).

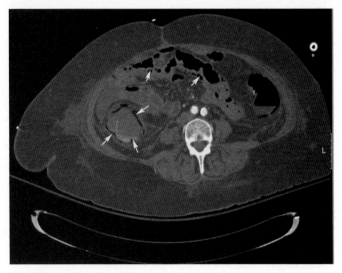

**FIGURE 45-3** Axial image from computed tomographic (CT) scan of the abdomen showing pneumatosis involving the small intestines and the right colon (white arrows).

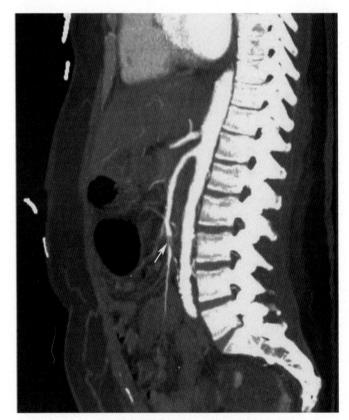

**FIGURE 45-4** Sagittal image from computed tomographic (CT) scan of the abdomen showing embolus within superior mesenteric artery (SMA) (white arrow) with reconstitution of flow distally.

- Malodorous peritoneal fluid or frank spillage of visceral contents may be present due to advanced intestinal necrosis and perforation. In this setting, bowel resection without re-establishment of continuity should be performed first to prevent further contamination of the peritoneal cavity.

- The SMA is located at the root of the mesentery by lifting the transverse colon or mesocolon upwards. A transverse arteriotomy is performed and Fogarty balloon catheter thromboembolectomy is performed distally and proximally (Figure 45-8). Good back-flow and in-flow should be established prior to closure of the arteriotomy with fine, interrupted, monofilament sutures. This avoids narrowing the SMA at the repair site.

- On-table mesenteric angiogram should be performed to assess mesenteric perfusion and for identification of any other lesions that require intervention.

- If thromboembolectomy is successful, the intestine is allowed to reperfuse and the resected ends are evaluated for viability.

- Mesenteric bypass may be necessary if inflow cannot be established. This can be performed in antegrade (supraceliac aorta to celiac and/or the SMA) or retrograde (distal abdominal aorta or common iliac artery to celiac and/or the SMA) fashion. See Chapter 47—Chronic Mesenteric Ischemia.

- Viability of the intestines is assessed by palpation of distal mesenteric arcade pulses, continuous-wave Doppler signal of perfusion on the intestinal antimesenteric border, return of intestinal color and peristalsis, and evaluation of perfusion with intravenous fluorescein under ultraviolet exposure (Wood lamp).[2,4,5]

- Intestinal reanastomosis should not be performed in the presence of hypotension, hypothermia, acidosis, blood-product transfusion requirement, or questionably viable tissue.

- Return to the operating room for a second look in 24 to 48 hours is highly recommended to confirm viability of the intestines and improve patient survival.

## SMA Thrombosis

- SMA thrombosis will likely exhibit absent pulses from the origin of the artery distally. The underlying atherosclerotic disease is palpable and the artery should be opened longitudinally.

- Thromboembolectomy with Fogarty balloon catheters should be performed distally and proximally.

- Local endarterectomy of the diseased segment of the SMA may be required to re-establish blood flow. The arteriotomy is closed with a patch angioplasty (Figure 45-9).

- Autologous patch material (autologous saphenous vein) is preferred if there is gross intra-abdominal contamination.

- Mesenteric bypass may be necessary if inflow cannot be established. SMA revascularization should precede the CA, as the former can be considered more of an end artery. Prosthetic conduits (Dacron or polytetrafluoroethylene [PTFE]) can be used in the absence of gross contamination. Choices of bioprosthetic conduits include autologous or cadaveric saphenous vein.

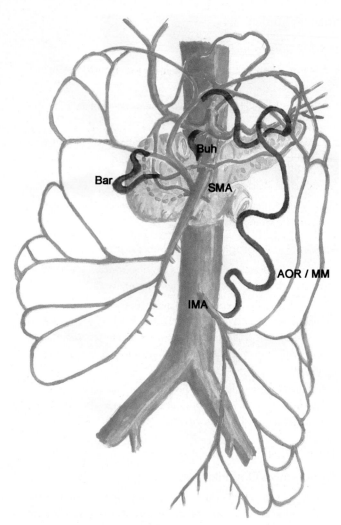

**FIGURE 45-5** Diagram depicting potential compensatory collateralization: arc of Riolan (AOR)—between superior mesenteric artery (SMA) and inferior mesenteric artery (IMA)—centrally located within mesenteric arcades. Also known as meandering mesenteric of Moskowitz (MM) when significantly hypertrophied; arc of Bühler (Buh)—between the celiac artery (CA) and SMA main trunks; arc of Barkow (Bar)—between the celiac artery and the SMA, from right and left gastroepiploic arteries to the middle colic artery or its branches.

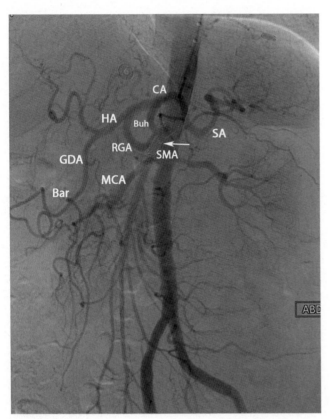

FIGURE 45-6 Mesenteric angiogram showing collaterals between the celiac artery (CA) and the superior mesenteric artery (SMA), arc of Bühler (Buh), arc of Barkow (Bar). Note the SMA stent (white arrow) for treatment of chronic mesenteric ischemia (CMI). Enlarged right gastric artery (RGA), middle colic artery (MCA), hepatic artery (HA), gastroduodenal artery (GDA), and splenic artery (SA). (*Image courtesy of Henry Baele, MD.*)

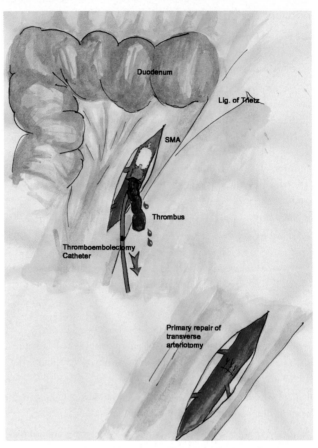

FIGURE 45-8 Superior mesenteric artery (SMA) balloon catheter thromboembolectomy and closure of the transverse arteriotomy.

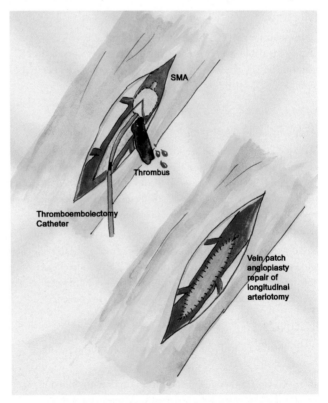

FIGURE 45-9 Longitudinal arteriotomy for thromboembolectomy of superior mesenteric artery (SMA) thrombosis and closure with great saphenous vein patch angioplasty.

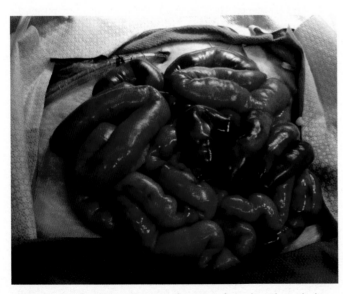

FIGURE 45-7 Patchy small intestinal necrosis from thromboembolism to the superior mesenteric artery (SMA).

### Endovascular Therapy

- In the absence of peritonitis or shock, mesenteric angiography may be useful in determining the extent of mesenteric occlusion, stenosis, and amenable revascularization options.

- Catheter-directed thrombolytic therapy may unmask culprit stenotic lesions once the thrombus burden resolves, and these lesions may be treated with balloon angioplasty or stenting.[6] The thrombolysis infusion catheter is directed into the mesenteric artery that is occluded or thrombosed. Typically, patients undergo continuous infusion of catheter-directed thrombolytics (eg, tissue plasminogen activator [tPA] at 0.5-1 mg/h) for 12 to 24 hours prior to follow-up imaging.

- Failure of thrombolytic therapy or worsening clinical status warrants expedient operative intervention. A high index of suspicion is required for progressive visceral ischemia leading to bowel necrosis, as the degree of ischemia cannot be reliably predicted by physical examination, laboratory testing, or current imaging tests.

### NOMI

- Mainstay of treatment for NOMI comprises cessation of the inciting agents (digitalis or alpha-adrenergic drugs) and catheter-directed vasodilators such as papaverine or nitroglycerin into the affected mesenteric artery.

- Patients should undergo systemic heparinization and hemodynamic optimization of other underlying conditions.

- Similarly, early operative intervention to resect gangrenous bowel rests on a high index of suspicion, along with a planned second-look operation.

### MVT

- Treatment for MVT includes fluid resuscitation, correction of hypercoagulable state, systemic anticoagulation, and resection of necrotic bowel. Venous thrombectomy has not been shown to be durable or effective.[7]

### Aortic Dissection With Malperfusion

- Malperfusion to the visceral arteries is a surgical emergency.

- Revascularization can be achieved by open aortic (intimal) fenestration and re-establishment of flow into the mesenteric true lumen by careful fine tacking sutures of the intima at the mesenteric ostia. The extremely friable nature of a dissected aorta renders any open surgical procedure as high risk and fraught with bleeding complications.

- Endovascular revascularization using angiography and intravascular ultrasound for confirmation of true luminal flow, and closure of the proximal aortic intimal tear with an endograft followed with mesenteric stenting may be amenable for selected patients.[8]

### PROGNOSIS

- AMI remains a lethal condition with a 30-day mortality rate in excess of 30%.[2]

- Poor prognosticators include multiorgan system dysfunction, age greater than 70 years, and recurrent mesenteric thrombosis.

- Longer-term survival is approximately 60% at 1 year and 30% at 2 years.

### PATIENT EDUCATION

- Post-hospitalization care involves management of the patient's underlying comorbidities. Compliance with anticoagulation and/or antiplatelet medications should be stressed in order to prevent recurrence. Surviving patients should be counseled on the signs and symptoms of short-bowel syndrome.

### PROVIDER RESOURCES

- http://emedicine.medscape.com/article/189146-overview
- http://www.uptodate.com/contents/acute-mesenteric-ischemia
- http://www.learningradiology.com/notes/ginotes/mesentericischemiapage.htm

### PATIENT RESOURCES

- http://www.nlm.nih.gov/medlineplus/ency/article/001156.htm
- http://my.clevelandclinic.org/heart/disorders/vascular/visceralischemiasyndrome.aspx

### REFERENCES

1. Stoney RJ, Cunningham CG. Acute mesenteric ischemia. *Surgery.* 1993;114:489-490.

2. Park WM, Gloviczki P, Cherry KJ, et al. Contemporary management of acute mesenteric ischemia: factors associated with survival. *J Vasc Surg.* 2002;35:445-452.

3. Siegelman SS, Sprayregen S, Boley SJ. Angiographic diagnosis of mesenteric arterial vasoconstriction. *Radiology.* 1974;112: 533-542.

4. Taylor LM, Moneta GL, Porter JM. Treatment of acute intestinal ischemia caused by arterial occlusions. In: Rutherford RB, ed. *Vascular Surgery*, 5th ed. Philadelphia, PA: WB Saunders; 2000: 1512-1518.

5. Ballard JL, Stone WM, Hallett JW, et al. A critical analysis of adjuvant techniques used to assess bowel viability in acute mesenteric ischemia. *Am Surg.* 1993;59:309-311.

6. McBride KD, Gaines PA. Thrombolysis of a partially occluding superior mesenteric artery thromboembolus by infusion of streptokinase. *Cardiovasc Intervent Radiol.* 1995;6:785-791.

7. Schwartz LB, McKinsey JF, Funaki B, et al. Visceral ischemic syndromes. In: Hallet JW, Mills JL, Earnshaw JJ, Reekers JA, eds. *Comprehensive Vascular and Endovascular Surgery*. Philadelphia, PA: Elsevier; 2004:603-615.

8. Slonim SM, Nyman UR, Semba CP, et al. True lumen obliteration in complicated aortic dissection: endovascular treatment. *Radiology.* 1996;201:161-166.

# 46 CELIAC AXIS COMPRESSION SYNDROME

Joseph Habib, MD
Bhagwan Satiani, MD, MBA, RPVI, FACS

## PATIENT STORY

A 22-year-old Caucasian woman presented to the vascular clinic with intense postprandial abdominal pain that occurred 20 to 30 minutes after eating. She also relayed a history of food fear along with occasional nausea and vomiting. She had experienced about a 25-lb weight loss over the last 6 months. Her past medical history was not significant for any chronic illnesses or conditions including absence of a psychiatric or drug abuse history. She stated that she had undergone an extensive gastrointestinal workup including upper and lower endoscopy and a right upper quadrant ultrasound, but no diagnosis had been established. On examination the patient appeared thin, in no acute distress. Her abdomen was soft, nontender, nondistended. On auscultation, an epigastric bruit that increased with expiration was found. A computed tomographic angiogram (CTA) was obtained that demonstrated extrinsic compression of the celiac axis by the median arcuate ligament of the diaphragm and poststenotic dilatation of the celiac artery (Figure 46-1).

This patient has the typical presentation of celiac axis compression syndrome (CACS), also known as median arcuate ligament syndrome.

## EPIDEMIOLOGY

- A significant number of individuals have narrowing of the celiac axis by the median arcuate ligament of the diaphragm, and full expiration seems to exacerbate this compression. It is still uncertain whether chronic intestinal ischemia can develop from compression of the celiac axis alone.

- Usually occurs in young, thin females.[1-3]

- Severe compression that persists during inspiration occurs in approximately 1% of patients.[3]

- Between 13% and 50% of patients may have some degree of compression and experience no symptoms.[3]

## ETIOLOGY AND PATHOPHYSIOLOGY

- First described by Harjola in 1963.[4]

- Also known as median arcuate ligament syndrome or celiac band syndrome.[2]

- Median arcuate ligament is a tendinous group of fibers that form an arch between the diaphragmatic crura.[3]

- Usually the ligament passes above the origin of the celiac axis, but in some individuals (10%-24%) it may cross the axis anteriorly leading to compression.[3]

- Compression of the axis may cause obstruction of blood flow resulting in symptoms.[3]

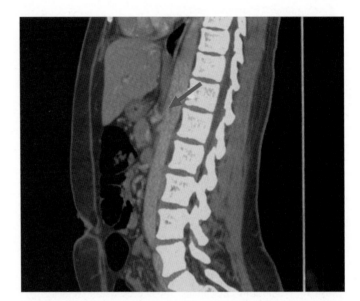

**FIGURE 46-1** Computed tomographic angiogram (CTA) sagittal plane view of a patient with median arcuate ligament syndrome. Red arrow indicates median arcuate ligament causing compression of the celiac artery with poststenotic dilatation.

- The superior mesenteric artery (SMA), which is the main source of blood flow to the bowel, forms a rich collateral network with the celiac artery (CA).[1]

## DIAGNOSIS

- Usually a diagnosis of exclusion, both clinical and radiographic features should be present.[1,3]
- Classic triad[2]
  1. Postprandial abdominal pain
  2. Epigastric bruit that increases with expiration (83%)
  3. Evidence of extrinsic compression of the celiac access by vascular imaging
- Most frequently seen in young, thin females.[2]
- Common symptoms include intense postprandial epigastric pain occurring 20 to 30 minutes after eating, food fear, nausea, vomiting, and weight loss.[2]
- Usually patients have undergone extensive gastrointestinal workups without a diagnosis being established.[2]

## LABORATORY TESTS

- No specific laboratory tests are necessary.

## IMAGING

- Duplex ultrasound—The criteria for celiac artery stenosis: greater than 50% stenosis includes an increase in peak systolic velocity greater than 180 cm/s at baseline.[2,5] The patient presented had elevated systolic velocities during inspiration (Figure 46-2), which further increased during expiration (Figure 46-3).
- CTA: good for assessing the proximal portion of the celiac access (Figure 46-1).[2,3]
- Magnetic resonance angiography (MRA): may also be used, no radiation risk.[2]
- Angiography: (gold standard) lateral projection showing compression of celiac access (hook sign) with poststenotic dilatation.[2,3]

## DIAGNOSIS

- Median arcuate ligament syndrome is truly a diagnosis of exclusion and patients have often been through an extensive gastrointestinal workup without the establishment of a diagnosis.[2]
- Peptic ulcer disease, gallbladder pathology, motility disorders of the stomach and esophagus, and inflammatory bowel disease should all be ruled out.
- Patients should also be screened for psychiatric disorders and drug abuse.[1]

## MANAGEMENT

- No medical treatment exists.
- Surgical division of the constrictive bands around the celiac access up to its origin on the aorta (may be performed open or laparoscopically).[2]
- Laparoscopic division of the constrictive celiac bands was first introduced in 2000 and has been shown to result in a shorter hospital stay, less postoperative pain, and faster recovery.[2]

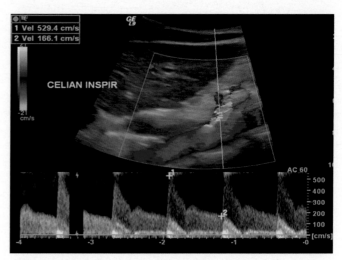

**FIGURE 46-2** Mesenteric color flow duplex ultrasound of the celiac artery in a patient with median arcuate ligament syndrome during inspiration. Baseline Doppler spectral velocities are elevated.

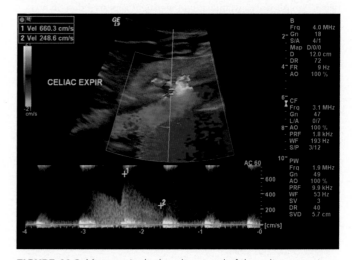

**FIGURE 46-3** Mesenteric duplex ultrasound of the celiac artery in a patient with median arcuate ligament syndrome during expiration. The Doppler spectral velocities are markedly elevated compared to inspiration.

- Celiac revascularization procedure may or may not be performed.
- Celiac artery revascularization procedures include[2]
  - Patch angioplasty of the celiac access
  - Aortoceliac bypass with vein or prosthetic graft
  - Reimplantation of the celiac trunk into the aorta
  - Endovascular angioplasty and stenting of the celiac artery

## FOLLOW-UP

In general, previous reports have observed that a large percentage of patients diagnosed with the syndrome were later found to have other gastrointestinal causes such as gallstones or peptic ulcer disease.[1] Therefore, even if the patient is treated with some form of intervention, it behooves the physician to look for recurrent symptoms and repeat the gastrointestinal workup.

In a series of 51 patients treated surgically, 68% experienced cure of their symptoms with a mean follow-up of 9 years. Patients were more likely to experience improvement if they had symptoms of postprandial pain, were between 40 and 60 years of age, or had experienced weight loss of 20 lb or more.[6]

### PROVIDER RESOURCES

- http://www.uptodate.com/contents/celiac-artery-compression-syndrome
- http://www.torna.do/s/The-celiac-axis-compression-syndrome-CACS-critical-review-in-the-laparoscopic-era/

### PATIENT RESOURCE

- http://www.torna.do/s/The-celiac-axis-compression-syndrome-CACS-critical-review-in-the-laparoscopic-era/

## REFERENCES

1. Huber TS, Lee WA. Mesenteric vascular disease: chronic ischemia. In: Cronenwett JL, Johnston KW, eds. *Rutherford's Vascular Surgery*. 7th ed. Philadelphia, PA: Elsevier; 2010:2287.

2. Cienfuegos JA, Rotellar F, Valenti V, et al. The celiac axis compression syndrome in the laparoscopic era. *Rev Esp Enferm Dig*. 2010;102:193-201.

3. Horton KM, Talamini MA, Fishman EK. Median arcuate ligament syndrome: evaluation with CT angiography. *RadioGraphics*. 2005;25:1177-1182.

4. Harjola PT. A rare obstruction of the celiac artery: report of a case. *Ann Chir Gynaecol Fenn*. 1963;52:547-550.

5. Sproat IA, Pozniak MA, Kennell TW. US case of the day: median arcuate ligament syndrome. *Radiographics*. 1993;13:1400-1402.

6. Reilly LM, Ammar AD, Stoney RJ, Ehrenfeld WK. Late results following operative repair of for celiac compression syndrome. *J Vasc Surg*. 1985;2:79-91.

# 47 CHRONIC MESENTERIC ISCHEMIA

John C. Wang, MD, MSc
Vikram S. Kashyap, MD

## PATIENT STORY

A 66-year-old woman with long-standing tobacco use presented with recurrent postprandial abdominal pain and food aversion for the last 18 months. An associated weight loss of 22 lb in addition to intermittent nausea, vomiting, and diarrhea was described as well. Physical examination was remarkable for a malnourished-appearing female with right carotid, epigastric, and bilateral femoral bruits. The femoral through pedal pulses were weak but palpable. Mesenteric duplex arterial ultrasonography identified 70% to 99% stenosis within the celiac and superior mesenteric arteries with abundant diffuse aortomesenteric plaque. A computed tomographic angiogram (CTA) of the abdomen confirmed the above findings and documented a meandering mesenteric artery of Moskowitz. A diagnosis of chronic mesenteric ischemia (CMI) was made.

## EPIDEMIOLOGY

- Overall incidence is quite low, patients between 40 and 70 years of age, common in women.[1]
- Etiology is atherosclerosis, usually affecting mesenteric arteries at the ostia or "spill-over" disease from the abdominal aorta.
- Most patients are smokers and hypertensive.

## PATHOPHYSIOLOGY

- Celiac artery (CA), superior mesenteric artery (SMA), and inferior mesenteric artery (IMA) usually have good pre-existent collaterals; therefore, usually two of three arteries must be critically stenosed or occluded before symptoms arise.
- Single arterial disease may become symptomatic if there is no good collateral circulation.
- CMI can lead to intestinal malabsorption, inanition, bowel infarction, and ultimately death.

## CLINICAL PRESENTATION

### Symptoms

- Classic triad of abdominal pain, food fear, and weight loss.
- Almost all patients develop central abdominal pain, the onset of which is usually 30 minutes postprandial, lasting minutes to hours. Patients learn to associate pain with food and hence develop food fear. Poor dietary intake leads to malnutrition and weight loss.
- Ischemic ulcerations in the stomach, duodenum, or colon may cause epigastric pain, nausea, emesis, gastrointestinal bleeding, or change in bowel habits resultant of colonic strictures.

### Signs

- Patients are generally thin, underweight, with a scaphoid abdomen. Muscle wasting is seen in advanced cases.
- However, not all patients appear emaciated as CMI can affect morbidly obese patients where a 20- to 30-lb weight loss is not readily noticeable.
- Abdominal bruit and tenderness may be present, but peritoneal signs are typically absent.
- Two-thirds of patients have evidence of atherosclerosis in other vascular beds (cerebrovascular, coronary, renal, and lower extremities) such as carotid bruits, coronary artery bypass or stents, and absent pedal pulses.[2]

## DIAGNOSIS

### Laboratory Testing

- Nonspecific

### Imaging Studies

#### Duplex Ultrasound Scan

- Elevated peak systolic velocities (PSVs) of greater than 200 cm/s in the CA and greater than 275 cm/s in the SMA are indicative of greater than 70% stenosis (Figures 47-1 and 47-2).[3] Elevated end diastolic velocities (EDVs) of 55 cm/s and 45 cm/s in the CA and the SMA, respectively, may also indicate greater than 50% stenosis.[4] PSV greater than 275 cm/s in the IMA suggests greater than 70% stenosis (Figure 47-3).
- Duplex ultrasound scan is limited by the presence of intestinal gas; therefore, patients need to fast overnight for this study.

#### Upper and Lower Endoscopy and CT Scan of Abdomen and Pelvis

- Due to similar clinical presentations, comprehensive radiographic and endoscopic imaging are required to rule out intra-abdominal malignancies such as pancreatic or gastrointestinal neoplasms, or other causes of gastric outlet obstruction such as peptic ulcer disease.

#### Angiography

- Advances in imaging technology rendered by CTA and magnetic resonance angiography (MRA) provide attractive diagnostic alternatives to formal mesenteric angiography.
- CTA enables visualization and quantification of the extent of disease in the aorta and its visceral branches. Axial images can also be reconstructed to three-dimensional images (Figures 47-4A-D and 47-5A, B).
- Formal mesenteric angiography remains the gold standard for diagnosis of CMI, along with the possibility of therapeutic endovascular

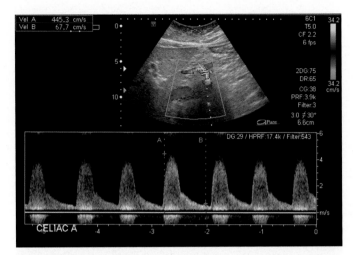

FIGURE 47-1 Duplex ultrasound scan with color flow Doppler. Celiac artery (CA) stenosis > 70% with peak systolic velocity (PSV) of 445 cms⁻¹ and elevated end diastolic velocity (EDV) of 68 cms⁻¹.

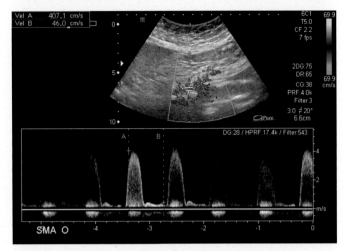

FIGURE 47-2 Duplex ultrasound scan with color flow Doppler. Superior mesenteric artery (SMA) stenosis > 70% with peak systolic velocity (PSV) of 407 cms⁻¹ and elevated end diastolic velocity (EDV) of 46 cms⁻¹.

intervention. Angiographic information is crucial when considering open revascularization options.

- Oblique or lateral projections are required for viewing the mesenteric arteries due to their ventral origin from the abdominal aorta (Figure 47-6).

- Other clues to significant CMI are presence of prominent compensatory collateral circulation between the CA and the SMA (arc of Bühler, arc of Barkow), and the SMA and the IMA (arc of Riolan or meandering mesenteric of Moskowitz) (Figure 47-7A, B).

## TREATMENT

- Open surgical revascularization should be offered to patients with symptomatic CMI who have acceptable risk profiles.

- Percutaneous revascularization with mesenteric angioplasty and/or stenting appears to be an attractive option, especially for patients with CMI who are typically malnourished. However, due to its slightly higher symptomatic recurrence rate, endovascular therapy should be offered to high-risk, older patients who are otherwise unfit for open surgery.[5]

### Mesenteric Bypass

- Open revascularization can be performed in antegrade or retrograde fashion.

- There is controversy about the number of mesenteric arteries that should be revascularized. Primary treatment aim is to revascularize the most symptomatic mesenteric vascular bed and potential secondary optimization of other diseased arteries.

### Antegrade Bypass

- Aortoceliac and/or SMA bypass can be achieved transabdominally via a midline laparotomy, or through bilateral subcostal incisions.

- The supraceliac aorta is accessed by entering the lesser sac, mobilization of the left liver lobe, and incising the left diaphragmatic

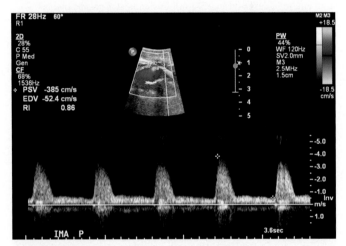

FIGURE 47-3 Duplex ultrasound scan with color flow Doppler. Inferior mesenteric artery (IMA) stenosis > 70% with peak systolic velocity (PSV) of 385 cms⁻¹.

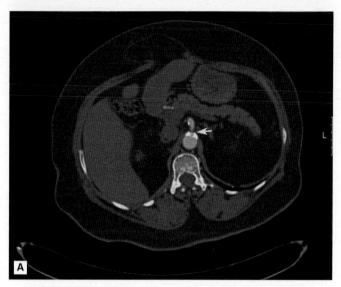

FIGURE 47-4A Computed tomographic (CT) scan with contrast of a patient with heavy tobacco use and chronic mesenteric ischemia (CMI); axial image of celiac artery (CA) stenosis and ostial calcific plaque (small white arrow).

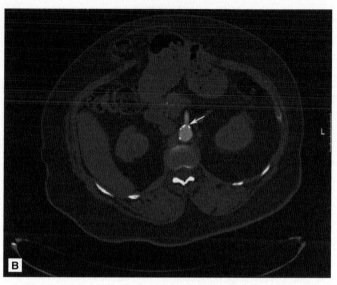

FIGURE 47-4B Axial image of superior mesenteric artery (SMA) stenosis and ostial calcific plaque (small white arrow).

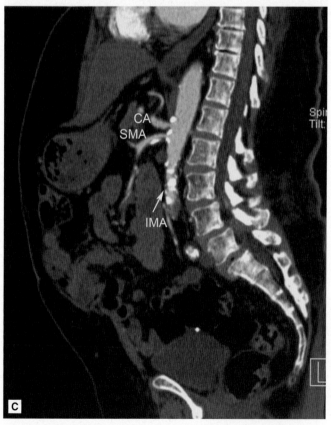

FIGURE 47-4C Computed tomographic (CT) scan sagittal image of celiac artery (CA) and superior mesenteric artery (SMA) stenosis, and occluded inferior mesenteric artery (IMA) (white arrow) with distal reconstitution.

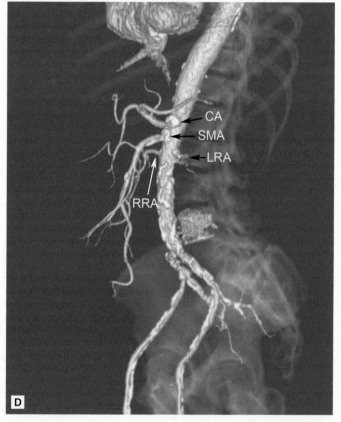

FIGURE 47-4D Three-dimensional reconstruction computed tomographic angiogram (CTA) image showing heavy ostial calcification of the celiac artery (CA), superior mesenteric artery (SMA), and occluded nonvisualization of the inferior mesenteric artery (IMA), right renal artery (RRA), left renal artery (LRA). Note paucity of collateralization.

crura. The stomach is retracted gently caudad and esophagus to the patient's left. Three to four inches of the supraceliac aorta can be isolated for creation of the proximal anastomosis.

- Within the lesser sac, the CA and its proximal branches (hepatic and splenic) are isolated for the celiac anastomosis. Simultaneous SMA bypass can be achieved with bifurcated prosthetic (Dacron or polytetrafluoroethylene [PTFE]) grafts (Figure 47-8A, B) or creation of pantaloon great saphenous vein grafts.

- Nonsynthetic graft conduits are used if there is intraperitoneal contamination of bacteria from bowel contents from either perforation or intestinal resection of nonviable bowel.

- The SMA is isolated at the base of the small bowel mesentery after taking down the ligament of Treitz. The bypass limb to the SMA is tunneled retropancreatically (Figure 47-8C).

- The patient is fully heparinized prior to aortic or arterial cross-clamping and creation of the anastomoses. Mannitol and furosemide may be given intraoperatively for renal protection during temporary aortic cross-clamp. Impaired cardiac function and heavy circumferential supraceliac aortic calcification are contraindications to antegrade mesenteric bypass. Retrograde mesenteric bypass is recommended for these patients.

## Retrograde Bypass

- A 3- to 4-cm SMA segment is isolated at its most proximal portion at the root of the small bowel mesentery as described earlier. The bypass can be constructed using prosthetic grafts, either in a short-conduit configuration or as a long C-loop (Figure 47-9A, B).

- The most important technical aspect is avoidance of graft kinking when the bowel (and SMA) is returned to its anatomic position on closure of laparotomy.

- The distal anastomosis on the SMA is constructed first. Proximal anastomosis can be from the distal infrarenal aorta, or proximal right or left common iliac arteries. The decision on choice of inflow depends on the lay of the graft and absence of circumferential calcification.

- Typically, only the SMA is revascularized as access to the CA is problematic. If the CA requires revascularization, a retrograde bypass to the hepatic artery can be constructed via a retropancreatic retroduodenal tunnel.

## Transaortic Mesenteric Endarterectomy

- Local endarterectomy of the paravisceral aorta and the mesenteric arteries is a useful alternative if mesenteric bypass is not amenable such as in the setting of a hostile abdomen, for example, intraperitoneal bacterial contamination from bowel perforation, previous radiation therapy with extensive changes, or gigantic ventral hernias.

- The paravisceral aorta can be accessed through a midline laparotomy or thoracoabdominal retroperitoneal approach. The aorta is exposed with a medial visceral rotation with the left kidney remaining in its renal fossa. The supraceliac to infrarenal aorta, CA, SMA, and bilateral renal arteries are isolated for vascular control (Figure 47-10A).

- The aorta is cross-clamped after full systemic anticoagulation and administration of mannitol or furosemide for renal protection.

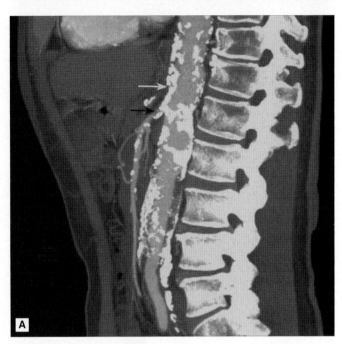

**FIGURE 47-5A** Computed tomographic (CT) scan with contrast of a patient with chronic mesenteric ischemia (CMI) and remote history of aortobifemoral bypass. Sagittal image of severe superior mesenteric artery (SMA) ostial stenosis and heavy "spill-over" aortic atherosclerotic plaque (black arrow). The celiac artery (CA) is occluded (small white arrow) and the inferior mesenteric artery (IMA) is not visualized. Note scaphoid abdomen associated with weight loss. (*Image courtesy of Henry Baele, MD.*)

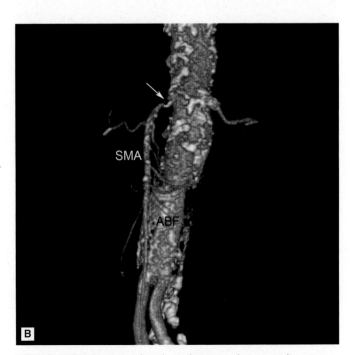

**FIGURE 47-5B** Corresponding three-dimensional computed tomographic angiogram (CTA) reconstruction with severe proximal stenosis (white arrow) and distal reconstitution of the superior mesenteric artery (SMA). Aortobifemoral graft (ABF). (*Image courtesy of Henry Baele, MD.*)

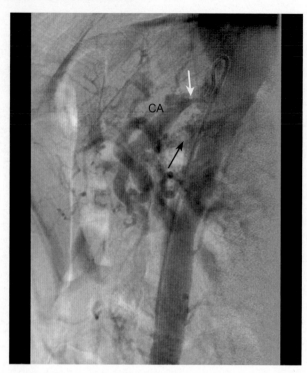

**FIGURE 47-6** Mesenteric angiogram, lateral view: severe celiac artery (CA) stenosis (white arrow), occlusion of superior mesenteric artery (SMA) (black arrow) with heavy calcification. (*Image courtesy of Henry Baele, MD.*)

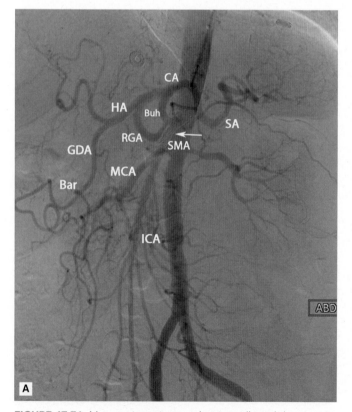

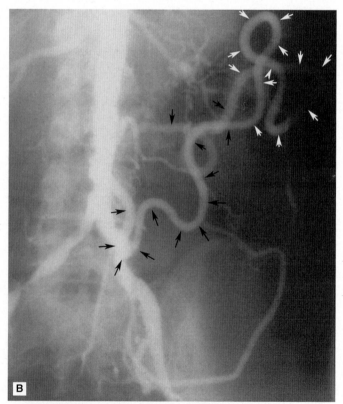

**FIGURE 47-7A** Mesenteric angiogram showing collaterals between the celiac artery (CA) and the superior mesenteric artery (SMA), arc of Bühler (Buh), arc of Barkow (Bar). Note the SMA stent (white arrow) for treatment of chronic mesenteric ischemia (CMI). Hepatic artery (HA), splenic artery (SA), hypertrophied right gastric artery (RGA), gastroduodenal artery (GDA), middle colic artery (MCA), ileocolic artery (ICA). (*Image courtesy of Henry Baele, MD.*)

**FIGURE 47-7B** Prominent arc of Riolan also known as the meandering mesenteric artery of Moskowitz (black/white arrows) communicating between the superior mesenteric artery (SMA) and the inferior mesenteric artery (IMA). (*Image courtesy of Jerry Goldstone, MD.*)

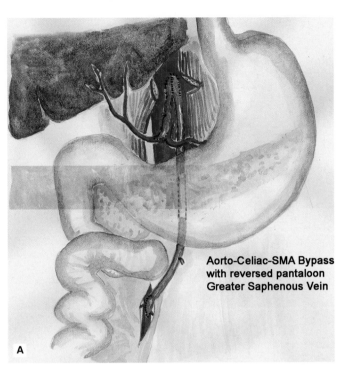

**FIGURE 47-8A** Diagram of aortoceliac and aorto-SMA bypass with a pantaloon reversed greater saphenous vein graft.

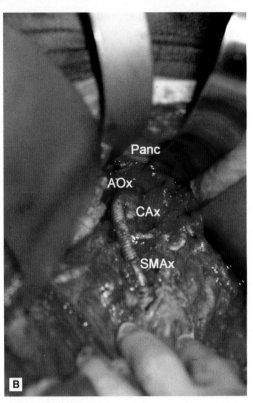

**FIGURE 47-8B** Intraoperative image of transabdominal aortoceliac-SMA bypass with bifurcated Dacron graft (DG). Proximal aortic anastomosis (AOx), celiac anastomosis (CAx), SMA anastomosis (SMAx), pancreas (Panc). (*Image courtesy of Jerry Goldstone, MD.*)

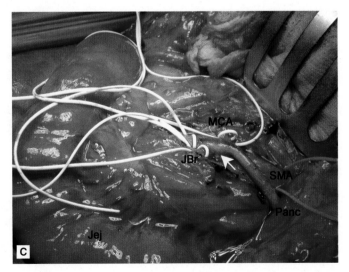

**FIGURE 47-8C** Intraoperative image of aorto-SMA bypass distal anastomosis (white arrow) with reversed great saphenous vein. Sialastic vessel loops are around superior mesenteric artery (SMA), jejunal branches (JBr), middle colic artery (MCA), inferior border of pancreas (Panc), and proximal jejunum (Jej).

- A trap door aortotomy is performed and endarterectomy of the aorta, CA, SMA is performed, down to the level of the renal arteries (Figure 47-10B, C). Renal endarterectomy can be included if there is concomitant disease. Intimal fixation with fine tacking sutures is placed at the aortic distal endpoint to prevent dissection.

- The aortotomy is usually closed primarily (Figure 47-10D). CA endarterectomy usually ends at the celiac trunk bifurcation to hepatic and splenic arteries. More extensive SMA endarterectomy can be performed through a second longitudinal arteriotomy of the proximal SMA for distal disease. The SMA is then closed with a vein or synthetic patch.

## Endovascular Revascularization

- Mesenteric angioplasty and stenting is an attractive alternative to open surgical revascularization due to its minimally invasive nature and lesser physiologic toll on CMI patients who are usually malnourished and have multiple other comorbidities.

- Mesenteric angioplasty has good short-term symptomatic relief but limited durability. Approximately a third of patients require reintervention for recurrent disease. Mesenteric stenting has better durability than angioplasty alone but remains inferior to open revascularization in the long term.[5]

- Endovascular revascularization should be offered to CMI patients who are not candidates for open surgery (Figure 47-11A-C).

## PROGNOSIS

- Patients are admitted to the intensive care unit for fluid management and hemodynamic optimization for 24 to 48 hours postoperatively. Fluid shifts are expected, and patients are monitored closely for bypass graft thrombosis and resultant intestinal ischemia or infarct, evidenced by increased abdominal pain, hypotension, tachycardia, leukocytosis, and deteriorating renal function. High index of suspicion and early return to the angiography suite or surgery for exploration is necessary for diagnosis and definitive treatment.

- Return of bowel function may be prolonged, especially if intestinal villus atrophy has ensued, and early feeding can be associated with malabsorptive diarrhea. Parenteral nutrition and stool bulking agents may be required. Food fear is a learned behavior and may take time to resolve, as opposed to physiologic intolerance to diet.

- Overall perioperative mortality is approximately 5% for mesenteric bypass. Patient survival is approximately 83% at 1 year and 55% at 8 years. Symptom-free survival at 5 years is in excess of 90%.[2]

- Patients should be followed with duplex ultrasound scan or CT scan for bypass graft surveillance at 6 and 12 months postoperatively, and annually thereafter.

## PATIENT EDUCATION

Patients should be advised on the critical importance of aggressively modifying their lifestyle as it relates to atherosclerosis. Medication compliance should be stressed and tobacco use must cease.

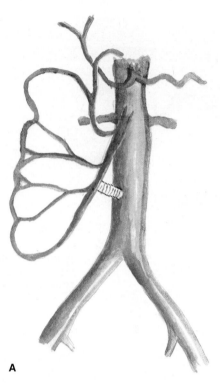

**FIGURE 47-9A** Retrograde bypass to the superior mesenteric artery (SMA) via a short conduit.

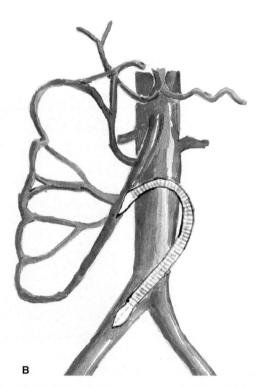

**FIGURE 47-9B** Right iliac-SMA bypass in a gentle C-loop configuration.

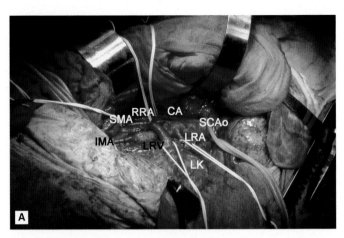

**FIGURE 47-10A** Retroperitoneal paravisceral aortic exposure for endarterectomy. Supraceliac aorta (SCAo), celiac artery (CA), superior mesenteric artery (SMA), right renal artery (RRA), left renal artery (LRA), left renal vein (LRV), left kidney (LK), inferior mesenteric artery (IMA). (*Image courtesy of Jerry Goldstone, MD.*)

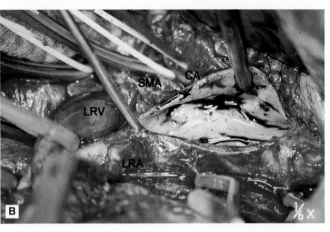

**FIGURE 47-10B** Transaortic mesenteric endarterectomy via trap door aortotomy. Celiac artery (CA), superior mesenteric artery (SMA), left renal artery (LRA), left renal vein (LRV). (*Image courtesy of Jerry Goldstone, MD.*)

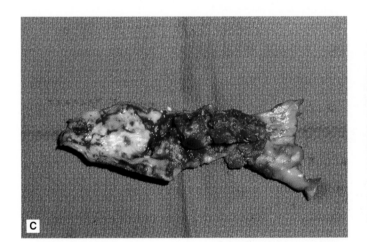

**FIGURE 47-10C** Aortomesenteric plaque. (*Image courtesy of Jerry Goldstone, MD.*)

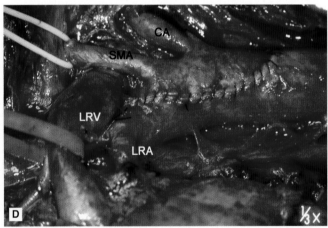

**FIGURE 47-10D** Primary repair of trap door aortotomy. Celiac artery (CA), superior mesenteric artery (SMA), left renal artery (LRA), left renal vein (LRV). (*Image courtesy of Jerry Goldstone, MD.*)

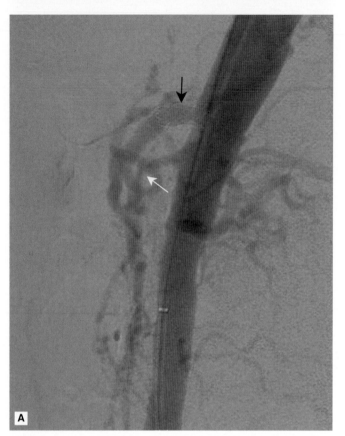

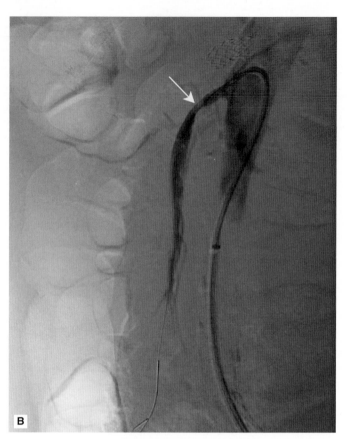

**FIGURE 47-11A** Celiac stenosis (same patient in Figure 47-6) treated with stent (black arrow) shows no residual stenosis. Superior mesenteric artery (SMA) is stenosed (white arrow). (*Image courtesy of Henry Baele, MD.*)

**FIGURE 47-11B** Superior mesenteric artery (SMA) occlusion recanalization and identification of further stenosis (white arrow). (*Image courtesy of Henry Baele, MD.*)

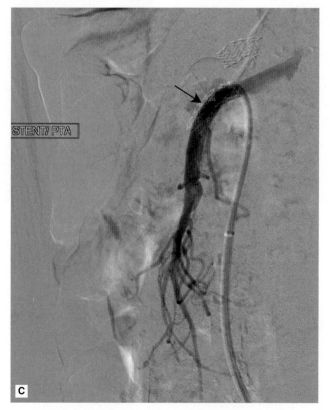

**FIGURE 47-11C** Superior mesenteric artery (SMA) stent (black arrow) and no residual stenosis. (*Image courtesy of Henry Baele, MD.*)

## FOLLOW-UP

Regularly scheduled postinterventional surveillance duplex arterial ultrasonography is recommended.

### PROVIDER RESOURCES

- http://emedicine.medscape.com/article/183683-overview
- http://www.vascularweb.org/vascularhealth/Pages/mesenteric-ischemia.aspx

### PATIENT RESOURCES

- http://www.vascularweb.org/vascularhealth/Pages/mesenteric-ischemia.aspx
- http://my.clevelandclinic.org/heart/disorders/vascular/visceralischemiasyndrome.aspx

## REFERENCES

1. Taylor LM, Moneta GL, Porter JM. Treatment of chronic visceral ischemia. In: Rutherford RB, ed. *Vascular Surgery*. 5th ed. Philadelphia, PA: WB Saunders; 2000:1532-1541.

2. Park WM, Cherry KJ, Chua HK, et al. Current results of open revascularization for chronic mesenteric ischemia: a standard for comparison. *J Vasc Surg*. 2002;35:853-859.

3. Moneta GL, Lee RW, Yeager RA, et al. Mesenteric duplex scanning: a blinded prospective study. *J Vasc Surg*. 1993;17:79.

4. Bowersox JC, Zwolak RM, Walsh DB, et al. Duplex ultrasonography in the diagnosis of celiac and mesenteric artery occlusive disease. *J Vasc Surg*. 1991;14:780.

5. Kasirajan K, O'Hara PJ, Gray BH, et al. Chronic mesenteric ischemia: open surgery versus percutaneous angioplasty and stenting. *J Vasc Surg*. 2001;33:63-71.

# 48 BUDD-CHIARI SYNDROME

Scott P. Albert, MD
Mark Bloomston, MD

## PATIENT STORY

A 34-year-old woman on oral contraceptive pills presents with vague right upper quadrant abdominal pain and worsening abdominal distention for the past 1 month. On examination, she has right upper quadrant tenderness with hepatomegaly. Her liver function panel shows slightly elevated serum aspartate (AST) and alanine aminotransferase (ALT) but normal bilirubin and coagulation profile. A right upper quadrant ultrasound shows hepatic venous occlusion and a moderate amount of ascites. She is started on anticoagulation as well as diuretics to manage her ascites. Her oral contraceptive pills are stopped and a hypercoagulable workup is initiated. A computed tomographic (CT) scan of her abdomen is undertaken to delineate the extent of hepatic venous thrombosis and further liver pathology. She will require close follow-up to monitor her liver dysfunction and potential intervention with percutaneous or surgical procedures in the future. Figures 48-1 to 48-3 demonstrate typical images of a patient with long-standing hepatic outflow occlusion.

## EPIDEMIOLOGY

- Rare condition that is more common in females than males and has a median age of presentation at 33 years.[1]

- The annual incidence of the syndrome is approximately 0.8 per 1 million population.[2]

- The syndrome can have a variety of presentations including fulminant, acute, subacute, and chronic forms depending on the extent and rapidity of the venous obstruction.[3]

## ETIOLOGY AND PATHOPHYSIOLOGY

- Most often related to hepatic vein thrombosis, but can also be secondary to inferior vena cava (IVC) obstruction at the level of the hepatic veins, extrinsic compression from tumor, or intrinsic congenital venous membranous webs.

- The syndrome should be distinguished from veno-occlusive disease, which involves obliteration of the microvasculature within the liver parenchyma.

- Underlying hematologic disorders are the most common cause and can be acquired or congenital. Polycythemia vera and paroxysmal nocturnal hemoglobinuria are the two most common hereditary conditions, whereas oral contraception usage and postpartum states are the most common acquired conditions.[1,3]

- Numerous other disease states are associated with this condition, including trauma, connective tissue disorders, and intrinsic membranous webs, which are more common in Japan and China.[1,4]

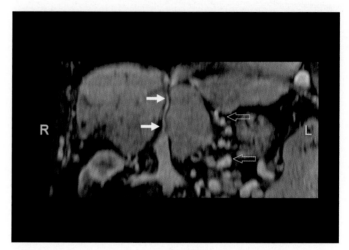

**FIGURE 48-1** Magnetic resonance imaging (MRI) T1-weighted coronal image showing severely narrowed inferior vena cava (IVC) (solid arrows) and no evidence of hepatic veins. There are extensive intra-abdominal venous collaterals (open arrows) consistent with long-standing hepatic outflow and vena cava obstruction.

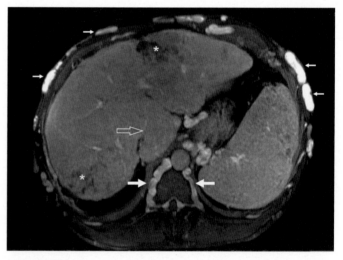

**FIGURE 48-2** Magnetic resonance imaging (MRI) T1-weighted axial image showing an occluded inferior vena cava (IVC) and an enlarged caudate lobe (open arrow). There are extensive venous collaterals, including large lumbar veins (large solid arrows) and large subcutaneous veins (small solid arrows). Also seen is multifocal hepatocellular carcinoma (*) secondary to long-standing cirrhosis from Budd-Chiari syndrome.

- Tumors such as adrenal carcinoma, hepatocellular carcinoma, and retroperitoneal sarcomas can cause extrinsic compression on the hepatic veins and vena cava, leading to liver outflow obstruction.

- Venous outflow obstruction leads to increased liver sinusoidal pressure, which results in centrilobular necrosis. Chronic regeneration can lead to fibrosis and ultimately cirrhosis with resultant liver failure.[3]

- Liver function can be maintained if sinusoidal pressures can be reduced either by the creation of portosystemic shunt or by collateral development between the portal and system circulation provided the outflow obstruction has developed over a time.

- Most cases are subacute in nature, with symptoms developing over weeks to months. Occasionally the presentation can take on a rapidly fulminant course or a more indolent chronic course, especially in cases of partial venous obstruction.[5]

## DIAGNOSIS

### Clinical Features

- The clinical presentation can be fulminant, acute, subacute, or chronic. Patients can present with abdominal distention secondary to ascites, vague abdominal pain, fatigue, splenomegaly, and jaundice.[3]

- In subacute and chronic cases, collateral venous channels have an opportunity to develop, thereby reducing the degree of symptoms. Orloff and colleagues have shown in a series of 60 patients that all presented with abdominal pain, distention, anorexia, and weakness, and about half of patients were jaundiced. On evaluation, all patients had massive ascites, hepatomegaly, splenomegaly, and generalized wasting. In the 19 cases of hepatic vein and IVC obstruction, 74% had significant lower extremity edema.[6] Therefore, clinical assessment of the presence and extent of lower extremity swelling may help define the level of the venous obstruction.

- Serum AST and ALT are often significantly elevated in more acute presentations.

- Abnormalities in alkaline phosphatase and bilirubin levels are variable and correlate with the degree of hepatic fibrosis or cirrhosis.

- The serum-ascitic fluid albumin gradient is usually high.

### Imaging

- Doppler ultrasound is frequently the first imaging test used for diagnosis and correlates with venography findings 80% of the time.[7]

- CT and magnetic resonance imaging (MRI) have become standard for liver imaging. Both modalities can demonstrate patency of hepatic veins, IVC, and portal veins. Figures 48-1 and 48-2 show typical MRI findings in Budd-Chiari syndrome. The MRI findings include caudate lobe hypertrophy, enlarged spleen, heterogeneous liver enhancement, and extensive venous collaterals.

- A hypercoagulable workup, percutaneous liver biopsy, and hepatic angiography are often included in the management.[3,4]

- If considering surgical shunting, hepatic angiography with pressure measurements of the hepatic veins and IVC are beneficial. A pre-shunt pressure gradient of greater than 10 mm Hg between the portal vein and IVC is related to improved outcomes after shunting.[6]

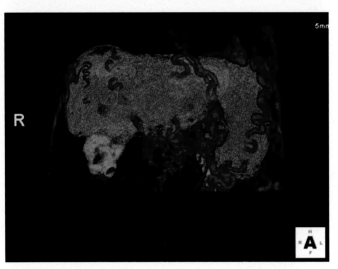

**FIGURE 48-3** Magnetic resonance imaging (MRI) with three-dimensional (3D) reconstruction highlighting the extensive perihepatic and subcutaneous venous collaterals (blue) that have developed with long-standing inferior vena cava (IVC) occlusion. The green denotes the kidneys.

## CLINICAL MANAGEMENT

### Medical

- The mainstay of medical management is anticoagulation followed by supportive management for underlying liver dysfunction. A heparin drip is initiated once the diagnosis is suspected, followed by transition to warfarin therapy with a goal international normalized ratio (INR) of 2 to 3.[3]

- The management of liver dysfunction includes sodium restriction, diuretics, and paracentesis for massive ascites. Diuretics include titrating spironolactone and furosemide for ascites management. Medical therapy alone might be all that is necessary in patients with few symptoms, minimal abnormalities in liver function tests, and no evidence of hepatic necrosis. Aggressive anticoagulation can prevent the propagation of venous thrombosis; however, thrombosis usually remains within the hepatic veins and/or IVC.

### Percutaneous Interventions

- Percutaneous interventional techniques include stenting of an obstruction in the hepatic veins or IVC, catheter-directed thrombolysis, or creation of a portosystemic shunt (eg, transjugular intrahepatic portosystemic shunt [TIPS]).

- The goal of interventional therapy is to help alleviate the elevated sinusoidal pressures by improving liver outflow or by creating a new portosystemic shunt.

- Catheter-directed thrombolysis has a greater chance of success if a thrombosis is diagnosed in the acute setting, particularly if the thrombus does not completely occlude the lumen.[8]

- Angioplasty and stenting are especially effective in cases involving occlusion of the IVC.[9] Percutaneous angioplasty has a short-term success rate of 90%, as evidenced by a significant reduction in hepatic venous pressures and symptom improvement.[10]

### Surgery

- Surgical shunts provide the most durable decompression of the liver and are indicated in patients with reversible liver injury.

- It is important to determine whether the IVC below the hepatic veins is patent before considering a surgical shunt. If the IVC is occluded or severely stenosed then consideration of a mesoatrial or cavoatrial shunt is necessary, since portocaval or mesocaval shunting will not adequately decompress the liver through the infrahepatic IVC. A very large caudate lobe may also make a portocaval shunt more difficult.[6,9]

- If a patient is being considered for liver transplantation then previous hilar dissection for a portocaval shunt can make the transplant operation more challenging.

- Liver transplant is an option in patients with progressive liver cirrhosis, with a failed portosystemic shunt, or who present with acute fulminant liver failure. The 5-year survival for patients being transplanted for Budd-Chiari syndrome has been reported to be between 45% and 95%.[3]

## PATIENT EDUCATION

- Long term surveillance for hepatocellular carcinoma is advisable.

- Routine monitoring of anticoagulation is typically required.

## FOLLOW-UP

Budd-Chiari syndrome is a rare condition requiring long-term follow-up and management. A multidisciplinary approach is required and includes surgeons, hepatologists, and interventional radiologists.

### PROVIDER RESOURCES

- http://emedicine.medscape.com/article/184430-overview
- http://www.uptodate.com/contents/clinical-manifestations-diagnosis-and-treatment-of-the-budd-chiari-syndrome

### PATIENT RESOURCES

- http://79.170.44.126/britishlivertrust.org.uk/wp-content/uploads/2012/12/BCS0208_lowres1.pdf1.pdf
- http://health.nytimes.com/health/guides/disease/hepatic-vein-obstruction-budd-chiari/overview.html

## REFERENCES

1. Slakey DP, Klein AS, Venbrux AC, et al. Budd-Chiari syndrome: current management options. *Ann Surg*. Apr 2001;233(4): 522-527.

2. Rajani R, Melin T, Bjornsson E, et al. Budd-Chiari syndrome in Sweden: epidemiology, clinical characteristics and survival—an 18-year experience. *Liver Int*. Feb 2009;29(2):253-259.

3. Menon KV, Shah V, Kamath PS. The Budd-Chiari syndrome. *N Engl J Med*. Feb 2004;350(6):578-585.

4. Horton JD, San Miguel FL, Ortiz JA. Budd-Chiari syndrome: illustrated review of current management. *Liver Int*. Apr 2008; 28(4):455-466.

5. Mancuso A. Budd-Chiari syndrome management: lights and shadows. *World J Hepatol*. Oct 2011;3(10):262-264.

6. Orloff MJ, Orloff MF, Orloff SL. Budd-Chiari syndrome and veno-occlusive disease. In: Blumgart LH, Belghiti J, Jarnagin WR, et al., eds. *Surgery of the Liver, Biliary Tract, and Pancreas*. 4th ed. Philadelphia, PA: Saunders Elsevier; 2007:1654-1692.

7. Orloff MJ, Dailey PO, Orloff SL, et al. A 27-year experience with surgical treatment of Budd-Chiari syndrome. *Ann Surg*. Sept 2000;232(3):340-352.

8. Millener P, Grant EG, Rose S, et al. Color Doppler imaging findings in patients with Budd-Chiari syndrome: correlation with venographic findings. *AJR*. 1993;161(2):307-312.

9. Sharma S, Texeira A, Texeira P, et al. Pharmacological thrombolysis in Budd Chiari syndrome: a single-center experience and review of the literature. *J Hepatol*. Jan 2004;40(1):172-180.

10. Li T, Zhai S, Pang Z, et al. Feasibility and midterm outcomes of percutaneous transhepatic balloon angioplasty for symptomatic Budd-Chiari syndrome secondary to hepatic venous obstruction. *J Vasc Surg*. Nov 2009;50(5):1079-1084.

# 49 SPLENIC VEIN THROMBOSIS

Lawrence A. Shirley, MD
Mark Bloomston, MD

## PATIENT STORY

A 55-year-old man with a history of chronic alcoholism and recurrent bouts of pancreatitis presented with new onset of hematemesis and hematochezia. He complained of an acute exacerbation of his usual chronic left-sided abdominal pain. Vital signs showed tachycardia with a heart rate of 115 bpm and a blood pressure of 95/62 mm Hg. Physical examination was remarkable for epigastric and left upper quadrant tenderness without stigmata of cirrhosis. Laboratory work was significant for hemoglobin of 7.5 g/dL, a hematocrit of 22.2%, an amylase of 397 IU/L, and a lipase of 264 U/L. Hepatic function panel was within normal limits. After initial resuscitation, upper endoscopy was undertaken, showing actively bleeding gastric varices, but no evidence of esophageal varices. Hemostasis was obtained endoscopically. Subsequent computed tomography (CT) imaging demonstrated an atrophic calcified pancreas with occlusion of the splenic vein, splenomegaly, and multiple perigastric collaterals. No tumor was seen in the pancreas, and there was no evidence of cirrhosis. The patient subsequently underwent a laparoscopic splenectomy prior to discharge. Figures 49-1 to 49-3 show representative imaging of a patient with splenic vein thrombosis (SVT).

## HISTORY AND EPIDEMIOLOGY

- SVT was first recognized over 80 years ago as a cause of gastrointestinal (GI) bleeding.[1]

- The exact incidence of SVT is unknown as the majority of patients are asymptomatic. It is also unknown how many patients with isolated SVT later go on to develop gastric varices.

- Between 45% and 72% of patients initially present with gastric variceal bleeding, with most of them requiring splenectomy.[2]

- SVT complicates pancreatitis or pancreatic pseudocysts in 7% to 20% of patients.[3,4]

- Patients with incidentally discovered gastric varices may have a lower risk of bleeding. The risk of variceal hemorrhage is 5% for patients with CT-identified varices compared to 18% for endoscopically identified varices. Of those, only 4% develop variceal hemorrhage and/or require splenectomy.[5]

- Partial occlusion of the splenic vein is considerably more common than complete occlusion, with 54% to 89% of patients with SVT demonstrating only partial occlusion.[6,7]

- The reported frequency has increased with the improved sensitivity of imaging modalities such as CT, magnetic resonance imaging (MRI), and ultrasound (US).

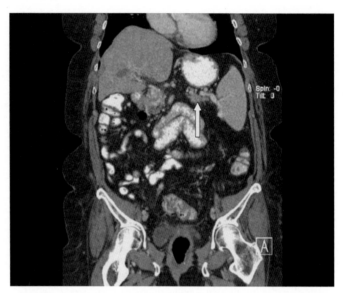

**FIGURE 49-1** Coronal computed tomography (CT) imaging of a patient with splenic vein thrombosis (SVT). The point of thrombosis near an area of pancreatic inflammation is noted with the white arrow.

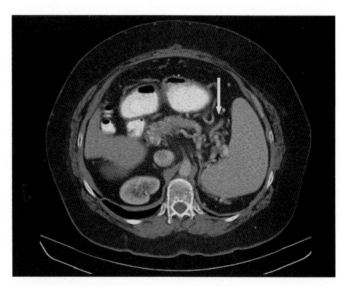

**FIGURE 49-2** Axial computed tomography (CT) imaging of a patient with splenic vein thrombosis (SVT). Cross-sectional imaging of patients with SVT can reveal splenomegaly as well as multiple enlarged perisplenic collateral vessels. Collaterals are noted with the white arrow.

## ETIOLOGY

- Causes of SVT include both acute and chronic pancreatitis, pancreatic malignancies, adenopathy from metastatic disease or lymphoma, idiopathic retroperitoneal fibrosis, and iatrogenic causes such as after splenectomy, gastrectomy, or a splenorenal shunt.[2,8,9]

- Although early reports found pancreatic carcinoma to be the most common cause of SVT, more recent reviews have noted pancreatitis as the inciting event in up to 60% of cases.[2,9]

- It is unknown if SVT is more likely in patients with alcoholic pancreatitis, as opposed to pancreatitis due to other causes.

## PATHOPHYSIOLOGY

- The path to development of SVT differs depending on the disease process that initiates the thrombosis.

- In acute pancreatitis, SVT is initiated by local prothrombotic inflammatory changes in the vascular endothelium of the splenic vein as it courses along the posterior aspect of the pancreatic tail, putting it in direct contact with peripancreatic inflammatory tissue.[10]

- Extrinsic compression from a pseudocyst, low pancreatic perfusion, or later development of pancreatic fibrosis may lead to SVT.[5]

- Enlarged lymph nodes, whether from malignant or inflammatory causes in the retroperitoneal, pancreatic, or perisplenic areas can compress the splenic vein, leading to obstruction.[2]

- Once occlusion of the splenic vein occurs, the most common collateral pathways use the short gastric veins for decompression. This ultimately leads to increased pressure within the submucosal veins of the fundus, resulting in gastric varices.[8]

- Anatomic variants and less common collateral pathways can lead to variations in the location of varices. If the coronary vein joins the splenic vein proximal to the obstruction, isolated esophageal varices can occur.[11] Additionally, the left gastroepiploic vein can collateralize with the left colic and inferior mesenteric veins, leading to colonic varices.[7] The incidence of both variations is rare.

## DIAGNOSIS

### Clinical Features

- Most patients with SVT are asymptomatic at the time of diagnosis and have normal liver function.[12]

- SVT should be suspected in patients with a history of pancreatitis and new onset of GI bleeding.

- Patients who have splenomegaly without a diagnosis of portal hypertension, cirrhosis, or hematologic diseases should be evaluated for SVT.

- Patients with isolated gastric varices on upper endoscopy should be suspected of having SVT. The first clinical manifestation of SVT is often acute or chronic GI bleeding. This can have a variety of presentations, ranging from chronic anemia to melena to hematemesis with hemodynamic instability.

- Approximately 25% of patients present with abdominal pain, which can be caused by multiple factors, including pancreatitis, pseudocyst, carcinoma, or splenomegaly.[2,9]

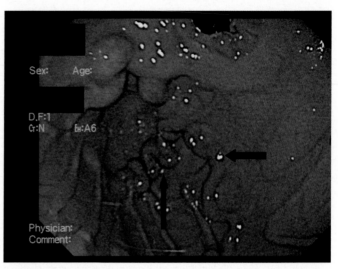

**FIGURE 49-3** Endoscopic imaging of isolated gastric varices in a patient with splenic vein thrombosis (SVT). The varices are noted with black arrows.

- Despite the fact that up to 71% of patients with SVT have splenomegaly, they rarely develop splenic pain, leukopenia, or thrombocytopenia.[9]

## Imaging Studies

- SVT is best seen with a high-quality CT scan with the appropriate venous contrast phase. The diagnosis may be made with nonvisualization of the splenic vein on CT.[5]

- MRI is also useful in diagnosing SVT. As opposed to invasive studies like venography, CT and MRI can help elucidate the etiology of SVT by imaging the stomach and pancreas.

- Ultrasound (US) can be used as a preliminary noninvasive test. Although SVT is difficult to diagnose using US, a normal-appearing splenic vein makes the diagnosis of SVT unlikely.[13,14]

- Endoscopic ultrasound (EUS) has been used more recently as an adjunct for the diagnosis of SVT. It can be used to make the diagnosis when the cause of gastric varices has not been elucidated by other imaging modalities.[15] EUS also has the potential to diagnose concurrent pancreatic carcinoma.

- Historically, other imaging studies used to diagnose SVT included splenoportography and venous phase angiography. However, these tests have largely been abandoned due to their invasive nature and the improved sensitivity of noninvasive studies.

## DIFFERENTIAL DIAGNOSIS

- There are a myriad of other causes of GI bleeding in patients with chronic pancreatitis, including pseudoaneurysms, pseudocysts, hemosuccus pancreaticus, peptic ulcer disease, gastritis, and Mallory-Weiss tears.

## MANAGEMENT

- Traditionally, the finding of SVT led to the recommendation that the patient should undergo routine splenectomy in order to prevent future gastric variceal bleeding, since a 1985 review documented that 50% of patients with SVT bled from gastric varices.[2]

- Splenectomy is the treatment of choice for patients with SVT and a history of bleeding gastric varices, as it decompresses the surrounding varices. Recurrent hemorrhage rates are exceedingly low after splenectomy.[2,8,9]

- Additional procedures to treat the underlying pathology may need to be undertaken simultaneously, including partial or total pancreatectomy, pseudocyst drainage, or partial gastrectomy.[2]

- For gastric varices themselves, sclerotherapy is less successful than for esophageal varices, with recurrent bleeding occurring in over half of the patients treated. Banding may prove more successful, but there is a lack of long-term follow-up for treatment of isolated gastric varices with this procedure. Thus, urgent splenectomy is recommended for acutely bleeding varices.[16]

- If due to simple compression by a pseudocyst, SVT may resolve after drainage of the associated pseudocyst.[5]

- Asymptomatic SVT secondary to pancreatitis identified by CT carries a risk of gastric variceal hemorrhage of only 4%.[5] As such, routine splenectomy is likely unnecessary, especially when gastric varices are not present.

- Splenectomy in patients with concomitant cirrhosis should be avoided if possible, as the subsequent development of portal vein thrombosis may complicate or even eliminate the opportunity for liver transplantation in future.

- Splenic artery embolization is a nonoperative alternative option for treatment of SVT with bleeding gastric varices. However, this treatment typically results in extensive splenic infarction, leading to splenic abscess in up to 25% of patients.[17] Additionally, there is no opportunity to treat the underlying pathology that caused SVT. Thus, this treatment is often limited to patients who are poor surgical candidates and/or in patients with advanced cancer.

- Given the low likelihood of complications from SVT as noted in recent literature, anticoagulation is not recommended, especially since it could possibly initiate bleeding from gastric varices.

## PATIENT EDUCATION

- If expectant management is to be pursued for SVT, especially for those with endoscopic evidence of gastric varices, patients must be educated about the risk of bleeding and possible need for urgent intervention.

## FOLLOW-UP

- Patients with known SVT, especially those with varices seen on CT, should undergo upper endoscopy at regular intervals to monitor the development and progression of gastric varices.

### PROVIDER RESOURCES

- http://en.diagnosispro.com/disease_information-for/splenic-vein-thrombosis/19807.html

- https://www.medify.com/conditions/splenic-vein-thrombosis

### PATIENT RESOURCE

- http://treato.com/Splenic+Vein+Thrombosis/?a=s

## REFERENCES

1. Hirschfeldt H. Die Erkankungen der Milz: Die Hepatolineal Erkankungen. *J Springer Verlag Berlin*. 1920;384.

2. Moosa A, Gadd M. Isolated splenic vein thrombosis. *World J Surg*. 1985;9:384-390.

3. Sakorafas G, Sarr M, Farle D, et al. The significance of sinistral portal hypertension complicating chronic pancreatitis. *Am J Surg*. 2000;179:129-133.

4. Mortele K, Mergo P, Taylor H, et al. Splenic and perisplenic involvement in acute pancreatitis: determination of prevalence and morphologic helical CT features. *J Comput Assist Tomogr*. 2001;25:50-54.

5. Heider TR, Azeem S, Galanko J, et al. The natural history of pancreatitis-induced splenic vein thrombosis. *Ann Surg*. 2004;239:876-882.

6. Leger L, Lenriot JP, Lemaigre G. L'hypertension et la stase portales segmentaires dans les pancreatites chroniques. A propos de 126 cas examines par splenoportographie et spleno-manometrie. *J Chir*. 1968;95:599-608.

7. Burbige EJ, Tarder G, Carson S, et al. A complication of pancreatitis with splenic vein thrombosis. *Am J Dig Dis*. 1978;23: 752-755.

8. Evans GRD, Yellin AE, Weaver FA, et al. Sinistral (left-sided) portal hypertension. *Am Surg*. 1990;56:758-763.

9. Madsen MS, Petersen TH, Sommer H. Segmental portal hypertension. *Ann Surg*. 1996;204:72-77.

10. Bernades P, Baits A, Levy P, et al. Splenic and portal venous obstruction in chronic pancreatitis. *Dig Dis Sci*. 1992;37:340-346.

11. Little AG, Moossa AR. Gastrointestinal hemorrhage from left-sided portal hypertension. *Am J Surg*. 1981;141:153-158.

12. Weber SM, Rikkers LF. Splenic vein thrombosis and gastrointestinal bleeding in chronic pancreatitis. *World J Surg*. 2003;27:1271-1274.

13. Webb LJ, Berger LA, Sherlock S. Grey scale ultrasonography of portal vein. *Lancet*. 1977;1:675-677.

14. Verbanck JJ, Rutgeerts LJ, Haerens MH, et al. Partial splenoportal and superior mesenteric venous thrombosis: early sonographic diagnosis and successful conservative management. *Gastroenterology*. 1984;86:949-952.

15. Wiersema MJ, Hawes RH, Lehman GA, et al. Prospective evaluation of endoscopic ultrasonography and endoscopic retrograde cholangiopancreatography in patients with chronic abdominal pain of suspected pancreatic origin. *Endoscopy*. 1993;25:555-564.

16. Trudeau W, Prindiville T. Endoscopic injection sclerosis in bleeding gastric varices. *Gastrointest Endosc*. 1986;32:264-268.

17. Lewis JD, Faigel DO, Morris JB, et al. Splenic vein thrombosis secondary to focal pancreatitis diagnosed by endoscopic ultrasonography. *J Clin Gastroenterol*. 1998;26:54-56.

# 50 MESENTERIC VENOUS THROMBOSIS

Alan Nadour, MD, FSVM
Raghu Kolluri, MD, FACP, FSVM

## PATIENT STORY

A 76-year-old Caucasian man presented with acute onset of intense periumbilical abdominal pain associated with nonbloody diarrhea. His past medical history was significant for portal vein thrombosis diagnosed 2 years earlier. At that time thrombophilia workup was unremarkable except for JAK2 V617F mutation. Subsequent bone marrow studies showed no evidence of myeloproliferative disease (MPD). Other comorbidities included coronary artery disease, atrial fibrillation, hypertension, and dyslipidemia. His Coumadin treatment was interrupted 1 week prior to the admission for a tooth extraction and was not resumed. His vital signs were normal except for mild tachycardia. The abdominal pain was severe and seemed to be out of proportion to the physical findings. The abdomen was soft with predominantly midline tenderness and mild guarding. The remainder of the physical examination was unremarkable.

Comprehensive laboratory evaluation was only remarkable for an elevated white blood cell (WBC) count to 21,000 cells per cubic millimeter with normal differential. Contrast-enhanced computed tomographic (CT) scan of the abdomen showed acute superior mesenteric vein (SMV) thrombosis, thickening of small bowel loops, and presence of collateral vessels at the porta hepatis (Figures 50-1 to 50-3).

Adequate anticoagulation was achieved with unfractionated heparin. However, the following day his abdominal pain was worse and WBC count increased to 34,000 per cubic millimeter. An exploratory laparotomy revealed an ischemic ileum that necessitated a small bowel resection with primary anastomosis. After a prolonged hospitalization, the patient recovered and was discharged home on Coumadin.

## BACKGROUND

- Mesenteric venous thrombosis (MVT) refers to thrombosis of the splanchnic veins draining the intestine (superior mesenteric, inferior mesenteric, portal, and splenic veins).

- Venous obstruction induces bowel edema and distension that ultimately impedes the arterial inflow leading to intestinal ischemia.

- JW Elliot first recognized MVT as a cause of intestinal ischemia in 1895.

- The high-mortality rates formerly encountered in patients with MVT have been attributed to its insidious course, late presentation, and missed diagnosis.

- Wide availability of CT venography (CTV) and magnetic resonance venography (MRV) has led to a decline in the mortality rates from acute MVT from early diagnosis.[1]

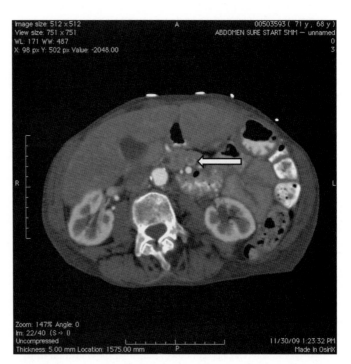

**FIGURE 50-1** Computed tomography (CT) image shows intraluminal filling defect in the superior mesenteric vein (SMV) consistent with acute thrombus (arrow).

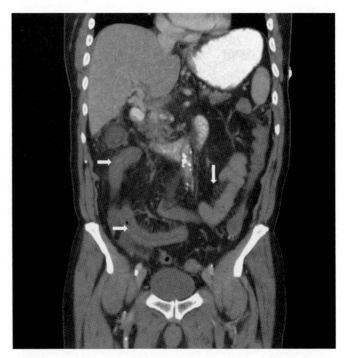

**FIGURE 50-2** Computed tomography (CT) image shows multiple loops of small intestine wall thickening (arrows).

- The SMV, which drains the small intestine, cecum, ascending colon, and transverse colon, is most commonly affected, whereas the inferior mesenteric vein (IMV) draining the descending colon, the sigmoid colon, and the rectum is rarely involved.

## EPIDEMIOLOGY

- The average age of presentation ranges from 45 to 60 years with an overall slightly higher male gender predominance.[2,3]

## ETIOLOGY AND PATHOPHYSIOLOGY

- MVT can be primary (without any underlying etiology) or secondary.
- Numerous causes of secondary MVT have been identified (Table 50-1).[4]
- The extent of the thrombotic event, rate of thrombus expansion, size of the vessel involved, and the depth of intestinal wall ischemia determine the degree of intestinal injury.
- Ischemic injury restricted to mucosa leads to abdominal pain and diarrhea, while transmural ischemia or necrosis can lead to gastrointestinal bleeding and peritonitis.
- Hypercoagulable states lead to thrombosis arising in the small veins (intramural venules, vasa recta, and venous arcades), which then propagates to involve the large veins. In contrast, thrombosis due to intra-abdominal causes (such as surgery or pancreatitis) begins in the large veins and then progresses distally to the small veins.
- Contrary to arterial causes of bowel ischemia, the transition from ischemic segment to normal bowel is usually gradual with no clear demarcation separating viable and nonviable tissues.

## CLINICAL FEATURES

- MVT symptoms are usually vague and nonspecific with insidious onset. The hallmark is abdominal pain out of proportion to the physical findings.[5]
- The severity, location, and duration of pain vary and depend on the rate of thrombus formation and extension.
- Mesenteric venous thrombosis can be acute, subacute, or chronic.
- Acute mesenteric venous thrombosis is associated with increased risk of bowel infarction and peritonitis and may mandate immediate surgical evaluation. Most patients present with the symptoms described above, but more than half may present with nonspecific signs and symptoms, such as fever, chills, nausea, vomiting, diarrhea, and anorexia.[5]
- Patients with the subacute form present with abdominal pain for days or weeks without bowel infarction or gastrointestinal bleeding.
- Chronic MVT may be asymptomatic due to the presence of adequate collateral venous drainage that prevents the development of bowel infarction and may present with complications of portal vein, splenic vein, or SMV thrombosis such as ascites and esophageal variceal bleeding.

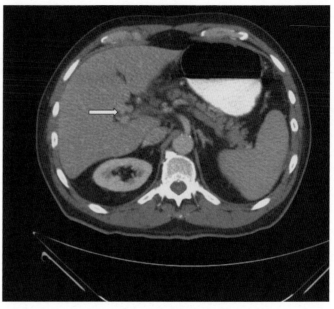

**FIGURE 50-3** Portal vein collaterals indicate chronic portal vein thrombosis (arrow).

## DIAGNOSIS

- Diagnosis must begin with a good history, physical examination, and high degree of suspicion.
- Laboratory findings such as lactic acidosis, leukocytosis, or thrombocytopenia are neither sensitive nor specific but are used to assess the overall severity of illness.

### Imaging Studies

- Plain abdominal radiographic films have limited value, but thumb printing, portal venous air, pneumatosis intestinalis (gas in the bowel wall), and free intraperitoneal air may be present in bowel infarction.
- Barium contrast studies interfere with visualization on angiography and should be avoided.
- Duplex ultrasonography is a noninvasive, widely available, and relatively inexpensive modality that can be rapidly performed. It may demonstrate venous flow abnormalities or thrombus in the mesenteric veins (Figures 50-4 to 50-6). Limitations of this technique include body habitus and bowel gas.
- CTV has sensitivity and specificity and accuracy of greater than 90%[6] and should be performed as the initial diagnostic test for MVT. In acute MVT, CTV may reveal intraluminal-filling defects, enlarged vein size, and sharply defined vein wall (Figure 50-7). Other findings include bowel wall edema and presence of layered pattern of enhancement (known as the target sign) indicating hyperemia in the mucosa and muscularis propria. Persistent venous obstruction leads to transmural intestinal infarction manifesting as homogeneous enhancement pattern with decreased bowel wall density. Intestinal pneumatosis (intramural gas), portal or mesenteric venous gas, bowel dilatation, and free intraperitoneal air resulting from perforation of the infracted bowel may also be present. Dilated fluid-filled loops of small bowel can be seen if small bowel obstruction develops (Figure 50-8). Collateralization in the mesentery indicates a thrombotic event of more than a few weeks duration.[7,8]
- Magnetic resonance angiography (MRA)—Gadolinium-enhanced MRA has also been shown to be highly accurate for the diagnosis of MVT with sensitivity and specificity reported to be 90% to 100% and 100%, respectively. Nevertheless, it is not as practical as CT due to the cost, longer scanning time, and suboptimal special resolution (Figure 50-9).
- Invasive mesenteric angiography imparts excellent anatomic details of the splanchnic vasculature and allows definitive distinction between occlusive and nonocclusive forms of mesenteric ischemia, but this is rarely needed for diagnosis of MVT.

## MANAGEMENT

- Effective treatment of MVT is based on identifying and treating the underlying predisposing condition, preventing progression to intestinal infarction, and initiating efficient supportive measures such as fluid resuscitation, nasogastric decompression, bowel rest, broad-spectrum antibiotics, and pain control.
- Heparin—On diagnosis of acute or subacute MVT, prompt anticoagulation with intravenous heparin should be commenced to prevent thrombus propagation, even in the presence of

**TABLE 50-1** Predisposing Factors and Conditions for MVT

| Inherited Thrombophilias |
| --- |
| Antithrombin III deficiency |
| Protein C deficiency |
| Protein S deficiency |
| Factor V Leiden mutation |
| Prothrombin G20210A mutation |
| Hereditary hemorrhagic telangiectasia |
| Dysfibrinogenemia |
| JAK2 V16F mutation |
| Plasminogen deficiency |
| Sickle cell disease |
| **Acquired Thrombophilias** |
| Antiphospholipid antibodies |
| Anticardiolipin antibodies |
| Beta-2 glycoprotein-1 antibodies |
| Heparin-induced thrombocytopenia |
| Disseminated intravascular coagulation |
| Myeloproliferative disease |
| Malignancy |
| Polycythemia vera |
| Essential thrombocythemia |
| Hyperhomocysteinemia |
| Monoclonal gammopathy |
| Nephrotic syndrome |
| Oral contraceptive use |
| Paroxysmal nocturnal hemoglobinuria |
| Decompression sickness |
| Sickle cell disease |
| Pregnancy |
| **Intra-abdominal Causes** |
| Cirrhosis and portal hypertension |
| Inflammatory bowel diseases |
| Intra-abdominal infection |
| Pancreatitis |
| Diverticulitis |
| Postoperative states |
| Intestinal volvulus |
| Congenital venous anomaly |
| Blunt abdominal trauma |
| Idiopathic |

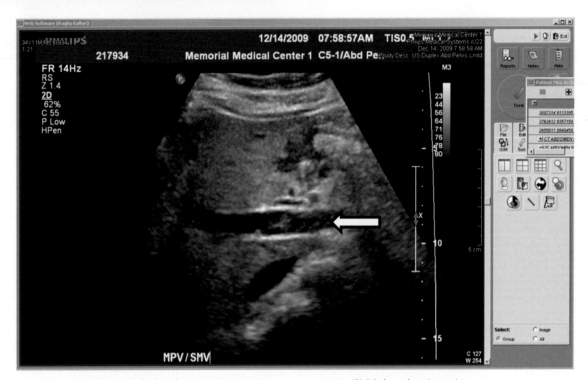

**FIGURE 50-4** Abdominal duplex demonstrates superior mesenteric vein (SMV) thrombus (arrow).

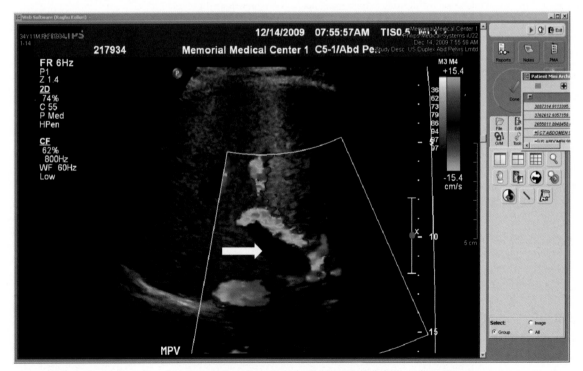

**FIGURE 50-5** Abdominal duplex shows no flow in the splenic vein consistent with thrombus (arrow).

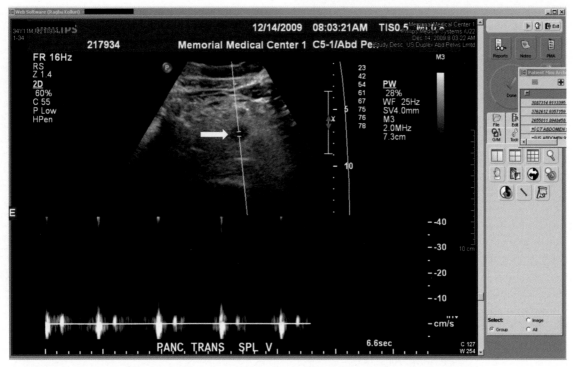

FIGURE 50-6 Abdominal duplex shows no flow in the splenic vein consistent with thrombus (arrow).

gastrointestinal bleeding, when the benefit of preventing intestinal infarction outweighs the risk of bleeding.[1]

- Warfarin—Once oral feeds are initiated, warfarin must be initiated along with heparin.

- Duration of anticoagulation—Patients with reversible or time-limited risk factors should be treated with warfarin for 3 to 6 months, whereas those with continuing risk factors such as persistent hypercoagulability should be considered for indefinite warfarin treatment.[5]

- Endovascular therapy—Percutaneous mechanical thrombectomy and catheter-directed thrombolysis have been employed as nonsurgical alternatives in the treatment of patients with extensive portal or SMV thrombosis with persistent or worsening symptoms while on anticoagulation.

- Surgery—Surgical intervention is not required for all patients with acute or subacute MVT. The strategy of withholding early operative approach holds the benefit of avoiding unnecessary bowel resection and potential subsequent short bowel syndrome.[9] Unstable patients presenting with signs of peritonitis or bowel infarction require immediate surgical exploration either by laparotomy or laparoscopy. Resection of the nonviable bowel segment should be undertaken with conservation of potentially viable intestine, followed by a second-look operation 24 to 48 hours after the initial resection to reassess the questionable bowel viability and the need for further resection.[10] Postoperative heparin therapy should be initiated when bleeding risk subsides.

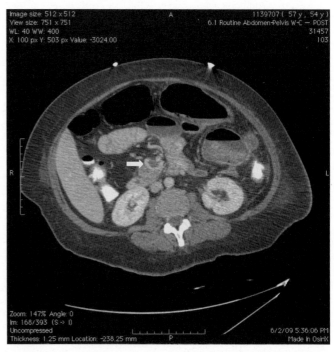

FIGURE 50-7 Contrast-enhanced computed tomography (CT) image demonstrates acute superior mesenteric vein (SMV) thrombus (arrow).

• Chronic MVT—Treatment is aimed at control of gastrointestinal bleeding from varices secondary to portal hypertension. Asymptomatic patients benefit from prophylactic pharmacologic therapy with propranolol. The use of anticoagulation in the setting of chronic MVT has been shown to prevent thrombosis recurrence and improve survival.[5]

## REFERENCES

1. Alvi AR, Khan S, Niazi SK, et al. Acute mesenteric venous thrombosis: improved outcome with early diagnosis and prompt anticoagulation therapy. *Int J Surg*. Jun 2009;7(3): 210-213.

2. Acosta S, Alhadad A, Svensson P, Ekberg O. Epidemiology, risk and prognostic factors in mesenteric venous thrombosis. *Br J Surg*. 2008;95:1245-1251.

3. Abu-Daff S, Abu-Daff N, Al-Shahed M. Mesenteric venous thrombosis and factors associated with mortality: a statistical analysis with five-year follow-up. *J Gastrointest Surg*. 2009;13: 1245-1250.

4. Primignani M, Mannucci PM. The role of thrombophilia in splanchnic vein thrombosis. *Semin Liver Dis*. 2008;28: 293-301.

5. Harnik IG, Brandt LJ. Mesenteric venous thrombosis. *Vasc Med*. 2010;15(5):407-418.

6. Acosta S, Alhadad A, Ekberg O. Findings in multi-detector row CT with portal phase enhancement in patients with mesenteric venous thrombosis. *Emerg Radiol*. 2009;16:477-482.

7. Lee SS, Ha HK, Park SH, et al. Usefulness of computed tomography in differentiating transmural infarction from non-transmural ischemia of the small intestine in patients with acute mesenteric venous thrombosis. *J Comput Assist Tomogr*. 2008;32:730-737.

8. Ofer A, Abadi S, Nitecki S, et al. Multidetector CT angiography in the evaluation of acute mesenteric ischemia. *Eur Radiol*. Jan 2009;19(1):24-30.

9. Cenedese A, Monneuse O, Gruner L, Tissot E, Mennesson N, Barth X. Initial management of extensive mesenteric venous thrombosis: retrospective study of nine cases. *World J Surg*. 2009;33(10):2203-2208.

10. Thomas RM, Ahmad SA. Management of acute post-operative portal venous thrombosis. *J Gastrointest Surg*. 2010;14(3):570-577.

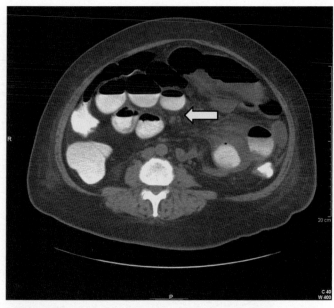

**FIGURE 50-8** Computed tomography (CT) image shows fluid-filled loops of dilated small bowel consistent with small intestine obstruction (arrow).

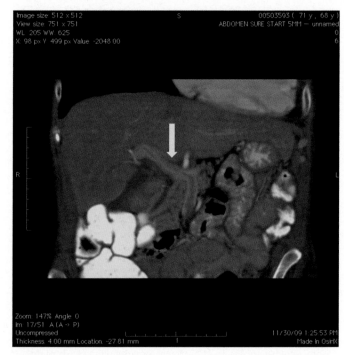

**FIGURE 50-9** Gadolinium-enhanced magnetic resonance venography (MRV) demonstrates thrombus in the superior mesenteric vein (SMV) (arrow).

# PART 7

# VENOUS DISEASES

# 51 ACUTE SUPERFICIAL VENOUS THROMBOSIS: EVALUATION AND TREATMENT

Teresa L. Carman, MD

## PATIENT STORY

A 74-year-old man presents with acute erythema, pain, and tenderness along the medial aspect of his thigh and knee. He was recently hospitalized with proximal calf cellulitis, but the pain and distribution of these clinical findings are different. He has a history of calf deep venous thrombosis (DVT) approximately 10 years ago. Duplex ultrasound demonstrates thrombus within the great saphenous vein (GSV). He is initially managed conservatively with nonsteroidal agents. On repeat duplex ultrasound, he is found to have proximal propagation into the common femoral vein junction. Anticoagulation is initiated for approximately 3 months. He does well and ultimately undergoes GSV ablation.

## EPIDEMIOLOGY

### Superficial Venous Thrombosis

- Affects approximately 125,000 people in the United States per year, but the true annual incidence is likely unknown due to under-recognition and under-reporting.
- Is reported in approximately 3% to 11% of the population.[1]
- Occurs more frequently in women than in men.
- Increases with age; mean age of presentation is 60 years.[2]
- Is associated with clinical features of obesity, immobility, and varicose veins.
- Occurs most commonly in the GSV (60%-80% of cases); the small saphenous vein and tributary varicosities are less frequently involved.
- Is associated with concomitant DVT in up to 40% of patients at the time of diagnosis.[3]
- Is associated with symptomatic pulmonary embolism (PE) in up to 12% of patients.[3]

### Upper Extremity SVT

- Differs from lower extremity SVT in that it is frequently associated with an indwelling catheter (PICC) or device.
- Is usually related to the size and location of the indwelling device.

## ETIOLOGY AND PATHOPHYSIOLOGY

Superficial venous thrombosis (SVT), also referred to as thrombophlebitis, typically has both thrombotic and inflammatory components.

- Inflammatory changes without thrombosis are termed as phlebitis.
- 60% to 80% of cases have associated varicose veins.

- There are common associations with external vein trauma, internal vein trauma, hemorheologic changes, and vein inflammation.[4]
- The role of thrombophilia has not been well defined, but prothrombotic conditions such as myeloproliferative disorders or underlying malignancy should be considered.[1,4]

### Lower Extremity SVT

- Is associated with prolonged immobilization, obesity, trauma, oral contraceptives and hormonal therapy, malignancy, inflammatory stimuli, autoimmune disease or vasculitis, and thromboangiitis obliterans.[4]

### Upper Extremity SVT

- Is usually related to indwelling catheters, phlebotomy, or intravenous infusion.

## DIAGNOSIS

### Clinical Findings

- Patients typically present with warmth, erythema, induration, and tenderness along the vein (Figure 51-1).[1,4]
- A palpable cord or thrombus within the vein is the most identifiable clinical finding.
- The pain may be out of proportion to the clinical findings.
- Patients may have associated varicose veins or skin changes of chronic venous disease.
- The presence of local trauma, inflammation or infection, or indwelling access should be noted.
- The presence of swelling is variable.
- Patients should be clinically assessed for signs and symptoms of PE.
- The uncommon presentations of Mondor disease (superficial thrombosis on the breast, abdominal wall, dorsal vein of the penis) or migratory SVT (Trousseau syndrome) are often indicative of an underlying malignancy and require thorough evaluation.

### Diagnostic Imaging

- Identification of noncompressible or partially compressible hypoechoic thrombus on duplex ultrasound within the vein is diagnostic (Figure 51-2).

- Duplex ultrasound is also warranted to document the extent of the SVT and to exclude DVT.[3] DVT may occur due to proximal extension of the SVT into a deep vein at the common femoral junction (Figure 51-3) or at the level of the popliteal vein. Extension through perforating veins into the deep system has also been demonstrated.

- In patients with signs and symptoms of PE, computed tomography angiography (CTA) or ventilation-perfusion nuclear imaging should be performed according to local standards.

- Venography is rarely warranted for SVT diagnosis.

## Laboratory Studies

- There is no laboratory testing that is sensitive or specific for SVT.

- Similar to patients with DVT, baseline complete blood count (CBC), comprehensive metabolic panel (CMP), and coagulation studies are appropriate in SVT.

- Given the association with malignancy, all patients should be up to date on age- and gender-appropriate cancer screening according to prevailing guidelines.

- Additional laboratory studies may be considered to evaluate clinical concerns found on history, physical examination, and a comprehensive review of systems.

- Thrombophilia testing for genetic disorders is rarely warranted.

- Testing for antiphospholipid antibodies should be considered in appropriate cases.

## DIFFERENTIAL DIAGNOSIS

- Infectious, inflammatory, and musculoskeletal conditions should be considered in the differential diagnosis.[1,5]

- Infection related to lymphangitis or focal cellulitis should be considered since the management will be significantly altered.

- Primary dermatologic considerations include acute lipodermatosclerosis or erythema nodosum.

- Inflammatory processes such as vasculitis or cutaneous polyarteritis nodosum should be considered.

- Muscle rupture, soft tissue hematoma, Baker cyst, or gout may also be contemplated.

- DVT should be excluded by duplex ultrasound.

## MANAGEMENT

- Since SVT has historically been regarded as a benign disease, many practitioners do not recognize the need for active management of SVT. Thus, management is frequently by "gestalt" or by default.

- The rationale for management of SVT is similar to that for DVT: to prevent proximal propagation to the deep system and assist with symptom resolution.

- Few randomized controlled trials are available to guide management of lower extremity SVT. These trials range from medical management with anticoagulants to the use of nonsteroidal agents to surgical management.[6] However, these trials frequently enroll small numbers of patients and are fraught with methodologic weaknesses that make comparison difficult.

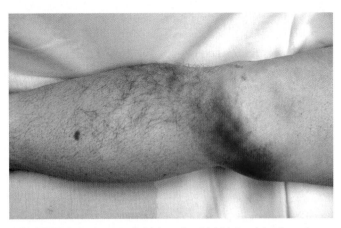

FIGURE 51-1 Acute superficial thrombophlebitis involving branch varicosities off the great saphenous vein (GSV). (*Image courtesy of Steven Dean, DO.*)

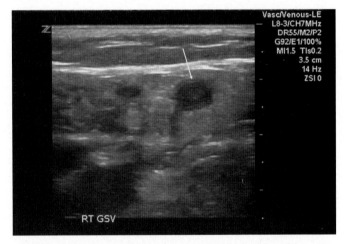

FIGURE 51-2 The great saphenous vein (GSV) lying within the saphenous sheath—noted by the arrow—is noncompressible and filled with hypoechoic thrombus.

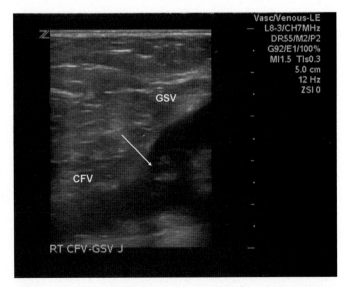

FIGURE 51-3 Thrombus (white arrow) extending from the great saphenous vein (GSV) into the common femoral vein (CFV) junction.

- Recommendations specifically applicable to upper extremity SVT are lacking.

- Historically, thrombus identified within 10 cm of the saphenofemoral junction dictated more aggressive therapy to prevent propagation. This notion was confirmed by the CALISTO trial.[7] In a similar fashion, upper extremity SVT within 5 cm of the subclavian vein may require more aggressive management.

- The 2012 American College of Chest Physicians (ACCP) guidelines have identified factors that favor the use of anticoagulants in SVT including extensive SVT; involvement of the GSV; above the knee SVT, especially in proximity to the saphenofemoral junction; a history of prior SVT or venous thromboembolism (VTE); active malignancy; or recent surgery.

## General Recommendations

- Oral or topical nonsteroidal agents may be used to relieve symptoms associated with SVT. But they do not impact risk for propagation and recurrence.

- Patients with SVT above the knee should undergo duplex ultrasound to exclude involvement of the deep veins.

- The ACCP guidelines have specifically recommended the use of fondaparinux 2.5 mg daily for 45 days over no anticoagulation for SVT 5 cm or greater in length (Grade 2B recommendation).[8] This recommendation is based on the CALISTO trial that compared fondaparinux 2.5 mg daily for 45 days to placebo in 3000 patients.[7]

- Other authorities recommend treating SVT involving either the upper or lower extremities similarly to DVT with respect to the use and duration of therapeutic anticoagulation—in effect acknowledging the high risk for associated DVT, propagation of the SVT, and risk for recurrence based on the clinical setting.[9]

- Compression stockings may be helpful to reduce inflammation and control edema but are not well studied with respect to propagation.

- Surgical ligation has been historically used, yet may carry a higher risk for proximal DVT and has mostly been abandoned.

- Patients presenting with Mondor disease or migratory SVT should be anticoagulated and fully evaluated for an associated malignancy.

## PROGNOSIS

- In general, the prognosis for isolated SVT is good. Most patients will have resolution of the thrombus without residual manifestations.

- Patients may experience some persistent staining or discoloration of the skin (Figure 51-4). Some patients will have a persistently palpable nodularity or "cord" at the site of the SVT.

## PATIENT EDUCATION

- Patients may be at increased risk for recurrent SVT or VTE and should be made aware of associated symptoms and clinical findings that direct further evaluation.

## FOLLOW-UP

- Repeat duplex ultrasound to determine resolution or persistence of the SVT may be helpful. This can establish a new baseline on which to evaluate recurrent symptoms.

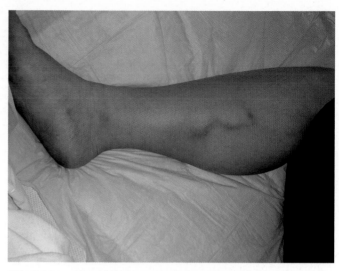

**FIGURE 51-4** Typical skin staining that may persist following resolution of superficial venous thrombosis (SVT).

- Routine clinical follow-up should be consistent with the extent of the underlying venous disease and requirements for preventative management (ie, maintaining compression and managing skin care issues as needed).

## PATIENT AND PROVIDER RESOURCES

- PubMed Health: http://www.ncbi.nlm.nih.gov/pubmedhealth/PMH0001248/
- Medscape Reference: http://emedicine.medscape.com/article/463256-overview
- Thrombophlebitis-Mayo Clinic: http://www.mayoclinic.com/health/thrombophlebitis/DS00223

## REFERENCES

1. Cesarone MR, Belcaro G, Agus G, et al. Management of superficial vein thrombosis and thrombophlebitis: status and expert opinion. *Angiology.* 2007;58(suppl 1):7S-15S.

2. Décousus H, Bertoletti L, Frappé P, et al. Recent findings in the epidemiology, diagnosis and treatment of superficial-vein thrombosis. *Thromb Res.* 2011;127(suppl 3):S81-S85.

3. Quéré I, Leizorovicz A, Galanaud JP, et al. Superficial venous thrombosis and compression ultrasound imaging. *J Vasc Surg.* 2012;56:1032-1038.

4. Litzendorf ME, Satiani B. Superficial venous thrombosis: disease progression and evolving treatment approaches. *Vasc Health Risk Manag.* 2011;7:569-575.

5. ten Cate-Hoek AJ, van der Velde EF, Toll DB, et al. Common alternative diagnoses in general practice when deep venous thrombosis is excluded. *Neth J Med.* 2012;70:130-135.

6. Di Nisio M, Wichers IM, Middeldorp S. Treatment for superficial thrombophlebitis of the leg. *Cochrane Database Syst Rev.* 2012; 3:CD004982.

7. Décousus H, Prandoni P, Mismetti P, et al. Fondaparinux for the treatment of superficial-vein thrombosis in the legs. *N Engl J Med.* 2010;363:1222-1232.

8. Kearon C, Akl EA, Comerota AJ, et al. Antithrombotic therapy for VTE disease. *Antithrombotic Therapy and Prevention of Thrombosis,* 9th ed: American College of Chest Physicians Evidence-Based Clinical Practice Guidelines. *Chest.* 2012;141(suppl 2): e419S-e494S.

9. Kitchens CS. How I treat superficial venous thrombosis. *Blood.* 2011;117:39-44.

# 52 EVALUATION AND TREATMENT OF CALF VEIN THROMBOSIS

Joshua A. Beckman, MD, MS

## PATIENT STORY

A 49-year-old man returns from a 1-week trip to Hong Kong and reports right calf cramping that started after picking up his luggage. Over the next 2 days the cramping persists, is made worse by walking, and the right calf becomes swollen (Figure 52-1). He sees his primary care physician, who refers the patient for a lower extremity duplex ultrasound examination. The examination reveals no evidence for proximal deep vein involvement, but he does have acute peroneal and posterior tibial vein thrombosis. Low–molecular weight heparin therapy is initiated and the patient is transitioned to warfarin anticoagulation for a 3-month therapeutic course.

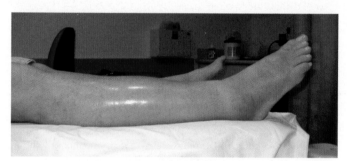

FIGURE 52-1 The edematous, erythematous right calf of a 49-year-old man. The calf was warm and tender to touch. Duplex ultrasound revealed thrombosis in the peroneal and posterior tibial veins.

## EPIDEMIOLOGY

- Two vessel types may develop thrombosis and be described as distal deep vein thrombosis (DVT): the muscular soleal and gastrocnemius veins and the paired deep calf posterior tibial, peroneal, and anterior tibial veins.

- In a prospective series of 855 consecutive patients with suspected pulmonary embolism, DVT was noted in approximately 20% of the subjects, with distal DVT accounting for approximately half of the venous thromboembolism (VTE).[1]

- In a retrospective review of the combination of the Cardiovascular Health Study and the Atherosclerosis Risk in Communities Study, 21,680 subjects were followed for nearly 8 years and evaluated for VTE.[2] The subjects were over the age of 45 years and lived in six different communities. In this cohort, the age-standardized incidence was 1.9 cases per 1000 subject-years. Men developed VTE more frequently than women, and in both groups the incidence increased with age. Nearly half of the cases had a well-demarcated antecedent to increase the risk of VTE (bedrest, trauma, surgery, cancer) and half were idiopathic. In this cohort, isolated distal VTE was noted in only 7% of the total VTE cases.

## ETIOLOGY AND PATHOPHYSIOLOGY

- Rudolf Virchow's triad remains the basis for our understanding of the factors that cause proximal and distal DVT. The components of the triad include stasis, hypercoagulability, and vascular injury. Table 52-1 lists the congenital and acquired risk factors by type.

- In the at-risk vascular bed, injury incites the liberation of fibrin, which binds red blood cells, platelets, and white blood cells. In the setting of a hypercoagulable state or stasis, the thrombus may propagate, both proximally and distally, or embolize to the pulmonary arteries.

**TABLE 52-1.** Inciting VTE Factors

| Stasis | Hypercoagulability | Vascular Injury |
|---|---|---|
| Surgery | Factor V Leiden | Indwelling catheter |
| Trauma | Prothrombin gene mutation | Pacemaker |
| Medical illness | Hyperhomocysteinemia | Chemotherapeutic agents |
| Immobilization (cast) | Protein C or S deficiency | Trauma |
| Air/car travel | Dysfibrinogenemia | Surgery |
| | Antiphospholipid antibodies | |
| | Malignancy | |
| | Inflammatory bowel disease | |
| | Heparin-induced thrombocytopenia | |

## DIAGNOSIS

- The challenge of calf vein thrombosis diagnosis lies in the poor predictive value of any specific symptom or sign for VTE. As a result, many physicians will apply a clinical decision rule to generate a probability of disease and indication for further blood and ultrasonographic testing.

### Clinical Decision Rules

- The most utilized clinical decision tool for lower extremity DVT is the Wells score.[3] The components of the score and their assigned values are listed in Table 52-2. Patients with a score of 3 or greater are considered at high risk for DVT, while those with a score of 0 or less are considered at low risk.

### Fibrin D-Dimer

- Fibrin D-dimer, commonly referred to as D-dimer, is one of the several fibrinogen cleavage products of plasmin. D-dimer is comprised of two D domains from adjacent fibrin monomers now cross-linked by activated factor XIII.

- D-Dimer's origin from fibrin, and not fibrinogen, permits elevated plasma levels to be interpreted as recent or continual intravascular coagulation.

- D-Dimer's formation is not particular to VTE, and elevated levels can be seen in patients with septicemia, active bleeding, recent surgery, and cancer. As a result, elevated levels of D-dimer do not accurately predict the presence of DVT, but a low level carries a very high negative predictive value as high as 99%.[4]

### Duplex Ultrasonography

- Duplex ultrasound is the most common and most reliable method of distal DVT detection.

- Duplex ultrasound examination relies on three components to make a diagnosis: noncompressibility of the imaged vein (Figure 52-2), abnormal blood flow as measured by Doppler pulse wave analysis, abnormal color Doppler imaging.

**TABLE 52-2.** Wells Score Components

| Clinical Component | Score |
|---|---|
| Active cancer | 1 |
| Paralysis or recent lower extremity casting | 1 |
| Recent major surgery or being bedridden >3 days | 1 |
| Tenderness localized to deep venous system | 1 |
| Full leg swelling | 1 |
| Calf swelling of >3 cm compared to contralateral leg | 1 |
| Pitting edema | 1 |
| Collateral superficial veins | 1 |
| Likely alternative diagnosis | −2 |

- Nascent thrombosis is echolucent (Figure 52-3), so the inability to compress a vessel without obvious intravascular occlusion is strongly indicative of acute venous thrombosis.
- The sensitivity and specificity of duplex ultrasonography for the diagnosis of proximal DVT are estimated at 95% and 98%, respectively.[5]
- The diagnosis of thrombosis in the calf veins is more challenging than in the proximal veins. The veins are smaller and are more difficult to locate with presentations of severe swelling (Figure 52-4).
- Well-trained technologists can adequately insonate these veins 80% to 90% of the time and, when well imaged, the sensitivity and specificity are above 90%. Others have reported a lower sensitivity and specificity for calf vein thrombosis.
- Most reviews suggest a high sensitivity and specificity when calf veins are visualized, but a frequency of indeterminate studies ranging from 9% to 82%.[6]

## Other Methods

- Angiographic evaluation of the calf veins is rarely necessary or performed anymore. Invasive contrast venography, formerly the gold standard evaluation, exposes the patient to heightened risks from radiation, contrast exposure, and the procedure itself.
- Magnetic resonance venography, rarely the first-line evaluation, is improving as a non invasive method to diagnose calf DVT. Recent data suggests a below-knee thrombosis identification sensitivity of 68% and specificity of 94%.[7]

## DIFFERENTIAL DIAGNOSIS

- The differential diagnosis for calf vein thrombosis is broad, for the symptoms are nonspecific (so nonspecific clinical decision rules are needed to decide on testing). Despite this, there are a range of diagnoses that should be considered for each patient who presents with calf swelling, discomfort, and/or erythema. The common diagnoses in patients with manifestations similar to calf DVT can be divided into venous and nonvenous causes.

### Common Venous Causes

- Superficial venous thrombosis—Venous thrombosis of the great or small saphenous veins or varicose veins may present with the same manifestations. Anticoagulation is rarely needed, for the risk of pulmonary embolism or proximal deep vein progression is very low.
- Chronic venous insufficiency—Impaired venous valve function and/or venous dilation facilitates venous pooling, diminishes venous return, increases intravascular venous pressure, and causes edema.
- Post-thrombotic syndrome (PTS)—It is found in up to half of all patients with a history of DVT. PTS is characterized by leg heaviness, pruritus, cramping, and, less commonly, ulceration. The difference between venous insufficiency and PTS lies in the persistent obstruction to flow found in the latter condition.

### Nonvenous Causes

- Baker cyst—A Baker cyst or popliteal cyst commonly results in the setting of knee inflammation, such as with a cartilaginous tear or arthritis causing excess fluid production and possible impingement on venous return.

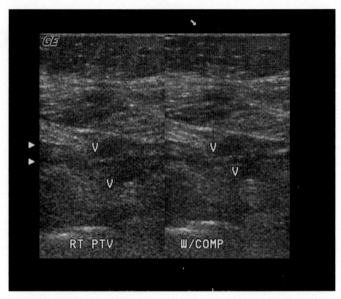

FIGURE 52-2 Compression ultrasound of the right posterior tibial veins. Acute thrombosis has the same ultrasonographic profile as flowing blood and remains echolucent. The lack of compression (right panel) of the veins indicates the presence of thrombosis.

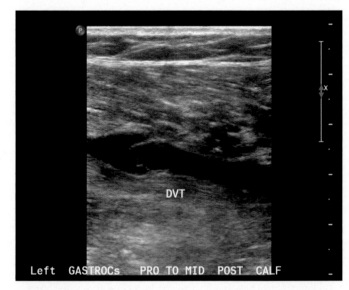

FIGURE 52-3 Duplex ultrasonography of a diffusely dilated and incompressible left gastrocnemius vein consistent with acute muscular vein thrombosis. (*Photograph courtesy of Dr. Steven M. Dean.*)

- Hematoma

- Gastrocnemius muscle tear—It may present with a characteristic layering below the malleolus of blood displaced by gravity from the tear called a "scimitar sign."

- Lymphedema—As a result of lymphatic absence, degeneration, or interruption, lymph may extrude from the lymphatics and present with lower extremity swelling. The edema is typically different from venous edema, presenting with swelling that extends into the foot. Over time, proteinaceous lymphedema is less responsive to compression and leg elevation.

- States of volume retention (ie, congestive heart failure or nephrotic syndrome).

## MANAGEMENT

- The management of calf vein thrombosis varies from the management of proximal DVT only in duration of anticoagulation. Therapeutic anticoagulation is commonly initiated with a heparin, intravenous unfractionated heparin (UFH), or subcutaneous low–molecular weight heparin (LMWH) for 5 to 7 days followed by 6 to 12 weeks of warfarin anticoagulation.

- In contrast to the 50% risk of pulmonary embolism in proximal DVT, calf vein thrombosis is expected to propagate approximately 20% of the time.[8]

- The American College of Chest Physicians Antithrombotic Guidelines recommend 3 months of therapy for patients with a reversible risk factor for venous thromboembolism.[9]

- In contrast to the recommendation for patients with an idiopathic proximal DVT for indefinite anticoagulation, the guidelines suggest that 3 months of anticoagulation is sufficient for distal DVT.

- For patients with a second unprovoked calf DVT, indefinite anticoagulation is recommended.

- The choice of agent is affected by the presence of cancer. Treatment of malignancy-related calf DVT should be with 3 to 6 months of LMWH and subsequent warfarin or LMWH until the cancer is resolved.[10]

- Patients should elevate their legs above the level of their heart until the swelling resolves.

- Graded compression stockings may be used to prevent venous insufficiency and PTS.

## PATIENT EDUCATION

- The risk associated with calf DVT is low compared to proximal DVT.

- Patients should be reassured and understand that anticoagulation is likely to be limited.

- Patients need to understand the risks of anticoagulation and symptoms associated with hemorrhagic events.

- They should be cautioned to ensure reporting of this event to other physicians and when in situations that may heighten the risk of VTE.

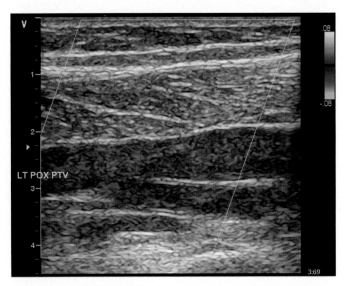

**FIGURE 52-4** Mildly echolucent acute thrombus is ultrasonographically illustrated in this dilated proximal posterior tibial vein. (*Photograph courtesy of Dr. Steven M. Dean.*)

## FOLLOW-UP

- Patients should be re-evaluated in the office toward the end of anticoagulation therapy to ensure a reduction in symptoms.
- Return to employment for most occupations may occur within a week, particularly with resolution of symptoms.
- Repeat ultrasonography is not required.

## PATIENT AND PROVIDER RESOURCES

- http://www.vdf.org
- http://circ.ahajournals.org/content/106/12/1436.full
- http://www.heart.org
- http://www.surgeongeneral.gov/topics/deepvein/

## REFERENCES

1. Righini M, Le Gal G, Aujesky D, et al. Complete venous ultrasound in outpatients with suspected pulmonary embolism. *J Thromb Haemost*. 2009;7(3):406-412.

2. Cushman M, Tsai AW, White RH, et al. Deep vein thrombosis and pulmonary embolism in two cohorts: the longitudinal investigation of thromboembolism etiology. *Am J Med*. 2004; 117(1):19-25.

3. Wells PS, Anderson DR, Ginsberg J. Assessment of deep vein thrombosis or pulmonary embolism by the combined use of clinical model and noninvasive diagnostic tests. *Semin Thromb Hemost*. 2000;26(6):643-656.

4. Wells PS, Owen C, Doucette S, Fergusson D, Tran H. Does this patient have deep vein thrombosis? *JAMA*. 2006;295(2):199-207.

5. Mattos MA, Londrey GL, Leutz DW, et al. Color-flow duplex scanning for the surveillance and diagnosis of acute deep venous thrombosis. *J Vasc Surg*. 1992;15(2):366-375; discussion 375-376.

6. Gottlieb RH, Widjaja J, Tian L, Rubens DJ, Voci SL. Calf sonography for detecting deep venous thrombosis in symptomatic patients: experience and review of the literature. *J Clin Ultrasound*. 1999;27(8):415-420.

7. Cantwell CP, Cradock A, Bruzzi J, Fitzpatrick P, Eustace S, Murray JG. MR venography with true fast imaging with steady-state precession for suspected lower-limb deep vein thrombosis. *J Vasc Interv Radiol*. 2006;17(11 pt 1):1763-1769.

8. Lagerstedt CI, Olsson CG, Fagher BO, Oqvist BW, Albrechtsson U. Need for long-term anticoagulant treatment in symptomatic calf-vein thrombosis. *Lancet*. 1985;2(8454):515-518.

9. Kearon C, Kahn SR, Agnelli G, et al. Antithrombotic therapy for venous thromboembolic disease: American College of Chest Physicians Evidence-Based Clinical Practice Guidelines (8th Edition). *Chest*. 2008;133(suppl 6):S454-S545.

10. Lee AY, Levine MN, Baker RI, et al. Low-molecular-weight heparin versus a coumarin for the prevention of recurrent venous thromboembolism in patients with cancer. *N Engl J Med*. 2003;349(2):146-153.

# 53 MEDICAL MANAGEMENT OF FEMOROPOPLITEAL DEEP VENOUS THROMBOSIS

Marcelo P. Villa-Forte Gomes, MD, FSVM

## PATIENT STORY

A 44-year-old Caucasian woman presented to the emergency department with a 2-week-history of right-leg pain and edema involving the lower thigh to the ankle. One week prior to her emergency room visit, she developed increasing fatigue associated with pleuritic chest pain, exertional dyspnea, and palpitations. Her leg symptoms began within 2 weeks after she was discharged from the hospital after undergoing a 4-day stay for surgery for breast cancer. Her medical history is significant for vasculitis (granulomatosis with polyangiitis/Wegener granulomatosis) and mild iron deficiency anemia. She stopped taking a birth control pill a few weeks prior to surgery. Physical examination demonstrates blood pressure of 138/68 mm Hg, heart rate of 102 bpm, body mass index of 34, regular heart rate and rhythm, and lungs clear to auscultation. The right lower extremity has soft pitting edema with negative Homan sign. There is no cyanosis in the extremities, and distal lower extremity pulses are intact and symmetrical. Acute deep venous thrombosis (DVT) is suspected. The quantitative D-dimer level is 1200 mg/dL, and a venous duplex ultrasound reveals acute DVT involving the common femoral (Figure 53-1), femoral, and popliteal veins.

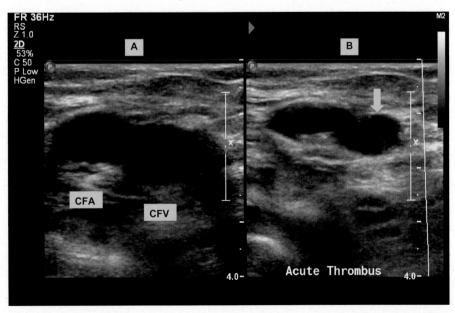

**FIGURE 53-1** Transverse view of gray-scale ultrasound imaging of the right upper thigh, depicting the common femoral artery (CFA) and common femoral vein (CFV). Panel A shows the ultrasound image of the vascular structures without compression. Panel B shows a noncompressible CFV (arrow) due to acute thrombus when pressure is applied to the skin directly above the vein by the operator.

## EPIDEMIOLOGY

- Venous thromboembolic disease, including acute DVT and acute pulmonary embolism (PE), is the third most common cardiovascular disease in the United States.

- Approximately two-thirds of all venous thromboembolic events (VTE) are related to hospitalization.

- It is estimated that over a million cases of VTE are diagnosed each year in the United States alone.

- The absolute risk of DVT or PE in the population (all ages) is estimated at 1% to 3% per year.

- The incidence of DVT or PE increases with age. The estimated age-associated incidence of VTE increases approximately from 1 case per 100,000 person-years (1/100,000) in teenagers (estimated absolute risk of 0.001% per year) to 1/100 person-years over the age of 75 (estimated absolute risk of 1% per year).[1]

## ETIOLOGY AND RISK FACTORS

- Acute DVT or PE is a multifactorial disease. The greater the number of risk factors present, the more likely a patient is to develop acute DVT.

- In addition to increasing risk with age, risk factors for DVT or PE can be classified as situational, acquired, or inherited (Table 53-1).[1-3]

- Situational risk factors can be defined as transient clinical circumstances that increase the risk of VTE while they are present and for a short period (from a few weeks to a few months) after they have resolved.

- Acquired risk factors consist of medical conditions that interfere with normal hemostasis or plasma viscosity. Due to their relapsing or remitting clinical course, these conditions tend to increase the risk of VTE periodically. For example, a patient with a

**TABLE 53-1** Risk Factors for Venous Thromboembolic Disease

| Situational | Acquired | Inherited |
|---|---|---|
| • Surgery | • Cancer | • Factor V Leiden |
| • Prolonged immobility (including long-haul flights) | • Antiphospholipid antibodies | • Prothrombin gene G20210A mutation |
| • Bony fractures or leg casts | • Hyperhomocysteinemia | • Antithrombin deficiency |
| • Pregnancy | • Vasculitis | • Protein C deficiency |
| • Oral contraceptives | • Systemic lupus erythematosus | • Protein S deficiency |
| • Hormone replacement therapy | • Inflammatory bowel disease | • Factor VIII excess |
| • Adjuvant hormonal therapy for breast cancer | • Nephrotic syndrome | • Factor IX excess |
| • Chemotherapy | • Myeloproliferative disorders | • Factor XI excess |
| • Obesity | • Monoclonal gammopathies | • Other point mutations in the genes that encode for factor V and prothrombin genes |
| • Central venous catheters | • Hyperviscosity syndromes | |
| • Heparin-induced thrombocytopenia (HIT) | • Paroxysmal nocturnal hemoglobinuria | |
| | • Factor VIII excess | |

vasculitis (such as granulomatosis with polyangiitis) has a significantly increased risk of VTE during a flare of disease activity, but the risk is reduced when the disease is in remission.

- Inherited risk factors represent congenital thrombophilias, that is, genetic mutations and polymorphisms that increase the risk of thrombosis by causing specific changes in the delicate balance of normal hemostasis that ultimately result in greater thrombin generation and clinical thrombosis.

## PATHOPHYSIOLOGY

- Rudolph Virchow was a 24-year-old pathologist when he postulated that thrombus formation was influenced by the presence of three conditions (triad): venous stasis, vascular injury, and changes in the blood itself (ie, hypercoagulability of blood). Those conditions, alone or in combination, were invariably present in patients who had DVT diagnosed during autopsy.

- Modern understanding of the multifactorial pathophysiology of DVT suggests that, in any given individual, one or several clinical risk factors may cause one or more of the conditions postulated in Virchow triad, hence leading to abnormal thrombus formation. For example, a patient with cancer may have venous stasis (from direct tumor invasion of a vein or by extrinsic venous compression resulting in venous obstruction), vascular injury (by direct invasion of a vein by tumor itself or metastasis), and hypercoagulability due to cancer cell–mediated synthesis of prothrombotic proteins or by increasing plasma tissue factor levels.

- Most acute DVT results from thrombus formation that begins in venous valves and/or in calf veins, followed by cranial propagation.[4]

- Acute DVT is defined as proximal if it involves the veins at or above the knee level, that is, popliteal, femoral, common femoral, and/or iliac veins. Acute DVT is defined as distal if it involves the calf veins (peroneal, posterior tibial, soleal, gastrocnemius—Figure 53-3).

- Approximately 40% to 50% of patients with symptomatic, proximal lower extremity acute DVT without any chest symptoms have evidence of (asymptomatic) PE by pulmonary angiography or ventilation-perfusion scintilography (V/Q scan).[5]

- Of all patients with symptomatic acute PE, between 40% and 70% will have a concomitant acute DVT (that may be symptomatic or not) by venous duplex ultrasound of the lower extremities. Two-thirds of these DVTs will be proximal DVTs, while one-third will be isolated calf DVTs.[6]

## DIAGNOSIS

- Clinical diagnosis of acute DVT is insensitive and nonspecific.[5]

- The severity of signs and symptoms does not necessarily correlate with the extension or location of the acute DVT.

- The Homan sign was originally described as calf discomfort elicited by passive dorsiflexion of the ankle of a limb with suspected DVT. It has poor sensitivity (<50%) and unreliable specificity (40%-90%) for the diagnosis of acute DVT.[7]

- A concomitant, underlying acute DVT is present in as many as 30% of patients with a clinical diagnosis of acute superficial thrombophlebitis in the lower extremities.

- Because clinical diagnosis of DVT is unreliable, objective confirmation by imaging tests is imperative.[5]

- Venous duplex ultrasonography is the method of choice for objective diagnosis of an acute femoropopliteal DVT, with sensitivity and specificity greater than 95% to 99%. Duplex implies the use of both gray-scale imaging ultrasound combined with analysis of blood flow by Doppler. The single most accurate and reliable sonographic criterion to diagnose acute DVT is lack of vein compressibility (Figure 53-1, panel B). If a vein is free of thrombus, it will become completely compressible when external pressure is applied directly over the vein (Figure 53-2, panel B). This sonographic maneuver is performed and observed by interrogation of lower extremity veins using gray-scale ultrasound in transverse view (Figure 53-3).

- Other imaging methods that can objectively diagnose an acute DVT include computed tomography (CT) with venous-phase contrast, magnetic resonance (MR) venography, and contrast venography.

- A normal plasma D-dimer result has a high negative predictive value (approaching 100%) and a very low negative likelihood ratio (approaching zero), thus being a powerful and simple laboratory tool to exclude the diagnosis of acute DVT in patients with a low pretest clinical probability. However, an elevated (positive) D-dimer level has a low positive predictive value and cannot be used to diagnose acute DVT.[8]

- Although the clinical diagnosis of acute DVT is not reliable, validated clinical scores can and should be used when evaluating a patient with suspected DVT. These clinical scores usually classify patients into low, moderate, or high pretest clinical probability of DVT.[9] In patients with a low pretest clinical probability of DVT, a normal quantitative D-dimer essentially rules out acute DVT without the need for imaging studies. However, in patients with a moderate or high pretest clinical probability, an imaging diagnostic test such as duplex ultrasonography should always be used for objective confirmation or exclusion of acute DVT, regardless of D-dimer level.

## NATURAL HISTORY

### Short-Term Complications

- Acute PE

- Early DVT recurrence—Estimates derived from clinical studies suggest that in patients who cannot be treated with anticoagulation therapy during the first 3 months following a diagnosis of acute proximal DVT, the incidence of recurrent thrombosis may approach 50% on the first month and 15% per month for each of the subsequent 2 months.[10]

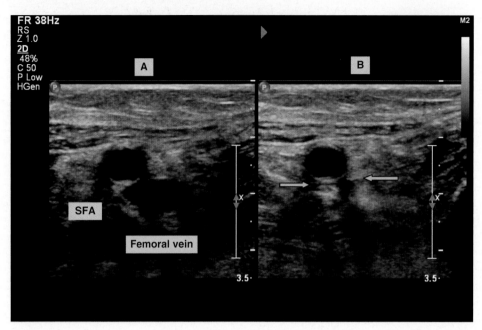

**FIGURE 53-2** Transverse view of gray-scale ultrasound imaging of the right mid-thigh, depicting the superficial femoral artery (SFA) and femoral vein. Panel A shows the ultrasound image of the vascular structures without compression. Panel B shows a fully compressible femoral vein when pressure is applied to the skin directly above the vein by the operator (arrows).

- Phlegmasia cerulea dolens—It is reported to occur in less than 1% of all patients with proximal DVT, and typically in patients with iliofemoral thrombosis. The pathophysiology consists of severe venous hypertension leading to secondary arterial ischemia at tissue level, sometimes resulting in venous limb gangrene (Figure 53-4).

## Long-Term Complications

- Long-term VTE recurrence
- Post-thrombotic syndrome (PTS)
- Chronic thromboembolic pulmonary hypertension (CTEPH)
- Increased risk of cardiovascular events

### Long-Term VTE Recurrence

- The risk of recurrent VTE varies depending on the nature of the original DVT event.
- The risk of VTE recurrence is as low as 2% to 3% during the first year following cessation of warfarin for provoked (situational) DVT, and as high as 12% to 15% during the first year following cessation of warfarin for an unprovoked (idiopathic) DVT.[10]
- The cumulative risk of VTE recurrence can be as high as 30% to 45% within 5 years of warfarin cessation.[11]

### Post-thrombotic Syndrome

- Consists of chronic, intermittent leg pain and edema in patients with a previous or recent history of DVT.
- The risk of PTS appears to be influenced by two intrinsically related factors: early patency of the deep veins and venous valvular dysfunction.

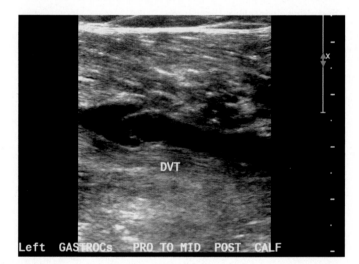

**FIGURE 53-3** Longitudinal view of gray-scale ultrasound imaging of acute occlusive calf DVT within a gastrocnemius vein. The vein is diffusely dilated and incompressible. (*Photograph courtesy of Steven M. Dean, DO.*)

- PTS occurs in 20% to 79% of patients following acute lower extremity DVT, with most cases developing within the first 2 years after the DVT.[4,12]

- Some patients may develop PTS symptoms as long as 5 years after the original DVT event.

- The risk of PTS is higher with more extensive, proximal DVT.

- The incidence of PTS is increased sixfold after ipsilateral recurrent DVT.

- Treatment of PTS consists of prescription of graded, elastic compression stockings.

- Three prospective trials of knee-high compression stockings (of 20-30 mm Hg or 30-40 mm Hg strength) demonstrated an approximately 50% to 70% risk reduction in the development of PTS, and a similar reduction in the severity of PTS symptoms, with those wearing elastic stockings being more likely to develop milder forms of PTS as opposed to those not wearing any compression.[12]

### Chronic Thromboembolic Pulmonary Hypertension

- The cumulative incidence of CTEPH is in the range of 2% to 3.8% within 2 years after a first event of acute pulmonary embolism.[4,13]

- Patients develop progressively worse symptoms that resemble congestive heart failure.

- Pulmonary angiography is considered the diagnostic method of choice for diagnosing CTEPH. CT angiography in multidetector row CT scanners has also been reported as accurate for diagnosing CTEPH.

- Treatment consists of surgical pulmonary thromboendarterectomy under cardiopulmonary bypass (CPB).

### Increased Risk of Cardiovascular Events

- There is mounting evidence that patients with DVT, especially unprovoked (idiopathic) VTE, have an increased long-term risk of cardiovascular events.

- One population-based longitudinal cohort study in over 6000 individuals aged 20 to 64 years showed that the cumulative, 10-year incidence of acute myocardial infarction and cardiovascular mortality was significantly higher in individuals who had a diagnosis of VTE compared to same-age individuals without a history of VTE in the previous 10 years.[14]

## MANAGEMENT

- Goals of DVT therapy consist of (a) reduction in the risk of short- and long-term recurrence, (b) prevention of DVT extension, (c) prevention of acute PE, (d) restoration of venous patency and preservation of venous valvular function, as well as (e) prevention of the PTS.

- Management of DVT can be divided into short-term and long-term management.

### Short-Term Management

- Once the diagnosis of an acute femoropopliteal DVT is confirmed (and even if there is a high index of clinical suspicion), anticoagulation therapy should be started immediately. Current best available

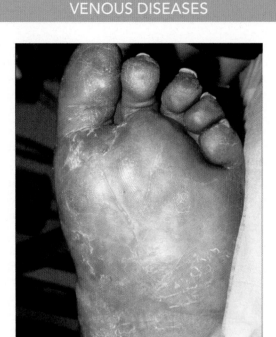

**FIGURE 53-4** Venous limb gangrene is a rare and devastating consequence of acute deep venous thrombosis (DVT) complicated by phlegmasia cerulea dolens. Like many with phlegmasia, this patient had metastatic cancer. (*Photograph courtesy of Steven M. Dean, DO.*)

evidence supports the following anticoagulation strategies as Level 1A options for acute-phase DVT therapy: intravenous (IV) unfractionated heparin (UFH), subcutaneous (SC) low-molecular-weight heparin (LMWH), SC UFH (by fixed or weight-based dosing), or SC fondaparinux (Table 53-2).[15-17]

- Oral anticoagulation with warfarin should *not* be employed without a concomitant parenteral anticoagulant with an acute thromboembolic event.

- Patients should have a baseline activated partial thromboplastin time (aPTT), prothrombin time (PT), platelet count, hemoglobin or hematocrit, and serum creatinine obtained prior to initiation of parenteral anticoagulation.

- If IV UFH is used, it should be administered by a weight-based nomogram (80 U per kg IV bolus followed by 18 U per kg per hour infusion) with the goal of achieving a therapeutic target of aPTT within less than 24 hours of initiation of therapy. The therapeutic target range for the aPTT during IV UFH therapy should be the aPTT range (in seconds) that corresponds to a plasma anti-Xa activity of 0.3 to 0.7 U for UFH, and may vary among different hospitals. Because different aPTT assays use different sources of partial thromboplastin in vitro, assays may have different sensitivities to the effects of similar plasma concentrations of UFH. Thus, in one hospital the therapeutic range of aPTT for IV UFH therapy may be 60 to 90 seconds, whereas this range may be 80 to 120 seconds in another hospital.

- If the patient's calculated creatinine clearance is greater than 30 mL/min, the use of therapeutic-intensity (weight-based) SC LMWH for acute DVT treatment can be considered. Indeed, this is the preferred form of initial DVT therapy in many countries. One of the practical advantages of SC LMWH over IV UFH is the fact that LMWH can be used both in the inpatient and outpatient settings.

- Meta-analyses have demonstrated that the use of SC LMWH for the initial treatment of acute femoropopliteal DVT has similar efficacy and safety compared to IV UFH.

- Oral anticoagulation with warfarin should be initiated in parallel to parenteral anticoagulation with a heparin-like agent. Overlap between UFH (or LMWH) and warfarin should be continued for at least 5 days and until the target international normalized ratio (INR) is achieved. The target INR for acute VTE therapy is 2.5 (accepted range is between 2 and 3).

- Although there is no formal consensus, it is prudent to obtain a platelet count at least once or twice during heparin exposure.

- Placement of inferior vena cava (IVC) filters should not be considered in the initial management of acute femoropopliteal DVT. Current guidelines recommend against the use of IVC filters in the absence of a strong indication.

- The two absolute indications for IVC filter placement are (1) presence of a concomitant, absolute contraindication for anticoagulation therapy (eg, ongoing major bleeding at the time of DVT diagnosis), and (2) development of an absolute contraindication to anticoagulation (ie, major hemorrhage) during administration of anticoagulation therapy.

**TABLE 53-2** Evidence-Based Options for Initial Anticoagulation Therapy in Patients With Acute Femoropopliteal DVT

Intravenous unfractionated heparin (UFH)

Subcutaneous UFH (fixed- or weight-based dosing)

Subcutaneous low-molecular-weight heparins (LMWHs)

Subcutaneous fondaparinux

- Systemic thrombolytic therapy via peripheral intravenous infusion should not be used for DVT therapy because of increased risk of major bleeding without any significant improvement in any of the goals of DVT therapy. Moreover, superior and safer venous recanalization is achieved by catheter-based thrombolytic therapy.

- Phlegmasia cerulea dolens represents the only absolute indication for invasive, endovascular treatment of a proximal lower extremity DVT.

- The term *pharmacomechanical* therapy is a contemporary definition for endovascular DVT therapy that implies the use of catheter systems that can perform mechanical thrombectomy combined with the use of catheter-directed infusion of fibrinolytic agents.

- At present, there is insufficient data to recommend routine pharmacomechanical therapy for an acute femoropopliteal DVT. A prospective, randomized, NIH-sponsored trial of endovascular therapy versus anticoagulation therapy alone for the treatment of acute femoropopliteal DVT is ongoing.

- Once anticoagulation therapy is initiated, patients can be allowed to ambulate as tolerated. There is no need for absolute bed rest. If patients are in the postoperative setting of orthopedic surgery, they should be allowed to undergo physical therapy within 24 hours of initiation of anticoagulation therapy.

- All patients diagnosed with an acute lower extremity DVT should be fitted for knee-high graded elastic compression stockings (20-30 mm Hg or 30-40 mm Hg strength) as soon as possible.

- Studies indicate that early ambulation and use of graded elastic compression stockings do not increase the risk of acute PE in patients who are adequately anticoagulated.

- Prior to hospital discharge (or prior to releasing the patient from clinic, in those being treated exclusively as outpatients), patients should be thoroughly educated with regard to the rationale for warfarin monitoring, as well as diet-drug and drug-drug interactions pertinent to warfarin.

## Long-Term Management

- Options for long-term anticoagulation therapy in patients with femoropopliteal DVT include oral warfarin, SC LMWH, and SC UFH.

- Warfarin is the most commonly used and the preferred method for anticoagulation in the majority of patients with lower extremity acute DVT.[18]

- Optimal duration of anticoagulation therapy for patients with provoked (ie, postoperative) DVT is 3 months.

- Patients with unprovoked (idiopathic) DVT should be treated for a minimum of 3 to 6 months, and perhaps indefinitely.

- Current guidelines from the American College of Chest Physicians (ACCP) recommend that indefinite anticoagulation should be considered in patients with unprovoked DVT who do not have an underlying increased risk of major bleeding.

- The use of SC LMWH monotherapy should be strongly considered in patients who develop acute DVT in the setting of active malignancy because long-term SC LMWH therapy is associated with a significant reduction (as high as 45%) in the risk of recurrent VTE compared to warfarin in that special patient population.

- Because warfarin is associated with significant risk of fetal malformations in the first trimester of pregnancy, as well as increased risk of bleeding late in the third trimester (due to peripartum hemorrhage), the use of SC LMWH is typically preferred and highly recommended for pregnant women who develop an acute DVT.

- The use of long-term SC UFH has fallen out of favor because of inferior pharmacokinetics and pharmacodynamics compared to SC LMWH, and also because long-term SC UFH is associated with significant risk of osteoporosis (which has not been observed in patients using SC LMWH).

## COMPLICATIONS OF ANTICOAGULATION THERAPY

### Hemorrhage

- Major hemorrhage occurs in approximately 5% of patients treated with heparin(s). The rates of major hemorrhage associated with warfarin use increase with age, but are estimated at 2% to 3% per year in patients with long-term warfarin use.

### Heparin-Induced Thrombocytopenia

- Occurs in 1% to 5% of patients exposed to UFH, and in 0.1% to 1% of those exposed to LMWH.[19]

- This complication should be suspected when the platelet count falls (a) greater than 50% from baseline and (b) greater than 30% from baseline with new thrombotic event despite ongoing UFH or LMWH therapy.

- Typical-onset heparin-induced thrombocytopenia (HIT) is defined as thrombocytopenia that occurs between days 4 and 14 of heparin exposure.

- Rapid-onset HIT is defined as thrombocytopenia that occurs within 24 hours of heparin exposure in patients with recent heparin exposure (usually within the previous 3 months).

- Principles of management of HIT include immediate cessation of any and all forms of UFH or LMWH exposure, as well as initiation of anticoagulation therapy with an intravenous direct thrombin inhibitor such as argatroban, lepirudin, or bivalirudin.

### Elevation of Transaminases

- Reported in as many as 4% of patients receiving either UFH or LMWH. It is usually mild and transient.

## FOLLOW-UP

- Patients with femoropopliteal DVT should ideally be followed at 30 days, 3 months, and 6 months after a diagnosis of DVT, and yearly thereafter.

- Follow-up visits provide opportunities to (a) monitor the development of PTS and/or CTEPH, (b) fit patients properly for graded elastic compression stockings, (c) reassess bleeding risk as well as the risks and benefits of ongoing anticoagulation therapy, and (d) continuously educate patients regarding warfarin drug-drug and drug-dietary interactions.

- The 3-month and 6-month visits represent a key opportunity to make a formal decision regarding the appropriateness of discontinuation of anticoagulation therapy.

## PATIENT EDUCATION

- The critical importance of compliance with regular appointments to monitor anticoagulation must be emphasized.
- Patients need to be aware of the signs and symptoms of recurrent venous thromboembolic disease and to immediately seek medical attention if they develop.

### PROVIDER RESOURCES

- http://emedicine.medscape.com/article/1911303-overview
- http://www.uptodate.com/contents/deep-vein-thrombosis-dvt-beyond-the-basics

### PATIENT RESOURCES

- http://www.nursingcenter.com/lnc/journalarticle?Article_ID=1197498
- http://www.emedicinehealth.com/blood_clot_in_the_legs/article_em.htm

## REFERENCES

1. White RH. The epidemiology of venous thromboembolism. *Circulation.* 2003;107:I-4-I-8.
2. Weinmann EE, Salzman EW. Deep-vein thrombosis. *New Engl J Med.* 1994;331:1630-1641.
3. Deitcher SR, Gomes MPV. Hypercoagulable state testing and malignancy screening following venous thromboembolic events. *Vasc Med.* 2003;8:33-46.
4. Kearon C. Natural history of venous thromboembolism. *Circulation.* 2003;107:I-22-I-30.
5. Hull RD, Raskob GE, LeClerc JR, et al. The diagnosis of clinically suspected venous thrombosis. *Clin Chest Med.* 1984;5:439-456.
6. Moser KM, Fedullo PF, LitleJohn JK, et al. Frequent asymptomatic pulmonary embolism in patients with deep venous thrombosis. *JAMA.* 1994;271:223-225.
7. McGee S. *Evidence-Based Physical Diagnosis.* 3rd ed. New York, NY: Saunders; 2012.
8. Bates SM, Kearon K, Crowther M, et al. A diagnostic strategy involving a quantitative latex D-dimer assay reliably excludes deep vein thrombosis. *Ann Intern Med.* 2003;138:787-794.
9. Wells PS, Anderson DR, Rodger M, et al. Evaluation of D-dimer in the diagnosis of suspected deep-vein thrombosis. *New Engl J Med.* 2003;349:1227-1235.
10. Kearon C, Hirsch J. Management of anticoagulation before and after elective surgery. *New Engl J Med.* 1997;336:1506-1511.
11. Heit JA, Mohr DN, Silverstein MD, et al. Predictors of recurrence after deep vein thrombosis and pulmonary embolism. *Arch Intern Med.* 2000;160:761-768.
12. Bernardi E, Bagatella P, Frulla M, et al. Postthrombotic syndrome: incidence, prevention, and management. *Semin Vasc Medicine.* 2001;1:71-79.
13. Pengo V, Lansing AWA, Prins MH, et al. Incidence of chronic thromboembolic pulmonary hypertension after pulmonary embolism. *New Engl J Med.* 2004;350:2257-2264.
14. Spencer FA, Ginsberg JS, Chong A, et al. The relationship between unprovoked venous thromboembolism, age, and acute myocardial infarction. *J Thromb Haemost.* 2008;6:1507-1513.
15. Holbrook A, Schulman S, Witt DM, et al. Antithrombotic therapy and prevention of thrombosis. American College of Chest Physicians Evidence-Based Clinical Practice Guidelines. *Chest.* 2012;141: S152-S184.
16. Kearon C, Akl EA, Comerota AJ, et al. Antithrombotic therapy for VTE disease. American College of Chest Physicians Evidence-Based Clinical Practice Guidelines. *Chest.* 2012;141:S419-S494.
17. Garcia DA, Baglin TP, Weitz JI, et al. Parenteral anticoagulants. American College of Chest Physicians Evidence-Based Clinical Practice Guidelines. *Chest.* 2012;141:S24-S43.
18. Ageno W, Gallus AS, Wittkowsky A, et al. Oral anticoagulant therapy. American College of Chest Physicians Evidence-Based Clinical Practice Guidelines. *Chest.* 2012;141:S44-S88.
19. Arepally GM, Orthel TL. Clinical practice. Heparin-induced thrombocytopenia. *New Engl J Med.* 2006;355:809-817.

# 54 PERCUTANEOUS ENDOVENOUS INTERVENTION IN FEMOROPOPLITEAL DEEP VENOUS THROMBOSIS

Mohsen Sharifi, MD, FACC, FSCAI, FSVM

## PATIENT STORY

A 36-year-old previously healthy man presents with a swollen and painful right calf 1 week after returning from a trip to Europe. On examination, the affected calf is tender, slightly warm, and swollen. A venous duplex ultrasound documents acute occlusive deep venous thrombosis (DVT) involving the posterior tibial, popliteal, and femoral veins. The common femoral vein is patent. The patient has no history of bleeding problems. In order to reduce the lifelong risk of the post-thrombotic syndrome (PTS), percutaneous endovenous intervention is undertaken.

## RATIONALE FOR THROMBOREDUCTIVE STRATEGIES

- The pathophysiology of sequelae of DVT excluding those related to embolization is due to venous obstruction and reflux.

- Persistence of thrombus has been shown to be associated with valvular damage and resultant reflux.[1]

- Thrombus acts as a nidus for further propagation.[2]

- Anticoagulation alone does not dissolve the formed thrombus but merely reduces new thrombus formation and the risk of embolization.

- The body's fibrinolytic system has to dissolve the formed thrombus, a process that may take weeks to months, hence the ineffectiveness of anticoagulation alone to prevent permanent valvular damage.

- In a recent randomized trial of acute iliofemoral DVT patients who were treated with regional thrombolysis within 3 weeks of symptom onset, reflux continued to develop in 60% of patients at 6 months.[3]

- There is a limited time window to intervene to prevent venous reflux beyond which permanent valvular would occur.

- The combination of venous obstruction and reflux work in synergy to initiate a cascade of acute and chronic inflammatory changes at the microcellular level.

- Ambulatory venous hypertension leads to edema, inflammatory cellular mobilization and activation, hemosiderin deposition, hypoxic injury, fibrosis, lipodermatosclerosis, loss of muscle pump function, venous claudication, and ultimately ulceration.[4,5]

- Rarely phlegmasia cerulea dolens may occur with a high mortality and morbidity.[6]

## FEMOROPOPLITEAL DVT

- The majority of the interventional literature has focused on treatment of iliac DVT with caudal extension to the common femoral vein.

- There is a paucity of data on percutaneous endovenous intervention (PEVI) in the femoropopliteal vein alone.

- Approximately half of the patients who present with "first-time" acute femoropopliteal DVT exhibit venographic evidence of previous and often recurrent DVT without even knowing about it.[7]

- The "20% rule" applies to patients with femoropopliteal DVT: 20% have a known history of previous DVT, 20% have concomitant symptomatic PE on admission, 20% have asymptomatic DVT on the contralateral side (if unprovoked), and 20% have DVT in the iliac veins.[7]

- The currently available thromboreductive modalities are applicable in both femoropopliteal and iliofemoral DVT.

- The efficacy and success of treatment depends on several factors: (1) extent of thrombus, (2) chronicity of thrombus, (3) presence of venous stenosis or sclerosis, and (4) preservation of venous anatomy.

- There is a spectrum in the venographic appearance of DVT with important clinical implications. On one side of the spectrum is the first-time DVT with preserved venous anatomy, which is quite responsive to regional thrombolysis and thrombectomy (Figure 54-1). On the other side of the spectrum is distorted venous anatomy with venosclerosis and stenosis and minimal thrombus burden, which is highly resistant to thrombolysis. Here a "venous conduit" needs to be reconstructed, often times with the use of stents. Balloon venoplasty alone is less effective due to the high elastic recoil and perivenous fibrosis. Frequently, in-between forms exist, that is, acute on chronic DVT (Figure 54-2).

## DEVICE SELECTION

- A number of devices are currently available that may be used in the femoropopliteal vein. They use a combination of thrombolysis and aspiration. Use of ultrasound has been claimed to accelerate the process of clot dissemination.

- The available devices include (1) Angiojet (Possis Medical, Minneapolis, MN), (2) Trellis (Covidien, Mansfield, Mass), (3) Ekos Endowave (Ekos, Bothell, WA), (4) Helix Clot Buster (ev3, Plymouth, MN), (5) Hydrolyser (Cordis, Warren, NJ), (6) Eliminator (IDev Technologies, Houston, TX), and (7) Arrow Trerotola (Teleflex, Limerick, PA). The first two have been used more frequently (Figure 54-3).

- In general, acute DVT responds favorably to any of the above modalities, whereas chronic DVT and venosclerosis are highly resistant. The color of the aspirate in the suction tubing of the Angiojet device is a predictor of success. Effective clot lysis is expected when the aspirate color is dark as compared to bright red (Figure 54-4).

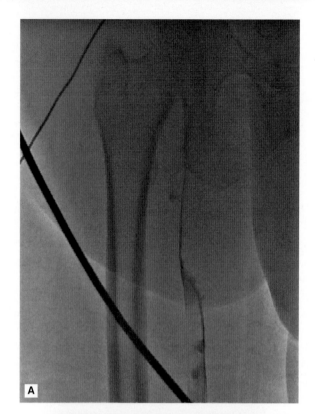

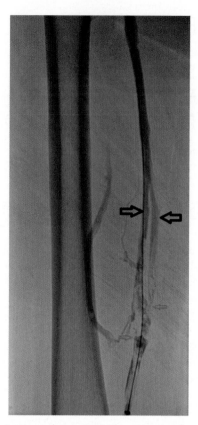

FIGURE 54-2 Acute on chronic DVT. There is a dual femoral venous system at the mid-thigh level with deep venous thrombosis (DVT) in both (black arrows). Note presence of venous stenosis (red arrows) in addition to fresh thrombus.

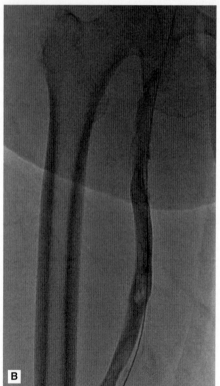

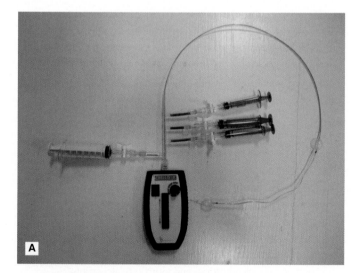

FIGURE 54-1 A. Fresh thrombus in femoropopliteal vein. Note pre-served venous anatomy with no venosclerosis or stenosis. B. Same vessel after two thrombectomy runs with Angiojet device. Substantial resolution of thrombus has occurred.

FIGURE 54-3 A. Trellis device in vitro. (Continued)

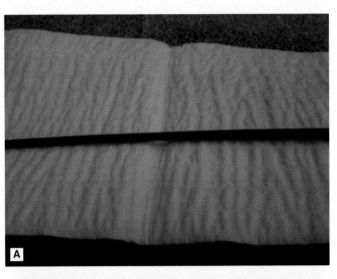

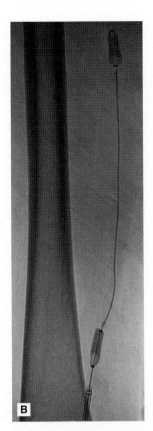

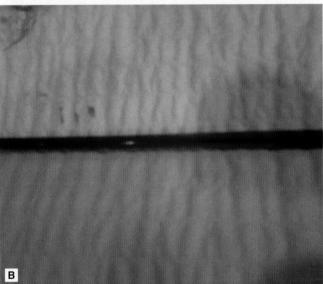

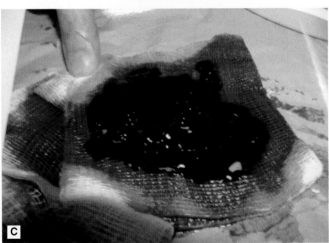

FIGURE 54-4 A. Dark color of the aspirate through the Angiojet device is a predictor of effective thrombus extraction. B. Brightly colored aspirate indicates absence of fresh thrombus and presence of venosclerosis.

FIGURE 54-3 (Continued) B. Trellis device placed in the femoropopliteal vein. (C) Aspirated thrombus after device activation.

## ACCESS SITE

- The desired access site for PEVI for femoropopliteal DVT is the popliteal vein.

- Working in a cephalad direction is far more effective than working caudally. The venous side branches are more numerous and larger than their arterial counterparts, rendering the caudal approach very difficult.

- Entry to the vein should be sonographically visualized. Inadvertent arterial access can thus be easily avoided. The use of a micropuncture needle is preferred.

- Initial venography should be performed through the sheath to delineate the cephalad course of the vein. Segmental venography is then performed by moving a soft-tip 5 F catheter cephalad. The patient should be made ambulatory after 1 hour of bed rest. This is our routine practice and cannot be overemphasized.[7] Early mobility activates the muscle pump and reduces the likelihood of recurrence.

## ANTICOAGULATION AND THROMBOLYTIC THERAPY

- Patients can undergo PEVI while fully anticoagulated. There is no need to withhold anticoagulation as is usually required when intervening in the arterial system.

- Bleeding complications are negligible if proper technical skill and use of an appropriate anticoagulation regimen are applied. Older bleeding complication rates of as high as 11% are simply not acceptable in the contemporary era.[8]

- Major bleeding is exceedingly rare, and minor bleeding can be expected in around 2% of cases.[7]

- It is important to modify the dose of heparin if thrombolysis is given overnight.

- In our practice, tissue plasminogen activator (tPA) is given at 1 mg/h through the infusion catheter and heparin (via the side port of the popliteal sheath) at 8 to 12 U/kg/h followed by initiation of rivaroxaban at 20 mg daily in 2 hours after completion of lysis.

- The maximum weight considered for heparin dose calculation should not exceed 100 kg even in patients exceeding this weight.

- The activated partial thromboplastin time of 1.5 to 2× the baseline level (and always below 100 seconds) should be maintained.

- Aspirin is given at 81 mg daily for 1-6 months in addition to the oral anticoagulant. We have found a favorable response in the reduction of PTS with aspirin which is very similar to the reduction in recurrent venous thromboembolism rate recently reported with this drug.[9]

## BALLOON VENOPLASTY AND STENTING

- Until recently, stenting in the femoropopliteal vein was not reported. The fear of stenting in this segment is not based on concrete data but on hypothetical assumptions and the finding of 4 out of 5 stent closures in an old venous registry.[8]

- We have shown that stenting is safe and effective in the femoropopliteal vein with excellent midterm outcomes comparable to stents placed in the iliac veins.[10]

- Stenting is performed for venous stenosis (Figure 54-5) or when a new venous conduit has to be created due to distortion of normal

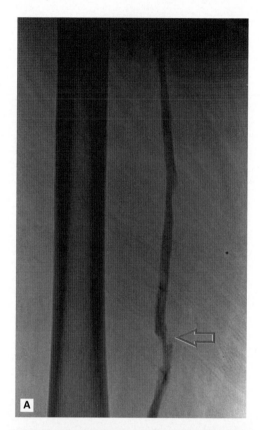

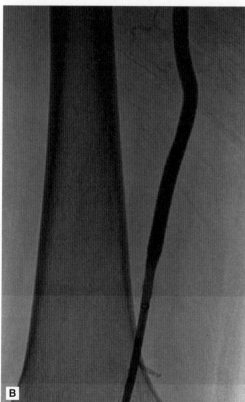

**FIGURE 54-5** A. High-grade stenosis in the popliteal vein after regional thrombolysis and before stenting (red arrow). B. Same region after deployment of a Viabahn 6×100-mm stent.

anatomy in chronically scarred and venosclerotic segments. The use
of multiple stents may become necessary (Figure 54-6). Stenting is
not performed for thrombus alone.

- The usual stent diameter is 6 to 10 mm. For the popliteal vein we
  use Viabahn stents (Gore, Flagstaff, AZ) with the theoretic assumption that such stents may better resist stress forces at the knee level.

- The natural history of stenting in the venous circulation is funda-
  mentally different than that seen in the arterial system, requiring a
  shift in the paradigm of expectations.[10]

- An intriguing observation derived from intravascular ultrasound
  (IVUS) imaging is the lack of neointimal hyperplasia (NIH) as a
  cause of stent closure that is distinctly different from that seen in
  arterial stents in which NIH is the major etiology (Figure 54-7).

- This may be due to the lower venous pressure, oxygen tension, and
  pH; absence of pulsatile flow; and higher compliance of the veins.
  The thinner media and adventitia and presence of a lower number
  of inflammatory cells may be other contributing factors.[7,10]

- Stent thrombosis, however, occurs in 4% of cases at an approxi-
  mate mean follow-up of 14 months. It does not occur independently and is usually an extension of DVT in the adjacent venous segments with high-grade stenosis (in-flow or out-flow obstruction).

- External compression is an important factor in preventing full stent
  expansion, which is seen in extensive venosclerosis and contributes
  to stent closure, usually in the presence of some degree of thrombosis, but not NIH (Figure 54-8).[10]

- Contrary to its arterial counterpart, stent thrombosis is often
  asymptomatic or mildly symptomatic. It is not associated with
  significant sequelae and is amenable to re-do PEVI.[10]

- Postimplant surveillance of stent patency in the femoropopliteal
  vein can be successfully performed with venous duplex imaging,
  even for covered stents (Figure 54-9).

- Balloon venoplasty alone is seldom enough to effectively treat high-
  grade stenosis or a venosclerotic segment (Figure 54-10). This is
  due to the increased elastic recoil and perivenous fibrosis. It should
  be used for postdilatation of stents and to macerate the clot as an
  adjunct to thrombectomy devices (Figure 54-11).

## MANAGEMENT OF PERFORATION OF THE FEMOROPOPLITEAL VEIN

- Occasionally, perforation of the femoropopliteal vein may occur as
  a result of instrumentation (Figure 54-12).

- This complication is exceedingly rare when intervening in acute
  DVT with preserved venous architecture. It predominantly occurs
  in chronic DVT with venosclerosis and calcification.

- Caution should be exerted in the deployment of the proximal
  balloon of the Trellis device in a venosclerotic portion of the
  popliteal vein, as it may lead to perforation (Figure 54-12).

- Almost always the perforation can be managed conservatively
  with manual pressure alone without major sequelae. The affected
  extremity should be elevated and an external blood pressure cuff
  applied over the site and inflated just over the venous pressure for
  10 to 20 minutes.

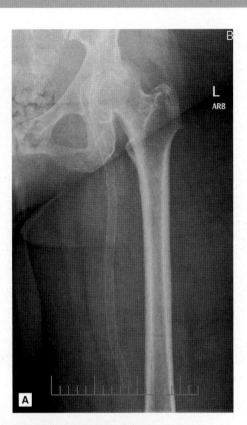

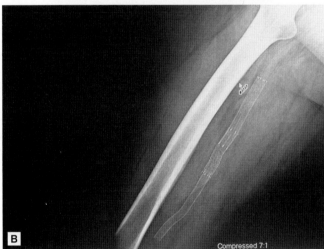

**FIGURE 54-6** A. Reconstruction of a long segment of the femoral vein
with two 8×150-mm Viabahn stents in severe venosclerosis. B. Placement of two Protege and one Viabahn stent in the femoral vein.

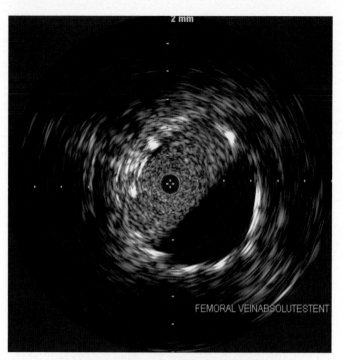

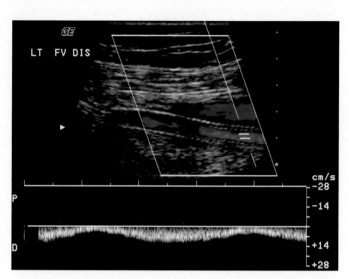

FIGURE 54-9 Venous duplex imaging of a Viabahn stent in the distal femoral vein 3.5 years after implantation. Note stent patency, normal flow, and the expected variation of the spectral Doppler with the respiratory cycle.

FIGURE 54-7 Intravascular ultrasound (IVUS) imaging in an Absolute stent 14 months after implantation in the femoral vein. Note absence of neointimal hyperplasia despite development of moderate amounts of thrombus.

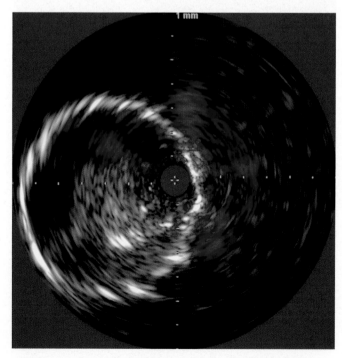

FIGURE 54-8 Intravascular ultrasound (IVUS) imaging with Chromaflo in a Viabahn stent in the popliteal vein 550 days postimplant. Note development of thrombus within the stent plus external compression from 12 to 6 o'clock. Again, no neointimal hyperplasia is noted.

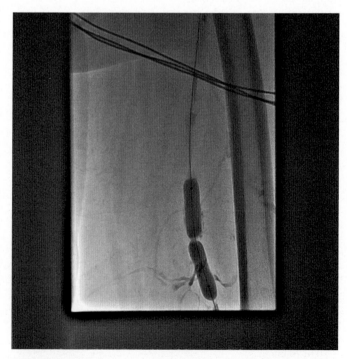

FIGURE 54-10 Balloon venoplasty in the popliteal vein showing significant stenosis.

- Usually there is no need for reversal of anticoagulation. The procedure may continue in the same setting if hemostasis is achieved.
- Endoluminal tamponade of the perforated site with a long balloon is very effective.
- A covered stent may also be used in more severe cases but is usually not required. We have not witnessed the necessity for blood transfusion or surgical intervention for femoropopliteal venous perforation.

## ROLE OF INFERIOR VENA CAVA FILTERS

- The purpose of inferior vena cava (IVC) filter placement is to prevent iatrogenic pulmonary embolism (PE) during PEVI.
- The frequency of PE during PEVI has varied between 0% and 45%.[3,11]
- In the TORPEDO trial, thrombus entrapment by the IVC filter post-PEVI was seen in 11% of the patients.[7]
- In a recent randomized trial of patients with DVT who underwent PEVI, the frequency of symptomatic PE was 11.3% in patients without an IVC filter versus 1.4% in those with an IVC filter.[12]
- There was no mortality benefit from IVC filter placement.
- A 4.2% rate of transient hemodynamic instability occurred during the procedure in patients with predictors of iatrogenic PE who did not receive a filter.
- These predictors were PE on admission, involvement of two or more adjacent venous segments with fresh thrombus, inflammatory form of DVT, and vein diameter 7 mm or greater with preserved architecture. If only catheter-directed thrombolysis is performed without other instrumentation, there would be no need for filter placement.[12]
- A selective approach may thus be exercised in the implantation of IVC filters during PEVI.[12]
- Filter removal beyond 1 month of implant is associated with macroscopic evidence of thrombus in one-third of the patients (Figure 54-13).

## CONCLUSION

DVT in the femoropopliteal vein can be quite symptomatic and associated with chronic complications of pulmonary hypertension, recurrent venous thromboembolism (VTE), and PTS. PEVI is safe and effective in the treatment of DVT in this venous bed. We believe that symptomatic femoropopliteal DVT should receive a higher vigor and intensity of treatment than is currently exercised.

## REFERENCES

1. Guyatt G, Akl E, Crowther M, et al. Antithrombotic therapy and prevention of thrombosis for venous thromboembolic disease: American College of Chest Physicians evidence-based clinical practice guidelines (9th edition). *Chest*. 2012;141(2-Suppl) 2S-801S.
2. Markel A, Manzo RA, Bergelin RO, Strandness DE. Valvular reflux after deep vein thrombosis: incidence and time of occurrence. *J Vasc Surg*. 1992;15:377-384.

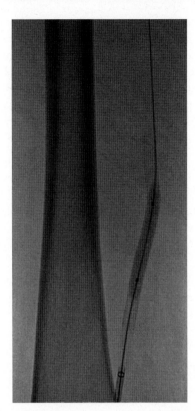

FIGURE 54-11 Postdilatation with an oversized balloon in a Viabahn stent placed in the popliteal vein.

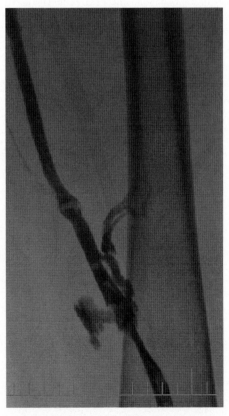

FIGURE 54-12 Perforation of the popliteal vein after use of the Trellis. The site of perforation is where the proximal device was deployed.

3. Enden T, Haig Y, Kløw NE, et al., on behalf of the CaVenT Study Group. Long-term outcome after additional catheter-directed thrombolysis versus standard treatment for acute iliofemoral deep vein thrombosis (the CaVenT study): a randomised controlled trial. *Lancet*. 2012;379:31-38

4. Araki CT, Back TL, Padberg FT, et al. The significance of calf muscle pump function in venous ulceration. *J Vasc Surg*. 1994;20:872-877.

5. Welkie JF, Comerota AJ, Katz ML, Aldridge SC, Kerr RP, White JV. Hemodynamic deterioration in chronic venous disease. *J Vasc Surg*. 1992;16:733-740.

6. Vahedian J, Sadeghipour A. Phlegmasia cerulea dolens of the upper extremity: a fatal complication after coronary artery bypass grafting—case report and review of the literature. *Iran Heart J*. 2008;8:63-68.

7. Sharifi M, Bay C, Mehdipour M, Sharifi J. Thrombus Obliteration by Rapid Percutaneous Endovenous Intervention in Deep Venous Occlusion (TORPEDO) Trial: Midterm Results. *J Endovasc Ther*. 2012;19:273-280.

8. Mewissen MW, Seabrook GR, Meissner MH, et al. Catheter-directed thrombolysis for lower extremity deep venous thrombosis: report of a national multicenter registry. *Radiology*. 1999;211:39-49.

9. Becattini C, Agnelli G, Schenone A, et al. Aspirin for preventing the recurrence of venous thromboembolism. *N Engl J Med*. 2012;366:1959-1967.

10. Sharifi M, Javadpour S, Bay C, Mehdipour M, Emrani F, Sharifi J. Outcome of stenting in the lower extremity venous circulation for the treatment of deep venous thrombosis. *Vasc Dis Mgmt*. 2010;7:E233-E239.

11. Kolbel T, Alhadad A, Acosta S, Lindh M, Ivancev K, Gottsater A. Thrombus embolization into IVC filters during catheter-directed thrombolysis for proximal deep venous thrombosis. *J Endovasc Ther*. 2008;15;605-613.

12. Sharifi M, Bay C, Skrocki L, Lawson D, Mazdeh S. Role of IVC filters in endovenous therapy for deep venous thrombosis: the FILTER-PEVI trial. *Cardiovasc Intervent Radiol*. 2012;35(6): 1408-1413.

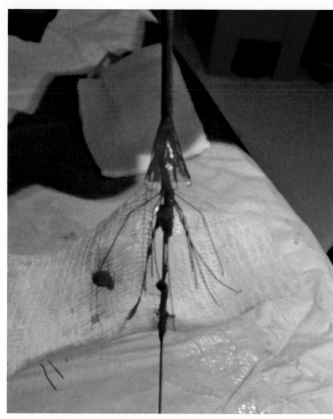

**FIGURE 54-13** An eclipse IVC filter removed 6 months after implantation. Note attached nonocclusive thrombus.

# 55 MAY-THURNER SYNDROME

Jonathan Forquer, DO
Mitchell Silver, DO, FACC, FSVM

## PATIENT HISTORY

A 35-year-old woman presented with a 2-day history of progressive left lower extremity pain and swelling. She had started oral contraceptives 4 months prior, and had flu-like symptoms that required her to stay home for the past week. Physical examination confirmed marked swelling extending from the left ankle to the groin. An erythrocyanotic appearance existed throughout the involved limb. Duplex ultrasonography revealed acute thrombosis within the calf, popliteal, femoral, and common femoral veins. The iliac vein was technically difficult to insonate. Due to suspicion of a coexistent iliac deep venous thrombosis (DVT), a left lower extremity venogram was obtained that confirmed acute thrombosis within the left iliac and common femoral veins (Figure 55-1). This presentation and clinical constellation of signs and symptoms was consistent with May-Thurner syndrome (MTS).

### EPIDEMIOLOGY

- A condition of predominantly left-sided DVT caused by compression of the left common iliac vein by the overlying right common iliac artery and underlying lumbar vertebrae (Figure 55-2).

- More commonly found in women in their second to fourth decades of life.[1-3]

- About 50% of patients with left iliac vein thrombosis have documented left iliac vein compression.[4]

- Hypercoagulable states are found in up to 67% of screened patients who have chronic iliac vein thrombosis.[2]

- Affected patients often have a superimposed thrombotic trigger including recent trauma, pregnancy, oral contraceptives, or protracted immobilization.

- Although the prevalence of MTS-associated DVT is unusually low (2%-3%), this statistic is probably a gross underestimation as the condition is frequently overlooked.

### ANATOMY AND PATHOPHYSIOLOGY

- Iliac vein compression was first described in the 19th century by Virchow.

- May and Thurner documented venous webs or "spurs" in 22% of the left iliac veins of cadavers.[1,4]

- Intimal proliferation and scarring (deposition of elastin and collagen) were attributed to compression of the left iliac vein by the pulsations of the overlying right common iliac artery.[2,4]

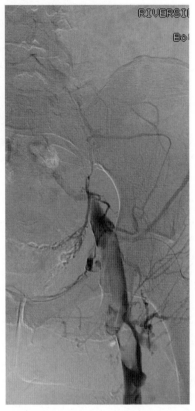

**FIGURE 55-1** Left lower extremity venogram demonstrating extensive left common femoral, external iliac, and common iliac deep venous thrombosis (DVT). Patient is in the supine position.

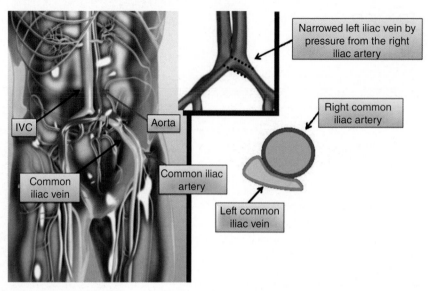

**FIGURE 55-2** Schematic depicting May-Thurner syndrome (MTS). Note the right common iliac artery compressing the left common iliac vein.

- Several other anatomic variants have been observed as the cause of compression thrombosis.[1,2]
  - ○ Left iliac vein compression by the left internal iliac artery
  - ○ Right iliac vein compression by the right internal iliac artery
  - ○ Inferior vena cava (IVC) compression by the right iliac artery

## DIAGNOSIS

### Clinical Features

- Young female patients presenting with unilateral, usually left-sided, lower extremity pain and edema.[1-3] These signs and symptoms involve not only the calf but the thigh as well.

- Left hemi-inguinal and flank pain may occur.

- May have signs of post-thrombotic syndrome (PTS) such as varicose veins, phlebitis, pigment deposition, recurrent skin ulcers, and chronic swelling (Figure 55-3).[1-3]

- Approximately half of MTS patients treated with conventional anticoagulation will ultimately develop lifestyle-limiting venous claudication.

- A prethrombotic stenotic variant exists that is associated with similar manifestations.

### Imaging Studies

- Gold standard remains conventional venography, which can be diagnostic and provide an option for endovascular therapy.[1-3]

- Duplex ultrasound is safe and effective for diagnosis of lower extremity DVT, but is limited in visualization of pelvic veins and cannot assess the degree of compression by the overlying iliac artery.[1,2,4]

- Computed tomography (CT) venography is sensitive and specific for the diagnosis of ileofemoral DVT. CT venography can determine the percentage of iliac vein compression in MTS. CT venography is limited by
  - ○ Kidney function—intravenous (IV) contrast administration[1-3]

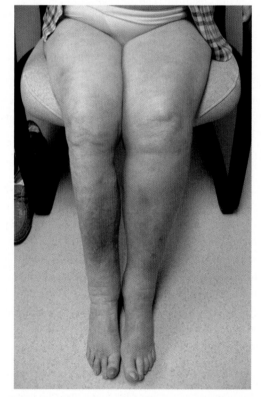

**FIGURE 55-3** A 58-year-old woman with left lower extremity post-thrombotic syndrome (PTS) from an iliofemoral deep venous thrombosis (DVT) treated with conventional anticoagulation 6 months prior. She has chronic pain, swelling, eczema, and venous claudication. The contralateral right leg displays classic post-thrombotic skin changes as well. (*Photograph courtesy of Dr. Steven M. Dean.*)

○ Volume status—overestimates degree of compression in dehydrated patients[2]

○ Technique—timing of scan during venous phase can be challenging[2]

- Magnetic resonance venography (MRV): Direct contrast-enhanced MR venography is over 90% sensitive and specific when compared to conventional venography.[5]

- Intravascular ultrasound (IVUS): IVUS is now considered to be an important adjunctive diagnostic tool that provides invaluable information to manage patients with MTS. Conventional venography may miss functional webs of the common iliac vein or residual mural thrombus. IVUS also provides valuable information when sizing vascular stents for the common iliac vein.

## Differential Diagnosis

- Chronic venous insufficiency (swelling, hyperpigmentation, eczema, varicosities, and ulcerations)

- Baker cyst (rupture, extension, or compression of the popliteal vein)

- Cellulitis

- Trauma

- Lymphedema (carcinoma, lymphoma, sarcoidosis, filariasis, retroperitoneal fibrosis)

- Reflex sympathetic dystrophy

- Tumor or fibrosis obstructing iliac vein

- True or false aneurysms

- Arteriovenous fistula

- Loiasis (Loa loa infection)

## MANAGEMENT

- Two-step approach: reducing clot burden and venous stenting[3,6] (Figure 55-4A-C)

- Reducing clot burden can be accomplished by
  ○ Catheter-directed thrombolysis
  ○ Percutaneous mechanical thrombectomy
  ○ Open surgical thrombectomy[3,6]

- Venous stenting, using flexible, self-expanding stents, after thrombectomy has been shown to be more effective than thrombectomy alone.[3] Patency rates have been reported between 73% and 100% after 1 year.[4,7]

- A minimum 6 months of anticoagulation with Coumadin (warfarin) is typically utilized. Other clinical features such as a hypercoagulable state or a concomitant pulmonary embolus may dictate a longer duration of anticoagulation (1 year or indefinitely).[1-3,7]

- Lower extremity graduated compression stockings play an important role in patients with MTS.

- Using only standard anticoagulation in patients with MTS is associated with an unacceptably high rate of disabling PTS. Thus, affected patients should be offered thrombolytic and endovascular therapy, assuming no contraindications exist.

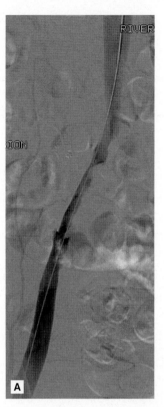

**FIGURE 55-4A** Venogram of the left common iliac vein illustrating thrombus and stricture in a patient with May-Thurner syndrome (MTS). Patient is in prone position.

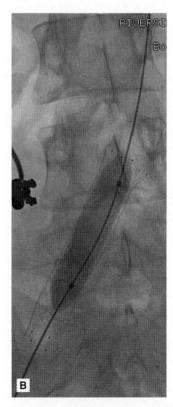

**FIGURE 55-4B** Venogram demonstrating post balloon dilation of self-expanding nitinol stent within the left common iliac vein following successful catheter-directed thrombolysis and thrombectomy. Patient is in prone position.

## PATIENT EDUCATION

- Patients should be educated on the importance of graduated compression stocking compliance.

- Information on anticoagulation risks and management should be provided.

- Strategies for high-risk situations including long-duration travel, need for surgery, and pregnancy should be reviewed in detail.

## FOLLOW-UP

- Follow-up venous duplex ultrasound is done at 6 months and at 1 year to follow stent patency. Annual venous duplex ultrasound is then recommended for 5 years.[3,7]

- Maintenance of a healthy body mass index (BMI) is important.

### PROVIDER RESOURCE

- http://www.angiologist.com/venous-disease/may-thurner-syndrome/

### PATIENT RESOURCES

- http://my.clevelandclinic.org/disorders/vascular
  _abnormalities/vs_may-thurner_syndrome.aspx

- http://patientblog.clotconnect.org/2011/01/10/may-thurner-syndrome/

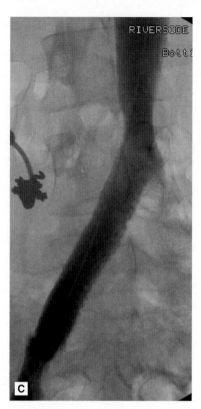

**FIGURE 55-4C** Completion venogram of the left common iliac vein in the patient presenting with May-Thurner syndrome (MTS) following successful catheter-directed thrombolysis, thrombectomy, and venous stenting. Patient is in prone position.

## REFERENCES

1. Fazel R, Froehlich JB, Williams DM, Saint S, Nallamothu BK. A sinister development. *N Engl J Med.* 2007;357:53-59.

2. Al-Nouri O, Milner R. May-Thurner syndrome. Available at: http://vasculardiseasemanagement.com/content/may-thurner-syndrome. Accessed March 2011.

3. Silver M, Ansel G. Venous intervention. In: Topol E, Teirstein P, eds. *Textbook of Interventional Cardiology.* 6th ed. Philadelphia, PA: Elsevier-Saunders; 2012:563-575.

4. Kibbe MR, Ujiki M, Goodwin A, et al. Iliac vein compression in an asymptomatic patient population. *J Vasc Surg.* 2004;937-943.

5. Gurel K, Gurel S, Karavas E, Buharalioglu Y, Daglar B. Direct contrast-enhanced MR venography in the diagnosis of May-Thurner Syndrome. *Euro J Radiology.* 2011;80:533-536.

6. Mickley V, Schwagierek R, Rilinger N, Gorich J, Sunder-Plassmann L. Left iliac venous thrombosis caused by venous spur: treatment with thrombectomy and stent implantation. *J Vasc Surg.* 1998;28:492-497.

7. Moudgill N, Hager E, Gonsalves C, Larson R, Lombardi J, DiMuzio P. May-Thurner syndrome: case report and review of the literature involving modern endovascular therapy. *Vascular.* 2009;17:330-335.

# 56 PAGET-SCHROETTER SYNDROME

Jonathan Forquer, DO
Mitchell Silver, DO, FACC, FSVM

## PATIENT STORY

A previously healthy 22-year-old man presents with a 3-day history of right upper extremity swelling and pain. He is a competitive cross fit athlete and performs vigorous upper body weight lifting several days per week. On examination the right forearm and brachium are diffusely swollen with an overlying erythrocyanotic appearance. A venous duplex ultrasound identifies acute thrombosis within the axillary and subclavian veins. In preparation for catheter-directed thrombolysis, a right upper extremity venogram is performed. Figures 56-1A and B venographically illustrate diffuse intraluminal filling defects consistent with acute brachial and axillosubclavian deep vein thrombosis (DVT).

## EPIDEMIOLOGY

- Primary effort-related thrombosis of the subclavian vein caused by compression within the thoracic outlet (Figure 56-2A).

- Provocative arm positioning includes repetitive hyperabduction and external rotation of the upper extremity or posterior and inferior shoulder rotation.

- Absence of other causes, such as extrinsic mass or indwelling catheter.

- Male-to-female ratio is approximately 2:1.[1]

- Mostly in third and fourth decades of life.[1,2]

- Young, healthy athletes after vigorous upper extremity exercise and in patients who do frequent overhead maneuvers (painters, construction workers, wood choppers, auto repair workers).[1]

- Involves the dominant arm in 80% of cases.

## ANATOMY AND PATHOPHYSIOLOGY

- The subclavian vein passes through the thoracic outlet bounded by the clavicle and subclavius muscle anteriorly, the anterior scalene muscle laterally, the first rib posterior-inferiorly, and the costoclavicular ligament medially (Figure 56-2B).

- Extrinsic compression of the subclavian vein by the first rib and the clavicle.[1-3]

- Hypertrophy of the anterior scalene muscle and/or the subclavius muscle can decrease the size of the outlet and compress the subclavian vein.[1]

- Multifactorial pathophysiology that fulfills the Virchow triad including (1) anatomic changes listed above leading to stasis; (2) hypercoagulability in association with exercise-associated stress; (3) intimal tears within the vein wall in association with repetitive shoulder-arm movement.

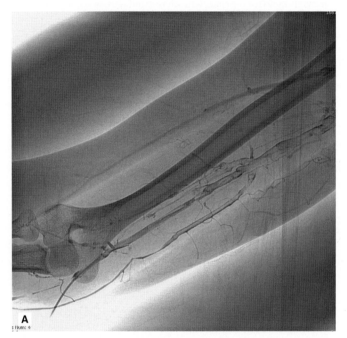

**FIGURE 56-1A** Right upper extremity venogram demonstrating acute right brachial deep venous thrombosis (DVT).

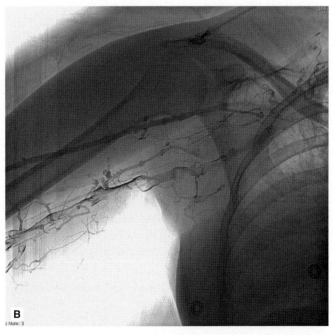

**FIGURE 56-1B** Right upper extremity venogram demonstrating acute right axillosubclavian vein deep venous thrombosis (DVT).

## DIAGNOSIS

### Clinical Features

- Young patient presenting with blue, heavy, swollen, painful arm.[1]
- History of vigorous exercise or activity with the affected extremity, usually within the previous 24 hours.[1,2]
- Dull aching pain within the affected arm and shoulder that is aggravated by activity yet relieved with rest and elevation.
- If symptoms are chronic, superficial collateral veins of the arm, neck, and chest may be present (Figure 56-3).[1]
- If the diagnosis is delayed, patients may rarely present with superior vena cava syndrome and associated plethora of the head or neck, visual changes, and periorbital edema.

### Differential Diagnosis

- Superior vena cava syndrome
- Noneffort-related subclavian vein thrombosis
- Lymphedema, for example, after mastectomy with lymph node dissection
- Obstructing lesions, for example, mediastinal masses, metastatic bone tumors, Pancoast tumor
- Cellulitis or fasciitis
- Muscle or tendon rupture
- Complex regional pain syndrome
- Septic bursitis of elbow

### Imaging Studies

- Duplex ultrasound is considered the best first-line diagnostic test for upper extremity DVT. Positive duplex ultrasound in the right clinical scenario is also so specific that additional imaging is not needed prior to conventional venography.[1] However, thrombi that are small and nonocclusive or proximally located and obscured by the claviculosternal region may be missed by duplex ultrasonography.
- Venography is the next step if noninvasive imaging is inconclusive or if initial testing is positive with plans for intervention.[1-3] Venography is performed with the arm in the neutral and abducted position to visualize possible compression or positional changes. Venous cannulation may be inhibited by associated arm swelling.
- The utility of computed tomography (CT) and magnetic resonance imaging (MRI) is emerging in Paget-Schroetter syndrome. These tests are showing improvements in resolution illustrating the degree of vein compression within the thoracic outlet. CT with coronal and sagittal reconstruction will likely play a major role in the diagnosis in the future.[1,3]
- A cervical spine x-ray is useful to assess for an associated cervical rib.

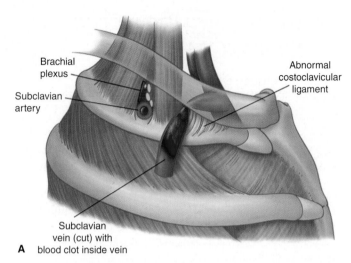

**FIGURE 56-2A** Schematic of subclavian vein deep venous thrombosis (DVT) caused by compression from abnormal costoclavicular ligament.

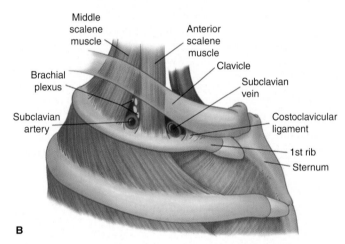

**FIGURE 56-2B** Schematic of normal anatomy of the thoracic outlet.

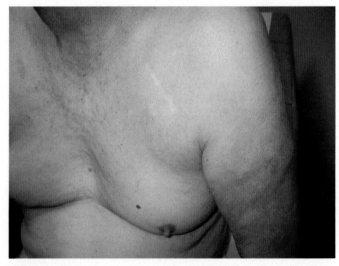

**FIGURE 56-3** Dilated subcutaneous veins in a patient with a chronically occluded left subclavian vein. (*Photograph courtesy of Dr. Steven M. Dean.*)

## MANAGEMENT

- There are two main goals to treating primary, effort-induced thrombosis. First is to restore venous patency and preserve venous anatomy. Second is to prevent secondary events, such as pulmonary embolism (caused by the migration or propagation of the thrombus), recurrent DVT, or post-thrombotic syndrome (PTS).[1-3]

- Thrombolytics serve to restore venous patency and reduce the risk of debilitating post-thrombotic symptoms. Symptoms that are present for more than 14 days present a challenge for thrombolysis because there has been sufficient time for the thrombus to organize.[3] Ideally patients should undergo thrombolysis within 1 to 2 weeks of symptom onset.

- Catheter-directed thrombolytic techniques demonstrate good results and low complication rates. A catheter can be placed directly within the thrombus, maximizing drug delivery and decreasing total dose, which ultimately decreases bleeding risk (Figure 4A-C).[2]

- Percutaneous mechanical thrombectomy can be used in combination with thrombolytics to help restore venous flow quickly, allow for lower doses of thrombolytic agents, and decrease thrombolytic infusion times.[2]

- After the acute thrombus is resolved with thrombolytic therapy, the patient should be started on therapeutic anticoagulation. Imaging of the thoracic outlet using MRI or CT is then performed to identify any underlying anatomic defects. Once the anatomic defect is identified, thoracic outlet surgery should be considered that may involve removal of a cervical rib, transaxillary resection of the first rib, or resection of the costoclavicular ligament.[1,3,4]

- The use of standard anticoagulation alone in patients with Paget-Schroetter syndrome has a high rate of PTS.[1]

## PATIENT EDUCATION

- These young, active patients will need counseling from both their physician and coach regarding the risk of continued sporting activities. The risk–benefit of thoracic-outlet release surgery needs to be at the forefront of long-term planning.

## FOLLOW-UP

- A minimum of 3 to 6 months of anticoagulation with Coumadin (warfarin) is generally recommended. Other clinical features such as concomitant pulmonary embolus or hypercoagulable state may dictate a longer duration of anticoagulation (1 year or indefinite).[1,3]

- Repeat ultrasound and physical examination are recommended at 1 and 6 months, then yearly, or with any recurrent symptoms.[1]

- A comprehensive physical therapy program aimed at stretching and loosening the scalene and subclavius muscles is important in the prevention of recurrent symptoms. Other lifestyle changes that can help prevent recurrence include weight loss and maintenance of a healthy body mass index (BMI).[3]

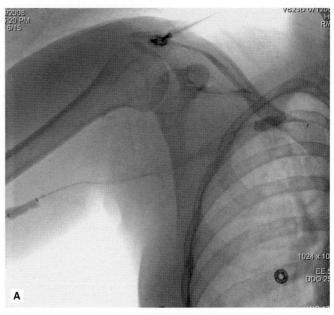

**FIGURE 56-4A** Venogram illustrating the use of Trellis catheter (Bacchus Vascular, Santa Clara, CA) for direct drug delivery into a right upper extremity axillosubclavian deep venous thrombosis (DVT).

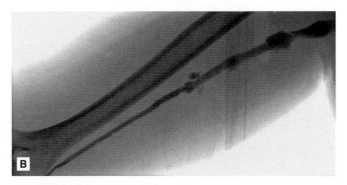

**FIGURE 56-4B** Venogram of a widely patent right brachial vein illustrating resolution of thrombus.

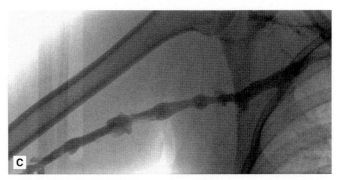

**FIGURE 56-4C** Venogram of a right axillosubclavian vein illustrating dissolution of thrombus following catheter-directed thrombolysis.

## PROVIDER RESOURCES

- http://emedicine.medscape.com/article/462166-overview
- http://www.angiologist.com/venous-disease/paget-schroetter-syndrome/

## PATIENT RESOURCES

- https://www.medify.com/conditions/paget-schroetter-syndrome
- http://www.hopkinsmedicine.org/news/publications/cardiovascular_report/cardiovascular_report_winter_2013/effort_thrombosis_an_unusual_disease_in_athletes

## REFERENCES

1. Illig KA, Doyle AJ. A comprehensive review of Paget-Schroetter syndrome. *J Vasc Surg*. 2010;51:1538-1547.

2. Silver M, Ansel G. Venous intervention. In: Topol E, Teirstein P, eds. *Textbook of Interventional Cardiology*. 6th ed. Philadelphia, PA: Elsevier-Saunders; 2012:563-575.

3. Doyle A, Wolford HY, Daves MG, et al. Management of effort thrombosis of the subclavian vein: today's treatment. *Ann Vasc Surg*. 2007;21:723-729.

4. Urschel HC, Patel AN. Surgery remains the most effective treatment for Paget-Schroetter syndrome: 50 years' experience. *Ann Thorac Surg*. 2008;28:254-260.

# 57 BENIGN ACUTE BLUE FINGER

Ido Weinberg, MD
Michael R. Jaff, DO

## PATIENT STORY

A 35-year-old Caucasian man was referred for evaluation of recurrent upper extremity digital ischemia. He had experienced three discrete episodes of acute right finger discoloration over the previous 2 years. The first episode involved a spontaneous, painless purple mass that appeared at the base of the right fourth finger without antecedent trauma. A two-dimensional transthoracic echocardiogram (TTE) performed to assess for a cardiogenic source of emboli was normal. The finger discoloration resolved within several days. Computed tomographic angiography (CTA) of the aortic arch and left upper extremity arteries was performed and was normal. He was ultimately diagnosed with benign blue finger.

### EPIDEMIOLOGY

• The epidemiology of benign acute blue finger (BABF) is unknown.

### ETIOLOGY AND PATHOPHYSIOLOGY

• The pathophysiology of BABF is unrecognized.

• A mechanism of subcutaneous ecchymosis due to spontaneous rupture of a small digital venule has been suggested[1] and this syndrome has been referred to as "spontaneous venous hemorrhage."

### DIAGNOSIS

The diagnosis of BABF is clinical. A comprehensive history and physical examination must be performed to exclude other potential etiologies, as this is a diagnosis of exclusion.

### Clinical Features

• A thorough history should be obtained from any patient presenting with an acute blue finger. The history should be aimed at risk factors for cardiogenic sources of emboli (eg, prior myocardial infarction, atrial fibrillation, valvular heart disease), atherosclerotic risk factors, thoracic outlet syndrome, or toxin ingestion (cocaine, methamphetamines [ie, Adderall], ergotamines). History suggestive of rheumatologic diseases should be pursued.

• BABF is often isolated to one finger (Figures 57-2 and 57-3). It may recur in different locations.[2,3]

• An important, yet not mandatory (Figure 57-4), physical finding is sparing of bluish discoloration of the fingertip. Physical examination must not reveal embolic phenomena.[4]

### Laboratory and Imaging Studies

• There is no need for laboratory or imaging studies in patients who present with BABF, as this is a clinical diagnosis. Testing should only be performed to exclude other potential diagnoses.

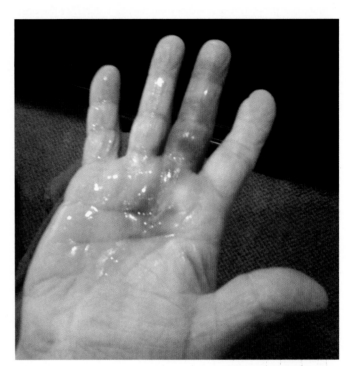

FIGURE 57-1 Purple-blue discoloration of the palmar surface of the third digit on the right hand. Notice the tip of the finger is not involved. (*Photograph courtesy of Dr. Bruce Mintz.*)

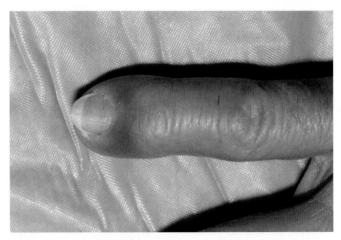

FIGURE 57-2 Acute benign blue finger involving the right third digit. The patient was initially misdiagnosed with Raynaud phenomenon. (*Photograph courtesy of Dr. Bruce Mintz.*)

- Patients presenting with BABF often undergo unnecessary evaluation for other cause of acute blue finger.[2,3]

## Differential Diagnosis

- The causes for blue fingers can be mechanistically divided into obstruction of arterial circulation, vasospasm, impaired venous outflow, and abnormal circulating blood elements (Table 57-1).[5]

- Emboli to the fingers arise either from the heart, aorta, or proximal arm arteries. Cardiac sources include the left atrial appendage, diseased or mechanical cardiac valves, or a dysfunctional or aneurysmal left ventricle. Artery-to-artery emboli arise from atheromatous lesions or aneurysms. Aneurysms may be idiopathic or result from thoracic outlet syndrome, hypothenar hammer syndrome, or, rarely, fibromuscular dysplasia. Clinically, emboli present as painful, discrete lesions, typically at the tip of the finger. Embolic distribution attests to their source. Unilateral distribution suggests a proximal arterial source, while bilateral distribution suggests a more proximal source from the heart or the aortic arch. Finally, emboli can be composed of thrombus or tumor.

- Thromboangiitis obliterans is a segmental inflammatory condition that affects small and medium-sized arteries, veins, and nerves. It is typically a disease of young people, usually under the age of 50 years, who abuse tobacco. Clinical manifestations include pain in a digit or extremity, digital ischemia, Raynaud phenomena, distal digital ulcerations, and extremity claudication. Treatment consists of complete abstinence from tobacco or nicotine.[6]

- Raynaud phenomenon is manifest by a biphasic or triphasic color change of the fingers and toes from white to blue to red. It occurs in as many as 5% of the general population.[7] Raynaud phenomena can be primary, which is painless and rarely associated with tissue ulceration, or secondary,[8] which is associated with many rheumatologic and noninflammatory conditions. The most common disorder associated with secondary Raynaud phenomena is scleroderma.[9] Treatment includes tobacco cessation, thermal protection of the extremities, and avoidance of digital injury. Vasoconstrictors must be avoided. Pharmacologic treatment with vasodilators is the next step. Dihydropyridine calcium channel blockers are the most widely used.

- Acrocyanosis is characterized by a symmetric bluish discoloration of the hands and less commonly the feet and face. It can be primary and benign or secondary, which may be asymmetric and can result in tissue loss.[10] Multiple systemic conditions have been described in association with secondary acrocyanosis. Examples include hypoxemia, stroke, myocardial infarction, systemic infection, various pulmonary diseases, connective tissue disease, anorexia nervosa and starvation, malignancy, hematologic conditions, drugs and toxins, psychiatric conditions, and heritable conditions such as Ehlers-Danlos syndrome. Treatment of acrocyanosis should first include general measures to protect and warm the affected limbs. Pharmacologic treatment has been described with minoxidil, bromocriptine, and reserpine.[11]

- Pernio, also known as chilblains, manifests as inflammatory cutaneous lesions after exposure to nonfreezing cold weather. Presentation is more common during late winter or early spring. Pernio may be recurrent. The lesions are typically painful, pruritic, and

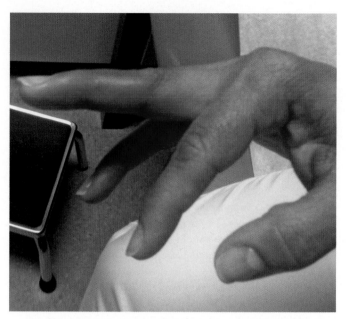

**FIGURE 57-3** Diffuse palpably warm cyanotic right third finger is displayed in a classic representation of acute benign blue finger. (*Photograph courtesy of Dr. Bruce Mintz.*)

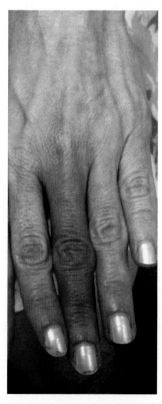

**FIGURE 57-4** Purplish discoloration along the distal portion of the finger illustrating an exception to the rule in this case of acute benign blue finger. (*Photograph courtesy of Dr. Bruce Gray.*)

erythrocyanotic in color. A misdiagnosis as vasculitis or an embolic event may lead to an elaborate and expensive workup.[12] Treatment consists of skin protection and refraining from cold exposure.

- Hematologic disorders can cause ischemic fingers in several mechanisms including hyperviscosity (multiple myeloma, polycythemia vera), immune-complex precipitation (cryoglobulinemia), and thrombosis.

- Venous thrombosis can result in blue fingers. The mechanism is reduced blood outflow and cyanosis secondary to deoxygenation.

- Factitious blue fingers have been described, for example, in a patient that used blue dye.[13]

## MANAGEMENT

- Treatment for BABF is supportive with reassurance of the benign nature of the syndrome, with knowledge that this usually resolves spontaneously.

- Anticoagulation should be avoided.

## PATIENT EDUCATION

Once other conditions have been ruled out, reassurance that BABF is self-limited is the most important information to communicate to the patient.

## FOLLOW-UP

- Follow-up of patients with BABF is clinical. Some patients develop similar lesions over ensuing months and years.[2-5]

## REFERENCES

1. Cowen R, Richards T, Dharmadasa A, Handa A, Perkins JMT. The acute blue finger: management and outcome. *Ann R Coll Surg Engl.* 2008;90:557-560.

2. Deliss LJ, Wilson JN. Acute blue fingers in women. *J Bone Joint Surg Br.* 1982;64(4):458-459.

3. Khaira HS, Rittoo D, Vohra RK, Smith SRG. The non-ischemic blue finger. *Ann R Coll Surg Engl.* 2001;83:154-157.

4. Weinberg I, Jaff MR. Spontaneous blue finger syndrome: a benign process. *Am J Med.* 2012;125(1):e1-e2.

5. Hirschmann JV, Raugi GJ. Blue (or purple) toe syndrome. *J Am Acad Dermatol.* 2009;60(1):1-20.

6. Piazza G, Creager MA. Thromboangiitis obliterans. *Circulation.* 2010;121(16):1858-1861.

7. Wigley FM. Clinical practice. Raynaud's phenomenon. *N Engl J Med.* 2002;347(13):1001-1008.

8. Herrick AL. Pathogenesis of Raynaud's phenomenon. *Rheumatology (Oxford).* 2005;44(5):587-596.

**TABLE 57-1.** Differential Diagnosis of Acute Benign Blue Finger

| Obstruction of Flow |
| --- |
| Emboli from proximal source—left ventricle, left atrial appendage, mechanical valve, rheumatic heart disease, atheromatous plaque, arterial aneurysm (with or without arterial thoracic outlet syndrome, hypothenar hammer syndrome, or fibromuscular dysplasia), vascular tumor |
| Arterial dissection |
| Thromboangiitis obliterans |
| **Vasospasm** |
| Raynaud phenomena |
| Acrocyanosis |
| Paraneoplastic phenomena |
| Vibration induced |
| Medication (eg, 5-fluorouracyl) |
| Illicit drugs (eg, cocaine) |
| Frostbite |
| **Abnormal Blood Components** |
| Hyperviscosity (eg, immunoglobulins, polycythemia, myeloma) |
| Cryoglobulinemia |
| Disseminated intravascular coagulation |
| Thrombosis secondary to polycythemia or thrombocythemia |
| Antiphospholipid antibody syndrome |
| **Impaired Venous Outflow** |
| **Other Causes** |
| Large vessel vasculitis—Takayasu and giant cell arteritis |
| Pernio |
| Wegener granulomatosis |
| Factitious |

9. Block JA, Sequeira W. Raynaud's phenomenon. *Lancet*. 2001;357(9273):2042-2048.

10. Kurklinsky AK, Miller VM, Rooke TW. Acrocyanosis: the Flying Dutchman. *Vasc Med*. 2011;16(4):288-301.

11. Morrish DW, Crockford PM. Acrocyanosis treated with bromocriptine. *Lancet*. 1976;2(7990):851.

12. Prakash S, Weisman MH. Idiopathic chilblains. *Am J Med*. 2009;122(12):1152-1155.

13. Serinken M, Karcioglu O, Turkcuer I, Bukiran A. Raynaud's phenomenon—or just skin with dye? *Emerg Med J*. 2009;26(3): 221-222.

# 58 PHLEGMASIA CERULEA DOLENS

Nikos Tsekouras, MD
Anthony J. Comerota, MD, FACS, FACC

## PATIENT STORY

A 65-year-old gentleman was referred with left lower extremity phlegmasia cerulea dolens (PCD) 1 day following an exploratory laparotomy. Postoperatively he developed painful diffuse swelling of his left lower extremity with bluish discoloration (Figure 58-1). On arrival, he underwent a venous duplex that demonstrated thrombosis of his tibial, popliteal, femoral, common femoral, and external iliac veins. Computed tomographic angiography (CTA) scan with contrast of the head, chest, abdomen, and pelvis was performed. The patient had bilateral, asymptomatic pulmonary emboli (Figure 58-2), and mediastinal, retroperitoneal, and pelvic lymphadenopathy (Figure 58-3), which subsequently proved to be lymphoma. The patient was brought to the interventional radiology suite and an ascending phlebogram was performed. The phlebogram confirmed extensive venous thrombosis from the calf veins through the iliac veins (Figure 58-4). With the patient in the supine position and under ultrasound guidance, access to the posterior tibial vein was obtained through which an EKOS Lysus (EKOS Corp, Bothell, WA) catheter was positioned. The patient was then placed in the prone position. Under ultrasound guidance, the popliteal vein was entered and a sheath advanced through which a Trellis (Covidien, Mansfield, MA) catheter was used (Figure 58-5).

Isolated segmental pharmacomechanical thrombolysis was performed with the Trellis catheter (Covidien, Medrad, MA) using 2 to 3 mg of recombinant plasminogen activator (rt-PA) in 10 cc of saline between the two balloons. The catheter was activated to macerate the thrombus for 15 to 20 minutes. After several runs, the Trellis catheter was removed, the sheath was advanced, and liquefied thrombus was aspirated (Figure 58-6). The femoral and iliac veins showed early and marked thrombus resolution (Figure 58-7). Infrapopliteal, popliteal vein, and residual iliofemoral thrombus was treated overnight with catheter-directed thrombolysis using the EKOS Lysus catheter, infusing rt-PA at 1 mg per hour. The following morning, an ascending phlebogram was performed, indicating both intrinsic stenosis and external compression of the external iliac vein. This was dilated and stented. The completion phlebogram (Figure 58-8) demonstrated patent veins providing unobstructed venous drainage into the vena cava.

Sixteen months post-treatment, he was asymptomatic (Figure 58-9). A complete noninvasive venous evaluation demonstrated that all veins were patent with normal venous valve function.

## EPIDEMIOLOGY

- Extensive deep vein thrombosis (DVT) presenting with the classical triad of extremity edema, cyanosis, and pain.

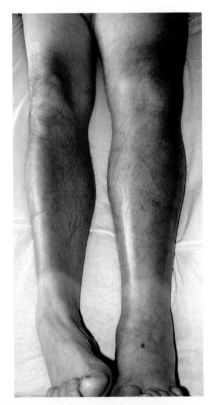

**FIGURE 58-1** Phlegmasia cerulea dolens of the left lower extremity. Photo illustrates swelling and cyanosis. The patient experienced continuous discomfort.

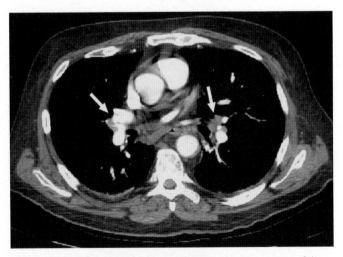

**FIGURE 58-2** Computed tomographic (CT) scan with contrast of the chest shows (right arrow) asymptomatic pulmonary emboli and (left arrow) mediastinal lymphadenopathy.

- Majority of cases occur in the lower extremity where extensive DVT commonly involves the iliofemoral segment and occludes the single venous outflow channel.

- PCD is not a rare entity, contrary to what is often stated in the literature.

- PCD is associated with severe post-thrombotic morbidity[1-3] and high recurrence rates if treated with anticoagulation alone.[4]

- Typically, younger patients with PCD are females. Once patients reach their fifth and sixth decades, gender distribution is equal.

- Left lower extremity is most commonly affected.[5]

- Up to 5% of the cases occur in the upper extremity.[6]

- Rarely can lead to venous gangrene, especially in patients with underlying malignancy.

- The rare occasion of venous gangrene carries a 20% to 50% risk of amputation with a mortality rate of about 20% to 40%.[7]

- Can be rapidly reversed if clot is eliminated.

## ETIOLOGY AND PATHOPHYSIOLOGY

- Extensive DVT involving the major deep venous channels that leads to severe and often sudden venous hypertension. There can be profound translocation of fluid into the interstitial space, resulting in massive edema and marked increase of compartment pressures.[8]

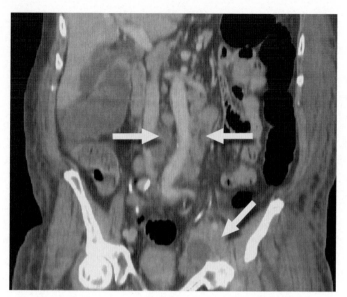

**FIGURE 58-3** Computed tomographic (CT) scan of the abdomen and pelvis demonstrates extensive retroperitoneal and pelvic lymphadenopathy (arrows).

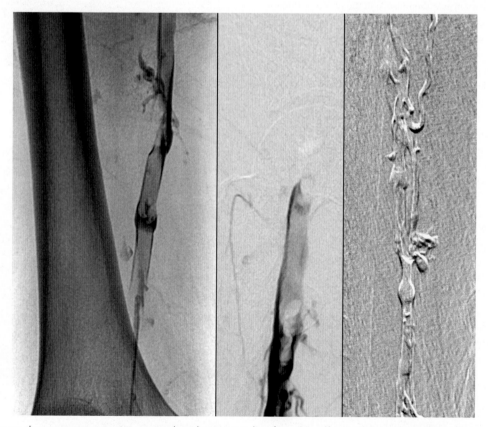

**FIGURE 58-4** Venogram demonstrates extensive venous thrombosis extending from the calf veins through the pelvic veins.

Patients can suffer hypotension as a result of third space fluid sequestration.[5]

- Factors affecting severity may include a dysregulation of homeostasis between coagulation and fibrinolysis, as well as circulatory collapse and shock from the loss of venous return.[9]

## DIAGNOSIS

The diagnosis of PCD is clinical, supported by ultrasound findings of acute DVT.

## Clinical Features

Patients typically present with a painful, cyanotic, and swollen extremity (Figure 58-10). These findings often start distally and extend proximally at varying rates, from a few hours to several days. Pain is due to the associated venous hypertension and elevated compartment pressures. Although arterial compromise is unusual, when it occurs the pain is usually unremitting and of a different character. Blistering of the skin indicates particularly high tissue pressures that can result in partial-thickness necrosis (early venous gangrene) if the venous return is not rapidly re-established. Full thickness skin necrosis is considered venous gangrene.

Pedal pulses are palpable in most patients with PCD. Patients rarely lose their distal pulses; however, Doppler signals generally remain intact. Sensory or motor deficit is a rarity. If observed, venous gangrene is imminent and indicates a poor prognosis regarding the viability of the limb. If either arterial or neural compromise exists or if skin blistering is observed, methods to remove the thrombus and restore venous return should be undertaken immediately.

## Laboratory Studies

Despite the fact that clinical presentation is characteristic, Doppler ultrasonography should be used to confirm the diagnosis. It is important to assess the inferior vena cava (IVC) for thrombus as it may alter treatment. CTA, magnetic resonance venography (MRV), or standard venography may be used. MRV is more time-consuming compared to CTA, but eliminates radiation and avoids the use of nephrotoxic, iodinated agents that can cause complications in the setting of severe volume depletion. However, if catheter-based treatment will be used to eliminate thrombus, a venographic study of the IVC can be performed at that time.

Thrombophilia evaluations are often suggested in patients presenting with PCD. Such evaluations are not helpful in patient management, either acutely or over the long term, and need not be performed. In patients with an idiopathic venous thrombosis, a thrombophilia evaluation of first-degree female relatives of childbearing potential is indicated.

## DIFFERENTIAL DIAGNOSIS

- Acute arterial occlusion has historically been confused with PCD. An appropriate history and physical examination should quickly point to the proper diagnosis.

- Phlegmasia alba dolens is characterized by painful swelling of the entire extremity without cyanosis.

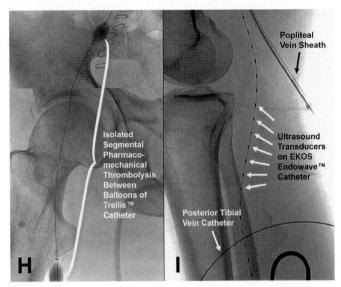

**FIGURE 58-5** X-rays showing the Trellis catheter positioned in the iliofemoral location and the EKOS Lysus catheter positioned in the femoral, popliteal, and tibial vein location.

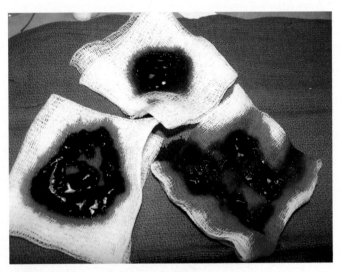

**FIGURE 58-6** Thrombus aspirated after treatment with Trellis catheter.

## MANAGEMENT

- PCD should be treated with a strategy of thrombus removal. Successful management will eliminate thrombus, reduce recurrence,[10,11] and reduce or avoid post-thrombotic morbidity.[12,13]

- Initial management includes therapeutic anticoagulation, elevation of the affected limb when in bed, snug compression bandaging of the limb from toes to upper thigh, appropriate fluid resuscitation, and ambulation.

- Surgical thrombectomy with or without an arteriovenous fistula is effective.[14] A multicenter randomized trial has shown that venous thrombectomy is superior to anticoagulation alone. In general, catheter-based strategies of thrombus removal are preferred over thrombectomy.

- Catheter-directed thrombolysis can be performed with success rates in the 85% to 95% range.[15-17] When combined with mechanical techniques the amount of clot removed is greater over a short period of time using a lower dose of lytic agent.[18,19]

- 30 to 40 mm Hg compression stockings worn from the morning until returning to bed at night.

- Long-term oral anticoagulation with warfarin to a target international normalized ratio (INR) of 2 to 3.

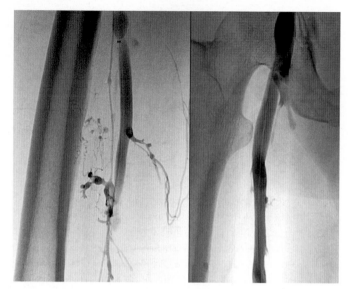

**FIGURE 58-7** Venogram demonstrates early thrombus resolution following several runs of the Trellis catheter.

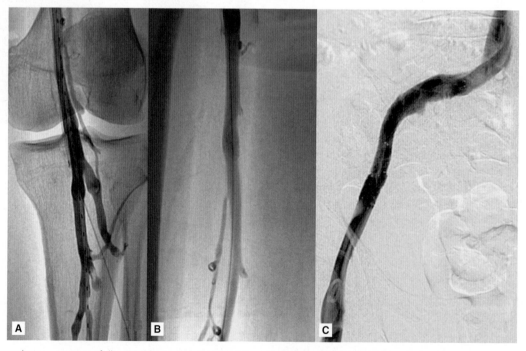

**FIGURE 58-8** Completion venogram following pharmacomechanical thrombolysis, overnight recombinant plasminogen activator (rt-PA) infusion, and venoplasty and stenting of the iliac veins. The tibioperoneal trunk, popliteal, femoral, common femoral, and iliac veins are now widely patent.

## SUMMARY

Phlegmasia cerulea dolens is the clinical presentation of a painful, edematous, and cyanotic extremity as a result of an extensive DVT most commonly involving the iliofemoral segment. It is an easily recognized clinical entity, with ultrasound being the imaging examination of choice to confirm the diagnosis. The key to proper management in the majority of patients is successful clot removal and correction of any underlying venous stenosis. 30 to 40 mm Hg gradient compression stockings will control swelling, and long-term therapeutic anticoagulation will avoid recurrence.

## PATIENT EDUCATION

- Counsel the patient on the critical importance of regular visits to an anticoagulation clinic or their physician's office to ensure a therapeutic INR.

- Instruct patients on the manifestations of recurrent venous thromboembolic disease and to seek medical attention immediately if they occur.

### PROVIDER RESOURCE

- http://emedicine.medscape.com/article/461809-overview

### PATIENT RESOURCE

- http://www.drugs.com/enc/phlegmasia-cerulea-dolens.html

## REFERENCES

1. Delis KT, Bountouroglou D, Mansfield AO. Venous claudication in iliofemoral thrombosis: long-term effects on venous hemodynamics, clinical status, and quality of life. *Ann Surg.* 2004;239(1):118-126.

2. Akesson H, Brudin L, Dahlstrom JA, Eklof B, Ohlin P, Plate G. Venous function assessed during a 5 year period after acute ilio-femoral venous thrombosis treated with anticoagulation. *Eur J Vasc Surg.* 1990;4(1):43-48.

3. Kahn SR, Ginsberg JS. Relationship between deep venous thrombosis and the postthrombotic syndrome. *Arch Intern Med.* 2004;164(1):17-26.

4. Douketis JD, Crowther MA, Foster GA, Ginsberg JS. Does the location of thrombosis determine the risk of disease recurrence in patients with proximal deep vein thrombosis? *Am J Med.* 2001;110(7):515-519.

5. Perkins JM, Magee TR, Galland RB. Phlegmasia cerulea dolens and venous gangrene. *Br J Surg.* 1996;83(1):19-23.

6. Mousa A, Henderson P, Dayal R, Bernheim J, Kent KC, Faries PL. Endoluminal recanalization in a patient with phlegmasia cerulea dolens using a multimodality approach. *Vascular.* 2005;13(5):313-317.

7. Oguzkurt L, Tercan F, Ozkan U. Manual aspiration thrombectomy with stent placement: rapid and effective treatment for phlegmasia cerulea dolens with impending venous gangrene. *Cardiovasc Intervent Radiol.* 2008;31(1):205-208.

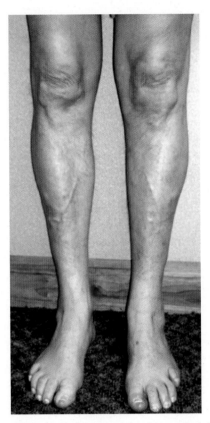

**FIGURE 58-9** Photograph of a patient's leg 16 months following treatment. The patient was asymptomatic; the veins were patent and had normal valve function. Chemotherapy for the patient's lymphoma was successful and he was in complete remission.

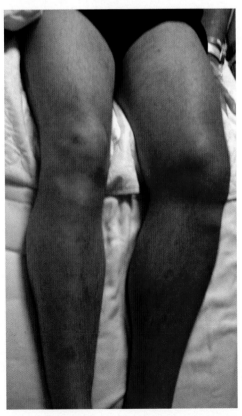

**FIGURE 58-10** Stereotypical painful, swollen, cyanotic leg characteristic of phlegmasia cerulea dolens.

8. Saffle JR, Maxwell JG, Warden GD, Jolley SG, Lawrence PF. Measurement of intramuscular pressure in the management of massive venous occlusion. *Surgery*. 1981;89(3):394-397.

9. Hood DB, Weaver FA, Modrall JG, Yellin AE. Advances in the treatment of phlegmasia cerulea dolens. *Am J Surg*. 1993;166(2):206-210.

10. Aziz F, Chen JT, Comerota AJ. Catheter-directed thrombolysis of iliofemoral DVT reduces DVT recurrence. Abstract presented at the American Venous Forum, 2011 February 24.

11. Baekgaard N, Broholm R, Just S, Jorgensen M, Jensen LP. Long-term results using catheter-directed thrombolysis in 103 lower limbs with acute iliofemoral venous thrombosis. *Eur J Vasc Endovasc Surg*. 2010;39(1):112-117.

12. Comerota AJ, Grewal N, Martinez J, et al. Postthrombotic morbidity correlates with residual thrombus following catheter-directed thrombolysis for iliofemoral DVT. *J Vasc Surg*. 2012;55(3):768-773.

13. Grewal N, Martinez J, Andrews L, Comerota AJ. Quantity of clot lysed after catheter-directed thrombolysis for iliofemoral deep venous thrombosis correlates with post-thrombotic morbidity. *J Vasc Surg*. 2010;51(5):1209-1214.

14. Sarwar S, Narra S, Munir A. Phlegmasia cerulea dolens. *Tex Heart Inst J*. 2009;36(1):76-77.

15. Mewissen MW, Seabrook GR, Meissner MH, Cynamon J, Labropoulos N, Haughton SH. Catheter-directed thrombolysis for lower extremity deep venous thrombosis: report of a national multicenter registry. *Radiology*. 1999;211(1):39-49.

16. Bjarnason H, Kruse JR, Asinger DA, et al. Iliofemoral deep venous thrombosis: safety and efficacy outcome during 5 years of catheter-directed thrombolytic therapy. *J Vasc Interv Radiol*. 1997;8(3):405-418.

17. Comerota AJ, Kagan SA. Catheter-directed thrombolysis for the treatment of acute iliofemoral deep venous thrombosis. *Phlebology*. 2000;15:149-155.

18. Martinez J, Comerota AJ, Kazanjian S, DiSalle RS, Sepanski DM, Assi Z. The quantitative benefit of isolated, segmental, pharmacomechanical thrombolysis for iliofemoral DVT. *J Vasc Surg*. 2008;48(6):1532-1537.

19. Lin PH, Zhou W, Dardik A, et al. Catheter-direct thrombolysis versus pharmacomechanical thrombectomy for treatment of symptomatic lower extremity deep venous thrombosis. *Am J Surg*. 2006;192(6):782-788.

# 59 PANNICULITIS

Benjamin H. Kaffenberger, MD

## PATIENT STORY

A 26-year-old Caucasian woman presents for evaluation of painful, red nodules on her bilateral shins that started several days ago. The nodules were initially bright red. They are now turning darker and becoming flatter. She had a similar occurrence several months ago where she developed a bruise-like discoloration for several weeks that resolved without scarring. Her review of systems is positive for a low-grade fever, malaise, and some joint pains. Additionally, she admits to intermittent bouts of abdominal pain, as well as a few episodes of bloody diarrhea.

This patient was ultimately diagnosed with erythema nodosum that was found to be associated with inflammatory bowel disease. Figures 59-1 and 59-2 demonstrate characteristic erythema nodosum on the classic locations. She was prescribed rest and nonsteroidal anti-inflammatory drugs, and was referred to a gastroenterologist. After initiating treatment for Crohn disease, the nodules healed without scarring and did not recur.

### EPIDEMIOLOGY

#### Erythema Nodosum

- The most common panniculitis that is typically seen in young women between the ages of 20 and 40. Erythema nodosum is seen 3 to 6 times more frequently in women than men. An underlying cause can be found in approximately two-thirds of cases.[1]

- In children, it is most commonly associated with streptococcal pharyngitis or perianal infection.

- In adults, it is most commonly associated with drug ingestion, sarcoidosis, or upper respiratory tract infection. Table 59-1 presents the most common associations seen in teenagers and adults.

#### Panniculitis Associated With Systemic Disease

- Lupus panniculitis (or lupus profundus)—may be seen in up to 2% to 3% of patients with systemic lupus.[2] It may also be seen independently of systemic lupus. Similar but less frequent panniculitides may be seen in dermatomyositis and scleroderma.

- Pancreatic panniculitis—occurs in 2% to 3% of patients with pancreatic disease.[3]

- Alpha-1-antitrypsin deficiency—this manifestation is less frequent than the characteristic liver and lung disease.[4]

#### Infectious Panniculitis

- Occurs primarily in patients who are immunocompromised. This panniculitis is usually the result of hematogenous spread with seeding of organisms into the subcutaneous fat.

#### Traumatic and Factitial Panniculitis

- Traumatic panniculitis—prevalence is difficult to assess. In adults this is most commonly seen as a tender breast mass that resolves

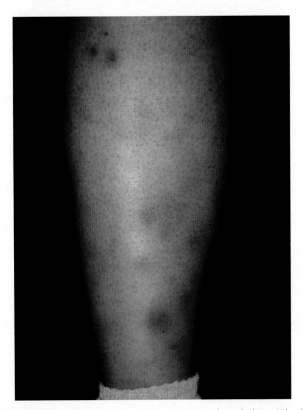

FIGURE 59-1 Erythema nodosum in a patient with underlying Kikuchi disease. (*Photograph courtesy of Matthew Zirwas, MD.*)

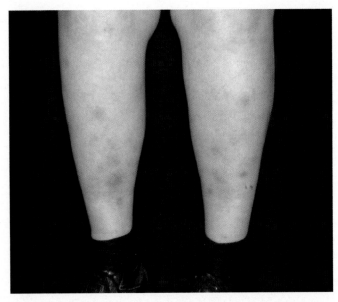

FIGURE 59-2 Erythema nodosum in a patient with no underlying abnormality. (*Photograph courtesy of Matthew Zirwas, MD.*)

**TABLE 59-1.** Common Associations of Erythema Nodosum and Clinical Pearls

| Common Associations of Erythema Nodosum | Frequency Seen in 106 Consecutive Patients Older Than 14 Years of Age Diagnosed in Spain[1] | Clinical Pearl |
|---|---|---|
| Idiopathic | 34.3% | Treatments: First line: nonsteroidal anti-inflammatory drugs + rest Second line: corticosteroids |
| Sarcoidosis | 22% | Lofgren syndrome: Erythema nodosum, hilar lymphadenopathy, and arthritis Most patients with this presentation will undergo remission |
| Upper respiratory infection | 12.7% | Check throat culture and antistreptolysin-O titer. |
| Upper respiratory infection + drug | 6.9% | If possible, stop recent drugs |
| B-hemolytic streptococcal infection | 6.9% | Most common cause in children |
| Tuberculosis | 4.9% | Chest x-ray, PPD, especially in high-risk individuals |
| Inflammatory bowel disease | 3% | Crohn disease slightly more common than ulcerative colitis |
| Drugs alone | 2.9% | Numerous drugs have been associated with this condition[9] |
| Other | 6.4% | Geographic variants exist. Coccidioidomycosis and histoplasmosis can frequently be associated with erythema nodosum in acute infections |

without treatment. Cold panniculitis occurs in cold weather and is associated with low-grade trauma, classically in horseback riders corresponding to the areas of the thighs that rest on the saddle.

- Factitial panniculitis—occurs after the injection of exogenous substances into the subcutaneous fat.

## ETIOLOGY AND PATHOPHYSIOLOGY

### Erythema Nodosum

- Hypersensitivity reaction to an underlying inflammatory state.

### Panniculitis Associated With Systemic Disease

- Lupus panniculitis—a specific autoimmune inflammatory condition that may be partially related to sensitization from traumatized subcutaneous fat.
- Pancreatic panniculitis—associated but not fully explained by lipase release into the blood stream from an inflamed pancreas.
- Alpha-1-antitrypsin deficiency—triggered by unopposed activity of numerous catabolic enzymes.

## Infectious Panniculitis

- Caused by hematogenous spread of infection, resulting in thrombosis of deep subcutaneous vasculature and extension of organisms into the deep subcutaneous fat. In hematogenous cases, the primary entry point for the organism is via the lungs.

## Traumatic and Factitial Panniculitis

- Traumatic panniculitis—initiated by abrupt vascular insufficiency, and results in an inflammatory response to encapsulate necrotic adipocytes.

- Factitial panniculitis—induced by inflammatory histiocytes attempting to encapsulate foreign material.

## DIAGNOSIS

- There are no pathognomonic clinical findings; consequently, an accurate diagnosis of all cases of panniculitis requires an early deep incisional or punch biopsy containing copious subcutaneous fat (Figure 59-3).

## CLINICAL FEATURES

### Erythema Nodosum

- Classically presents with rapid onset of painful, vaguely defined, erythematous, warm nodules that may be associated with low-grade fever, malaise, and arthralgias. After several days, the erythema resolves with an ecchymotic appearance. Ulceration does not occur. All skin findings should fully resolve in 3 to 6 weeks without scarring. Erythema nodosum may recur. Table 59-1 lists some of the common associations of erythema nodosum.

### Panniculitis Associated With Systemic Disease

- Lupus panniculitis—deep subcutaneous nodules sometimes with overlying features of discoid lupus. May be seen with or without systemic lupus. Atrophy of skin and fat occurs frequently after resolution. Figures 59-4 and 59-5 show typical fat atrophy of lupus panniculitis.

- Pancreatic panniculitis—most commonly seen in patients with acute and chronic pancreatitis. Rarely, it may be seen with pancreatic carcinoma. It presents as erythematous nodules that may ulcerate.

- Alpha-1-antitrypsin deficiency—rarely can be the presenting sign of homozygous disease. Usually, patients already manifest emphysema, hepatitis, or cirrhosis. Presents as subcutaneous nodules that frequently ulcerate and drain necrotic adipocytes. Scars frequently form after resolution.

### Infectious Panniculitis

- Multiple erythematous nodules usually found in immunocompromised patients that result from direct inoculation of the subcutaneous fat via local extension of a deeper or superficial infection. Hematogenous dissemination of infection into the subcutaneous tissue may occur. Bacteria, fungi, parasites, or viruses are responsible.

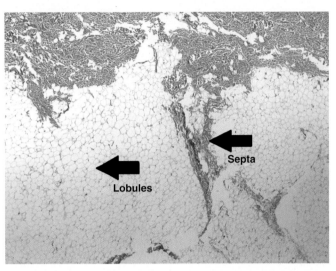

**FIGURE 59-3** Demonstration of fat architecture that underlies the primary classification of panniculitis. Inflammation is classified as predominantly lobular or septal. (*Photograph courtesy of Rebecca Ziegler, MD.*)

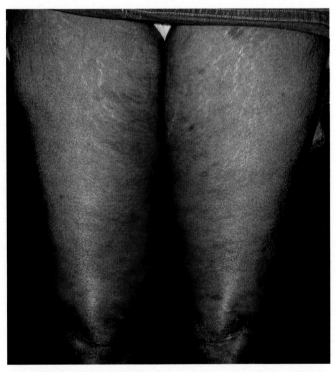

**FIGURE 59-4** Lupus panniculitis with associated postinflammatory hyperpigmentation and lipoatrophy. (*Photograph courtesy of Matthew Zirwas, MD.*)

## Traumatic and Factitial Panniculitis

- Traumatic panniculitis—erythematous nodule at the site of isolated or repetitive trauma with or without cold exposure. Figure 59-6 shows a panniculitis at the site of a frequently traumatized area in a young woman.
- Factitial panniculitis—may include patients with psychiatric pathology injecting substances in the fat. May also be seen in healthcare workers or patients of unlicensed practitioners attempting to augment the breasts, buttocks, or genitalia, or to improve facial wrinkles.

## TYPICAL DISTRIBUTION

### Erythema Nodosum

- Usually symmetrically located on the shins.

### Panniculitis Associated With Systemic Disease

- Lupus panniculitis—location is distinct from other panniculitides. It most frequently occurs on the proximal arms, shoulders, buttocks, or face.
- Pancreatic panniculitis—most commonly seen on distal shins and ankles.
- Alpha-1-antitrypsin deficiency—usually on the lower extremities.

### Infectious Panniculitis

- It can occur anywhere on the body. Direct extension can arise from the thorax or abdominal cavities. It may occur at sites of invasive catheters.

### Traumatic and Factitial Panniculitis

- Traumatic panniculitis—may involve the breasts due to low-grade trauma from the associated weight. Sometimes seen over areas of frequent trauma such as the shins.
- Factitial panniculitis—often appears in areas that are cosmetically sensitive including face, breasts, groin, and buttocks.

## LABORATORY STUDIES

### Erythema Nodosum

- Obtain cultures, rapid streptococcal antigen, antistreptolysin-O, consider chest x-ray for sarcoidosis and tuberculosis (TB), purified protein derivative (PPD), evaluation for underlying medical conditions. Biopsy results: septal inflammation without vasculitis.

### Panniculitis Associated With Systemic Disease

- Lupus panniculitis—obtain antinuclear antibody (ANA). Biopsy results: lymphocytic lobular infiltrate with possible superficial changes of discoid lupus. Minimal necrosis. Consider direct immunofluorescence to assist with diagnosis.[5]
- Pancreatic panniculitis—check amylase and lipase levels. Lipase is more frequently elevated. Biopsy results: focal lobular panniculitis with "ghost cells" and necrosis of adipocytes.[6]
- Alpha-1-antitrypsin deficiency—an alpha-1-antitrypsin phenotype test can quantify levels in the serum, and deoxyribonucleic acid (DNA) testing is available for definitive diagnosis. Biopsy results: lobular panniculitis with variable cellular infiltrate and necrosis of adipocytes.[7]

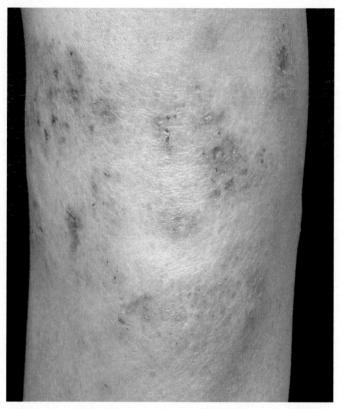

FIGURE 59-5 Lupus panniculitis on the arm. Note the characteristic overlying scarring. (*Photograph courtesy of Katya Harfmann, MD.*)

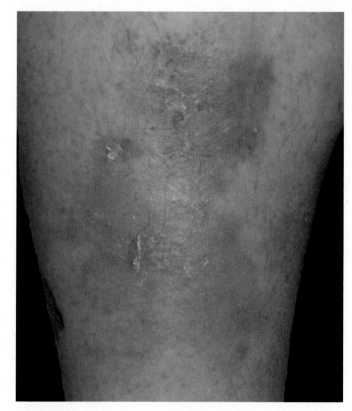

FIGURE 59-6 Traumatic panniculitis in a young female.

## Infectious Panniculitis

- Medically appropriate cultures. Biopsy result: neutrophil dominant inflammation of lobular adipocytes and organisms seen on periodic acid-Schiff (PAS), gram, or acid-fast bacillus (AFB) stains.

## Traumatic and Factitial Panniculitis

- Traumatic panniculitis—no laboratory tests needed unless the diagnosis is in doubt. Biopsy results: traumatic fat necrosis, lobular necrosis of adipocytes, fat microcysts interspersed.[8]
- Factitial panniculitis—biopsy results: lobular panniculitis with granulomatous inflammatory infiltrate. Polarization may reveal foreign material. Tissue culture and microbial stains should be performed.

## MANAGEMENT

### Erythema Nodosum

- First line: Treat infections, evaluate for other underlying causes, and stop any new drugs.
- If no underlying cause identified, treatment consists of nonsteroidal anti-inflammatory drugs, rest, and elevation. Potassium iodide solution, 120 to 300 mg three times daily, is effective although contraindicated during pregnancy. Systemic corticosteroids are also effective.

### Panniculitis Associated With Systemic Disease

- Lupus panniculitis—trial of topical corticosteroids. If there is no improvement, treatment with systemic corticosteroids or hydroxychloroquine can be considered.
- Pancreatic panniculitis—manage acute pancreatitis. If elevated lipase without abdominal pain or history of pancreatitis exists, consider abdominal computed tomography (CT) for evaluation of possible pancreatic carcinoma.
- Alpha-1-antitrypsin deficiency—dapsone is effective for mild disease. Severe cases will require exogenous enzyme replacement or liver transplantation. Avoidance of trauma is important.

### Infectious Panniculitis

- Start systemic antibiotics immediately and modify if needed after sensitivities from tissue culture are known. Evaluate the patient for an immunocompromised state.

### Traumatic and Factitial Panniculitis

- Traumatic panniculitis—avoidance of overt and low-grade trauma, avoidance of cold in some cases.
- Factitial panniculitis—treat coexisting infection if present. Implanted material may need to be removed. Discuss psychiatric treatment with the patient, as the patient may be resistant to a psychiatric referral.

## PATIENT EDUCATION

### Erythema Nodosum

- Education on recurrence risk and need for evaluation of underlying cause. It typically responds well to treatment. The lesions will heal without scarring.

### Panniculitis Associated With Systemic Disease

- Lupus panniculitis—education on the need for continued follow-up, and the need for a complete evaluation for systemic lupus. There is a risk of new lesions with trauma. The patient likely will scar.
- Pancreatic panniculitis—education on alcohol avoidance and other factors exacerbating pancreatitis.
- Alpha-1-antitrypsin deficiency—education on codominant inheritance patterns, familial testing, and systemic features of disease.

### Infectious Panniculitis

- Education on wound care, consequences of immunosuppression.

### Traumatic and Factitial Panniculitis

- Traumatic panniculitis—education on avoidance of trauma. Lesions may heal with atrophy.
- Factitial panniculitis—education on psychiatric pathology, risks of procedures from unlicensed practitioners, and the risks involved with the injection of foreign materials.

## FOLLOW-UP

### Erythema Nodosum

- Follow-up in 4 to 6 weeks to ensure resolution. Will need regular follow-up afterward to ensure that no other systemic signs develop. Thoroughly evaluate other systemic complaints, for example, abdominal pain, diarrhea, menstrual irregularities, and lymphadenopathy.

### Panniculitis Associated With Systemic Disease

- Lupus panniculitis—follow-up for topical or systemic treatments as well as a history and laboratory evaluation of systemic lupus.
- Pancreatic panniculitis—follow-up with gastroenterology or primary care physician. Control and prevention of pancreatitis should resolve the panniculitis.
- Alpha-1-antitrypsin deficiency—referral to the following specialists should be considered: genetics, transplant hepatology, and pulmonology.

### Infectious Panniculitis

- Long-term antibiotics and follow-up care are required for likely systemic infection. Strongly consider an infectious disease referral. Length of antibiotic use depends on causative organism and response to therapy.

### Traumatic and Factitial Panniculitis

- Traumatic panniculitis—no follow-up needed unless lack of improvement.
- Factitial panniculitis—may require treatment for psychiatric pathology or follow-up for infected material.

**PROVIDER RESOURCES**

- http://dermnetnz.org/dermal-infiltrative/panniculitis.html
- http://www.uptodate.com/contents/panniculitis-recognition-and-diagnosis

**PATIENT RESOURCES**

- http://www.patient.co.uk/leaflets/idiopathic_lobular_panniculitis.htm
- http://rarediseases.info.nih.gov/gard/7879/nodular-nonsuppurative-panniculitis/resources/1

## REFERENCES

1. García-Porrúa C, González-Gay MA, Vázquez-Caruncho M, et al. Erythema nodosum: etiologic and predictive factors in a defined population. *Arthritis Rheum*. 2000;43(3):584-592.

2. Diaz-Jouanen E, Dehoratius R, Alarcon-Segovia D, et al. Systemic lupus erythematosus presenting as panniculitis (lupus profundus). *Ann Intern Med*. 1975;82:376-379.

3. Sibrack L, Gouterman I. Cutaneous manifestations of pancreatic diseases. *Cutis*. 1978;21(6):763-768.

4. Lyon MJ. Metabolic panniculitis: alpha-1 antitrypsin deficiency panniculitis and pancreatic panniculitis. *Dermatol Ther*. 2010;23(4): 368-374.

5. Sánchez NP, Peters MS, Winkelmann RK. The histopathology of lupus erythematosus panniculitis. *J Am Acad Dermatol*. 1981;5(6):673-680.

6. Dahl PR, Su WPD, Cullimore RC, et al. Pancreatic panniculitis. *J Am Acad Dermatol*. 1995;33(3):413-417.

7. Valverde R, Rosales B, Ortiz-de Frutos FJ, Rodríguez-Peralto JL, Ortiz-Romero PL. Alpha-1-antitrypsin deficiency panniculitis. *Dermatol Clin*. 2008;26(4):447-451.

8. Moreno A, Marcoval J, Peyri J. Traumatic panniculitis. *Dermatol Clin*. 2008;26(4):481-483.

9. Requena L, Yus ES. Panniculitis. Part I. Mostly septal panniculitis. *J Am Acad Dermatol*. 2001;45(2):163-183.

# 60 STASIS DERMATITIS

Georgann Anetakis Poulos, MD
Lana Alghothani, MD

## PATIENT STORY

A 55-year-old-woman was admitted to the hospital to rule out bilateral lower extremity cellulitis. She presented with lower extremity edema and sharply demarcated pretibial erythema that extended just above the medial malleolus bilaterally (Figure 60-1). She was afebrile, and complete blood count (CBC) was within normal limits. The patient was diagnosed with classic stasis dermatitis, a condition commonly misdiagnosed as bilateral lower extremity cellulitis.

### EPIDEMIOLOGY

- The prevalence is estimated to be greater than 1% of the population.[1]
- Slight female preponderance reported.[1]
- Prevalence increases with age.
  - Estimated prevalence of 6% to 7% in patients older than 50 years.[2]

### ETIOLOGY AND PATHOPHYSIOLOGY

- Stasis dermatitis likely occurs secondary to the chronic inflammation and microangiopathy that result from chronic venous insufficiency.[1]
  - Disruption in function of the venous valve system in the deep and perforating venous tributaries of the legs causes backflow into the superficial venous system, yielding venous hypertension.[1]
    - Valvular dysfunction results from increasing age or can be the result of specific events, including deep vein thrombosis, pregnancy, surgery, or history of a lower extremity injury.[1]
  - Venous hypertension decreases the flow of blood in the microvasculature and allows for an increase in the capillary permeability, resulting in the extravasation of erythrocytes and the passage of fluid and plasma proteins into the tissue, consequently leading to microangiopathy.[1]
    - Proteins, most commonly fibrin, are deposited perivascularly, forming a hyaline cuff and inhibiting oxygen diffusion.[1,2]
    - Decreased blood flow causes an upregulation of intercellular adhesion molecule-1 (ICAM-1) and vascular cell adhesion molecule (VCAM-1), thus activating neutrophils and macrophages.[1,2]
    - Activated neutrophils release inflammatory mediators, free radicals, and proteases, causing pericapillary inflammation.[1]

### DIAGNOSIS

#### Clinical Features of Stasis Dermatitis

- Often first manifests as lower extremity edema.
- Scaling, xerosis, and pruritus are often present within the mid and distal medial calf (Figure 60-2). Less often, similar manifestations affect the lateral calf.

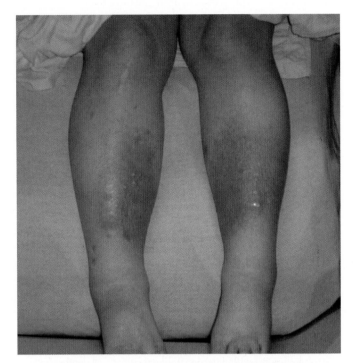

**FIGURE 60-1** Lower extremity edema and pretibial erythema consistent with stasis dermatitis. This is commonly misdiagnosed as bilateral lower extremity cellulitis.

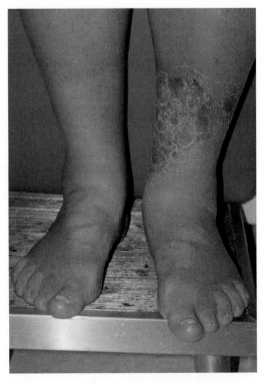

**FIGURE 60-2** Scaling, xerosis, and pruritus are often present in the medial lower extremity. (*Photograph courtesy of Dr. Steven M. Dean.*)

- Hemosiderin deposition often leads to the classic brown discoloration seen in stasis dermatitis (Figure 60-3).

- Erythema, scaling, and diffuse dermatitis can result in a weepy appearance with oozing and crusting (Figure 60-4).

- When stasis dermatitis is present chronically, fibrosis of the underlying tissues progresses to lipodermatosclerosis. A constricting band forms around the distal calf causing the classic "inverted wine bottle appearance" of the lower extremity (Figure 60-5).

- Chronic stasis dermatitis can also present with violaceous papules, plaques, and nodules mimicking Kaposi sarcoma. This entity is known as pseudo-Kaposi sarcoma or acroangiodermatitis.[2]

## Typical Distribution

- Most evident in the medial supramalleolar region, the site of major communicating veins and therefore the region where microangiopathy is most intense.[1]

- Patches of dermatitis occur commonly over dilated varicose veins.[1]

- Can occur unilaterally when the lower extremity has been injured via trauma or surgery.

## Laboratory Studies

- Clinical diagnosis based on appearance and history of chronic venous insufficiency.

- If suspecting cellulitis or sepsis, appropriate blood work is warranted (CBC with differential, blood cultures, wound cultures).

- If stasis dermatitis is secondary to venous thrombosis, consider an evaluation for an underlying hypercoagulable state.

- A venous duplex ultrasound is critical in order to assess for acute and/or remote deep venous thrombosis. Importantly, this examination can identify the anatomic location of venous reflux, which may facilitate subsequent corrective intervention.

## COMPLICATIONS

- Allergic contact dermatitis affects 58% to 86% of patients with venous ulcers.[3]
  - This can be secondary to the use of topical therapies, including creams, antibiotics, and antiseptics.[3] Topical antibiotics such as neomycin and bacitracin were the culprits in superimposed allergic contact dermatitis in a sensitized patient (Figure 60-6).

- Stasis dermatitis can lead to secondary dissemination, with patches of eczema arising in symmetric and distant distribution patterns.[1] This is known as autosensitization dermatitis or Id reaction.[1]

- A coexisting irritant dermatitis secondary to wound or venous ulcer secretions can occur.[1]

## DIFFERENTIAL DIAGNOSIS

- Asteatotic eczema—also known as eczema craquele. This condition involves xerotic skin with superficial cracks resembling a "dried river bed."

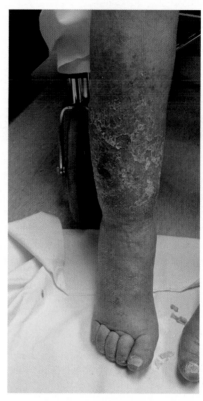

**FIGURE 60-3** Hemosiderin deposition often leads to the classic brown discoloration seen in stasis dermatitis. (*Photograph courtesy of Dr. Steven M. Dean.*)

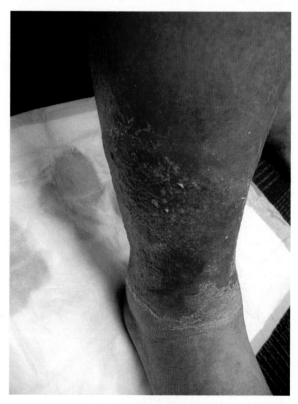

**FIGURE 60-4** Erythema, scaling, and diffuse dermatitis can lead to a weepy appearance with oozing and crusting. (*Photograph courtesy of Dr. Steven M. Dean.*)

- Atopic dermatitis—typically the patient has a history significant for eczema, asthma, or seasonal allergies.

- Allergic contact dermatitis—associated with stasis dermatitis since venous leg ulcer patients often have contact sensitivities to medicaments used in the management of the ulcers. Commonly reported allergens include topical antibiotics, fragrances, Balsam of Peru, lanolin alcohol, topical corticosteroids, and rubber accelerators.[3]

- Irritant contact dermatitis—often due to exudate from venous ulcers that cause inflammation and irritation of the skin.[1]

- Pretibial myxedema—infiltrative plaques of the pretibial region often associated with Graves disease.

- Cellulitis—often unilateral. May be accompanied by constitutional symptoms such as fever. White blood cell count may be elevated. Stasis dermatitis can be seen along with cellulitis (Figure 60-7).

- Psoriasis—sharply demarcated erythematous plaques with characteristic scale. Patient typically presents with plaques at common sites such as scalp, extensor surfaces of extremities, umbilicus, and lower back.

- Mycosis fungoides—skin biopsy for histologic assessment can be helpful in the appropriate clinical situation.

- Deep venous thrombosis.

## MANAGEMENT

- Underlying varicosities and saphenous vein insufficiency should be addressed, with treatment aimed at improving venous return and decreasing edema.
  - Compression therapy, including Unna boots and various other pressure wraps or compression stockings.
  - Leg elevation above heart level several times per day.
  - Lifestyle changes, including exercise and weight loss.
  - Surgical ligation or thermal ablation of incompetent communicating veins may be indicated if stasis dermatitis persists despite correcting saphenous vein reflux.

- The eczematous dermatitis and pruritic component can be treated with mid-potency topical corticosteroids.[1,4]

## PATIENT EDUCATION

- Patients should be educated about the underlying cause of stasis dermatitis, as well as the necessary treatments for the underlying venous insufficiency.

- Encourage daily use of compression devices as prescribed.

## FOLLOW-UP

- Patients with long-standing but stable stasis dermatitis can manage the condition on an outpatient basis.

- Acute exacerbations should be closely observed by a physician to prevent the formation of nonhealing ulcers and infection.

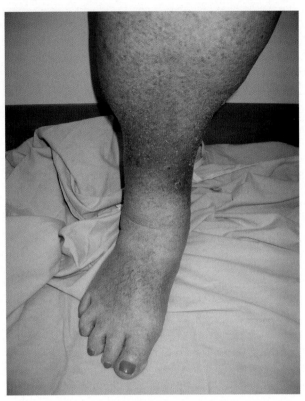

FIGURE 60-5 The classic "inverted wine bottle appearance" of lipodermatosclerosis. (*Photograph courtesy of Dr. Steven M. Dean.*)

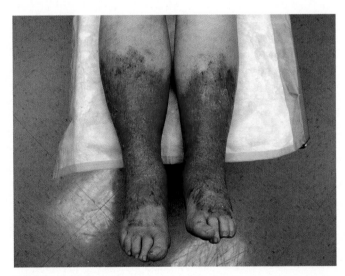

FIGURE 60-6 Stasis dermatitis along with allergic contact dermatitis in a patient previously sensitized to topical neomycin. (*Photograph courtesy of Dr. Steven M. Dean.*)

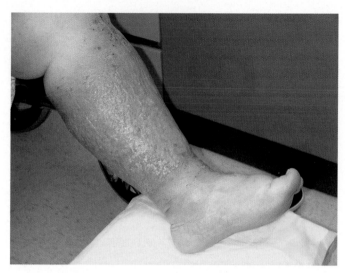

**FIGURE 60-7** Lower extremity cellulitis can be present along with stasis dermatitis.

## REFERENCES

1. Bolognia JL, Rapini RP, Jorizzo JL. *Dermatology*. 2nd ed. Chicago, IL: Mosby; 2003.

2. Flugman S. Stasis Dermatitis. Available at: http://emedicine. medscape.com/article/1084813-overview. Accessed January 14, 2012.

3. Tavadia S, Bianchi J, Dawe RS, et al. Allergic contact dermatitis in venous leg ulcer patients. *Contact Dermatitis*. 2003;48:261-265.

4. James WD, Berger TG, Elston DM. *Andrews' Diseases of the Skin, Clinical Dermatology*. 10th ed. Philadelphia, PA: Saunders Elsevier; 2006.

# 61 PSEUDO-KAPOSI SARCOMA (ACROANGIODERMATITIS)

Essa M. Essa, MBBS
Michael Davis, MD, FSVM

## PATIENT STORY

A 54-year-old man with a history of Klippel-Trenaunay syndrome (KTS) presented with unilateral left lower extremity painless skin lesions that had been increasing in size for the past several years (Figure 61-1). He first noticed several purplish raised areas that transformed into nodules that slowly and progressively increased in size. Biopsy revealed a regular pattern of small blood vessel proliferation, fibroblasts, extravasated erythrocytes, and hemosiderin deposition within the dermis. No endothelial cell atypical mitoses or vascular slits were identified. Polymerase chain reaction (PCR) analysis for human herpesvirus 8 (HHV 8) was negative. A diagnosis of acroangiodermatitis or pseudo-Kaposi sarcoma was made.

## INTRODUCTION

Acroangiodermatitis of Mali, which is also referred to as simply acroangiodermatitis or pseudo-Kaposi sarcoma, is a rare vascular phenomenon with skin manifestations characterized by violaceous nodules or plaques arising from hyperplasia of pre-existing vasculature due to severe chronic venous insufficiency (CVI) and associated venous hypertension. The term *pseudo-Kaposi sarcoma* originated from clinical similarities and histologic characteristics of the cancerous condition Kaposi sarcoma.[1] The term *acroangiodermatitis* was first described by Mali and Kuiper in 1965, who described 18 patients with mauve-colored macules, papules, and/or nodules predominantly over the extensor surface of feet with underlying chronic venous insufficiency.[2] In 1967, morphologically similar lesions were described independently by Stewart as well as by Bluefarb and Adams on the legs of patients with arteriovenous malformations (AVMs) and coined Stewart-Bluefarb syndrome.[3]

## EPIDEMIOLOGY

- Pseudo-Kaposi sarcoma is a unique vasoproliferative disorders of pre-existing vasculature with fewer than 100 cases reported.

## ETIOLOGY AND PATHOGENESIS

- Acroangiodermatitis is reported in patients with CVI,[2] paralyzed extremities,[4] amputation stumps (especially with poor-fitting suction-type prostheses),[5] iatrogenic arteriovenous fistula (AVF),[6] and in association with KTS,[7] homozygous activated protein C resistance,[8] and 20210A prothrombin gene mutation carriers.[9]

- Acroangiodermatitis associated with CVI is hypothesized to be a direct effect of severe venous valvular incompetence with or without insufficiency of the calf muscle pump. Sustained venous

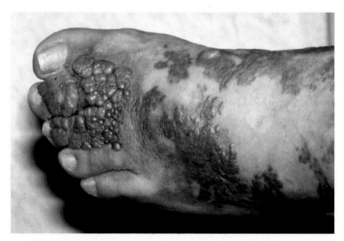

**FIGURE 61-1** Acroangiodermatitis (pseudo-Kaposi sarcoma) presenting as dark purplish verrucous nodules on the dorsum of the distal foot and toes with proximal papules and plaques. (*Photograph courtesy of Steven M. Dean, DO*).

hypertension leads to elevation of the capillary pressure and chronic tissue hypoxia that triggers neovascularization and fibroblast proliferation.[10]

- Stewart-Bluefarb syndrome is clinically and histologically similar to pseudo-Kaposi sarcoma and is associated with AVMs. The inciting event may be different from pseudo-Kaposi sarcoma and triggered by stimulation of endothelial growth from the resultant increase in venous pressure from associated AVMs.[11] Reports postulate that the inciting mechanism is related to an increase in endothelial growth factor signaling proteins from local ischemia induced by the AVMs.[12]

## DIAGNOSIS

### Clinical Features

- A history of a predisposing underlying condition (CVI, AVMs, or limb prosthesis) is usually present.

- Lesions usually manifest as painless macules and papules involving the extensor surfaces of the lower extremities that evolve slowly into purplish plaques and nodules.

- Predisposition for the toe and ankle, including the malleolus, but on occasion they may involve the anterior and posterior leg (Figure 61-2).[13]

- The color characteristics of the lesions range from red to brown and purplish in color with the majority of end-stage lesions demonstrating a dark purple to violet hue.

- Painful, refractory ulcerations may occur (Figure 61-3).

### Physical Examination

- Attention to physical examination findings may highlight other vascular conditions that are associated with acroangiodermatitis or pseudo-Kaposi sarcoma and aid the clinician in the correct diagnosis. Other entities include intravenous (IV) drug abuse with needle tracks, KTS, and dermatoses of a paralyzed or amputated limb.

- Acroangiodermatitis associated with CVI is usually bilateral with surrounding features of venous hypertension such as stasis dermatitis and lipodermatosclerosis, while unilateral limb involvement is seen in patients with KTS or other vascular malformations.

- Acroangiodermatitis associated with AVMs or Stewart-Bluefarb syndrome presents early in life with unilateral purple-blue macules and papules. The involved leg usually shows increase in length or girth, and an audible bruit and/or a palpable thrill is usually present with the presence of AVMs.

### Laboratory Studies

- Complete blood count (CBC) and chemistry usually reveal no abnormalities. Human immunodeficiency virus (HIV) infection should be ruled out, especially if Kaposi sarcoma is suspected. Tissue biopsy is indicated to histologically differentiate from Kaposi sarcoma. HHV 8 is associated with Kaposi sarcoma, and PCR testing for this virus may be indicated.

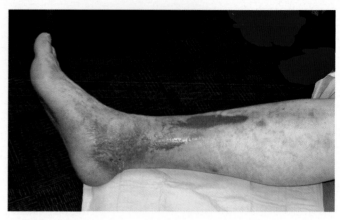

**FIGURE 61-2** Acroangiodermatitis (pseudo-Kaposi sarcoma) presenting as dark purplish plaques involving the anteromedial distal leg associated with stasis dermatitis and a medial malleolus venous ulcer in a patient with marked venous insufficiency. (*Photograph courtesy of Steven M. Dean, DO.*)

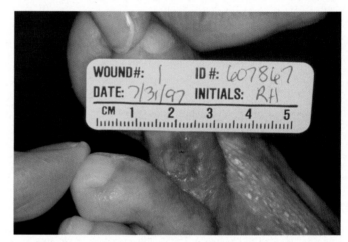

**FIGURE 61-3** Ulcerative acroangiodermatitis along the second toe of a male with a hemolymphatic vascular malformation (Klippel-Trenaunay syndrome [KTS]). The toe was ultimately amputated as the ulceration would not heal despite appropriate therapy. (*Photograph courtesy of Steven M. Dean, DO.*)

## Imaging Studies

- Venous duplex ultrasound to detect underlying venous insufficiency, venous varicosities, and venous malformations or the presence of AVMs
- Arteriography in select cases for improved sensitivity and image acquisition, especially for high clinical probability of AVMs

## Histopathologic Features

- In acroangiodermatitis, biopsy shows dilated capillaries with plump endothelial cells, extravasated erythrocytes, and hemosiderin deposition surrounded by hyperplastic granulation tissue with perivascular mononuclear cells infiltrate in the upper dermis.[14] In Stewart-Bluefarb syndrome, the entire dermis is involved and in large specimens an AV shunt may also be present.
- The proliferating fibroblasts are positive for antifactor XIIIa antibody.[15]
- Immunostaining shows a strong labeling of endothelial cells of the hyperplastic vessels. However, in sharp contrast to Kaposi sarcoma, perivascular cells completely lack CD34 expression.[16]

## DIFFERENTIAL DIAGNOSIS

It is essential to distinguish pseudo-Kaposi sarcoma from similar-looking malignant conditions. The most important distinction is from Kaposi sarcoma that requires histopathologic comparison. Other clinical entities that are similar and may require a biopsy to differentiate are pigmented purpura, vasculitis, and lichen planus.[17]

- In Kaposi sarcoma—thin endothelial cell line, irregular jagged blood vessels align pre-existing vessels. There are characteristic vascular slits and polymorphous hyperchromatic spindle cells that are not seen in pseudo-Kaposi sarcoma.
- In Kaposi sarcoma, both endothelial cells and perivascular spindle cells are CD34 positive. In contrast, perivascular cells of pseudo-Kaposi sarcoma lack CD34 expression.[18]
- Pigmented purpuric dermatitis has dilated capillaries with the absence of plump endothelial cells, dermal fibroblasts, or eosinophils in dermal infiltrates, as seen in pseudo-Kaposi sarcoma.
- Stasis dermatitis differs from pseudo-Kaposi sarcoma by epidermal changes (parakeratosis and spongiosis), deeper dermal involvement, and greater hemosiderin deposition.

## MANAGEMENT

- Treatment is indicated to prevent ulceration, infection, and tissue loss requiring amputation. Therapeutic options should be directed to the primary underlying disorder.
- External compression is the best method and can be combined with topical antibiotics and corticosteroids. Lesion regression and symptomatic relief has been reported with combination manual compression and leg elevation.[13]
- Oral erythromycin and oral dapsone are reported as adjunctive therapeutic options.[14,19]
- Underlying vascular pathology like AVM can be surgically managed with elimination of the shunts and embolization of small fistulae.[20]
- Laser ablation can be used to clear some individual lesions.[21]

- In the case of limb prosthesis, evaluation of the mechanical effect on the stump is warranted.
- Depression screening may be indicated as some patients may be psychologically distressed by the appearance of their affected limb.

## PATIENT EDUCATION

- Education in regard to compression therapy and follow-up physician visits to enforce compliance are paramount to treating venous hypertension.
- Education about skin care and avoiding mechanical trauma that could induce ulceration or bleeding are essential.

## PROVIDER RESOURCES

- http://emedicine.medscape.com/article/1085635-overview
- http://www.piklive.com/?q=Acroangiodermatitis

## REFERENCES

1. Earhart RN, Aeling JA, Nuss DD, Mellette JR. Pseudo-Kaposi sarcoma. A patient with arteriovenous malformation and skin lesions simulating Kaposi sarcoma. *Arch Dermatol.* 1974;110: 907-910.

2. Mali JW, Kuiper JP, Hamers AA. Acro-angiodermatitis of the foot. *Arch Dermatol.* 1965;92:515-518.

3. Bluefarb SM, Adams LA. Arteriovenous malformation with angiodermatitis. Stasis dermatitis simulating Kaposi's disease. *Arch Dermatol.* 1967;96:176-181.

4. Landthaler M, Langehenke H, Holzmann H, Braun-Falco O. Mali's acroangiodermatitis (pseudo-Kaposi) in paralyzed legs. *Hautarzt.* 1988;39:304-307.

5. Sbano P, Miracco C, Risulo M, Fimiani M. Acroangiodermatitis (pseudo-Kaposi sarcoma) associated with verrucous hyperplasia induced by suction-socket lower limb prosthesis. *J Cutan Pathol.* 2005;32:429-432.

6. Kim TH, Kim KH, Kang JS, Kim JH, Hwang IY. Pseudo-Kaposi's sarcoma associated with acquired arteriovenous fistula. *J Dermatol.* 1997;24:28-33.

7. Lyle WG, Given KS. Acroangiodermatitis (pseudo-Kaposi's sarcoma) associated with Klippel-Trenaunay syndrome. *Ann Plast Surg.* 1996;37:654-656.

8. Scholz S, Schuller-Petrovic S, Kerl H. Mali acroangiodermatitis in homozygous activated protein C resistance. *Arch Dermatol.* 2005;141:396-397.

9. Martin L, MacHet L, Michalak S, et al. Acroangiodermatitis in a carrier of the thrombophilic 20210A mutation in the prothrombin gene. *Br J Dermatol.* 1999;141:752.

10. Lugovic L, Pusic J, Situm M, et al. Acroangiodermatitis (pseudo-Kaposi sarcoma): three case reports. *Acta Dermatovenerol Croat.* 2007;15:152-157.

11. Hueso L, Llombart B, Alfaro-Rubio A, et al. Stewart-Bluefarb syndrome. *Actas Dermosifiliogr.* 2007;98:545-548.

12. Requena L, Farina MC, Renedo G, Alvarez A, Yus ES, Sangueza OP. Intravascular and diffuse dermal reactive angioendotheliomatosis secondary to iatrogenic arteriovenous fistulas. *J Cutan Pathol*. 1999;26:159-164.

13. Pimentel MI, Cuzzi T, de Azeredo-Coutinho RB, Vasconcellos Ede C, Benzi TS, de Carvalho LM. Acroangiodermatitis (pseudo-Kaposi sarcoma): a rarely-recognized condition. A case on the plantar aspect of the foot associated with chronic venous insufficiency. *An Bras Dermatol*. 2011;86(4 suppl 1):S13-S16.

14. Mehta AA, Pereira RR, Nayak CS, Dhurat RS. Acroangiodermatitis of mali: a rare vascular phenomenon. *Indian J Dermatol Venereol Leprol*. 2010;76:553-556.

15. Murakami Y, Nagae S, Hori Y. Factor XIIIa expression in pseudo-Kaposi sarcoma. *J Dermatol*. 1991;18:661-666.

16. Kanitakis J, Narvaez D, Claudy A. Expression of the CD34 antigen distinguishes Kaposi's sarcoma from pseudo-Kaposi's sarcoma (acroangiodermatitis). *Br J Dermatol*. 1996;134:44-46.

17. Hung NA, Strack M, Van Rij A, North CJ, Blennerhassett JB. Spontaneous acroangiodermatitis in a young woman. *Dermatol Online J*. 2004;10:8.

18. Rao B, Unis M, Poulos E. Acroangiodermatitis: a study of ten cases. *Int J Dermatol*. 1994;33:179-183.

19. Rashkovsky I, Gilead L, Schamroth J, Leibovici V. Acro-angiodermatitis: review of the literature and report of a case. *Acta Derm Venereol*. 1995;75:475-478.

20. Agrawal S, Rizal A, Agrawal CS, Anshu A. Pseudo-Kaposi's sarcoma (Bluefarb-Stewart type). *Int J Dermatol*. 2005;44:136-138.

21. Rongioletti F, Rebora A. Cutaneous reactive angiomatoses: patterns and classification of reactive vascular proliferation. *J Am Acad Dermatol*. 2003;49:887-896.

# 62 HEPARIN-, LOW–MOLECULAR WEIGHT HEPARIN–, AND WARFARIN-INDUCED SKIN NECROSIS

Aditya M. Sharma, MD
John R. Bartholomew, MD, FACC, MSVM

## PATIENT STORY

A 53-year-old woman was treated with intravenous unfractionated heparin (UFH) for an acute pulmonary embolism. She was started on 10 mg of warfarin on her fourth day of heparin therapy. Her baseline platelet count was normal, but decreased to $86 \times 10^9/L$ by day 7 of treatment. Her international normalized ratio (INR) was 3.2 at that time and heparin was discontinued. A platelet factor 4 (PF 4)–heparin immunoassay was found to be positive, consistent with a diagnosis of heparin-induced thrombocytopenia (HIT). Three days later she developed a violaceous discoloration of both breasts that progressed to full-thickness skin necrosis and warfarin-induced skin necrosis was diagnosed (Figure 62-1). Warfarin was discontinued and the direct thrombin inhibitor (lepirudin) instituted as the platelet count dropped further to $22 \times 10^9/L$. She ultimately required extensive surgical debridement of both the breasts and reconstructive surgery. Warfarin was later resumed cautiously at 1 mg/d after full platelet recovery (overlapped with lepirudin) until the INR was therapeutic (>2) for two consecutive days.

## HEPARIN- AND LOW–MOLECULAR WEIGHT HEPARIN–INDUCED SKIN NECROSIS

### EPIDEMIOLOGY

- Severe anticoagulant-induced skin reactions that can develop following subcutaneous injection of heparin (UFH) or any of the low–molecular weight heparin (LMWH) preparations.[1-5] It can also be seen following intravenous UFH administration.[3,4,7]

- More commonly seen in patients receiving UFH than LMWH. It has been reported in most of the LMWH preparations including dalteparin, enoxaparin, tinzaparin, tedelparin, certoparin, and nadroparin.[4]

- Incidence likely underestimated due to either under-recognition and/or under-reporting.

- An uncommon manifestation of HIT.

- Most patients (50%-75%) will not develop thrombocytopenia despite the presence of heparin-dependent antibodies. However, if antibodies are present they are a marker for HIT.[2,4,5]

- Only 10% to 20% of patients who develop HIT antibodies during subcutaneous administration of UFH or LMWH will develop skin lesions.[2]

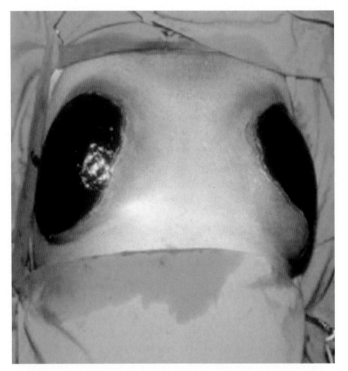

**FIGURE 62-1** This patient, described in the patient story, developed heparin-induced thrombocytopenia (HIT) following unfractionated heparin (UFH) administration for an acute pulmonary embolism. She was started on warfarin prior to correction of her platelet count and developed violaceous discoloration of both the breasts that progressed to full-thickness skin necrosis and eventual skin grafting. (With permission from the *Archives of Internal Medicine.* 2004;164:66-70.)

## ETIOLOGY AND PATHOPHYSIOLOGY

- Generally develops in conjunction with HIT, an immunologic reaction triggered by the binding of heparin to PF 4 resulting in the formation of heparin-dependent antibodies that can cause thrombocytopenia and venous and/or arterial thrombosis.[1,2,4,5]

- Patients often have other comorbid conditions such as hypertension, diabetes mellitus and obesity, underlying malignancy, or a connective tissue disease.[1]

## DIAGNOSIS

### Clinical Features

- Consider in any patient who develops a skin reaction while receiving subcutaneous UFH or LMWH or intravenous UFH (Figure 62-2).

- Lesions appear suddenly and vary from tender, local erythematous plaques to painful sharply delineated necrotic lesions with a cuff of erythema or violaceous discoloration surrounding the necrosis (Figure 62-3).[2,5,6]

- Lesions may be multiple.

- Skin manifestations have also been reported with other unusual presentations of HIT such as adrenal hemorrhagic infarction and severe acute anaphylactoid reaction.[2,5]

### Typical Distribution

- Most commonly found at the injection site, although they may be found at distal sites, especially regions with extensive subcutaneous fat tissue such as the buttocks, thighs, breasts, or abdomen.[4]

## LABORATORY STUDIES

- Thrombocytopenia, defined as a platelet count less than $150 \times 10^9/L$ or 50% or greater drop from preadministration levels in patients receiving UFH or LMWH who are considered at risk for HIT.

- Obtain heparin antibodies, an immunologic study (PF 4–heparin immunoassay), and/or a functional test (serotonin release assay).

- Majority of patients with heparin-induced skin necrosis (HISN) will have serologic confirmation of HIT.

- Skin biopsy demonstrates extensive focal epidermal necrosis with marked neutrophil infiltration and extensive fibrin deposition within the capillaries and venules of the dermis without any evidence of vasculitis.[1]

## DIFFERENTIAL DIAGNOSIS

- A number of conditions can mimic HISN (Table 62-1).[7]

- Important to recognize that HISN is similar in appearance to warfarin-induced skin necrosis (WISN), although several factors help differentiate these two[3]:
  - Timing—HISN generally develops between days 5 and 14, while WISN classically develops earlier between days 3 and 7.
  - There is no immunologic basis for WISN.
  - WISN does not induce thrombocytopenia, platelet aggregation, or arteriovenous thrombosis.

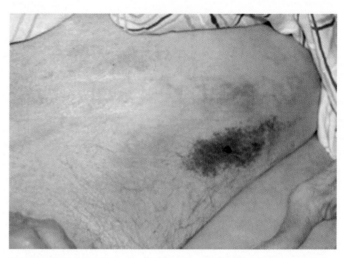

**FIGURE 62-2** Heparin-induced skin necrosis (HISN) seen in an elderly female at the site of a subcutaneous heparin injection. Note the erythematous border surrounding the central area of ischemia.

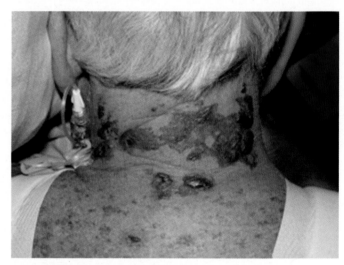

**FIGURE 62-3** An example of a heparin-induced skin reaction that did not result in necrosis. Although most commonly found at the subcutaneous heparin injection site, these multiple purpuric papules were found in the neck region of a patient receiving intravenous heparin.

## MANAGEMENT

- Instruct patients, nurses, and physicians to look for early cutaneous signs of intolerance (tender areas of erythema at the UFH or LMWH injection site) or anywhere on the skin.

- Particular attention should be made to any patient complaining of pain or erythema at UFH or LMWH injection sites.

- Immediate discontinuation of UFH or LMWH is mandatory once the diagnosis of HISN is suspected. Converting to LMWH for patients receiving UFH is not recommended because of cross-reactivity between these two anticoagulants.[1,2]

- Treatment using a direct thrombin inhibitor (DTI) such as lepirudin, bivalirudin, or argatroban or the low–molecular weight heparinoid, danaparoid (no longer available in the United States) is recommended.

- Avoid warfarin if the patient has HIT, until the platelet count has recovered to $150 \times 10^9$/L or greater.[8]

- Small necrotic lesions should be treated conservatively with topical agents. Large necrotic lesions usually require surgical debridement with or without skin grafting.

## WARFARIN-INDUCED SKIN NECROSIS

### EPIDEMIOLOGY

- Reported in patients taking vitamin K antagonists including any of the following preparations: warfarin, bishydroxycoumarin, phenprocoumon, and acenocoumarol.

- Estimated to occur in 0.01% to 0.1% of patients taking warfarin.

- Women are four times more likely to develop than men.[9]

- Predominantly seen in areas of increased subcutaneous fat including the breasts, buttocks, and thighs.[10,11]

### ETIOLOGY AND PATHOPHYSIOLOGY

- Warfarin can rarely cause WISN during its initial period of administration by decreasing the functional activity and synthesis of the vitamin K–dependent proteins II, VII, IX, and X and the natural anticoagulant proteins C and S. Depletion of protein C (which has a shorter half-life than the procoagulant factors II, IX, and X) may result in a transient hypercoagulable state that can cause thrombosis of cutaneous vessels and WISN.[12-14]

- Patients with protein C deficiency are at greater risk of developing WISN, although it has been reported in patients with a lupus anticoagulant, antithrombin, and protein S deficiencies and in patients who receive large loading doses of warfarin.

- Also associated in HIT, especially when warfarin has been initiated before the platelet count has recovered and in patients who develop a supratherapeutic INR during induction of warfarin therapy.[13,14]

- Most commonly develops in individuals being treated for a deep vein thrombosis or pulmonary embolism.

**TABLE 62-1.** The Differential Diagnosis for Anticoagulant-Induced Skin Reactions[7]

| |
|---|
| Warfarin-induced skin necrosis (WISN) |
| Heparin-induced skin necrosis (HISN) |
| Low–molecular weight heparin (LMWH) skin necrosis |
| Purpura fulminans |
| Pyoderma gangrenosum |
| Ecthyma gangrenosum |
| Necrotizing fasciitis |
| Infective endocarditis |
| Atheroembolism |
| Pressure ulcers |
| Calciphylaxis |
| Disseminated intravascular coagulation (DIC) |
| Cryofibrinogenemia |
| Antiphospholipid syndrome |
| Systemic vasculitis (cryoglobulinemia, systemic lupus erythematosus) |

## DIAGNOSIS

### Clinical Features

- Mainly affects obese, middle-aged women.
- Initial presentation consists of a painful pressure-like sensation or paresthesias followed by a petechial rash that progresses to an erythematous macule and blue-black ecchymosis. This rapidly evolves to hemorrhagic bullae and full-thickness skin necrosis.[9-11]
- Characteristically presents as single lesions occurring unilaterally; however, up to one-third of patients will have multiple lesions.[9,14]
- Usually occurs within the first 3 to 7 days of initiating warfarin therapy.

### Typical Distribution

- WISN typically occurs in areas of extensive subcutaneous fat such as the breasts, buttocks, abdomen, and thighs. It may be seen in other areas such as the face, arms, calves, back, and on the penis.[9,12]
- In the setting of HIT, may also present as venous limb gangrene, a condition defined as progression of a deep vein thrombosis to limb necrosis despite palpable or Doppler-identifiable arterial pulses.[13]

## LABORATORY STUDIES

- Evaluate protein C activity levels once the acute event has subsided and/or the patient is off warfarin. May also consider checking for the presence of a lupus anticoagulant, protein S, or antithrombin levels if protein C levels are normal.
- Determine the INR, check the platelet count, and measure anti-PF 4 or heparin antibodies, especially if the INR is supratherapeutic.
- Biopsies display cutaneous tissue necrosis, thrombosis of dermal veins, subcutaneous capillaries, venules, and deep veins with diffuse fat necrosis and interstitial hemorrhage.[12]

## DIFFERENTIAL DIAGNOSIS

- The differential diagnoses are the same as those for HISN[7] (Table 62-1).

## MANAGEMENT

- Awareness of this unusual adverse reaction to warfarin is extremely crucial as early recognition and management can be limb and/or lifesaving, especially in the patient with HIT.
- Clinicians and other health care givers must be attentive to patients complaining of localized skin discomfort or pain, especially in areas of extensive subcutaneous fat such as the breasts, thighs, or buttocks.
- Immediate cessation of warfarin therapy and reversal of its effects with fresh frozen plasma and vitamin K is mandatory.[8,13,14]
- Use of an alternate anticoagulant such as UFH or LMWH is recommended until the necrotic lesion heals, unless HIT is suspected or diagnosed.[1,9,10,12]
- Warfarin can be reintroduced but it should be used with extreme caution and initiated only at low doses (1-2 mg/d) in combination with a parenteral anticoagulant over an extended period of time up to 14 days.[1]

- Protein C concentrates have been used in patients with protein C deficiency. Prevention of the progression of the skin lesions and/or regression has been reported.[1,9,12]
- If HIT is diagnosed, a DTI should be initiated and warfarin should not be started until the patient improves clinically and the platelet count recovers to $150 \times 10^9/L$ or greater.[8,14,15] Once initiated, modest doses of warfarin should be used, avoiding an overshoot of the INR, and it should be overlapped with a DTI for a minimum of 5 days.[8,14]
- Small necrotic lesions are usually managed conservatively with topical agents. However, large necrotic lesions may require surgical debridement with or without skin grafting, and reconstructive surgery or amputation may be necessary.

## PATIENT EDUCATION

- Instruct patients about the potential for adverse skin reactions when using UFH, LMWH, or vitamin K antagonists such as warfarin.
- Reassure the patient that these conditions are usually self-limited if identified early.
- Patients should be educated to avoid UFH or LMWH preparations in the future and to inform all of their physicians of the complications they have experienced with warfarin, UFH, or LMWH.

## FOLLOW-UP

- Routine follow-up is necessary until the skin lesions have healed. Future recommendations regarding the use of anticoagulant therapy is essential.

### PROVIDER RESOURCES

- http://dermnetnz.org/reactions/warfarin-necrosis.html
- http://www.ncbi.nlm.nih.gov/pubmed/22315270

### PATIENT RESOURCE

- http://www.realself.com/answer/what-coumadin-induced-skin-necrosis-10-things-you-need-know

## REFERENCES

1. Harenberg, J, Hoffmann U, Huhle G, Winkler M, Bayerl C. Cutaneous reactions to anticoagulants. Recognition and management. *Am J Clin Dermatol.* 2001;2(2):69-75.
2. Warkentin TE, Roberts RS, Hirsh J, Kelton JG. Heparin-induced skin lesions and other unusual sequelae of the heparin-induced thrombocytopenia syndrome: a nested cohort study. *Chest.* 2005;127(5):1857-1861.
3. White PW, Sadd JR, Nensel RE. Thrombotic complications of heparin therapy: including six cases of heparin-induced skin necrosis. *Ann Surg.* 1979;190(5):595-608.
4. Handschin AE, Trentz O, Kock HJ, Wanner GA. Low molecular weight heparin-induced skin necrosis—a systematic review. *Langenbecks Arch Surg.* 2005;390(3):249-254.

5. Warkentin TE. Heparin-induced skin lesions. *Br J Haematol*. 1996;92(2):494-497.

6. Shelley WB, Sayen JJ. Heparin necrosis: an anticoagulant-induced cutaneous infarct. *J Am Acad Dermatol*. 1982;7(5): 674-677.

7. Denton MD, Mauiyyedi S, Bazari H. Heparin-induced skin necrosis in a patient with end-stage renal failure and functional protein S deficiency. *Am J Nephrol*. 2001;21:289-293.

8. Bartholomew JR. Transition to an oral anticoagulant in patients with heparin-induced thrombocytopenia. *Chest*. 2005;127(suppl 2): S27- S34.

9. Howard-Thompson A, Usery JB, Lobo BL, Finch CK. Heparin-induced thrombocytopenia complicated by warfarin-induced skin necrosis. *Am J Health Syst Pharm*. 2008;65:1144-1147.

10. Chan YC, Valenti D, Mansfield AO, Stansby G. Warfarin induced skin necrosis. *Br J Surg*. 2000;87(3):266-272.

11. Cole MS, Minifee PK, Wolma FJ. Coumarin necrosis—a review of the literature. *Surgery*. 1988(103):271-277.

12. Chacon G, Nguyen T, Khan A, Sinha A, Maddirala S. Warfarin-induced skin necrosis mimicking calciphylaxis: a case report and review of the literature. *J Drugs Dermatol*. 2010:9(7):859-863.

13. Warkentin TE, Elavathil LJ, Hayward CP, Johnston MA, Russett JI, Kelton JG. The pathogenesis of venous limb gangrene associated with heparin-induced thrombocytopenia. *Ann Intern Med*. 1997;127(9):804-812.

14. Srinivasan AF, Rice L, Bartholomew JR, et al. Warfarin-induced skin necrosis and venous limb gangrene in the setting of heparin-induced thrombocytopenia. *Arch Intern Med*. 2004; 164(1):66-70.

15. Warkentin TE, Greinacher A, Koster A, Lincoff AM. Treatment and prevention of heparin-induced thrombocytopenia. American College of Chest Physicians evidence-based clinical practice guidelines (8th edition). *Chest*. 2008;133:S340-S380.

# 63 OVERVIEW OF SPIDER, RETICULAR, AND VARICOSE VEINS

Sapan S. Desai, MD, PhD
Eric Mowatt-Larssen, MD

## PATIENT STORY

A 44-year-old man presents with a 5-year history of progressive right lower extremity pain, discomfort, swelling and prominent calf veins (Figure 63-1). His symptoms occur daily, and are worse with standing, particularly during his job as a nurse working 12-hour shifts in the emergency department. Overnight his symptoms improve. He has no other known past medical history, including that of venous thromboembolism. He is interested in an intervention to improve his quality of life. Physical examination is notable only for large medial calf varicose veins and mild pitting edema around the ankle.

## CLINICAL FEATURES

- Patients have symptoms that range from asymptomatic to severe pain or discomfort. Patients may also present with lower extremity swelling, a distal calf rash, or a leg ulcer.[1]

- Pain or discomfort is the most common symptom of chronic venous disease. The symptoms are usually described as achiness, cramping, fatigue, heaviness, itching, or throbbing. The pain and discomfort are often located at varicosity sites, at the medial extremity (for great saphenous vein reflux—Figure 63-2) or posterolateral calf (for small saphenous vein reflux).

- Pain, discomfort, and/or swelling are usually worse with dependence (eg, standing) and improve with extremity elevation or compression.

- Swelling and skin changes tend to start around the ankle, but can gradually progress proximally over years (Figure 63-3).

- Leg ulcers tend to occur around the ankle or medial or lateral foot (Figure 63-4).

- Physical findings are described using the CEAP (Clinical-Etiology-Anatomy-Pathophysiology) class (Table 63-1). Higher CEAP classes indicate more advanced venous disease.[2]

- Spider veins (Figures 63-5 and 63-6) are often, but not always, asymptomatic.

- Unlike varicose veins (Figure 63-7), reticular veins (Figure 63-8) typically do not protrude from the skin surface.

## EPIDEMIOLOGY AND RISK FACTORS

- 20% of adults have varicose veins. Prevalence increases with age.[3]

- 5% of adults have venous skin changes.

- 1% of adults have or have had a venous ulcer.

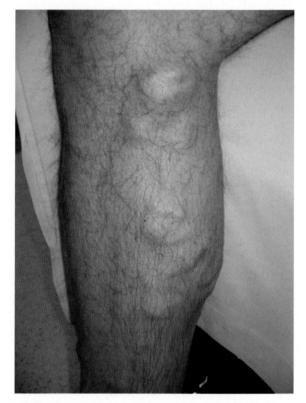

**FIGURE 63-1** This patient has classic varicose veins. Varicosities are blue, subcutaneous, tortuous veins over 3 mm in diameter.

- Risk factors for varicose veins are advanced age, positive family history, female gender, and multiparity.

- Risk factors for chronic venous insufficiency are advanced age, positive family history, and obesity.

## PATHOPHYSIOLOGY

- Lower extremity veins have bicuspid one-way valves to keep blood flowing toward the heart during dependence (eg, standing).[4]

- Reflux is abnormal retrograde flow of blood in the thigh and calf. It represents valve failure and is defined as an abnormally long valve closure time (0.5 second for most of the superficial lower extremity veins, except 1 second for femoropopliteal system).

- Reflux is the most common cause of chronic venous disease. Reflux spreads to proximal or distal segments over time. It is caused by vein wall and/or valve weakness.

- Veins can also become obstructed from chronic deep vein thrombosis (DVT) or anatomic obstruction (eg, May-Thurner syndrome or tumor compression). Chronic venous obstruction also causes chronic venous disease.

- Combined reflux and obstruction also occur, and usually result in worse signs and symptoms than either process alone.

- Chronic venous disease at all CEAP classes is commonly caused by saphenous reflux. More advanced venous disease (ie, CEAP classes C3-C6) tend to involve perforator and deep reflux as well.

- Patients in CEAP classes C3 to C6 have chronic venous insufficiency. These patients have ambulatory venous hypertension (AVH): inability to lower venous pressure when the lower extremity is dependent. Over time, AVH leads to edema, skin changes, and ulcers.

- The constant effect of AVH through the effects of gravity on a refluxing vein system leads to the accumulation of blood in the dependent extremities. This eventually leads to capillary outflow of fluid, contributing to the edema in the lower leg. The increased pressure stretches the vein wall, producing the red blood cell leakage, resulting in hyperpigmentation, and chronic skin inflammation.

## DIAGNOSIS

- Duplex ultrasound is the most important initial test since it accurately identifies venous reflux or obstruction. The saphenous, perforator, and deep systems are interrogated. A "rule out DVT" venous study is not sufficient to diagnose and treat chronic venous disease. Management of chronic venous disease is based on the map where reflux begins and ends.[5]

- Duplex ultrasound helps to identify the cause for venous disease, along with delineating the anatomy of the venous system. Duplex ultrasound uses a combination of color flow imaging and Doppler signals to determine the flow vectors and thereby identify sites of reflux.

- The differential diagnosis for the patient with extremity pain or discomfort includes peripheral arterial disease, neuropathy (often lumbar radiculopathy), muscle pain, and compartment syndrome.

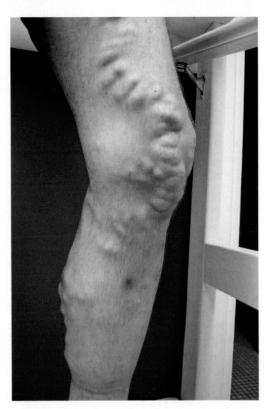

**FIGURE 63-2** Large protuberant varicose vein along the anteromedial thigh and medial calf. This represents a tributary of an underlying incompetent great saphenous vein.

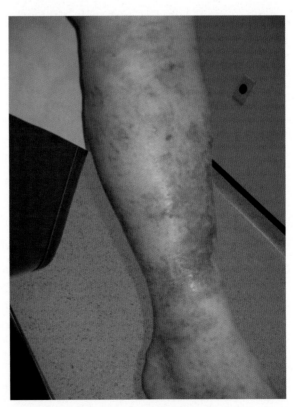

**FIGURE 63-3** Hyperpigmentation along the anteromedial calf with surrounding spider and small varicose veins.

- Causes of leg ulcer include peripheral arterial disease, neuropathy (especially diabetes mellitus), chronic mechanical compression (as in paraplegia), and skin cancer.

- None of the common skin changes seen are specific for chronic venous disease. Dermatology consult or further workup should be considered in patients with skin changes without significant vein diagnosis.

- Patients with unilateral leg edema may have lymphedema or proximal venous obstruction. Patients with bilateral lower extremity edema may also have congestive heart failure, lipedema, kidney disease, liver failure, or proximal venous obstruction.

- Patients with pelvic congestion syndrome can present with proximal thigh varicosities. They often have chronic pelvic pain and/or pelvic varicosities. Diagnosis of ovarian or other pelvic vein reflux can be made by transvaginal ultrasound, conventional venography, magnetic resonance venography (MRV), or computerized tomography venography (CTV), depending on the capabilities of the facility.

- Patients with venous-type symptoms out of proportion to findings on infrainguinal ultrasound or history of DVT may have iliocaval obstruction from anatomic obstruction (May-Thurner), thrombotic obstruction, or tumor. Imaging to check for these diagnoses

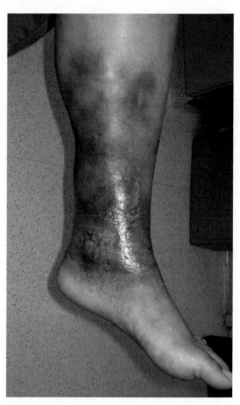

FIGURE 63-4 Severe venous stasis with a combination of hyperpigmentation, lipodermatosclerosis, eczematous crusting, and small stasis ulceration.

TABLE 63-1. CEAP Classes

| CEAP Class | Physical Finding | Definition |
|---|---|---|
| C0 | None | None |
| C1 | Spider veins | Dilated intradermal venules less than 1 mm in diameter (Figures 63-5 and 63-6) |
| C1 | Reticular veins | Dilated blue subdermal vein 1 to 3 mm in diameter, usually tortuous (Figure 63-7) |
| C2 | Varicose veins | Dilated subcutaneous vein greater than 3 mm in diameter, usually tortuous (Figures 63-1, 63-2, and 63-8) |
| C3 | Edema | Increase in skin and subcutaneous fluid volume, usually indents with pressure |
| C4a | Eczema | Erythematous dermatitis, can progress to weeping, blistering, or scaling |
| C4a | Hyperpigmentation | Localized brown skin discoloration (Figures 63-3 and 63-4) |
| C4b | Atrophie blanche | Localized, circular, white, and atrophic skin areas surrounded by dilated capillaries and sometimes hyperpigmentation |
| C4b | Lipodermatosclerosis | Localized chronic inflammation and fibrosis of skin and subcutaneous tissues, sometimes associated with contracture or scarring (Figure 63-4) |
| C5 | Healed venous ulcer | |
| C6 | Active venous ulcer | Full-thickness skin defect (Figure 63-4) |

Adapted from Eklöf B, Rutherford RB, JJ Bergan et al. By consensus, the patient CEAP class is the highest class physical finding. For example, a patient with spider veins, varicose veins, and lipodermatosclerosis is class C4b.

include intravascular ultrasound, transvaginal ultrasound, conventional venography, MRV, or CTV, depending on the capabilities of the facility.[6]

## TREATMENT

• Compression therapy is used for patients with any level of venous reflux. Compression improves venous hemodynamics and quality of life for patients with chronic venous disease, reduces edema and skin discoloration, and improves the venous ulcer healing rate.[7] The main contraindication to compression use is peripheral arterial disease, especially with ankle-brachial index (ABI) less than 0.5. Commercially available compression stockings are most often used.

• Inelastic compression, such as Unna boots, is also used in patients with active ulcers. Compression is also used after most other vein treatments, including surgery, thermal ablation, and sclerotherapy.

• Reflux is corrected in the following order: saphenous, epifascial, perforator, deep. The main contraindication to treatment of reflux is venous obstruction. Treating great saphenous reflux often corrects small saphenous vein, perforator, or deep venous reflux. Superficial reflux correction also carries less patient morbidity than deep venous reflux correction.[8]

• Correction of saphenous reflux in patients with varicose veins improves quality of life.

• Correction of saphenous reflux in patients with active or healed venous ulcers reduces ulcer recurrence risk by 25% absolute.

• Endovenous laser ablation (EVLA), radiofrequency ablation (RFA), ultrasound-guided foam sclerotherapy (UGFS), and great saphenous vein high ligation and stripping can be used to correct saphenous reflux. EVLA, RFA, and UGFS all cause eventual fibrosis of the treated vein. Heat is used to cause the fibrosis for EVLA and RFA, and chemical sclerosis in UGFS. The fibrosis results in ablation, or lack of blood flow, which is verified by postoperative ultrasound.[9]

• Sclerotherapy and ambulatory phlebectomy are used to correct epifascial veins.

• EVLA, RFA, UGFS, and subfascial endoscopic perforator surgery (SEPS) can be used to correct perforator reflux when indicated.

• Deep vein correction options include valvuloplasty, bypass, and other procedures, and are only performed in cases of severe disease at specialized centers.

**FIGURE 63-5** Small spider veins or telangiectasias.

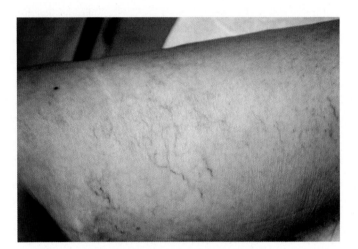

**FIGURE 63-6** Blue and red telangiectasias.

## REFERENCES

1. Caggiati A, Rosi C, Heyen R, et al. Age-related variations of varicose veins anatomy. *J Vasc Surg*. 2006;44:1291-1295.

2. Porter JM, Moneta GL. Reporting standards in venous disease: an update. International Consensus Committee on Chronic Venous Disease. *J Vasc Surg*. 1995;21:635-645.

3. Beebe-Dimmer JL, Pfeifer JR, Engle JS, et al. The epidemiology of chronic venous insufficiency and varicose veins. *Ann Epidemiol*. 2005;15:175-184.

4. Labropoulos N, Mansour MA, Kang SS, et al. New insight into perforator vein incompetence. *Euro J Vasc Surg*. 1999;18:228-234.

5. Neglen P, Egger JF, Olivier J, Raju S. Hemodynamic and clinical impact of ultrasound-derived venous reflux parameters. *J Vasc Surg*. 2004;40:303-310.

6. O'Meara S, Cullum NA, Nelson EA. Compression for venous leg ulcers. *Cochrane Database Syst Rev*. 2009;3:1-143.

7. Labropoulos N, Tiongson J, Pryor L, et al. Nonsaphenous superficial vein reflux. *J Vasc Surg*. 2001;34:872-877.

8. Shortell C, Rhodes JR, Johanssen M, et al. Radiofrequency ablation for superficial venous reflux: improved outcomes in a high volume university setting. Paper presented at: the SVS Annual Meeting; June 12, 2005; Chicago, IL.

9. Bergan J. Inversion stripping of the saphenous vein. In: Bergan JJ, ed. *The Vein Book*. New York, NY: Elsevier; 2007:231-237.

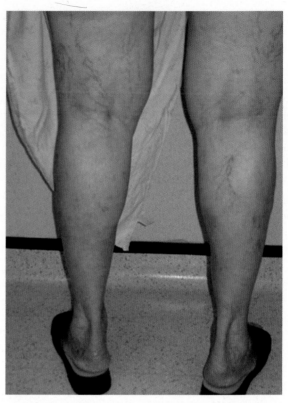

**FIGURE 63-7** A combination of spider and reticular veins along the posterior thighs and calves.

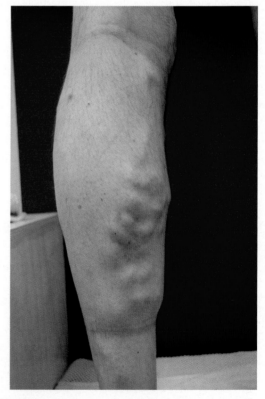

**FIGURE 63-8** Large varicose vein overlying the posterior calf. (*Copyright Eric Mowatt-Larssen, used with permission.*)

# 64 SCLEROTHERAPY

Bhagwan Satiani MD, MBA, RPVI, FACS

## PATIENT STORY

A 40-year-old otherwise healthy school teacher presented with disfiguring spider and reticular veins on the posterior-lateral aspect of her left thigh. Her spider veins appeared in her mid-twenties and worsened with each childbirth. She was concerned about the appearance of this area since she was starting to take her young children to the swimming pool in the summer months. She described no pain but experienced occasional burning and stinging.

Physical examination showed no large varicosities. Her left lateral thigh and popliteal area was covered with a number of 2- to 3-mm reticular veins and by clusters of spider veins. Foam sclerotherapy was chosen as the treatment with good results (Figure 64-1).

## PATHOPHYSIOLOGY

- An elevated venous pressure in the subdermal capillaries is blamed for spider veins. Valvular incompetence in the larger axial veins and pressure secondary to reflux of blood into the superficial cutaneous capillaries may also cause enlargement of reticular and spider veins.

- Other etiologic factors blamed for varicose and spider veins include aging, sun exposure, hormonal shifts, smoking, alcohol intake, obesity, occupation, heredity, pregnancy, and birth control hormonal medications.

- There is some speculation that endothelial cells and endothelin receptor density and distribution may play a role in the development of varicose veins.[1]

## CLINICAL FEATURES

- Spider and reticular veins are most often located on the legs and thighs in women, although they occur on the nose and face as well. Men can develop spider veins as well.

- Although asymptomatic for the most part, some patients with large reticular and extensive spider veins complain of burning, stinging, swelling, throbbing, cramping, and leg fatigue.

- A bluish subdermal reticular pattern of veins may be visible in patients with pale translucent skin.

## DIAGNOSIS

- A variety of small veins are visible on physical examination. These small vessels include telangiectasia, venulectasia, and reticular ecstasias.

- Telangiectasias are flat red vessels, very close to the skin surface, and less than 1 mm in diameter.

- Venulectasias are bluish in color, sometimes distended and barely above the skin surface, and less than 2 mm in diameter.

- Reticular veins have a dark bluish or cyanotic hue and are between 2 and 4 mm in diameter.

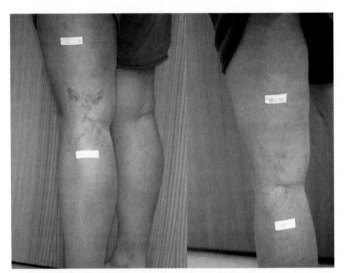

**FIGURE 64-1** Left: Pretreatment photograph of the thigh area with visible reticular and spider veins. Right: Posttreatment appearance of the thigh veins a few weeks following sclerotherapy.

- Varicose veins are generally larger (>3-4 mm in diameter), protrude above the skin surface, and compress easily with slight manual pressure.

## DIFFERENTIAL DIAGNOSIS

- Dermatologic conditions with or without pigmentation can be mistaken for small varicose veins.
- Capillary malformations associated with congenital venous malformations can also be confused with reticular and spider veins.
- Cellulitis.
- Stasis dermatitis.
- Osler-Weber-Rendu syndrome or hereditary hemorrhagic telangiectasia.

## INVESTIGATIONS

- Laboratory tests do not contribute anything to the management of spider and reticular veins.
- Doppler tests are also not usually indicated unless there is suspicion of saphenous vein or deep vein reflux. If there are large feeding veins or large branches originating from the great or small saphenous veins (GSVs or SSVs), a duplex ultrasound scan is needed to locate incompetence of valves in these large axial veins. In the presence of reflux in these axial veins, sclerotherapy of spider or reticular veins will fail or temporary success will be followed by recurrence.

## MANAGEMENT

- Sclerotherapy is used for superficial cutaneous or subdermal varicose veins, residual or recurring varicose veins following surgery, and spider or reticular veins.
- Sclerotherapy using liquids such as sodium tetradecyl sulfate (Sotradecol) or polidocanol have been used for many years to obliterate spider veins (<3 mm diameter) or reticular veins. Injection of these liquids leads to endothelial destruction and then fibrosis and reabsorption, leading to elimination of the superficial veins.
- Recent progress has been made in using foam sclerotherapy (air mixed with detergent solution to create foam) for sclerosing larger varicosities, recurrent veins, and even venous malformations.
- The best results are obtained in patients with competent large superficial axial veins (GSVs or SSVs). A recent Cochrane review supports the role of sclerotherapy for small veins or recurrent veins after surgery.[2]
- Foam sclerotherapy has been successfully utilizing various agents with obliteration of the GSV in 88%.[3] A small tuberculin syringe with a 30-gauge needle is used for reticular and spider veins.
- Magnification is essential in accurately injecting intraluminally and avoiding extravasation, which can be painful and cause skin necrosis.
- No anesthesia is required for sclerotherapy. Occasionally topical anesthesia is utilized for laser ablation of spider veins.

- Ultrasonographic guidance may prove useful when sclerotherapy is used for larger subdermal veins that are noted to feed the superficial spider veins.
- Other options include laser and intense-pulsed-light (IPL) therapy.
- Although the use of liquid or foam sclerotherapy in the treatment of the axial GSVs or SSVs has been controversial, an increasing number of studies have demonstrated its safety. Ultrasound-guided foam sclerotherapy for primary varicose veins or recurrent veins has shown good results with minimal complications, although follow-up sclerotherapy sessions may be required.

## COMPLICATIONS

- Besides unsuccessful obliteration of the veins, common side effects include hyperpigmentation, skin necrosis, matting, ulceration, and rarely anaphylactic or allergic reactions.
- Neurologic complications such as transient ischemic attacks or strokes are rare. Visual disturbances are often described with foam sclerotherapy. Occasional headaches or even migraine with an aura following treatment also occur. The overall incidence of all neurologic complications is reported to be around 0.9%.[4]
- Pulmonary embolism is extremely rare.

## PATIENT EDUCATION

- Patients must also be warned about unusual side effects such as transient neurologic symptoms including transient ischemic attacks, migraine-like headaches, or visual disturbances.
- Compulsive wearing of stockings post-therapy has been traditionally emphasized to decrease the incidence of hyperpigmentation or matting, which is an appearance of new small capillaries around the site of treatment.
- Patients must be informed prior to treatment with sclerotherapy or laser of the need for more than one treatment to successfully obliterate the veins.

## FOLLOW-UP

- Following sclerotherapy all patients must be followed up for inspection of the local area and detection of possible superficial or deep venous thrombosis and rarely systemic side effects.
- Compliance with stockings is repeatedly emphasized.
- Since hyperpigmentation occurs in 10% to 30% of patients, patients are instructed to avoid heavy sun exposure while the injected areas are healing.[5] In addition, evacuation of microthrombus inside the occluded and sclerosed veins is advised to reduce the chances of hyperpigmentation. Patients must therefore return, often more than once, as part of their treatment.
- In general, hyperpigmentation resolves in 6 to 12 months.[6] Superficial veins greater than 1 mm are more likely to leave pigmentation marks than small spider or deeper varicose veins.

## PROVIDER RESOURCES

- http:// onlinelibrary.wiley.com/doi/10.1002
  /14651858.CD001732. pub2/abstract; jsessionid
  = F623C8F725B9E48E8951D 04C10048054.d04t03.

- http://www.bidmc.org/Centers-and-Departments
  /Departments/Cardiovascular-Institute/Your-Cardiovascular-
  Health/~/media/Files/CentersandDepartments
  /CardioVascular%20Institute/Womens%20Event%202012
  /AlMahameed.ashx

## PATIENT RESOURCE

- http://www.webmd.com/skin-problems-and-treatments
  /cosmetic-procedures-spider-veins

## REFERENCES

1. Agu O, Hamilton G, Baker DM, Dashwood MR. Endothelin receptors in the aetiology and pathophysiology of varicose veins. *Eur J Vasc Endovasc.* 2002;23(2):165-171.

2. Tisi PV, Beverley C, Rees A. Injection sclerotherapy for varicose veins. Editorial Group: Cochrane Peripheral Vascular Diseases Group. Published online: 21 Jan 2009. Available at: http:// onlinelibrary.wiley.com/doi/10.1002/14651858.CD001732. pub2/abstract;jsessionid=F623C8F725B9E48E8951D 04C10048054.d04t03. Accessed December 25, 2011.

3. Smith PC. Chronic venous disease treated by ultrasound guided foam sclerotherapy. *Eur J Vasc Endovasc Surg.* Nov 2006;32(5): 577-583.

4. Bradbury AW, Bate G, Pang K, Darvall KA, Adam DJ. Ultrasound-guided foam sclerotherapy is a safe and clinically effective treatment for superficial venous reflux. *J Vasc Surg.* 2010;52:939-945.

5. Sarvananthan T, Shepherd AC, Willenberg T, Davies AH. Neurological complications of sclerotherapy for varicose veins. *J Vasc Surg.* 2012;55:243-251.

6. Guex J-J, Allaert F-A, Gillet, J-L, Chlier F. Immediate and midterm complications of sclerotherapy report of a prospective multi-center registry of 12,173 sclerotherapy sessions. *Dermatol Surg.* 2005;31:123-128.

# 65 ENDOVENOUS LASER ABLATION FOR VARICOSE VEINS

Bhagwan Satiani, MD, MBA, RPVI, FACS

## PATIENT STORY

A 35-year-old woman, mother of three, presented with a progressive increase in the size of the vein on the inside of her thigh during her pregnancies. She described aching, fatigue, and heaviness as the day wore on and experienced some relief with elevation. She initially related some relief with prescription stockings but steady worsening over the last year. She found it difficult to stand at work or during regular chores at home. Both her parents had intervention for varicose veins.

Her physical examination showed a very large great saphenous vein (GSV) from the mid calf to the groin with some tenderness along the course of the vein without any palpable thrombus. No ulceration or pigmentation was noted at the ankle. Her duplex venous ultrasound examination showed no deep or superficial venous thrombosis but a large-diameter GSV and significant reflux (retrograde flow during a Valsalva maneuver) down to the mid-calf (Figure 65-1).

After discussing various options she elected for ablation of her GSV with a laser (Figure 65-2).

## PATHOPHYSIOLOGY

- The prevalence of varicose veins in the Western population is about 20%.[1]

- The bicuspid venous valves are crucial in promoting unidirectional flow caudal to proximal, with the most important saphenous valve being close to the saphenofemoral junction.

- Most varicose veins probably have a multifactorial etiology, although an intrinsic structural weakness is a likely cause.

- Varicose veins can also occur following deep venous thrombosis or on a congenital basis.

## CLINICAL FEATURES

- Common symptoms of varicose veins include pain, heaviness, aching, burning, fatigue, throbbing, itchiness, and occasionally restless legs syndrome.

- Physical examination should mainly focus on the extremity involved with the patient standing as well as supine. The location, size, and general distribution of the varicose veins are noted and preferably marked on a diagram.

- Palpation as well as auscultation is also recommended to detect pulsatility, thrills, bruits, or any tenderness.

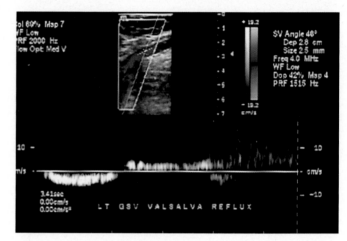

**FIGURE 65-1** Duplex ultrasound venous examination demonstrating reflux (retrograde flow) in the great saphenous vein (GSV).

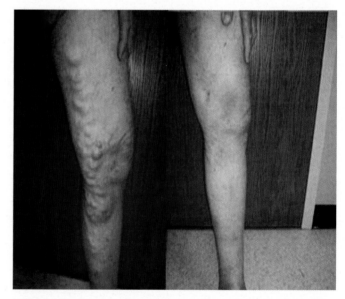

**FIGURE 65-2** Preoperative photograph of the enlarged varicose veins (left image) and a postoperative photograph (right image) following endovenous laser ablation and phlebectomies.

- Signs of chronic disease such as ulceration, skin changes, pigmentation, eczema, temperature changes, and edema should be noted.
- A record of palpable pulses is made.
- The traditional named tests such as Trendelenburg test or Perthes test are now rarely performed, and their utility today is questionable.

## DIAGNOSTIC EVALUATION

- Duplex venous scanning is performed to identify reflux or retrograde flow in the GSV, and to document the vein size and extent of the reflux.
- Normally, Doppler evaluation of the GSV during a Valsalva maneuver results in little retrograde flow through the first valve in a caudal direction. However, in patients with varicose veins due to saphenous vein incompetence, retrograde reflux is easily detected. Any reflux lasting longer than 0.5 ms and ideally greater than 1 ms is said to be diagnostic of valvular incompetence. In addition, measurement of the vein diameter and extent of the reflux is also important. A very large-sized saphenous vein, certainly greater than 20 mm in diameter, may lead to a high failure rate with ablation, although recent developments in technology may allow larger veins to be ablated.
- Venography or other imaging studies are generally not necessary.

## LABORATORY STUDIES

- Since most ablation procedures are performed either under local anesthesia or with light sedation, routine laboratory tests are not needed.
- If regional or general anesthesia is necessary for specific reasons, then hospital or ambulatory care policies will dictate tests such as a complete blood cell count or electrolyte panel.

## DIFFERENTIAL DIAGNOSIS

- The patient's unilateral symptoms of venous insufficiency are fairly typical in this age group. Other diagnoses to consider include rare arterial conditions causing intermittent claudication and neurologic conditions.
- The main differential diagnosis to be considered is varicosities due to a secondary cause such as deep venous obstruction. A previous history of deep venous thrombosis (DVT), pregnancies, and a family history of thrombotic disorders are relevant. A duplex ultrasound examination should eliminate this cause of varicose veins.
- Congenital causes of varicose veins are easily ruled out on history taking by the time of appearance of varicosities.

## MANAGEMENT

- Most patients with symptomatic varicose veins are treated successfully, although not cured, with compression stockings.
- Intervention is usually only indicated for symptoms not relieved by stockings or complications of varicose veins such as ulceration or bleeding.

- Surgical stripping of the GSV or small saphenous vein (SSV) with or without removal of the branches (phlebectomy) has been the most common procedure to treat varicose veins for decades.
- Liquid sclerotherapy or foam sclerotherapy is also an option in some patients.
- The recent option of an endovenous approach using radiofrequency ablation (RFA) or laser thermal ablation has become widespread as a less invasive alternative.[2]

## INDICATIONS

Most patients subjected to ablation will have had a trial of nonoperative regimen including compression stockings for longer than 3 months and sometimes much longer. There are no medications that are scientifically proven to benefit patients with large, symptomatic varicose veins.

## PROCEDURE

- Endovenous ablation using either laser or RFA is relatively recent as a less invasive option for the treatment of large axial varicose veins.
- The procedure is performed under ultrasound guidance with percutaneous entry into the below-knee GSV (Figure 65-3). A sheath and then a guidewire is threaded upwards near the saphenofemoral junction and positioned about 2 cm distal to the junction (Figures 65-4 and 65-5).
- Tumescent anesthesia is administered and with duplex ultrasound imaging, the RFA or laser catheter is slowly pulled back, heating and ablating the vein (Figure 65-6).
- The patient is discharged home with compression stockings or bandaging with instructions to ambulate frequently and elevate the extremity when sitting.

## RESULTS

- The short-term efficacy and safety of endovenous ablation with a laser or radiofrequency has been established.[3]
- Many randomized controlled trials as well as observational reports and a meta-analysis is available to assist clinicians in determining the best option for patients in need of intervention. Early success rates showing occlusion of the GSV range from 93% to 100%.[4]
- In a recent randomized report comparing 100 ablative procedures with traditional high ligation and stripping of the GSV showed no difference in symptom relief or quality of life. Hematomas occurred more frequently in the surgical cohort.[5] However, two GSVs were found completely recanalized and five were partially recanalized after laser ablation compared to none in the surgical group.
- Another similar randomized clinical trial showed no difference in pain score between the open surgical stripping versus ablation, but less bruising and edema after the latter.[6]
- It is also generally agreed that although the efficacy and disease-specific quality of life is the same, an earlier return to normal activity is reported after laser ablation.[7]

- In general, new techniques of minimally invasive stripping are comparable to ablation procedures with a slight increase in pain and a minimal increase in return to work time.

- However, ablation procedures can almost always be performed in the outpatient office under local anesthesia with or without sedation with great patient satisfaction.

## PATIENT EDUCATION

- The pathophysiology of varicose veins and the benign nature of the problem must be explained along with signs and symptoms of complications resulting from long-standing varicose veins.

- The beneficial effect of proper graduated compression stockings and the importance of compliance is an essential part of patient education.

- Following ablation procedures, ambulation is strongly advised to prevent venous stasis and subsequent DVT.

- Superficial venous thrombosis of the ablated GSV or SSV occurs occasionally, and the patient must be forewarned about symptoms of pain and swelling in the area associated with it.

## FOLLOW-UP

Although major complications such as acute DVT following ablation are rare (<1%), erythema, saphenous neuralgia, early and late hyperpigmentation, edema, and occasionally superficial venous thrombosis of tributaries does occur. Therefore, outpatients must be warned of symptoms of DVT. Repeat duplex ultrasound studies are performed in the first or second year to confirm closure of the GSV or if recurrent symptoms occur.

### PROVIDER RESOURCES

- http://www.ncbi.nlm.nih.gov/pubmed/20347542
- http://www.ncbi.nlm.nih.gov/pubmed/16175538

### PATIENT RESOURCE

- http://www.webmd.com/skin-problems-and-treatments /news/20110919/surgery-vs-laser-treatment-for-varicose-veins

## REFERENCES

1. Murad MH, Coto-Yglesias F, Zumaeta-Garcia M, et al. A systematic review and meta-analysis of the treatments of varicose veins. *J Vasc Surg*. 2011;53:S49-S65.

2. Gillespie DL, Gloviczki ML, Lohr JM, et al. The care of patients with varicose veins and associated chronic venous diseases: clinical practice guidelines of the Society for Vascular Surgery and the American Venous Forum. *J Vasc Surg*. 2011;53:S2-S48.

3. Rasmussen LH, Bjoern L, Lawaerts M, Blemings A, Lawaertz B, Eklof B. Randomized trial comparing endovenous laser ablation of the great saphenous vein with high ligation and stripping in patients with varicose veins: short-term results. *J Vasc Surg*. 2007;46: 308-315.

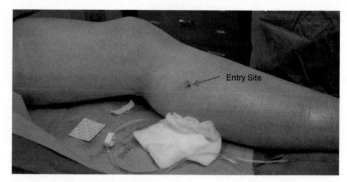

**FIGURE 65-3** The entry site is shown below the knee after removal of the sheath and laser catheter prior to placing an adhesive bandage (different patient).

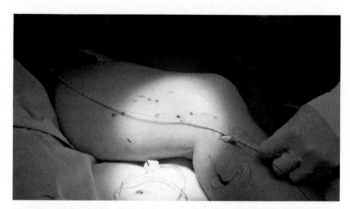

**FIGURE 65-4** Photograph demonstrating a sheath in place and the laser catheter placed on the outside prior to insertion (different patient).

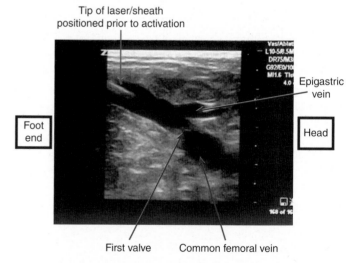

**FIGURE 65-5** Intraoperative duplex ultrasound picture demonstrating the tip of the laser catheter (red arrow), the epigastric vein, the common femoral vein, and the first valve at the great saphenous vein (GSV) and femoral vein junction (purple arrows).

4. Min RJ, Khilnani N, Zimmet SE. Endovenous EVL treatment of saphenous vein reflux: long-term results. *J Vasc Interv Radiol.* 2003;14:991-996.

5. Christenson JT, Gueddi S, Gemayel G, Bounameaux H. Prospective randomized trial comparing endovenous laser ablation and surgery for treatment of primary great saphenous varicose veins with a 2-year follow-up. *J Vasc Surg.* 2010;52(5):1234-1241.

6. Medeiros CAF, Luccas GC. Comparison of endovenous treatment with an 810 nm laser versus conventional stripping of the great saphenous vein in patients with primary varicose veins. *Dermatol Surg.* 2005;31:1685-1694.

7. Darwood RJ, Theivacumar N, Dellagrammaticas D, Mavor AID, Gough MJ. Randomized clinical trial comparing endovenous laser ablation with surgery for the treatment of primary great saphenous varicose veins. *Br J Surg.* 2008;95:294-301.

Post endo-venous laser

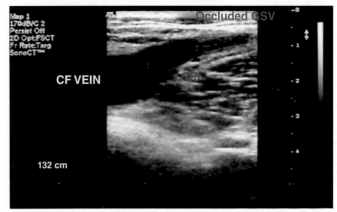

One day after procedure

**FIGURE 65-6** Postendovenous laser ablation duplex ultrasound picture showing the saphenofemoral junction with the great saphenous vein (GSV) ablated.

## PART 8

# LIMB SWELLING

# 66 PRIMARY AND SECONDARY LYMPHEDEMA

Ana Casanegra, MD
Suman Rathbun, MD

## PATIENT STORY

An 18-year-old woman seeks an opinion about swelling in her right leg. She first noticed it 1 year ago when her pants seemed to be tighter on that leg. She has no pain or discomfort; the edema does not improve after nocturnal rest.

On physical examination, the left leg is normal, and on the right the edema involves the toes, which look squared, along with nonpitting edema in the foot. The skin appears thickened, and there is a 4-cm difference in diameter between the legs measured in the calf. She has no adenopathy, and the abdominal examination is unremarkable. A diagnosis of lymphedema tarda is rendered.

## EPIDEMIOLOGY

- Lymphedema is an accumulation of lymphatic fluid in the interstitial tissues, most commonly in the limbs, resulting in edema.
- Incidence: primary lymphedema—1:6000 to 1:10,000; secondary lymphedema—varies among different populations; it can be as high as 30% in breast cancer patients after surgery and radiation therapy.[1,2]
- Primary lymphedema is more prevalent in females, 2.5 to 10:1.[2]
- Lymphedema can affect patients from birth (congenital lymphedema) to advanced age.
- Lymphedema rarely leads to death, but is a source of morbidity and affects body image.
- The natural history varies from minimal swelling to severe deformities in the limb.[1]

## ETIOLOGY AND PATHOPHYSIOLOGY

- Lymphatic vessels collect and drain the excessive interstitial fluid that escapes the capillary circulation. Lymphedema is the accumulation of this protein-rich lymphatic fluid in the tissues.
- Lymphedema occurs when the production of lymphatic fluid exceeds the transportation capacity of the lymphatic vessels.
- It can affect multiple areas, but most commonly involves the upper or lower extremities.
- In primary lymphedema there is an inherited defect in the lymphatic vessels that manifests at birth to the early 40s. Lymphedema can be the only manifestation, or it can be part of a syndrome (eg, yellow nail syndrome, lymphedema-distichiasis syndrome, Turner syndrome).[2]
- Secondary lymphedema is more common, caused by destruction or damage of the lymphatics or increased production of lymphatic fluid. Common causes include filarial infection (in tropical and subtropical regions of Asia, Africa, and Central and South America),[3] malignancy (involving lymph nodes or lymphatics), trauma (surgical damage or resection of lymphatics), chronic venous insufficiency (increased interstitial fluid), inflammatory diseases, recurrent bacterial infections, and chronic edema.[1,2]

## DIAGNOSIS

### History

- Lymphedema may present as unilateral, painless swelling with minimal change with elevation.
- The swelling usually starts distally and is more noticeable in fingers or toes.
- Recurrent cellulitis is a common complication.
- History of trauma, surgery, radiation therapy, and malignancy assists in confirming the diagnosis of secondary lymphedema.
- Congenital lymphedema is evident at birth or within the first 2 years of life; lymphedema praecox most commonly presents at puberty and lymphedema tarda after age 35.[1,4]
- Family history of lymphedema may be present.

### Physical Examination

- Most of the time the diagnosis is clinical, with no need for confirmatory imaging tests.[2]
- Edema may be pitting at early stages, but is nonpitting as the disease becomes chronic.[2,4]
- Squared-off toes are characteristic of primary lymphedema; the toes have a blunt, squared appearance (Figure 66-1).[1,2,4,5]
- Dorsal hump may occur, which presents as noticeable edema involving the dorsum of the foot (Figure 66-2).
- Stemmer sign is the inability to tent the skin at the base of the second toe.[1,2,4-6]
- Peau d'orange is a late-stage sign (Figure 66-3); dilated hair follicles with minimal pitting in the skin, cutaneous fibrosis.[2,5]
- Other skin involvement: hyperkeratosis (Figure 66-4), papillomatosis (Figures 66-5 and 66-6).[4]
- In infectious cellulitis (Figure 66-7), the skin appears erythematous, with increased temperature and lymphangitic streaks toward the lymph nodes.[4]
- Assess the area in between toes for tinea pedis, as it is a risk factor for cellulitis.[4]
- Surgical scars, masses, and other skin lesions can help with the diagnosis of secondary lymphedema.

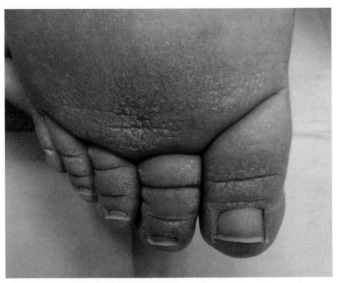

FIGURE 66-1 Squaring of the toes, increased skin folds, and hyperkeratosis consistent with lymphedema.

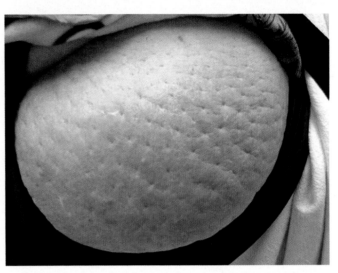

FIGURE 66-3 Classical "peau d'orange" or "skin of an orange" appearance signifies excessive cutaneous lymphatic fluid.

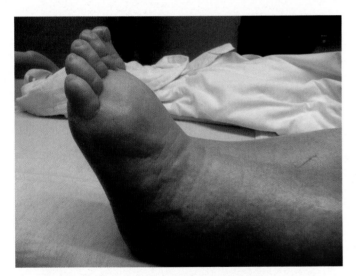

FIGURE 66-2 Dorsal pedal hump of lymphedema. Characteristic exaggerated skin folds at the ankle are also illustrated.

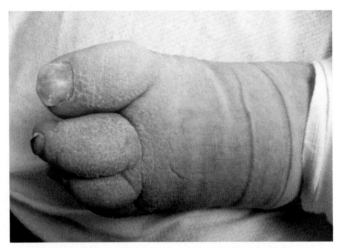

FIGURE 66-4 Lymphedema manifestations: hyperkeratosis of the skin. The edema affects the toes and foot predominantly. Note the marks of the elastic wrapping on the dorsum of the foot.

## Diagnostic Tests

- Lymphangiography, which involves the injection of iodinated contrast into cannulated lymphatics, is rarely used due to risk of worsening lymphedema.

- Lymphoscintigram (Figure 66-8): diagnostic method of choice. This nuclear scan follows the progression of a radiolabeled contrast injected in the subcutaneous tissues between toes or fingers. Diagnosis of lymphedema is suggested by delayed transport or backflow of the tracer, asymmetric or absent visualization of the vessels or nodes, and other abnormal patterns.[2,7]

- Duplex ultrasound can be useful to rule out other causes of edema such as venous insufficiency and deep venous thrombosis (DVT).

- Computed tomography (CT) can help diagnose causes for secondary lymphedema and assess volume discrepancies. Changes present in lymphedema are skin thickening, honeycomb pattern, and subcutaneous edema.[8]

- Magnetic resonance imaging (MRI) lymphography is promising but not widely available. Conventional MRI can show changes in the skin and subdermis.[9]

## DIFFERENTIAL DIAGNOSIS

- Chronic venous disease and post-thrombotic syndrome: edema, usually pitting; pain with prolonged standing; hyperpigmentation of the skin; varicose veins.[1]

- DVT presents acutely and needs to be excluded with duplex ultrasound.

- Lipedema affects mostly females; it is an abnormal bilateral deposition of subcutaneous fat. It spares the feet and involves calves. Stemmer sign is negative, and there are no skin lesions.[1]

- Myxedema can be localized or generalized. Usually bilateral, it is associated with generalized skin and adnexa changes such as thin hair, brittle nails, rough skin, and yellowish discoloration.[1]

- Systemic causes of edema (congestive heart failure, renal failure, volume overload, hypoalbuminemia): bilateral soft pitting edema with no skin changes, predominantly affecting the ankles and respecting the feet.

## MANAGEMENT

- Reduction of edema: Patients need to be referred to a physical therapist (PT) with training in manual lymphatic drainage (MLD), a special technique to reduce edema. The PT will also apply multilayer wraps between sessions to reduce edema and avoid reaccumulation of lymphatic fluid.[1,5]

- Maintenance: Compression stockings up to 40 to 60 mm Hg or sleeves 20 to 30 mm Hg need to be worn daily. Milder compression overnight and inelastic underwear are sometimes required. The compression garments need to be renewed regularly (every 3-6 months) as they lose elasticity.[1,4,5]

- Intermittent pneumatic compression: May be a helpful adjuvant for maintenance treatment.[1,4]

- Exercise is advised such as swimming, as it improves lymph flow.[4]

- Diuretics are generally not indicated.[2]

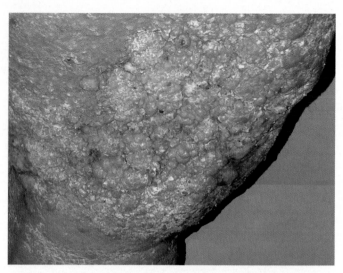

**FIGURE 66-5** Advanced skin changes in the calf of a patient with lymphedema. The papulonodular and hyperkeratotic appearance is also known as elephantiasis nostras verrucosa.

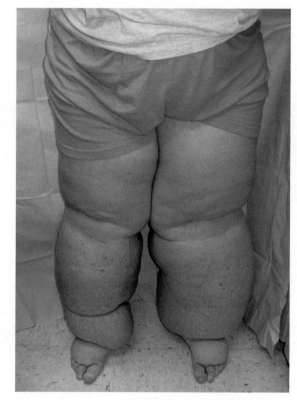

**FIGURE 66-6** A long-standing primary lymphedema patient with elephantiasis. The normal contour of the distal calves and malleoli have been lost consistent with an "elephantine" ankle. Other characteristic features include acral swelling with exaggerated skin creases, hyperkeratosis, and a papulonodular eruption in the background of profound leg swelling.

- Surgery is not usually recommended.[1,2]
- Complications
  - Cellulitis: *Streptococcus* and *Staphylococcus* are the most common agents. Cellulitis should be promptly treated with empiric antibiotics to prevent worsening of lymphedema. Recurrent cellulitis may need chronic antibiotic suppressive therapy.[1,4]
  - Cancer: Uncommonly lymphedema may undergo malignant degeneration (angiosarcoma or lymphangiosarcoma).

## PATIENT EDUCATION

- Compliance with the treatment is critical in this disease, as it requires lifelong management with a significant commitment from the patient.
- The patients or a family member should learn to perform MLD.
- Skin care: Patients should avoid wounds and cuts, and use protection for the affected limb: gloves for garden work, avoidance of walking barefoot. Skin moisturizing is advised, and periodic examination of the toe webs, with prompt treatment of tinea pedis.
- Cellulitis prevention: Patients should recognize the clinical signs and symptoms and promptly contact their physician while starting empirical antibiotics.

## FOLLOW-UP

- Initial frequent follow-up is helpful until the edema is well controlled, and to reinforce patient education, proper use of compression garments, and skin care.
- Long-term follow-up can be yearly if symptoms are well controlled and more often if complications arise.

### PATIENT AND PROVIDER RESOURCES

- http://www.lymphnet.org
- http://www.lymphedemaresources.org
- http://www.cancer.gov/cancertopics/pdq/supportivecare/lymphedema/Patient/page1
- http://www.ncbi.nlm.nih.gov/pubmedhealth/PMH0002106/
- http://www.mayoclinic.com/health/lymphedema/DS00609
- http://lymphaticresearch.org/main.php?content=home

## REFERENCES

1. Rockson SG. Lymphedema. *Am J Med.* 2001;110(4):288-295.

2. Rockson SG. Diagnosis and management of lymphatic vascular disease. *J Am Coll Cardiol.* 2008;52(10):799-806.

3. Taylor MJ, Hoerauf A, Bockarie M. Lymphatic filariasis and onchocerciasis. *Lancet.* 2010;376(9747):1175-1185.

4. Kerchner K, Fleischer A, Yosipovitch G. Lower extremity lymphedema update: pathophysiology, diagnosis, and treatment guidelines. *J Am Acad Dermatol.* 2008;59(2):324-331.

5. Rockson SG. Current concepts and future directions in the diagnosis and management of lymphatic vascular disease. *Vasc Med.* 2010;15(3):223-231.

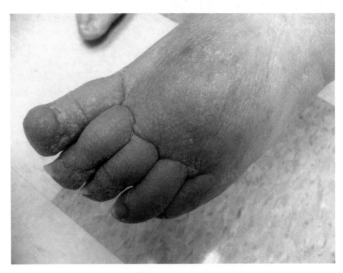

**FIGURE 66-7** Infectious cellulitis in a patient with lymphedema.

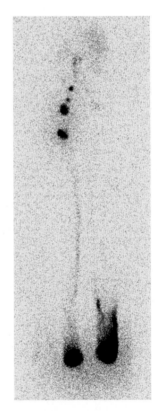

**FIGURE 66-8** Lymphoscintigram: posterior view at 4 hours shows dermal backflow in the right leg and absent lymphatic channels and lymph nodes on the right leg.

6. Stemmer R. [A clinical symptom for the early and differential diagnosis of lymphedema]. *Vasa*. 1976;5(3):261-262.

7. Jensen MR, Simonsen L, Karlsmark T, Bülow J. Lymphoedema of the lower extremities—background, pathophysiology and diagnostic considerations. *Clin Physiol Funct Imaging*. 2010;30(6): 389-398.

8. Monnin-Delhom ED, Gallix BP, Achard C, Bruel JM, Janbon C. High resolution unenhanced computed tomography in patients with swollen legs. *Lymphology*. 2002;35(3):121-128.

9. Astrom KG, Abdsaleh S, Brenning GC, Ahlström KH. MR imaging of primary, secondary, and mixed forms of lymphedema. *Acta Radiol*. 2001;42(4):409-416.

# 67 LOWER EXTREMITY CELLULITIS

Satish K. Sarvepalli, MD, MPH
Julie E. Mangino, MD

## PATIENT STORY

A 42-year-old man with morbid obesity, diabetes mellitus, congestive heart failure, and venous insufficiency presented with fever, pain, and swelling of his left lower extremity (LLE). He reported trivial trauma to his LLE after bumping into a table 2 weeks prior; the affected area progressed from mild redness to an open ulcer at the ankle. It eventually developed increased redness, warmth, and pain extending from the left ankle to the knee. At admission, he had an open ulcer with purulent drainage along with excoriation of the superficial layer of the skin (Figure 67-1). Given the purulent nature of the cellulitis and concern for methicillin-resistant *Staphylococcus aureus* (MRSA), he was started on intravenous vancomycin and received appropriate wound care. After initial improvement, he was switched to oral clindamycin to complete a total of 10 days of therapy. On a 2-week follow-up visit, his cellulitis had resolved.

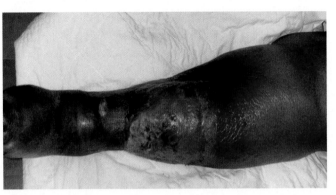

**FIGURE 67-1** Left lower extremity (LLE) cellulitis in a 42-year-old man with morbid obesity, diabetes, and venous insufficiency who suffered a minor abrasion that progressed into an open ulcer.

## EPIDEMIOLOGY

Cellulitis is a rapidly spreading infection of the skin involving the deeper dermis and the subcutaneous tissue.[1,2] It extends deeper than erysipelas,[3] which is in the differential diagnosis.

- A common infection seen by both hospital-based and primary care physicians.[4]
- Contributes to more than 600,000 hospitalizations each year.[4]
- Annual office visits for cellulitis and cutaneous abscess increased from 4.6 million to 9.6 million in 2005.[5]
- A lesion with exudate and purulent drainage, without an underlying drainable abscess, is defined as *purulent* cellulitis; it is predominantly due to *S aureus*.[4,6]
- Lesions without exudate, purulent drainage, or an underlying drainable abscess are defined as *nonpurulent* cellulitis, which is predominantly due to streptococcal species.[4]

## ETIOLOGY

### Common Pathogens

- Over the past decade, there has been an increase in purulent skin and soft tissue infections related to MRSA.[4]
- Most commonly caused by group A β-hemolytic *S aureus* and *Staphlycoccus aureus*.[3,4]

### Uncommon Pathogens

- Other β-hemolytic streptococci including groups B, C, and G[4]
- Fresh water exposure: *Aeromonas hydrophila*[1,4]
- Salt water exposure: *Vibrio vulnificus*[1,4] in those with cirrhosis

- Exposure to saltwater fish, shellfish, poultry, meat, and hides: *Erysipelothrix rhusiopathiae*, which can cause erysipeloid, mostly in the upper extremity[3]

- Cat or dog bites: *Pasteurella multocida* or *Capnocytophaga canimorsus*[1,4]

- Neutropenic hosts: *Pseudomonas aeruginosa* or other gram negatives[1,4]

- Human immunodeficiency virus (HIV): *Helicobacter cinaedi*,[1] rare cause, atypical appearance with no warmth, can be recurrent, multifocal, and can be associated with bacteremia

- Defective cell-mediated immunity: *Cryptococcus neoformans*[1]

## PATHOPHYSIOLOGY

Lower extremity cellulitis occurs when there is a portal of entry for micro-organisms through a disrupted cutaneous barrier.

### Predisposing Factors

- Trauma (Figure 67-1) to the lower extremity including puncture wound and abrasion.[3]

- Ulcers (Figure 67-1) and other skin lesions such as ecthyma, impetigo.[1,3]

- Fungal infection resulting in fissured toe webs (tinea pedis),[1] especially if it is complicated with bacterial colonization (Figure 67-2).[4]

- Obesity[4] and lower extremity edema from various other causes (Figure 67-3).[3]

- Saphenous venectomy for coronary artery bypass grafting resulting in changes to venous and lymphatic drainage.[3]

- Any underlying subcutaneous abscess or osteomyelitis with fistula tracking to the skin.[3]

- Alterations due to surgery, radiation, and neoplastic agents involving the pelvic lymph nodes leading to lower extremity lymphedema[3] (Figure 67-4).

- Rarely, secondary cellulitis from bacteremia can occur.[3]

## DIAGNOSIS

It is usually based on the clinical presentation and the examination findings.[1,4]

### Clinical Features

#### Local Findings

- Affected areas of the skin are usually warm, red, and tender.

- Borders are usually not well demarcated and elevated, unlike erysipelas.[3]

- Regional lymphadenopathy is usually seen.[3]

#### Systemic Findings

- Usually mild but can result in hypotension, tachycardia, fever, change in mental status, and increased white blood cell count.[1]

### Laboratory Studies

- Very low likelihood of positive blood cultures, but possible in very severe cases[1] and immunocompromised hosts; positive in less than 5% of the cases.[1]

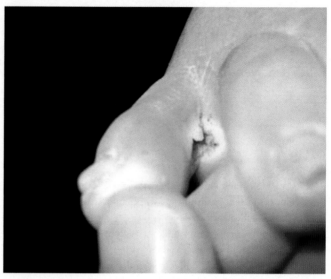

**FIGURE 67-2** Tinea pedis in a patient who had developed lower extremity cellulitis.

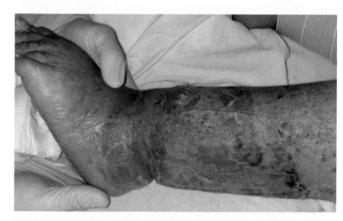

**FIGURE 67-3** Recurrent left lower extremity (LLE) cellulitis in a 54-year-old woman with long-standing LE ulcers, history of multiple deep vein thromboses (DVTs) in bilateral LE, and status post left ili-ofemoral thrombectomy.

- Biopsy or aspiration of the skin lesion considered in the following conditions:
  - When an unusual pathogen is suspected[3]
  - Failure to respond to initial therapy with antimicrobials[3]
  - Presence of fluctuant areas[3]
  - Immunodeficiency, neutropenia, diabetes mellitus, malignancy[1]
  - Immersion injury, animal bites[1]
- For nonpurulent cellulitis, which is mostly of streptococcal origin, consider acute and convalescent serologies of antistreptolysin O and anti-DNase B antibodies.[4]
- For a cutaneous abscess, incision and drainage is the primary treatment. Antibiotic therapy is recommended if severe or extensive disease (eg, involves multiple sites of infection) or rapid progression with associated cellulitis, signs or symptoms of systemic illness, associated comorbidities or immunosuppression, extremes of age, abscess in an area difficult to drain (eg, face, hand, and genitalia), associated septic phlebitis, lack of response to incision and drainage alone.[1] It is predominantly due to MRSA.

## Imaging Studies

- Ultrasound can be helpful with diagnosis and drainage when there is concern for underlying abscess.[2]
- When there is concern for adjacent osteomyelitis, consider plain-film or magnetic resonance imaging (MRI).[2,4]
- Computed tomography (CT) is more sensitive at showing soft tissue gas, and may additionally show deep fascial thickening or associated deep tissue abscesses.[4]
- MRI is the modality of choice for differentiating necrotizing fasciitis from cellultis.[4]
- The only way to definitively diagnose necrotizing soft tissue infections is by surgical exploration, which is recommended urgently for any case with substantial concern,[4] and if progression is suggestive, surgery should not be delayed.[2]

## DIFFERENTIAL DIAGNOSIS

- Acute dermatitis[3]
- Erysipelas[3] with well-demarcated borders
- Gout with cutaneous inflammation[2-4]
- Herpes zoster[3,4] grouped vesicles in a dermatomal distribution
- Venous stasis[4]
- Acute lipodermatosclerosis[3](LDS), a condition that affects the skin just above the ankle, usually on the inside surface, in patients with chronic venous insufficiency. LDS means "scarring of the skin and fat"; it is a slow process occurring over a number of years. Over time the skin becomes brown, smooth, tight, and often painful (Figure 67-5).
- Necrotizing fasciitis[2,4]: severe pain, swelling, and fever with hemorrhagic or bluish bullae, skin necrosis or ecchymosis, gas or crepitus, cutaneous anesthesia, edema that extends beyond the margin of erythema, and rapid progression.
- Erythema migrans[4] not painful, bull's eye appearance, tick exposure.
- Hypersensitivity reaction[4] pruritis.
- Fixed drug reaction[4] occurs temporally with drug ingestion.

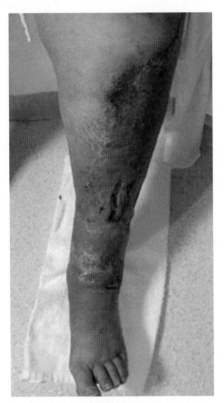

**FIGURE 67-4** Left lower extremity (LLE) cellulitis in 43-year-old woman with lymphedema, who had subsequent extension to the dorsum of the foot. She responded to intravenous (IV) vancomycin followed by oral doxycycline.

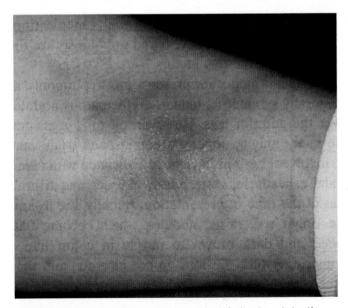

**FIGURE 67-5** Acute inflammation along the left distal medial calf in an obese middle-aged woman with long-standing leg swelling. The inflammatory plaque failed to improve despite several courses of antibiotics. She was ultimately diagnosed with acute lipodermatosclerosis. (*Photograph courtesy of Dr. Steven M. Dean.*)

• Deep venous thrombosis (DVT)[4] not typically associated with skin redness with exception of phlegmasia cerulea dolens.

## MANAGEMENT

### Outpatients With Purulent Cellulitis

• Empiric treatment for community-associated (CA) MRSA is recommended, pending culture data.[4,6]

• Available options: clindamycin, trimethoprim-sulfamethoxazole (TMP-SMX) (does not cover streptococcal species), doxycycline, minocycline, or linezolid.[6]

• Duration: 5 to 10 days, but is tailored based on the patient's clinical improvement.[6]

### Outpatients With Nonpurulent Cellulitis

• Treat empirically for β-hemolytic *Streptococcus*, pending culture data.[4,6]

• Oral therapy with activity against streptococci.[1] Agents include beta-lactams (dicloxacillin, cephalexin, and amoxicillin), clindamycin.[6]

• For cellulitis that fails to respond to beta-lactams[6] or is associated with trauma and underlying abscess, consider coverage for *S aureus*[1] (see purulent cellulitis).

• Duration: 5 to 10 days, but is tailored based on the patient's clinical improvement.[6]

### Hospitalized Cases

• Usually have complicated infections with comorbidities and empiric therapy for MRSA should be considered, in particular, CA-MRSA pending culture data.[4,6]

• Parenteral therapy with vancomycin, daptomycin, clindamycin, linezolid, or oral therapy with clindamycin, linezolid.[6]

• Can use parenteral therapy if intolerance to oral therapy.

• For nonpurulent cellulitis: parenteral beta-lactams like cefazolin, nafcillin (inactive against MRSA), and clindamycin.[6]

• If there is rapid progression or lack of response to therapy, consider necrotizing fasciitis, unusual pathogens, resistant organisms, or deeper contiguous infection.[1]

• For necrotizing infections due to clostridial and group A streptococcal organisms, addition of parenteral penicillin and clindamycin is recommended.[1] Overall mortality of necrotizing fasciitis ranges from 24% to 34% and surgical exploration should not be delayed.[3]

### Unusual Pathogens and Exposure

• Therapy is based on the type of exposure and the pathogen suspected.[2]

### Adjunctive Therapy and Preventive Measures

• Limit lower extremity edema by elevating the affected leg (Figure 67-6).[1]

• Appropriate use of diuretics based on the underlying conditions.[1]

• Treat the predisposing condition: for example, tinea pedis, trauma to the skin, stasis dermatitis.[1]

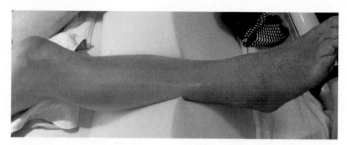

**FIGURE 67-6** Right lower extremity (RLE) cellulitis in a 46-year-old man following 48 hours of therapy. Note the receding margins of erythema that had extended up to the knee at admission.

- Skin emollients to avoid dryness and cracking.[1]
- Recurrent episodes can be prevented by decreasing lower extremity edema in appropriate clinical settings with pneumatic pressure pumps and compressive stockings.[1]

## FOLLOW-UP

- Usually responds to antibiotics; if worsens or does not improve, consider uncommon pathogens or other causes.
- Occasionally skin changes may worsen initially during therapy due to the inflammation resulting from the released toxins during pathogen destruction;[1] reinforce elevation.
- For recurrent infections, no clear recommendation for prophylactic antibiotics[1] but could be considered on case-by-case basis.
- For recurrent infections with MRSA, consider decolonization with nasal mupirocin (if nares are positive), topical antiseptic bathing with chlorhexidine gluconate soap, and avoiding sharing of towels, razors, etc.[6]

## PROVIDER RESOURCES

The practice guidelines prepared by the Infectious Disease Society of America (IDSA) are available on their website.

- For the treatment of cellulitis and other skin and soft tissue infections: http://www.idsociety.org/uploadedFiles/IDSA/Guidelines-Patient_Care/PDF_Library/Skin%20and%20Soft%20Tissue.pdf
- For the treatment of MRSA infections in adults and children: http://cid.oxfordjournals.org/content/early/2011/01/04/cid.ciq146.full

## PATIENT RESOURCES

- National Institute of Allergy and Infectious Diseases: www3.niaid.nih.gov/topics/cellulitisErysipelas/
- National Library of Medicine: www.nlm.nih.gov/medlineplus/ency/article/000855.htm

## REFERENCES

1. Stevens DL, Bisno AL, Chambers HF, et al. Practice guidelines for the diagnosis and management of skin and soft-tissue infections. *Clin Infect Dis*. 2005;41:1373-1406.
2. Swartz MN. Cellulitis. *N Engl J Med*. 2004;350:904-912.
3. Pasternack M, Swartz M. Cellulitis, necrotizing fasciitis, and subcutaneous tissue infections. *Princ Pract Infect Dis*. 2010;1:1289-1312.
4. Gunderson CG. Cellulitis: definition, etiology, and clinical features. *Am J Med*. 2011;124:1113-1122.
5. Hersh AL, Chambers HF, Maselli JH, Gonzales R. National trends in ambulatory visits and antibiotic prescribing for skin and soft-tissue infections. *Arch Intern Med*. 2008;168:1585-1591.
6. Liu C, Bayer A, Cosgrove SE, et al. Clinical practice guidelines by the Infectious Diseases Society of America for the treatment of methicillin-resistant *Staphylococcus aureus* infections in adults and children. *Clin Infect Dis*. 2011;52:e18-e55.

# 68 LEG SWELLING SECONDARY TO MUSCLE RUPTURE

Marcus D. Stanbro, DO, FSVM, RPVI
Stephen L. Chastain, MD, RVT

## PATIENT STORY

A 67-year-old man presented with spontaneous left-calf pain and swelling of 2-days duration. Four weeks prior, he had undergone percutaneous angioplasty of the left anterior descending artery (LADA), and was discharged on aspirin, warfarin, and clopidogrel. On examination, the left calf was swollen and tender with subtle erythematous changes. Posterior tibial and dorsalis pedis pulses were palpable. There were no ecchymoses or petechiae noted. A venous duplex showed a large, complex, mostly hypoechoic fluid collection beginning at the proximal posteromedial aspect of the calf, with distal extension to the medial mid calf (Figures 68-1 and 68-2). The collection was below the muscular fascia and consistent with an intramuscular hematoma. Due to progressive swelling and pain, he was taken to the operating room where a moderate amount of coagulum was removed from the gastrocnemius muscle. Although acute deep vein thrombosis (DVT) should be the predominant concern when anyone presents with acute unilateral pain and swelling, this was unlikely in this patient since he was therapeutically anticoagulated.

### EPIDEMIOLOGY

Acute unilateral leg swelling is a very common presentation to the vascular laboratory, emergency room, or the vascular specialist's office. The incidence of leg swelling secondary to muscle rupture is not known, but the clinical syndrome of strain or rupture of the medial head of the gastrocnemius muscle commonly known as "tennis leg" is not an uncommon presentation to the sports medicine specialist or emergency room physician. Medial calf injuries occur more commonly in men than in women, and these injuries usually afflict athletes and others in the fourth to sixth decades of life. Medial calf injuries are most commonly seen acutely, but up to 20% of affected patients report a prodrome of calf tightness several days before the injury, thus suggesting a potential chronic predisposition.[1]

### ETIOLOGY AND PATHOPHYSIOLOGY

#### Muscle Rupture

- Most commonly involves the medial head of the gastrocnemius muscle and is provoked by dorsiflexion of the ankle while the knee is extended. This so-called "tennis leg" often occurs during racquet sports.
- Tennis leg has also been reported in other sports-related activities such as running, basketball, football, skiing, and rugby.[2,3]
- Gastrocnemius ruptures occurring during daily activities such as stepping off a curb or climbing stairs have been reported.[3,4]

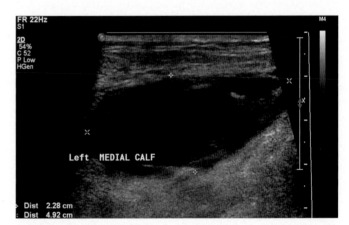

**FIGURE 68-1** Sagittal B-mode image of the proximal medial calf illustrating a complex hypoechoic fluid collection below the fascia, consistent with hematoma formation.

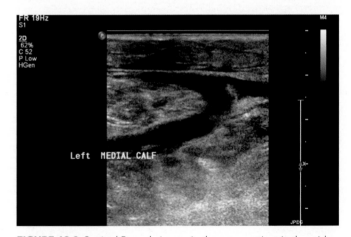

**FIGURE 68-2** Sagittal B-mode image in the same patient in the mid proximal medial calf showing fluid collection dissecting along the fascial planes.

- Ruptures or strains occurring in middle-aged or older patients may be associated with loss of flexibility or physiologic changes of muscle with aging.[5,6]

  Less commonly reported are injuries or ruptures to the soleus, plantaris, flexor hallucis longus muscles, and lateral head of the gastrocnemius muscle.[2]

## Calf Swelling

- Swelling is usually acute, and depending on the size, may be due to the hematoma itself with compression of adjacent structures.
- May be secondary to dissection of blood between muscles or deep within the muscles (ie, gastrocnemius and soleus).

## Calf Hematomas

- Can occur with direct trauma, muscle rupture, or spontaneously.
- Spontaneous intramuscular hematomas occur more commonly with anticoagulation.

## DIAGNOSIS

### History

- Commonly, the patient will complain of acute onset of pain in the proximal posterior calf related to a physical activity.[2] Patients often report a pop in the calf or a sensation of being kicked or shot in the calf, followed by increasing pain and swelling within 24 hours. Some patients will report the injury associated with daily activities such as climbing stairs, stepping off a curb, or getting up from namaz praying.[2,7]
- Individuals who are anticoagulated that experience a spontaneous or unprovoked muscle rupture or hematoma may report either a more gradual onset of symptoms or the simultaneous onset of discomfort and swelling with the rupture.

### Physical Examination

- The typical findings of tenderness to palpation, increased pain with passive dorsiflexion of the foot, and swelling may mimic DVT.
- The limb may display an erythrocyanotic appearance, but the presence of ecchymosis in the absence of trauma should alert the clinician to possible muscle rupture (Figure 68-3).
- The appearance of a semiarc of ecchymosis below the medial malleolus—resembling a scimitar—is indicative of a muscle rupture with blood dissecting down the calf and into the ankle. This physical finding may not appear for several days after the onset of symptoms. Figure 68-4 illustrates a rare scimitar sign along the lateral foot.
- If the rupture is close to the musculotendinous insertion, a defect may be palpable, signifying the presence of muscle retraction.[2]
- True muscle weakness may be evident, but usually is masked by the patient's discomfort and avoidance of aggravating movements or positions.

### Duplex Ultrasonography

- Given cost and easy availability, the initial test of choice for investigating acute limb swelling is duplex ultrasonography.

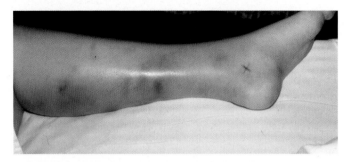

**FIGURE 68-3** Different patient with left calf muscle rupture misdiagnosed as calf vein thrombosis. Following anticoagulation, the left calf became very tense, painful, and ecchymotic.

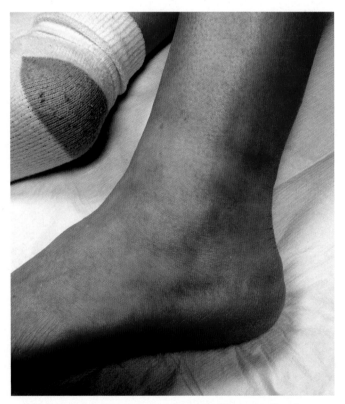

**FIGURE 68-4** "Scimitar sign" noted on the left lateral ankle. This physical finding is most commonly seen below the medial malleolus but can occur on the lateral side as well. Since it takes time for the blood to migrate distally, the scimitar sign is usually noted several days after the rupture.

- Ultrasound findings indicative of a muscle rupture may include a hypoechoic or anechoic mass or fluid collection that initially may have ill-defined borders.[8] The blood collection is usually heterogeneous in appearance,[9] but some authors have described more homogeneous fluid collections that may be associated with the age of the fluid collection. This collection may lie within the muscle compartment itself, or more commonly may appear between the gastrocnemius and soleus muscles in the case of medial head ruptures.

- Sonographic interrogation of the musculotendinous junction may reveal a partial or complete tear and is most helpful in cases where the medial head of the gastrocnemius muscle is involved.

- Even if a fluid collection suggesting a hematoma or muscle rupture is detected, careful interrogation of the deep veins is warranted since concomitant DVT can occur.[4]

- The most common duplex ultrasound findings in the assessment of the acutely swollen leg include[4,8]
  - DVT
  - Superficial thrombophlebitis
  - Venous insufficiency
  - Popliteal cysts (Baker cysts), with or without rupture
  - Hematomas
  - Lymphadenopathy
  - Joint effusions

- Less common duplex findings include
  - Soft tissue tumors
  - Popliteal artery or venous aneurysms
  - Hemorrhage into a popliteal cyst
  - Ganglion cysts

## Magnetic Resonance Imaging

Magnetic resonance imaging (MRI) offers excellent soft tissue imaging and is very useful in cases of diagnostic uncertainty or to assess bony structures and soft tissue structures not as easily identified on ultrasound. Ruptures to the anterior cruciate ligament; popliteus, plantaris, and soleus muscles; and the lateral head of the gastrocnemius muscle have been described.[2] Use is limited by cost and availability.

## DIFFERENTIAL DIAGNOSIS

- The presentation of leg swelling due to muscle rupture is most commonly confused with DVT and a ruptured Baker cyst.

- Since the clinical presentation of DVT can be indistinguishable from a muscle rupture, duplex imaging is essential. Although a complete discussion of the sonographic findings in DVT is beyond the scope of this chapter, the finding of dilated, noncompressible deep veins with absence or alteration of flow is diagnostic of DVT.

- A popliteal or Baker cyst without rupture is fairly easy to differentiate from a muscle rupture or hematoma based on the location in the popliteal fossa. Popliteal cysts are usually crescent shaped, well defined, and anechoic, but long-standing cysts may contain echogenic material and appear much more complex and heterogeneous. When a popliteal cyst ruptures and dissects distally into the calf, it is much more likely to present with acute limb swelling and pain. A Baker cyst is closely associated with the medial head of the gastrocnemius muscle, and therefore rupture of this cyst, especially if associated with hemorrhaging, may be challenging to differentiate from rupture of the medial head of the gastrocnemius muscle.[8]

- Causes for unilateral limb swelling are listed in Table 68-1.

## MANAGEMENT

Limb swelling secondary to muscle rupture is generally benign and self-limiting. Management depends on the cause and severity of the rupture and whether or not the patient requires anticoagulation. Understandably, individuals with partial tears or ruptures generally display a faster recovery and experience less pain and swelling.

- Treatment focuses on rest, ice packs, compression stockings or wraps, and elevation (RICE) and reassurance.

- Analgesics including nonsteroidal anti-inflammatories are the mainstay of therapy. Narcotic analgesics and muscle relaxants are frequently required.

- Discontinuation of antiplatelet agents or anticoagulation is often necessary and should be individualized, taking into consideration the severity of the muscle rupture, size of the hematoma, and presence of compartment syndrome.

- Severe or complete muscle ruptures may require a period of non-weight bearing or protected weight bearing with crutches.

- Calf muscle ruptures and even ruptured Baker cysts can rarely lead to acute compartment syndrome. Compartment syndrome is more common in anticoagulated patients and should be considered when the swollen leg is tense and the pain is described as severe or excruciating. Pain out of proportion to physical findings has been described. A high index of suspicion should be maintained and the neurovascular status followed closely. If there is no neurovascular compromise and time allows, compartment pressures may be obtained to assess the need for fasciotomy. Surgical evacuation of the fluid collection is occasionally required and is based on symptoms and the size of the fluid collection itself.

## PATIENT EDUCATION

Since the leg swelling is most commonly a benign, self-limiting condition, patients are reassured and followed clinically. Referral to a sports medicine specialist or physical therapist may be indicated to assess the severity of the muscle rupture and prescribe the appropriate stretching exercises, weight-bearing progression, cryotherapy, and physical rehabilitation.

## FOLLOW-UP

In addition to clinical follow up for leg swelling, compression therapy may be required for an extended period of time. Serial duplex examinations are not routinely performed but have been described in the literature to document regression of the fluid collection and the reparative process involving the muscle or musculotendinous rupture.

## REFERENCES

1. Saglimbeni AJ. Medial gastrocnemius strain. eMedicine. Available at: http://emedicine.medscape.com/article/91687-overview. Accessed December 27, 2011.

2. Campbell JT. Posterior calf injury. *Foot Ankle Clin N Am*. 2009;14:761-771.

3. Orchard J. Management of muscle and tendon injuries in footballers. *Aust Fam Physician*. 2003;32(7):489-493.

4. Delgado GJ, Chung CB, Lektrakul N, et al. Tennis leg: clinical US study of 141 patients and anatomic investigation of four cadavers with MR imaging and US. *Radiology*. 2002;224:112-119.

5. Ozcakar L, Solak HN, Yorubulut M. Tennis leg: a look from the geriatric side. *J Am Geriatr Soc*. 2005;53(2):356-357.

6. Zecher SB, Leach RE. Lower leg and foot injuries in tennis and other racquet sports. *Clin Sports Med*. 1995;14(1):223-239.

7. Yilmaz C, Orgenc Y, Ergenc R, et al. Rupture of the medial gastrocnemius muscle during namaz praying: an unusual cause of tennis leg. *Comput Med Imaging Graph*. 2008;32(8):728-731.

8. Zwiebel WJ. Nonvascular pathology encountered during venous sonography. In: Zwiebel WJ, Pellerito JS, eds. *Introduction to Vascular Ultrasonography*. 5th ed. Philadelpia, PA: Elsevier Saunders; 2005:501-510.

9. Bianchi S, Martinoli C, Abdelwahab IF, et al. Sonographic evaluation of tears of the gastrocnemius medial head ("tennis leg"). *J Ultrasound Med*. 1998;17:157-162.

**TABLE 68-1.** Causes of Unilateral Leg Swelling

| |
| --- |
| Deep vein thrombosis (DVT) |
| Superficial thrombophlebitis |
| Cellulitis |
| Lymphedema |
| Reperfusion edema |
| Factitial |
| Popliteal cyst, with or without rupture |
| Chronic venous insufficiency |
| Joint effusions |
| Abscess |
| Osteomyelitis |
| Popliteal artery aneurysm |
| Trauma |
| Soft tissue tumors |
| Muscle rupture |
| Hematoma |
| Acute Charcot arthropathy |
| Stress fractures |
| Hemihypertrophy |
| Vascular malformations |
| Arteriovenous fistula |

# 69 PRETIBIAL MYXEDEMA

Shane Clark, MD
Steven M. Dean, DO, FACP, RPVI

## PATIENT STORY

A 63-year-old woman presents for evaluation of unsightly erythematous-brown plaques on her anterior shins. The lesions appeared approximately 6 months ago and are occasionally itchy. She reports that she has delightfully but unintentionally lost 30 lb in the past year and her friends tell her she always looks "startled." On examination her skin is warm and flushed and her palms are sweaty, while her eyes are bulging with scleral show and proptosis of the upper eyelid. Examination reveals firm, nonpitting nodular red-brown plaques on her anterior shins and dorsal feet. She is diagnosed with hyperthyroidism with thyroid dermopathy. She is referred to endocrinology for further evaluation and definitive management of her hyperthyroidism and treated topically with daily application of a class 1 corticosteroid under occlusion; her skin lesions gradually resolve. Figures 69-1 and 69-2 show typical cases of pretibial myxedema (PTM), which is classically associated with Graves disease but can occur with other thyroid diseases.

## EPIDEMIOLOGY

- Localized myxedema or thyroid dermopathy is classically localized to the anterior shins; hence, it is more commonly known as PTM.

- PTM is rare and occurs in approximately 4.3% of patients with Graves disease.[1]

- PTM is nearly always associated with Graves disease but has been reported with Hashimoto thyroiditis as well as primary hypothyroidism and euthyroidism.[2]

- One-half of cases of thyroid dermopathy occur after the patient becomes euthyroid with treatment.[3]

- Peak incidence is in the fifth to sixth decades of life, but it can occur in children or at any age.[2]

- Females are more likely to be affected with a female-to-male ratio of 3.5:1.[2]

- The disease may regress spontaneously after months to years, persist indefinitely, or evolve into the most severe variant: elephantiasis nostras verrucosa (ENV).

## ETIOLOGY AND PATHOPHYSIOLOGY

- The exact cause and mechanism have yet to be determined.

- PTM is technically a misnomer, as edema is not a prominent feature of the disorder. Rather, the deposition of dermal mucin composed of glycosaminoglycans (GAGs), including hyaluronic acid and chondroitin sulfate, leads to the characteristic skin lesions.

- GAG deposition is thought to be due to fibroblast stimulation via activation by thyroid hormones or long-acting thyroid stimulator (LATS), an immunoglobulin G (IgG) antibody pathogenic in Graves disease.[2]

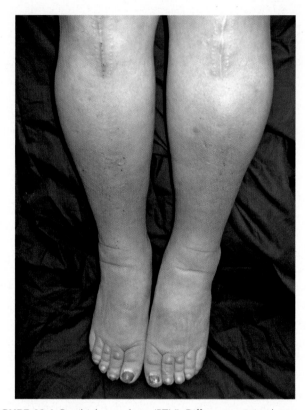

**FIGURE 69-1** Pretibial myxedema (PTM). Diffuse nonpitting brawny edema of the lower legs with characteristic involvement of the toes. (*Photograph courtesy of Steven M. Dean, DO.*)

- Pretibial and periorbital fibroblasts have been shown to share antigenic sites pathogenic in Graves disease, thus accounting for the development of myxedema even after destruction of the thyroid and establishment of euthyroidism.[3]

- Another theory proposes that thyroid hormones alter the metabolism of GAGs primarily through decreased degradation, thus accounting for their accumulation.[4]

- Mechanical trauma may contribute as well, given that localized myxedema may develop in areas of repetitive trauma.[5,6]

## DIAGNOSIS

- The diagnosis is typically clinical in the setting of the characteristic pretibial skin lesions with concurrent ophthalmopathy and a history of thyrotoxicosis.[7]

- A biopsy may be needed for confirmation in atypical cases, where the history is less clear, or when the patient has other confounding disease processes.

- The diagnosis is unlikely to be thyroid dermopathy if ophthalmopathy is not present.

- Patients with Graves disease will almost always have serologic evidence of autoimmune thyroid disease.[8]

## CLINICAL FEATURES

- While lesions may be morphologically variable (see Figures 69-1 to 69-6), the classical presentation consists of waxy, indurated, non-pitting, pebbly plaques that may have a peau d'orange appearance (Figure 69-3) on the anterior shins and dorsal feet. Alternatively, PTM may present as just a few skin-colored to purple-brown papules or nodules or appear as brawny nonpitting edema as in Figure 69-1. Pronounced infiltration of the dorsal toes with exaggerated skin creases is very characteristic of the disorder (see Figure 69-5).

- Less than 1% of cases evolve into ENV, which is characterized by coalescence of plaques and marked thickening and induration of the skin with a verruciform appearance (Figure 69-4).[9]

- PTM is often asymptomatic and only of cosmetic importance, but large plaques may be painful or pruritic.

- Rarely hypertrichosis or hyperhidrosis is present (limited to myxedematous skin).

- Patients often have other stigmata of Graves disease such as goiter, exophthalmos, and thyroid acropachy. Other signs of hyperthyroidism include cutaneous vasodilation causing facial flushing and palmar erythema, warm moist skin, fine soft hair, diffuse nonscarring scalp alopecia, nail changes including Plummer nails (onycholysis), or diffuse hyperpigmentation.

- PTM is found in up to 25% of patients with concurrent exophthalmos.[10]

- Patients typically manifest thyrotoxicosis first, followed by ophthalmopathy, and finally PTM (in cases where all three manifestations are present).[9]

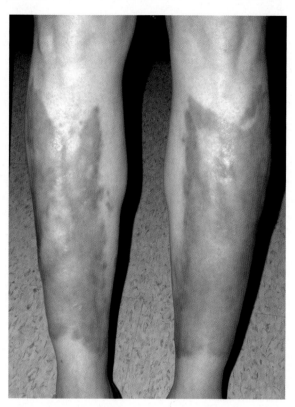

**FIGURE 69-2** Pretibial myxedema (PTM). Demarcated brownish-red plaques of the anterior shins consistent with PTM. (*Photograph courtesy of Matthew Zirwas, MD.*)

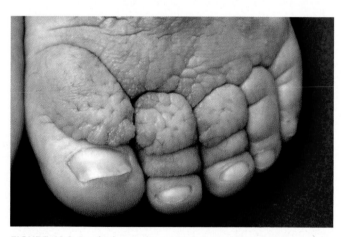

**FIGURE 69-3** Pretibial myxedema (PTM). Peau d'orange appearance on dorsal foot. (*Photograph courtesy of Matthew Zirwas, MD.*)

## TYPICAL DISTRIBUTION

- PTM (by virtue of its name) almost always affects the anterolateral leg and/or the dorsal foot and toes (Figure 69-6).
- Very rarely, localized myxedema may affect other parts of the body including shoulders, upper back, upper extremities, and pinnae.[11]

## LABORATORY STUDIES AND WORKUP

- A skin biopsy should be performed to rule out competing etiologies on the differential.
- Biopsy of PTM demonstrates a thickened dermis with increased dermal mucin limited to the reticular dermis with sparing of the papillary dermis. Collagen fibers are separated by mucin and appear reduced or wispy. Stellate fibroblasts may be present, but fibroblasts are normal in number. The epidermis often shows hyperkeratosis, papillomatosis, and acanthosis.[12]
- If the patient has undiagnosed thyroid disease, check thyroid studies including thyrotropin (thyroid-stimulating hormone), thyroxine ($T_4$), and triiodothyronine ($T_3$), as well as thyroid-receptor antibodies.

## DIFFERENTIAL DIAGNOSIS

- In all other diseases, ophthalmopathy and thyroid disease are typically absent.

### Lichen Simplex Chronicus

- Typically the patient gives a history of chronic pruritus.
- Pathology shows epidermal hyperkeratosis with a compact stratum corneum with irregular acanthosis. A stratum lucidum (typically limited to volar skin) may develop, giving the appearance of a "hairy palm."[12]
- No increased mucin is present.

### Lichen Amyloidosis

- This most often appears on the shins and is intensely pruritic, with lesions thought to be secondary to scratching.
- This can be seen in patients with multiple endocrine neoplasia type 2a (MEN 2a, also known as Sipple syndrome).
- Pathology demonstrates deposition of keratin-derived amyloid in the papillary dermis, as well as acanthosis and hyperkeratosis typical of lichen simplex chronicus.

### Scleromyxedema

- There are typically widespread lesions, and patients may have systemic and sclerodermoid features.
- The disorder may be associated with IgG paraproteinemia.
- Pathology demonstrates a thickened dermis with the triad of deposition of mucin, increased fibroblasts, and increased collagen.

### Stasis Dermatitis

- This appears most commonly in the setting of venous insufficiency as itchy brownish-red patches on the medial ankle that evolve to plaques and spread to the foot or calf.
- Mucin is restricted to the papillary dermis on pathology, and lesions will also display nodular angioplasia and hemosiderin deposition.

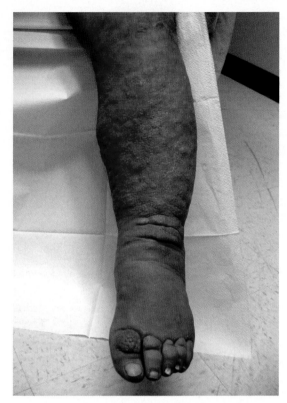

**FIGURE 69-4** Pretibial myxedema (PTM). PTM can rarely be nodular and elephantiasic. (*Photograph courtesy of Steven M. Dean, DO.*)

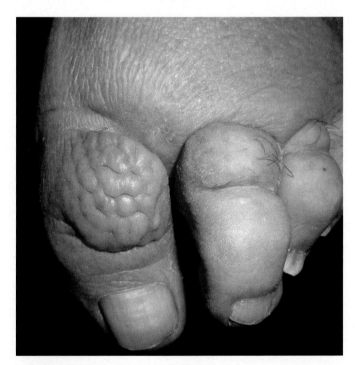

**FIGURE 69-5** Pretibial myxedema (PTM). Nodular with cerebriform plaque on great toe (close-up). (*Photograph courtesy of Matthew Zirwas, MD.*)

## Scleredema

- This is typically located on the upper back, neck, or face, but can involve the lower extremities.
- Depending on the type, it may be associated with a *Streptococcus* infection (type 1), a monoclonal gammopathy (type 2), or diabetes (type 3).
- Pathology demonstrates a thickened dermis with increased mucin most prominent in the reticular dermis. Fibroblasts are normal in number, and collagen bundles are normal but widely spaced with intervening mucin.[12]

## Hypertrophic Lichen Planus

- This presents with chronic, typically symmetric, extremely pruritic, thick hyperkeratotic plaques often on the anterior shins or dorsal feet.
- Pathology shows pronounced epidermal hyperplasia with acanthosis, papillomatosis, and elongated rete ridges without parakeratosis or eosinophils. A band-like infiltrate of lymphocytes is present at the epidermal-dermal junction with destruction of the basal layer.[12]
- This may be easily confused with well-differentiated squamous cell carcinoma on pathology.

## MANAGEMENT

- Normalizing thyroid function benefits the ophthalmopathy and may benefit the dermopathy.[13]
- Treatment is not needed unless the patient is symptomatic or bothered cosmetically. In a long-term study of 178 patients, only 54% required therapy.[8]
- Topical steroids are the standard of care—efficacy can be improved by occlusion (under Plastic Wrap).
- Long-term remission is dependent on severity of disease. After 25 years, 70% of mild untreated cases and 58% of more severe cases treated with local therapy had either a complete or partial remission.[8]
- Pentoxifylline may inhibit GAG synthesis and could be considered as an adjunctive therapy.[14]
- As PTM can result in secondary lymphedema, decongestive physiotherapy and compression may be helpful in certain cases.
- In the case of severe elephantiasis nostras verrucosa, consider surgical debridement.[15]

## PATIENT EDUCATION

- When other conditions have been ruled out, it is important to provide reassurance that the disease is often self-limited, infrequently symptomatic, and rarely a cause of any significant morbidity.

## FOLLOW-UP

- Periodic follow-up of monitoring for disease progression and for the prevention of complications related to therapy such as atrophy, telangiectasia, and striae related to topical corticosteroid therapy is appropriate.

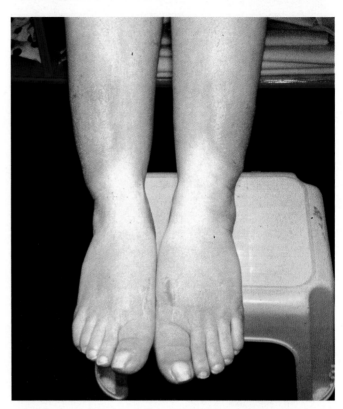

**FIGURE 69-6** Pretibial myxedema (PTM). Erythematous smooth plaques on anterior shins. (*Photograph courtesy of Steven M. Dean, DO.*)

## REFERENCES

1. Humbert P, Dupond JL, Carbillet JP. Pretibial myxedema: an overlapping clinical manifestation of autoimmune thyroid disease. *Am J Med.* 1987;83:1170-1171.

2. vonHilsheimer G. Pretibial myxedema. eMedicine. Available at: http://emedicine.medscape.com/article/1103765-overview. Accessed January 3, 2012.

3. Chung-Leddon J. Pretibial myxedema. *Dermatol Online J.* Feb 2001;7(1):18.

4. Komosinska-Vassev K, Winsz-Szczotka K, Olczyk K, Kozma EM. Alterations in serum glycosaminoglycan profiles in Graves' patients. *Clin Chem Lab Med.* 2006;44(5):582-588.

5. Davies TF. Trauma and pressure explain the clinical presentation of the Graves' disease triad. *Thyroid.* Aug 2000;10(8):629-630.

6. Singh SP, Ellyin F, Singh SK, et al. Elephantiasis-like appearance of upper and lower extremities in Graves' dermopathy. *Am J Med Sci.* Aug 1985;290(2):73-76.

7. Fatourechi V. Pretibial myxedema: pathophysiology and treatment options. *Am J Clin Dermatol.* 2005;6(5):295-309.

8. Schwartz KM, Fatourechi V, Ahmed DD, et al. Dermopathy of Graves' disease (pretibial myxedema): long-term outcome. *J Clin Endocrinol Metab.* Feb 2002;87(2):438-446.

9. Fatourechi V, Pajouhi M, Fransway AF. Dermopathy of Graves disease (pretibial myxedema). Review of 150 cases. *Medicine (Baltimore).* 1994;73:1-7.

10. Heymann WR. Cutaneous manifestations of thyroid disease. *JAAD.* 1992;25:885-906.

11. Noppakun N, Bancheun K, Chandraprasert S. Unusual locations of localized myxedema in Graves' disease. Report of three cases. *Arch Dermatol.* 1986;122:85-88.

12. Elston D, Ferringer T. Fibrous tumor. *Dermatopathology: Requisites in Dermatology.* Philadelphia, PA: Saunders; 2009: 313-344.

13. Wiersinga WM. Preventing Graves' ophthalmopathy. *N Engl J Med.* Jan 8 1998:338(2):121-122.

14. Chang CC, Chang TC, Kao SC, Kuo YF, Chien LF. Pentoxifylline inhibits the proliferation and glycosaminoglycan synthesis of cultured fibroblasts derived from patients with Graves' ophthalmopathy and pretibial myxedema. *Acta Endocrinol (Copenh).* Oct 1993;129(4):322-327.

15. Iwao F, Sato-Matsumura K, Sawamura D, Shimizu H. Elephantiasis nostras verrucosa successfully treated by surgical debridement. *Dermatol Surg.* 2004;30:939-941.

# 70 LIPEDEMA

Essa M. Essa, MBBS
Michael Davis, MD, FSVM
Steven M. Dean, DO, FACP, RPVI

## PATIENT STORY

A 50-year-old woman has noticed bilateral enlargement of her lower legs and buttocks since she was in her early 30s. She states that her feet appear normal and relates a marked size discrepancy between her upper body and lower body described as "my upper half is a size 8 and my lower half is a size 20." Her legs are extremely sore at the end of the day and bruise easily. Despite weight loss and exercise her swelling persists. She has been evaluated by several physicians in the past and had multiple negative venous duplex ultrasounds. Diuretics, compression stockings, and complex decongestive lymphatic physiotherapy were also prescribed without relief. After her last physician consultation she was given a diagnosis of "lymphedema" (Figure 70-1).

### EPIDEMIOLOGY

- The prevalence of lipedema is not well established. In two clinics specializing in lymphology and edema, 10% to 20% of clinic patients were diagnosed with lipedema, suggesting a prevalence of 0.06% to 0.07%.[1,2]

- A positive family history has been reported in 20% to 60% of patients diagnosed with lipedema, and current research suggests either X-linked dominant inheritance or, more likely, autosomal dominant inheritance with sex limitation.[3]

- Lipedema almost exclusively affects females, with only rare cases reported in men.[4]

- Onset of the disease is typically noticed between the ages of 10 and 30, but most patients present with this disease later in life or have had a substantial delay in diagnosis due to the under recognition of the condition.

### ETIOLOGY AND PATHOGENESIS

- Lipedema is a pathologic adverse deposition of fatty tissue, usually below the waist. It was first described by Dr. Edgar V. Allen and Dr. Edgar A. Hines in 1940 as a syndrome of subcutaneous symmetric deposition of fat in the buttocks and lower extremities and is often confused with obesity or lymphedema.[5]

- Lipedema is a chronic disease of lipid metabolism resulting in the symmetrical impairment of fatty tissue distribution and storage combined with hyperplasia and/or hypertrophy of individual fat cells.[6]

- The exact pathophysiologic cellular mechanism has not been clearly elucidated. It has been hypothesized that a correlation with an adverse hormonal axis exists due to lipedema's predilection for women as well as its onset around puberty. Other conditions of hormonal dysregulation such as cirrhosis underlie some cases, especially in men.[7]

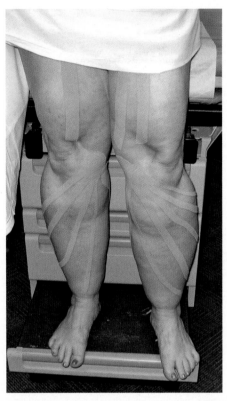

**FIGURE 70-1** Lipedema with sparing of the feet despite enlargement of the legs. Classic "ankle cut-off" sign is present with relatively symmetric deforming fat deposition in the upper thighs. The patient had been undergoing therapy for incorrectly diagnosed lymphedema.

- Additional mechanisms thought to play a role in the pathogenesis of lipedema include increased vascular permeability, excessive lipid peroxidation, and disturbances in adipocyte metabolism and cytokine production.[8]

- Lipedema is initially characterized by normal lymphatic function. However, as the disease progresses, some patients can develop lymphatic dysfunction and secondary lymphedema, a condition known as lipolymphedema. The majority of the patients with lipolymphedema are obese.

- Lipedema often runs a slow, progressive course over decades, but disease progression into lipolymphedema can accelerate suddenly.[9] Table 70-1 outlines a staging system to categorize disease progression.[10]

## DIAGNOSIS

The diagnosis of lipedema is a clinical one. Diagnostic tests are unhelpful but are sometimes used to identify associated conditions such as lymphedema or venous insufficiency.

## Clinical Features

### History

- The typical presentation of lipedema is one of symmetrical bilateral enlargement of the buttocks and lower extremities with sparing of the feet.[7]

- Involvement of the arms is less common but not rare. Most patients have a normal appearance from the waist up or a marked mismatch in fat deposition from the upper to lower body (Figure 70-2).

- Losing weight (including gastric bypass surgery) is usually not successful in reducing the size of the legs.

- The subcutaneous and adipose tissue is a source of persistent aching and tenderness, which is the genesis for the clinical synonym, the *painful fat syndrome*.[11]

- Patients with primary lipedema can have mild orthostatic edema, especially in warm weather. However, this superimposed edema is minimal and the overall size of the extremity is fixed and not alleviated by leg elevation and compression therapy.

- In contrast to patients with lymphedema, lipedema patients have a low incidence of cellulitis and other skin infections.

### Physical Examination

- The typical appearance of the lower extremities in lipedema is symmetrical enlargement of the bilateral legs with sparing of the feet (Figure 70-3).[12] The feet appear surprisingly normal, and the inability to pinch a fold of the dorsal skin at the base of the toes (Stemmer sign) is negative in lipedema.[9] In contrast, patients with lymphedema manifest swelling of the feet and toes.

- In early stages, the first sign is usually the disappearance of the concave spaces on both sides of the Achilles tendon (retromalleolar sulcus).[13] As the condition progresses, prominent perimalleolar fat pads form, creating the fat-pad sign. A sharp demarcation between normal and abnormal tissue at the ankle can often be observed, creating the classic "ankle cut-off" or "ankle cuff" sign (Figure 70-4).

**TABLE 70-1.** Grading of Lipedema

| Stage | Characteristics |
|-------|-----------------|
| I | The skin is still soft and regular, but nodular changes can be felt upon palpation. There are no color changes in the skin, and the subcutaneous tissues have a spongy feel, like a soft rubber doll. Tissue hyperesthesia may develop. |
| II | The subcutaneous tissue becomes tougher and nodular. Large fatty lobules begin to form on the medial, distal, and proximal thigh and the medial and lateral ankles just above the ankle bones. The skin may have a "cottage-cheese" or "mattress" appearance. The individual may report increased hypersensitivity over the skin area. Secondary lymphedema may develop with increased leg edema, color changes, and skin fibrosis. |
| III | Bulging protrusions of fat occur on the thighs and knees that can interfere with normal gait. The patient may transition into lipolymphedema with increasing lymphatic obstruction, progressive swelling, (sub)cutaneous fibrosis, and/or weeping skin erosions. The incidence of cellulitis is increased. |

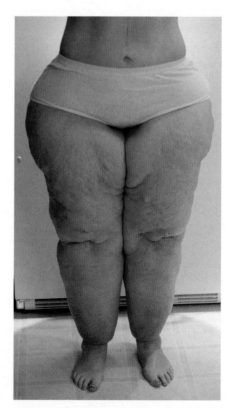

**FIGURE 70-2** Classic representation of the truncal–lower extremity mismatch that exemplifies lipedema.

- Nonpitting fatty edema exists in the early stages of lipedema; however, in long-standing lipedema, there may be lymphatic fluid accumulation with associated pitting edema.

- The subcutaneous adipose tissue is tender to palpation, and bruises may be identified from increased vascular permeability and blood vessel fragility.

- The skin examination in early stages of lipedema reveals a soft and regular appearance with mild nodularity when palpated. As the disease progresses, larger fat nodules form with skin mottling. This mottled appearance resembles a "mattress" or "walnut shell" (Figure 70-5).

- The final stage of lipedema is characterized by massively enlarged nodules and pendulous fat deposits resembling the "Michelin Tire Man" with associated progressive limb pain and gait disturbances (Figure 70-6).

- Severe lipolymphedema is associated with skin hardening and fibrosis often with weeping skin ulcerations. The feet and/or toes are swollen consistent with associated secondary lymphedema (Figure 70-7).

## Laboratory and Imaging Studies

Blood work and imaging studies are not routinely needed to establish a diagnosis for lipedema but to identify coexisting conditions. Vascular ultrasound can identify underlying venous pathology such as venous reflux in patients with lipedema, termed phlebolipedema, which can coexist and aggravate limb edema (Figure 70-8). Lymphoscintigraphy can confirm the diagnosis of coexistent lymphedema.[14,15] Magnetic resonance lymphangiography is a newer imaging modality that can be utilized to identify underlying lymphatic involvement.[15,16]

## Histopathologic Features

- Pathologically, the subcutaneous tissue seen in early lipedema patients is soft and lacks the fibrotic elements seen in patients with lymphedema.

- Histology usually reveals no specific abnormalities aside from edematous adipose cells with moderate hyperplasia and hypertrophy.[17]

## DIFFERENTIAL DIAGNOSIS

- Although lipedema can eventually lead to secondary lymphedema, it should not be mistaken for lymphedema in its early stages.

- Obesity is distinguished from lipedema by the distribution of the fatty deposition and by its response to diet and exercise. Additionally, obesity-associated swelling is not associated with the pain and tenderness found in lipedema.

- Table 70-2 summarizes the different clinical features of lipedema, lymphedema, and obesity.

## MANAGEMENT

- Gentle compression garments can be used to manage the orthostatic component of edema. There is limited benefit from aggressive compression bandaging and manual lymphatic drainage in the absence of secondary lymphedema.

- Diuretics are not overly beneficial and should be used sparingly if at all when secondary lymphedema develops.

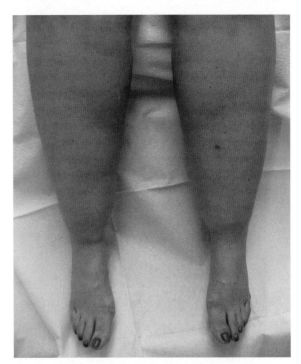

FIGURE 70-3 Lipedema with symmetric enlargement of the legs, sparing of the feet, and representative "ankle cut-off" sign. Note the ecchymotic area involving the left anterior tibial region from increased vascular permeability and blood vessel fragility. Stemmer sign is negative.

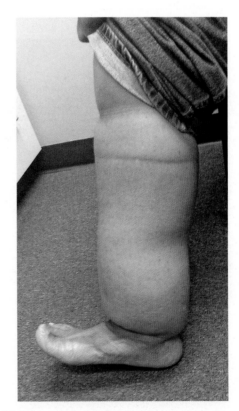

FIGURE 70-4 A rare male patient with lipedema and a "stove-pipe" appearing leg with ankle cut-off sign. The patient described several aunts who had skinny feet and large legs.

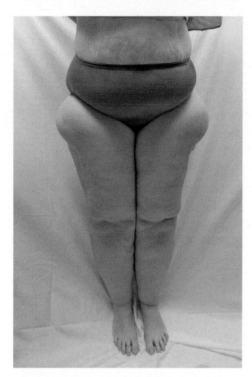

**FIGURE 70-5** Enlarged fatty nodules and a "walnut shell" appearance overlie the thighs of a patient with stage II lipedema.

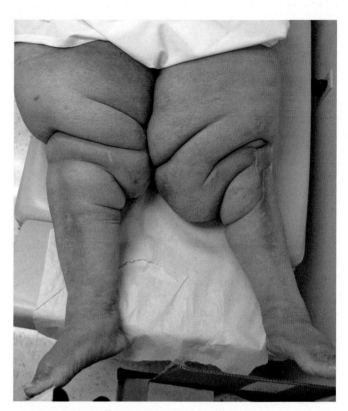

**FIGURE 70-7** Note the combination of massive proximal lipedema and milder distally located lymphedema or lipolymphedema.

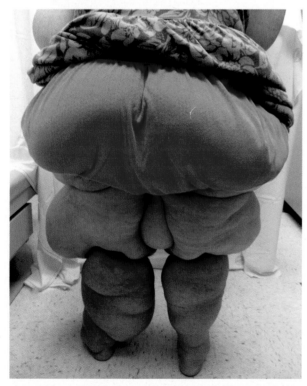

**FIGURE 70-6** Giant pendulous fat deposits exemplify stage III lipedema. Secondary lymphedema has swelved within the left calf as well, signifying lipolymphedema.

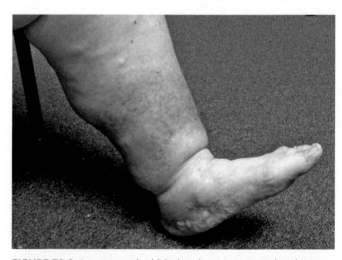

**FIGURE 70-8** A patient with phlebolipedema (coexisting lipedema and venous insufficiency). The lipedema heralded the venous changes by over a decade. Ankle cut-off sign is present with hyperpigmentation (bronzing) of the pretibial region with stasis dermatitis. Medial calf varicosities are also visualized.

**TABLE 70-2.** Clinical Features of Lipedema, Lymphedema, and Obesity

| Characteristic | Lipedema | Lymphedema | Obesity |
|---|---|---|---|
| Onset | Age 10 to 30 years | Childhood (primary) Adulthood (secondary) | Any age |
| Gender | Mostly female Rare cases male | Either sex | Either sex |
| Positive family history | Common | Only primary lymphedema variant | Common |
| Body area afflicted | Bilateral buttocks, thighs, and legs (sparing feet). Less commonly, arms (sparing hands) | Usually asymmetric, feet affected first followed by progressive leg involvement | All body parts |
| Effect of diet and weight loss | No effect | No effect | Positive effect |
| Leg pain (nonarthritic) | Yes | No | No |
| Easy bruising | Yes | No | No |
| Pitting edema | None/minimal | Absent until secondary lymphedema develops | Absent |
| Stemmer sign | Negative | Positive | Negative |

- Weight control and exercise are essential, especially in lipedema patients. Since pelvic and knee osteoarthritis is common due to excessive joint stress, water-based exercises are beneficial.

- Advanced cases of extreme pain, severe ambulatory disability, and distress from cosmetic appearance have been successfully treated with liposuction.[18-21]

## PATIENT EDUCATION

- Educating the patient about the condition is paramount since most patients have likely had a delay in diagnosis and previously performed therapies that were ineffective in improving their condition (diuretics, diet and weight loss therapy etc).

- Since the social and psychologic impact lipedema has on patients' lives can be demoralizing, attention to depression screening should be considered.

- Referral to psychologic counseling may be warranted in advanced cases to help patients deal with the entire clinical spectrum of lipedema.

- Education about skin care and avoiding mechanical trauma that could induce ulceration or bleeding is essential.

- Control of concomitant lymphedema with compression therapy and/or manual lymphatic drainage and pneumatic pumps can be effective.

- Weight loss and exercise in appropriate cases should be recommended.

## FOLLOW-UP

• Regarding lipedema, initial follow-up may be appropriate for control of symptoms, assurance of a stable disease course, and psychologic well-being. If lympholipedema is present, compliance with compression therapy should be monitored to prevent adverse lymphatic skin and tissue pathology.

### PATIENT AND PROVIDER RESOURCES

• http://www.curelipedema.org
• http://www.biglegwoman.com

## REFERENCES

1. Allen EV, Hines EA. Lipedema of the legs: a syndrome characterized by fat legs and orthostatic edema. *Proc Staff Mayo Clin.* 1940;15:184-187.

2. Herpertz U. Lipedema. *Z Lymphol.* 1995;19:1-11.

3. Gregl A. Lipedema. *Z Lymphol.* 1987;11:41-43.

4. Child AH, Gordon KD, Sharpe P, et al. Lipedema: an inherited condition. *Am J Med Genet A.* 2010;152A:970-976.

5. Chen SG, Hsu SD, Chen TM, Wang HJ. Painful fat syndrome in a male patient. *Br J Plast Surg.* 2004;57:282-286.

6. Macdonald JM, Sims N, Mayrovitz HN. Lymphedema, lipedema, and the open wound: the role of compression therapy. *Surg Clin North Am.* 2003;83:639-658.

7. Fonder MA, Loveless JW, Lazarus GS. Lipedema, a frequently unrecognized problem. *J Am Acad Dermatol.* 2007;57:S1-S3.

8. Foldi E, Foldi M, Tischendorf F. Adipositas, lipedema and lymphostasis. *Med Welt.* 1983;34:198-200.

9. Fife CE, Carter MJ. Lymphedema in the morbidly obese patient: unique challenges in a unique population. *Ostomy Wound Manage.* 2008;54:44-56.

10. Meier-Vollrath I, Schmeller W. [Lipoedema—current status, new perspectives]. *J Dtsch Dermatol Ges.* 2004;2:181-186.

11. Wold LE, Hines EA Jr, Allen EV. Lipedema of the legs; a syndrome characterized by fat legs and edema. *Ann Intern Med.* 1951;34:1243-1250.

12. Fife CE, Maus EA, Carter MJ. Lipedema: a frequently misdiagnosed and misunderstood fatty deposition syndrome. *Adv Skin Wound Care.* 2010;23:81-92; quiz 3-4.

13. Stutz JJ, Krahl D. Water jet-assisted liposuction for patients with lipoedema: histologic and immunohistologic analysis of the aspirates of 30 lipoedema patients. *Aesthetic Plast Surg.* 2009;33:153-162.

14. Pereira De Godoy JM, De Moura Alvares R, Simon Torati JL, De Fatima Guerreiro Godoy M. Clinical aspects of advanced stage lipo-lymphedema: case report. *G Ital Dermatol Venereol.* 2010;145:547-549.

15. Boursier V, Pecking A, Vignes S. [Comparative analysis of lymphoscintigraphy between lipedema and lower limb lymphedema]. *J Mal Vasc.* 2004;29:257-261.

16. Pecking AP, Desprez-Curely JP, Cluzan RV. [Tests and imaging of the lymphatic system]. *Rev Med Interne.* 2002;23(suppl 3):S391-S397.

17. Lohrmann C, Foeldi E, Langer M. MR imaging of the lymphatic system in patients with lipedema and lipo-lymphedema. *Microvasc Res.* 2009;77:335-339.

18. Bilancini S, Lucchi M, Tucci S, Eleuteri P. Functional lymphatic alterations in patients suffering from lipedema. *Angiology.* 1995;46:333-339.

19. Peled AW, Slavin SA, Brorson H. Long-term outcome after surgical treatment of lipedema. *Ann Plast Surg.* 2012;68(3):303-307.

20. Schmeller W, Meier-Vollrath I. Tumescent liposuction: a new and successful therapy for lipedema. *J Cutan Med Surg.* 2006;10:7-10.

21. Rapprich S, Dingler A, Podda M. Liposuction is an effective treatment for lipedema—results of a study with 25 patients. *J Dtsch Dermatol Ges.* 2011;9:33-40.

# 71 LIPOLYMPHEDEMA

Caroline E. Fife, MD
Marissa J. Carter, MA, PhD

## PATIENT STORY

A 44-year-old Caucasian woman with type I diabetes presented with massive localized lymphedema (MLL), a phenotype of lymphedema. She had been overweight most of her adult life, with most of her body weight being disproportionally distributed in her lower body. However, actual leg swelling had begun about 10 years ago. She was either scratched or bitten on the left calf and developed cellulitis with sepsis. The left leg edema continued to worsen even after the cellulitis resolved until it was profoundly enlarged, and gradually the right leg began to enlarge as well. The pendulous enlargements at the back of both thighs began slowly and continued to increase over the years until they began to affect her ability to walk. She had undergone a lap band for morbid obesity 2 years ago and had lost more than 45 kg, but this had little effect on her leg enlargement. Compression stockings would not fit.

On clinical examination she was found to have stage III lymphedema with elephantiasis and massive localized lymphedema on both the legs, the left being worse than the right (Figures 71-1 and 71-2). Her right foot was spared, but the left foot exhibited a positive Stemmer sign (the inability to pinch a fold of skin at the base of the second toe), which is diagnostic of lymphedema. The patient responded very well to standard treatment for lymphedema with complete decongestive physiotherapy (Figures 71-3 and 71-4). She was provided with custom garments and a pneumatic compression device to help her with long-term management.

It is common for patients to relate the onset of lymphedema to an episode of cellulitis. However, it can be difficult to determine whether the cellulitis was due to her lymphedema, or the other way around. Her age of onset, the fact that her foot was affected, and the severity of its progression are factors that suggest she might originally have had a form of primary lymphedema (lymphedema tarda), which presents about the age of 35. In other words, inherently inadequate lymphatic function may have predisposed her to cellulitis (a problem for which she was even at higher risk due to diabetes mellitus). The trigger for the development of clinically apparent lymphedema was likely the episode of cellulitis, with subsequent damage to the lymphatics after the cellulitis worsened lymphatic transport. Under these conditions a vicious cycle can develop, and this may result in recurrent episodes of cellulitis with continued worsening of lymphatic function and progressive edema. The patient also may have a genetic fatty deposition disorder called lipedema, which causes fat to be preferentially deposited below the waist. In some cases, patients with this type of leg enlargement progress to lymphedema. Most patients with lipedema have sparing of their feet until quite late. In patients like this, it can be challenging to determine whether they have primary (congenital) or secondary lymphedema, and these definitions may become obsolete, as better lymphatic imaging now suggests lymphatic transport

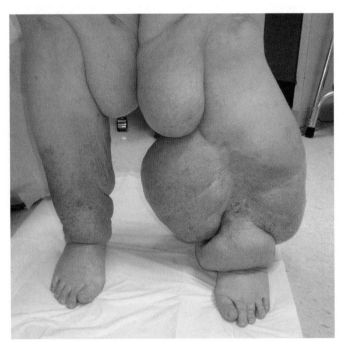

FIGURE 71-1 Anterior view of the patient at presentation.

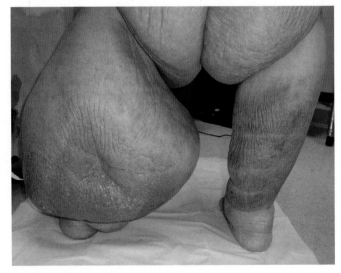

FIGURE 71-2 Posterior view of the patient at presentation.

capacity ranges along a continuum. Treatment differs little regardless of etiology.

## EPIDEMIOLOGY

### Lipedema

- Genetic disorder of fatty deposition, usually below the waist
- Usually presents in adulthood (typically 30 years onward)
- Progression is typically slow (period of years)
- Almost exclusively affects females so there is an assumed hormonal influence[1]

### Lipolymphedema

- Some patients with lipedema progress to develop lymphedema (thus, lipolymphedema), when swelling is persistent and the feet become affected (Figure 71-5). Cutaneous fibrosis suggests superimposed lymphedema has evolved as well.
- Rare, but may be increasing due to marked increase in obesity levels in Western populations.

### MLL

- Characterized by extreme localized enlargement of the limb (usually the thigh but can be the upper arm) due to lymphatic fluid and its associated inflammatory tissue changes.
- MLL is more common in morbidly obese patients.[2]
- Although lipolymphedema is rare in males, a substantial proportion of MLL patients are males.[2,3]
- Previously described in the literature as a rare disorder, in a clinic-based population of patients with lower extremity lymphedema, 1.3% had MLL.[4]

## ETIOLOGY AND PATHOPHYSIOLOGY

### Lipolymphedema

- Most common etiology appears to be initial lipedema with progression to secondary lymphedema, which can take as long as 17 years according to one study.[5,6] In this case, the lipedema—deposition of fat around the buttocks and legs but sparing of the feet (pantaloon appearance)—becomes more widespread as the lymphedema progresses. Although the mechanism for development of lipolymphedema is not fully understood, it is believed that in some instances the fat deposition from lipedema causes damage to lymphatic and capillary systems. A subclinical phenotype of primary lymphedema may also be present that predisposes the lower extremities toward lymphedema particularly after trauma or injury.[1]

### MLL

- Histologic findings of MLL consist of a thickened epidermis with expansion of the dermis, as well as lymphangiectasia in the absence of atypical stromal cells, adipocytes, or lymphoblasts.[2,3,7] Dilated lymphatic channels, dermal edema, and fibrosis are common.[8] Although pathogenesis is unclear, it might be that an initial localized lymphatic obstruction causes fluid to accumulate, thus stimulating tissue growth factor release with the emergence of hypertrophic chronic lymphedema.[9]

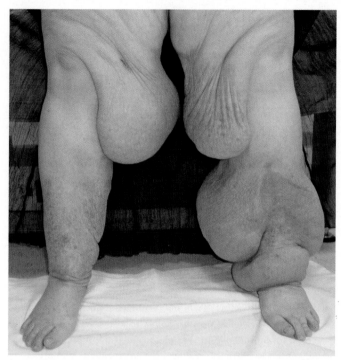

**FIGURE 71-3** Patient response after four weeks of intensive complex decongestive treatment.

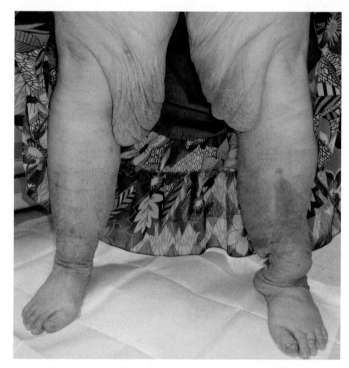

**FIGURE 71-4** Current view of lower extremities after eight weeks of intensive complex decongestive treatment.

## DIAGNOSIS

### Clinical Features

#### Lipedema

- The feet are spared initially, and orthostatic edema usually resolves with a night's rest.
- Affected tissue can be easily bruised, and pitting edema may be visible.[1]
- The legs are usually painful, often described as an aching dysesthesia.[1,10]

#### Lymphedema

- Skin inflammation.[10]
- Presentation tends to be bilateral if progressing from lipedema, but some asymmetricity in appearance does occur.[10]
- Peau d'orange skin changes or even "cobblestone" appearance with stage III.[2,8,9,11]
- Positive Stemmer sign (inability to pinch a fold of skin at the base of the toes).[1]

#### MLL

- Although single lymphedematous masses are the most common, multiple masses are frequently observed.
- Peau d'orange skin changes or even "cobblestone" appearance.[2,8,9,11]
- The degree of lymphedema associated with the MLL enlargements, sometimes referred to as "pseudosarcomas," in the lower extremities may vary from stage 0 to stage 3.

### Typical Distribution

#### Lipolymphedema

- Although the condition may initially affect the thighs, hips, and inguinal region, the feet become affected eventually (note that in this chapter we are only focusing on the lipolymphedema syndrome and not on congenital lymphedema, which can occur anywhere on the body, or lymphedema secondary to surgery, such as breast cancer).

#### MLL

- Usually localized to the medial aspect of the thigh, but also in the inguinal region and the dependent aspect of the abdomen (it has been described in the upper arm).[2,3,7]
- Masses ranging from 3 to 30 kg have been removed.

### Laboratory Studies

#### Lipedema

- There is no genetic test for this syndrome, and diagnosis is made on the basis of body habitus and history of the triad (easy bruising, aching dysesthesia, and orthostatic edema).

#### Lymphedema Associated With Lipedema (Lipolymphedema)

- In general, diagnostic tests are not needed as the diagnosis is usually made based on clinical findings (eg, Stemmer sign).

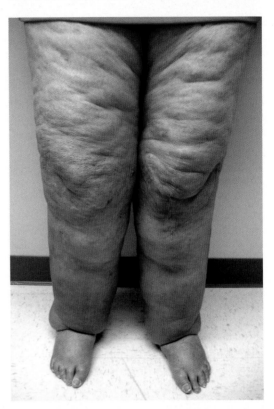

**FIGURE 71-5** A 59-year-old woman with a long-standing classic lipedema. Over the last 6 years, her feet have become swollen, suggesting evolution to lipolymphedema. (*Photograph courtesy of Steven M. Dean, DO.*)

- Currently available diagnostic tests are insufficient to distinguish primary from secondary lymphedema (eg, nuclear scintigraphy), but diagnostic studies under development may provide quantitative anatomic information (fluorescent indocyanine green), which could help determine whether the patient has a congenital lymphatic disorder or damage secondary to infection.[12] Magnetic resonance lymphangiography studies are helpful in defining lymphatic damage in lipolymphedema.[13] Venous duplex studies may be worthwhile to establish whether correctable venous disease is present.

## MLL

- MLL enlargements do not require biopsy as there have been no reports of angiosarcoma in the literature arising from MLL. However, angiosarcomas can arise from chronic lymphedematous tissue, so worrisome skin lesions may warrant biopsy. Often a biopsy is taken if the MLL is excised.

## DIFFERENTIAL DIAGNOSIS

### Differential Diagnosis of Limb Swelling

- Hypothyroidism and hyperthyroidism can both cause myxedema, which may mimic lymphedema (thyroid studies should be performed).

- Heart failure (right or left sided) and renal failure can cause severe peripheral edema, and compression may be dangerous to these patients until failure is controlled.

### Lipedema Versus Lymphedema

- Lipolymphedema can usually be differentiated from lipedema and secondary lymphedema by several factors (Table 71-1).

**TABLE 71-1.** Differential Diagnosis Between Lipolymphedema, Lipedema, and Secondary Lymphedema

| Attribute | Lipolymphedema | Lipedema | Secondary Lymphedema |
|---|---|---|---|
| Gender | Almost exclusively female | Almost exclusively female | Male or female |
| Trigger | Sometimes no trigger but can suddenly progress after injury, trauma, or surgery | Thought to be genetically mediated | Injury, trauma, or surgery |
| Time at onset and course | Usually 30 years onward; slow development | Usually 10 to 30 years; slow development | Adulthood; fast development in some cases |
| Family history positive | Sometimes | Common | No |
| Area affected | Legs, thighs, hips, but feet spared initially | Legs, thighs, hips, but feet spared | Typically arms, legs, thighs, but other areas can be affected |
| Effect of elevation | Helpful until fibrosis occurs | Minimal | None |
| Pitting edema | Often present | Minimal | Present until stopped by fibrosis |
| Bruises easily | Yes | Yes | No |
| Pain | Yes, legs | Yes, legs | Only in later stages |
| Stemmer sign | Present | Absent | Present |

## MLL

- It is important to rule out malignant lesions, such as well-differentiated liposarcoma, and a biopsy can be obtained when surgery takes place in cases of doubt.[11] However, many physicians and pathologists have difficulty identifying MLL, and it is sometimes mistaken for lipoma, lipomatosis, excess adipose tissue, lymphocoele, secondary lymphedema, atypical lipomatous tumor or well-differentiated liposarcoma (ALT or WDL), or some kind of neoplasm.[2] Gross examination of the specimen is the most accurate method to diagnose MLL.

## MANAGEMENT

### Lipolymphedema

- Lipedema, in the absence of actual lymphedema, does not respond to compression. If leg enlargement is due to uncomplicated fatty deposition, then light compression garments may provide relief from associated orthostatic edema.

- The lymphedema component of lipolymphedema usually responds to complete decongestive physiotherapy,[14] which comprises manual lymph drainage (MLD), compression bandaging, and skin care. Compression bandaging is provided with low-stretch washable, reusable cotton bandages that provide little elasticity when maximum tension is applied.[10] These have a low resting pressure on the skin but act as a shell against which the muscles contract (a high working pressure) during exercise. Bandaging is combined with MLD, a light, manual skin technique applied by certified lymphedema therapists to improve fluid removal from congested areas into lymph vessels and lymph nodes that are functioning.[15] The combination of bandaging, MLD, skin hygiene, and therapeutic exercise is referred to as complete decongestive physiotherapy (CDP).

- Custom garments may be necessary to fit patients with irregularly shaped extremities or patients who are obese.

- For obese patients who are not able to wear stockings, or for patients with very irregularly shaped extremities, a variety of semi-rigid devices, such as CircAid, LegAssist, or Farrow wraps, are available.[10]

- Use of intermittent pneumatic pumps can be helpful but are not a substitute for garments.[16]

- Long-term weight control is essential, either through diets or bariatric surgery for more obese patients. Some patients may benefit from liposuction.[1]

## MLL

- MLL masses are usually resected en bloc, although recurrence may occur in as many as 50% of cases.[7]

- After surgery, weight reduction, physical therapy, compression, MLD, and good skin hygiene will all help, although it is not known how successful these therapies are in reducing recurrence.[3,8,17]

## PATIENT EDUCATION

### Lipolymphedema

- It is important to communicate with the patient that this is a lifelong condition that at present cannot be cured but can be successfully managed through a variety of techniques. Most importantly, the initial phase of treatment of lymphedema will require cooperation from the patient and self-care.

## MLL

- Patients should be instructed to lose weight, have bariatric surgery if necessary, and maintain a healthy lifestyle with as much exercise as possible, as MLL is most associated with morbid obesity and has a high recurrence rate. MLL collections can be removed, but if weight is not controlled and compression is not maintained, they may return.

### PATIENT AND PROVIDER RESOURCES

- http://www.lymphedemapeople.com/thesite/lymphedema_lipodema.ht
- http://www.lipomadoc.org/

## REFERENCES

1. Fife CE, Maus EA, Carter MJ. Lipedema: a frequently misdiagnosed and misunderstood fatty deposition syndrome. *Adv Skin Wound Care*. 2010;23:81-94.

2. Manduch M, Oliveira AM, Nascimento AG, Folpe AL. Massive localised lymphoedema: a clinicopathological study of 22 cases and review of the literature. *J Clin Pathol*. 2009;62:808-811.

3. Farshid G, Weiss SW. Massive localized lymphedema in the morbidly obese: a histologically distinct reactive lesion simulating liposarcoma. *Am J Surg Pathol*. 1998;22:1277-1283.

4. Fife C, Carter M. Lymphoedema in bariatric patients. *J Lymphoedema*. 2009;4:29-37.

5. Pereira De Godoy JM, Augusto Dos Santos R, Vilela Filho RA, Guerreiro Godoy Mde F. Erysipelas and ulcer of the legs in patients with lipolymphedema. *Eur J Dermatol*. 2011;21:101-102.

6. Földi M, Idiazabal G. The role of operative management of varicose veins in patients with lymphedema and/or lipedema of the leg. *Lymphology*. 2000;33:167-171.

7. Wu D, Gibbs J, Corral D, et al. Massive localized lymphedema: additional locations and association with hypothyroidism. *Hum Pathol*. 2000;31:1162-1168.

8. Asch S, James WD, Castelo-Soccio L. Massive localized lymphedema: an emerging dermatologic complication of obesity. *J Am Acad Dermatol*. 2008;59(suppl 5):S109-S110.

9. Jensen V, Witte MH, Tatifi R. Massive localized lipolymphedema pseudotumor in a morbidly obese patient. *Lymphology*. 2006;39:181-184.

10. Fife CE, Carter MJ. Lymphedema in the morbidly obese patient: unique challenges in a unique population. *Ostomy Wound Manage*. 2008;54:44-56.

11. Berenji M, Kalani A, Kim J, Kelly K, Wallack MK. Massive localized lymphedema of the thigh in a morbidly obese patient. *Eur J Surg Oncol*. 2010;36:104-106.

12. Tan IC, Maus EA, Rasmussen JC, et al. Assessment of lymphatic contractile function after manual lymphatic drainage using near-infrared fluorescence imaging. *Arch Phys Med Rehabil*. 2011;92:756-764.e1.

13. Lohrmann C, Foeldi E, Langer M. MR imaging of the lymphatic system in patients with lipedema and lipo-lymphedema. *Microvasc Res*. 2009;77:335-339.

14. Foldi E. The treatment of lymphedema. *Cancer*. 1998;83(suppl American 12):2833-2835.

15. McNeely M. The addition of manual lymph drainage to compression therapy for breast cancer related lymphedema: a randomized controlled trial. *Breast Cancer Res Treat*. 2004;86:95-106.

16. Moseley AL, Carati CJ, Piller NB. A systematic review of common conservative therapies for arm lymphoedema secondary to breast cancer treatment. *Ann Oncol*. 2007;18:639-646.

17. Goshtasby P. Dawson J, Agarwal N. Pseudosarcoma: massive localized lymphedema of the morbidly obese. *Obes Surg*. 2006;16: 88-93.

# 72 PHLEBOLYMPHEDEMA

Peter M. Bittenbender, MD
Steven M. Dean, DO, FACP, RPVI

## PATIENT STORY

A 58-year-old morbidly obese woman presents for a second opinion regarding leg swelling. She describes bilateral lower extremity swelling and discoloration that has progressed over the past 4 years. Examination is remarkable for a body mass index (BMI) of 47 and severe nonpitting bilateral leg swelling involving the dorsal feet and toes with extension to the distal thighs. Atrophy is identified within hyperpigmented distal calves, which are diffusely indurated (Figure 72-1). Verrucous-appearing papules with deep creases overlie the distal calves. Although venous duplex ultrasonography does not indicate deep venous thrombosis (DVT), incompetent deep and superficial veins are identified bilaterally. The patient is ultimately diagnosed with a combination of chronic venous insufficiency (CVI) and lymphedema or phlebolymphedema.

### EPIDEMIOLOGY

- Because of the vast unawareness and underdiagnosis of phlebolymphedema[1,2] and the potentially confusing overlap in manifestations of CVI and lymphedema, there is little data in regard to the prevalence of this entity.

- CVI is estimated in up to 10% to 20% of the population, and up to 20% to 30% of patients with CVI will have associated lymphatic dysfunction.

- While the gender difference in phlebolymphedema is not reported, both CVI and lymphedema are more common among women. However, venous insufficiency is generally more severe in men.

- The emergence of venous insufficiency generally begins in the fourth or fifth decade and becomes more prevalent with advancing age.

### ETIOLOGY AND PATHOPHYSIOLOGY

- Phlebolymphedema is defined as combined insufficiency of both the venous and lymphatic systems.

- Although a preponderance of phlebolymphedema is secondary to severe CVI of various causes, primary cases in association with congenital lymphovenous defects exist. Klippel-Trenaunay syndrome is the classic example of primary phlebolymphedema (Figure 72-2).

- CVI is due to incompetent venous valves, venous obstruction (compression from an external mass or luminal obstruction from a venous thrombus), or both.

- CVI causes venous hypertension with subsequent excessive capillary filtration of fluid into the interstitial space. Lymphatic transport initially increases to compensate for this excess filtrate. If venous hypertension remains unabated, the lymphatic system is overwhelmed, eventuating in secondary lymphedema. Chronic

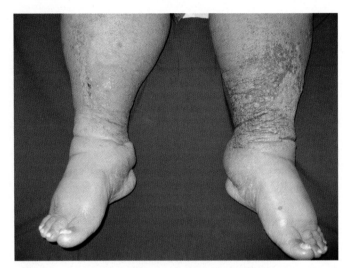

FIGURE 72-1 Classic example of secondary phlebolymphedema in a morbidly obese patient. Note the marked bilateral calf, foot and toe swelling consistent with lymphedema, yet associated relative distal calf atrophy and hyperpigmentation consistent with chronic stasis lipodermatosclerosis. The distal calf papulonodular and verrucous appearance is consistent with elephantiasis.

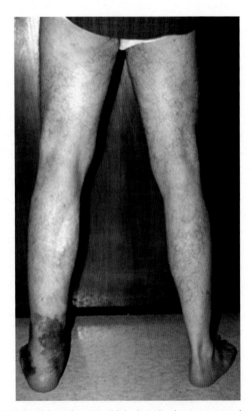

FIGURE 72-2 Although most phlebolymphedema is secondary to chronic venous insufficiency (CVI), congenital vascular malformations such as Klippel-Trenaunay syndrome are primary causes.

stasis-associated inflammation can lead to lymphangiothrombosis, which further impairs the lymphatic system.

- As in primary and secondary lymphedemas, the interstitial fluid in phlebolymphedema ultimately becomes protein rich, as opposed to the protein-poor fluid of uncomplicated venous insufficiency.

- The presence of high-protein lymphatic fluid in the interstitium stimulates fibroblasts, keratinocytes, and leukocytes, leading to the deposition of collagen and destruction of elastic fibers eventually yielding cutaneous and subcutaneous fibrosis.

- In severe cases, the lymphatic dysfunction becomes permanent, resulting in chronic lymphedema even if the underlying venous insufficiency is corrected.

- The aforementioned lymphovenous hypertension is more severe in the presence of morbid obesity.

- In a study of 21 patients with elephantiasis, 71% of the subjects had concurrent CVI, and all subjects were obese with a mean BMI of 56.[3]

## DIAGNOSIS

The diagnosis of phlebolymphedema is primarily based on history and physical examination.[4] However, duplex ultrasonography can document venous incompetency or obstruction. Nuclear lymphoscintigraphy may be performed to confirm the presence of concomitant lymphatic impairment, but is generally not necessary.

### Clinical Features

- Manifestations of both CVI and lymphedema coexist (Figures 72-3 and 72-4).

- Phlebolymphedema can be unilateral or bilateral.

- Early in the disease course, patients generally have pitting edema of the lower extremities, yet in protracted lymphovenous hypertension, the edema fails to pit due to associated (sub)cutaneous fibrosis.

- Signs of CVI include hyperpigmentation within the gaiter distribution, ectatic veins, eczema, and corona phlebectatica (ankle flair sign). Advanced venous hypertension is manifested by nonpitting woody edema, ulcerations, and lipodermatosclerosis with an "inverted bowling pin" appearance of the calves. The absence of foot swelling characterizes uncomplicated CVI (Figure 72-5).

- Signs of lymphedema include limb swelling that is pronounced distally including foot or toe involvement with an "elephantine" appearance to the ankles (Figure 72-6). Stemmer sign (the inability of the examiner to tent the skin over the dorsum of the second digit) is positive in advanced stages. With progressive lymphedema, hyperkeratosis, cutaneous fibrosis, and hypertrophic nodules with verrucous "cobblestoning" eventuate. Foul-smelling ulcerations may complicate elephantiasis.

- The majority of affected patients are obese or morbidly obese.

### Duplex Ultrasonography

Duplex ultrasonography is used to evaluate the deep veins of the lower extremity for thrombus or external compression, and is also used to evaluate the location and degree of venous reflux.

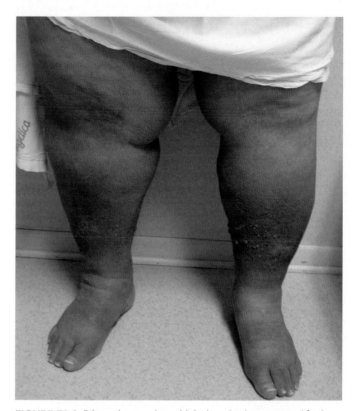

**FIGURE 72-3** Bilateral secondary phlebolymphedema exemplified by a combination of nodular elephantiasis and profound stasis hyperpigmentation. Woody induration and mild atrophy are present within the distal calves consistent with the "inverted bowling pin" appearance of long-standing lipodermatosclerosis.

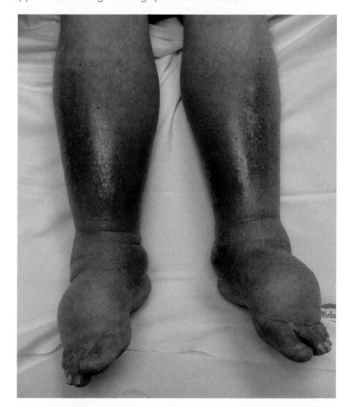

**FIGURE 72-4** Representative phlebolymphatic combination of diffuse stasis hyperpigmentation or dermatitis and pronounced lymphatic dorsal foot swelling or "buffalo humps." (*Reprinted with permission from Lippincott, Williams, Wilkins. Manual of Vascular Diseases. 2nd ed.*)

The presence of venous reflux is suggested by reversal of flow within the venous segment of a standing patient of greater than 0.5 seconds duration (for superficial and deep calf veins) or greater than 1 second (for femoropopliteal veins).

## Nuclear Lymphoscintigraphy

Nuclear lymphoscintigraphy illustrates lymphatic dysfunction including delayed, asymmetric, or absent visualization of regional lymph nodes and collecting trunks as well as dermal backflow. However, this study may not be overly helpful in the setting of known venous insufficiency.

## Other Diagnostic Modalities

Magnetic resonance imaging (standard, venographic, and/or lymphangiographic), contrast venography, and/or computed tomography (CT) with and without contrast can provide supplemental information about the iliac veins, soft tissues, and whether or not coexistent extratruncular vascular malformations are present.

## DIFFERENTIAL DIAGNOSIS

• CVI—See earlier description.

• Lymphedema (primary and nonvenous secondary)—See earlier description.

• Lipedema—a syndrome of symmetrical bilateral lower extremity enlargement caused by subcutaneous fat deposition. Extremity enlargement extends from the buttocks to the ankles and spares the feet. This entity almost exclusively affects females.

• Pretibial myxedema—rare dermopathy associated with Graves disease with bilateral calf, foot, and toe swelling. Pretibial skin manifestations include discoloration (pink to brown), plaques, and nodules. A rare variant with elephantiasis can occur. Nearly all patients have an associated ophthalmopathy.

• Medication-induced swelling—Swelling within the distal lower extremities is bilateral, soft, and pitting due to a low protein component. Easily reversible with limb elevation. Skin changes are rare.

• Central swelling (liver disease, cardiogenic)—Similar to medication-associated swelling.

## MANAGEMENT

• Ideally therapy should address both the lymphatic and venous hypertension.

• When venous occlusion is present, patency can sometimes be restored via balloon angioplasty and stenting.

• Significant superficial and/or perforating venous reflux can be corrected by using techniques such as endovenous laser therapy, radiofrequency ablation, or foam sclerotherapy.

• All patients should be treated with concomitant therapy aimed at mobilizing interstitial fluid. This includes leg elevation and gradient compression stockings. In more advanced cases sequential lymphatic pumps and complex lymphedema physiotherapy can be helpful.

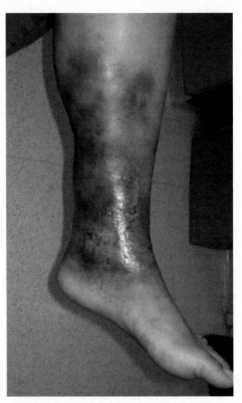

**FIGURE 72-5** Despite profound venous stasis hyperpigmentation and lipodermatosclerosis, there is no associated foot swelling suggestive of clinical lymphedema.

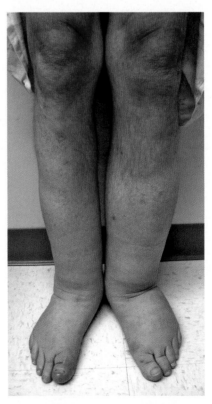

**FIGURE 72-6** Lymphedema within the bilateral lower extremities with distinctive swelling of the toes, feet, and calves. Note the "elephantine" appearance of the distal calves and the conspicuous absence of hyperpigmentation or the "inverted bowling pin" appearance of lipodermatosclerotic chronic venous insufficiency (CVI).

- Since most of the patients are significantly obese, weight loss is critical.
- Discontinuance of any medications known to exacerbate swelling (calcium channel blockers, nonsteroidal anti-inflammatory drugs [NSAIDs], thiazolidinediones, gabapentin, or pregabalin) if possible.

## PATIENT EDUCATION

- The importance of daily compliance with compression garments and similar devices should be stressed.
- Achieving an ideal body weight should be repeatedly emphasized.
- Fastidious skin care is important.
- Prompt notification of caregiver in the event of signs and symptoms of infection.

### PROVIDER RESOURCES

- http://www.medsourcellc.com/documents /PhlebolymphedemaManagementofDermalChangesandWounds.pdf
- http://www.angiologist.com/lymphatic-disease /lymphedema/2/

### PATIENT RESOURCES

- http://ocalamagazine.com/2011/06/13/edema-swelling-vs-lymphedema
- http://www.lymphedema-therapy.com/lymphedema-pictures .html

## REFERENCES

1. Bunke N, Brown K, Bergan J. Phlebolymphedema: usually unrecognized, often poorly treated. *Perspect Vasc Surg Endovasc Ther.* 2009;21(2):65-68.

2. Farrow W. Phlebolymphedema—a common underdiagnosed and undertreated problem in the wound care clinic. *J Am Coll Cert Wound Spec.* 2010;2(1):14-23.

3. Dean SM, Zirwas MJ, Horst AV. Elephantiasis nostras verrucosa: an institutional analysis of 21 cases. *J Am Acad Dermatol.* Jun 2011;64(6): 1104-1110.

4. Lee BB, Laredo J, Loose DA. Diagnosis and management of primary phlebolymphedema. *Lymphedema.* 2011;537-546.

# 73 FACTITIAL EDEMA

Clint Allred, MD
Mark Crandall, MD
Steven M. Dean, DO, FACP, RPVI

## PATIENT STORY

A 38-year-old woman presented with a persistently swollen left leg. The patient related that the swelling postdated a vague left calf injury incurred 6 months previously. Multiple physician evaluations (including repetitive emergency room visits) were inconclusive. Serial venous duplex ultrasonography, plain film tibial or fibular radiography, contrast venography, abdominopelvic computed tomography (CT), and a triple-phase bone scan were normal. Magnetic resonance imaging (MRI) was remarkable only for soft tissue swelling.

Examination revealed significant lymphedematous swelling of the left lower extremity. A peculiar fusiform swelling existed that abruptly terminated near the knee. Multiple horizontal indentations, depressions, and abrasions were identified along the popliteal fossa, proximal calf, and distal thigh (Figure 73-1). Factitial edema from a constricting band or tourniquet to the extremity was suspected.[1]

### EPIDEMIOLOGY

Factitial or factitious edema is a rare cause of upper or lower extremity swelling caused by the repetitive application of a constrictive band or tourniquet. It has also been called voluntary edema or artificial edema, and over time it can mimic true lymphedema. According to the Diagnostic and Statistical Manual of Mental Disorders, fourth edition, factitious disorders are characterized by the intentional production or feigning of physical or psychologic signs or symptoms and a need to assume a sick role.[2] Most patients with factitial edema present to multiple providers over a period of months to years and often undergo multiple diagnostic studies before eventual diagnosis.

It is usually unilateral, and patients often apply the tourniquet to the nondominant limb. Although typically affecting the lower extremity, factitious edema has been reported in the upper extremity. In one case report both the upper and lower extremities were involved.[3] There are only a few case reports in the literature, thus the true incidence of factitial edema is unknown.

### ETIOLOGY AND PATHOPHYSIOLOGY

With placement of a tourniquet, venous return is directly impaired, leading to increased hydrostatic pressure and fluid extravasation into adjacent soft tissue. Lymphatic return itself initially is normal or even increased,[4] though over time the lymph vessels can become fibrosed, especially directly under the site of the tourniquet placement.[5] It is conceivable that unabated increased hydrostatic pressure ultimately overwhelms lymphatic clearance and eventuates in clinical lymphedema. Reported associated psychologic issues include anxiety, depression, and conversion disorder. In contradistinction to malingering, which involves a conscious decision to self-harm, the factitial edema patient is unconsciously motivated.

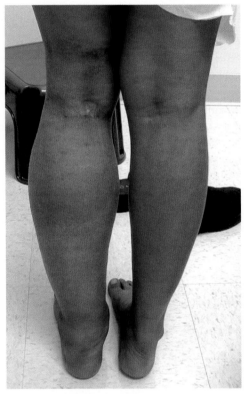

**FIGURE 73-1** Factitial edema of the left lower extremity. Multiple horizontal indentations, depressions, and abrasions exist along the popliteal fossa, proximal calf, and distal thigh. Note abrupt termination of the swelling at the level of the popliteal fossa. The contralateral extremity is normal.

## DIAGNOSIS

### Clinical Features

- The diagnosis of factitial edema is clinical.
- The hallmark sign is a sudden and abrupt onset of edema distal to the application site of a tourniquet. A visible demarcation between a normal-appearing proximal segment and an edematous segment distally exists.
- The clinician should carefully inspect the zone of demarcation for a burrowed tourniquet.
- Inspection of the epidermis may reveal linear abrasions or ring-like indentations (Figures 73-1 to 73-3), corresponding to a recently removed or visible tourniquet. In some case reports patients have been directly observed placing a tourniquet.[6]
- Factitial edema should be considered in patients who have undergone multiple evaluations for unilateral edema of no apparent etiology, especially when the contralateral limb is completely normal and there is suspicion of psychologic pathology.
- Careful attention should be given to the psychiatric assessment as the affected patient typically exhibits severe emotional conflict.

### Typical Distribution

- Usually unilateral, often affecting the nondominant limb.
- Typically involves one lower extremity.
- Rarely affects the upper extremity.

## DIFFERENTIAL DIAGNOSIS

- Chronic venous insufficiency (CVI)—Cutaneous manifestations in the gaiter distribution (telangiectasias, reticular veins, varicose veins, hyperpigmentation). Associated with cellulitis and ulcerations, especially in the medial malleolar region; typically no involvement of the toes. Long-standing factitial edema may exhibit some clinical features of CVI.
- Deep venous thrombosis—Usually unilateral, associated with erythrocyanosis and swelling. History of immobilization, recent surgery, or predisposing risk factors for thrombosis.
- Extrinsic venous compression—This can occur due to tumor, popliteal cyst, or an arterial aneurysm of the popliteal, femoral, or aortoiliac arteries. This can be unilateral or bilateral depending on the anatomic level of compression.
- Lymphedema—Most often unilateral, thick fibrosis of the skin, frequent recurrent cellulitis, also involves the foot and toes. Long-standing factitial edema can manifest a lymphedematous appearance.
- May-Thurner syndrome—Unilateral left lower extremity edema due to compression of the left common iliac vein by the right common iliac artery at the site of the L5 vertebral body. Because the level of compression is at the iliac level, edema is often present in the thigh.
- Cellulitis or lymphangitis—Associated limb swelling, erythema, heat, and tenderness. Regional lymphadenopathy may be present, and associated systemic symptoms may exist.

    Secondary cellulitis can complicate factitial edema.

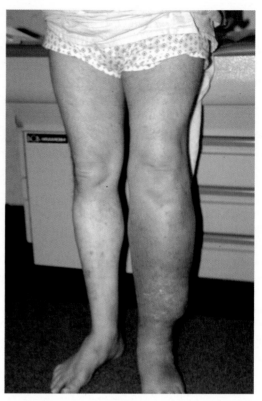

FIGURE 73-2 Severe long-standing factitial edema of the lower left extremity marked by severe infrageniculate swelling. Associated dermal hyperpigmentation with secondary fibrosis exists as well. Multiple depressed ring-like indentions were identified along his mid thigh yet his "hallmark sign" was prominent along the distal thigh (note tapered appearance). The right lower extremity is normal.

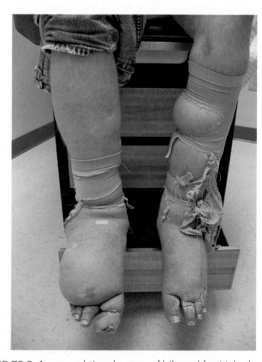

FIGURE 73-3 A rare and singular case of bilateral factitial edema from a variety of tourniquets that included using tattered pieces of compression hose. Severe, disfiguring, and disabling secondary lymphedema is present.

## MANAGEMENT

- If evidence of a tourniquet or constrictive band is identified, the patient should be confronted in a nonthreatening fashion and referral to psychiatry promptly arranged.

- A unique subset to note is the pediatric or mentally infantile population, who may innocently apply constrictive items without emotional instability.[7] Psychiatric intervention is not needed in this group.

- With cessation of the repetitive use of a tourniquet, factitial edema is completely reversible in mild and moderate cases.

## FOLLOW-UP

Without effective psychiatric intervention, it is unlikely that the patient's condition will improve.

## REFERENCES

1. Dean SM. Factial edema. *Vasc Med*. 2002;7:562.

2. American Psychiatric Association. *Diagnostic and Statistical Manual of Mental Disorders*. 4th text revision ed. Washington, DC: American Psychiatric Association; 2000.

3. Stoberl C, Musalek M, Partsch H. Artificial edema of the extremity. *Hautarzt*. 1994;45:149-153.

4. Kittner C, Kroger J, Rohrbeck R, et al. Lymphatic outflow scintigraphy in a case of artificial edema of the lower limb. *Nuklearmedizin*. 1994;33:268-270.

5. Browse NS, Burnarnd KG, Mortimer PS. Differential diagnosis of chronic swelling of the limbs. In: Browse N, Burnand KG, Mortimer PS, Peter S, eds. *Disease of the Lymphatics*. London, UK: Arnold; 2003:161-162.

6. De Godoy JM, Godoy MF, Spiandorin D, et al. Factitious lymphedema: case report and literature review. *J Vasc Br*. 2005;4(1):98-100.

7. McIver MA, Gochman RF. Elastic bands of the wrist: a not so "silly" complication. *Pediatr Emerg Care*. 2011;27(5):428-429.

## PART 9

# VASOSPASTIC AND VASCULITIC DISEASES

# 74 RAYNAUD PHENOMENON

Nicole C. Bundy, MD, MPH

## PATIENT STORY

A 21-year-old Caucasian woman with no past medical history presents with 9 months of painful color changes of her fingers upon cold exposure. She has no other complaints, and a thorough review of systems is negative. Her family history is significant for her mother having rheumatoid arthritis. She is a nonsmoker. Physical examination is normal other than dilated capillary loops and capillary dropout on nailfold capillary microscopy. Laboratory values reveal a positive antinuclear antibody (ANA) of 1:160 but are otherwise unremarkable. She is diagnosed with Raynaud phenomenon (RP).

RP is an exaggerated, reversible, vasospastic response of acral blood vessels upon exposure to cold or emotional stress. Clinically, it is characterized by sharply demarcated color changes of the digits often accompanied by pain or paresthesias (Figure 74-1).

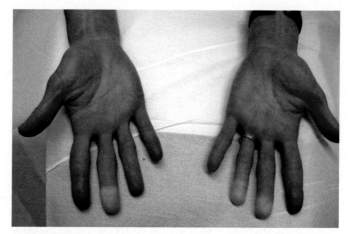

**FIGURE 74-1** Raynaud phenomenon (RP). Note the sharply demarcated color changes with some digits demonstrating pallor (ischemia) and others the blue-purple discoloration of deoxygenation. (*Photograph courtesy of Dr. Steven M. Dean.*)

## EPIDEMIOLOGY

The true prevalence of RP is difficult to establish because there is no gold standard diagnostic test.

- Estimated prevalence between 2% and 20% of the population.[1-4]
- Female-to-male ratio between 3:1 and 9:1.[1-4]
- More common in younger age groups; mean age of onset in second to third decades.
- Equal occurrence across races.

## ETIOLOGY AND PATHOPHYSIOLOGY

Primary RP (PRP) is the term used when there is no identifiable underlying disorder contributing to the vasospasm and there is no history of tissue damage from ischemia.

Secondary RP (SRP) occurs in the setting of an underlying disorder, most often a rheumatologic disease, and is often complicated by significant morbidity from digital ischemia (Table 74-1 and Figures 74-2 to 74-4). In severe disease with prolonged ischemic attacks, destruction of the distal phalanges may occur—a phenomenon known as acro-osteolysis (Figure 74-5).

The regulation of cutaneous blood flow involves complex interactions between structural components of blood vessels, neuronal signaling, and vasoactive chemical mediators. The precise ways in which this complicated system is disordered in RP have yet to be defined. Abnormalities in endothelial function, vascular reactivity, the secretion of vasoactive chemical mediators, and neurologic control of vasomotor tone have all been implicated in RP.[5] Several experiments have pointed to a central role of alpha-2 adrenergic receptors in RP,[6-8] possibly associated with increased protein tyrosine kinase activity.[9,10] Increased platelet activation via upregulation of the glycoprotein (GpIIb or IIIa) receptor was recently shown in patients with PRP.[11] While it appears that there is overlap in some of the functional impairments underlying PRP and SRP, the latter also involves intrinsic structural blood vessel abnormalities absent in PRP. Gross histologic examinations of digital arteries from patients with SRP have revealed intimal hypertrophy and fibrosis, vessel narrowing, and microthrombi, which are largely absent in PRP.

## DIAGNOSIS

The diagnosis of RP usually is made on the basis of a compelling history, as there are no gold standard diagnostic tests. Attempts to reproduce Raynaud attacks for purposes of confirming a diagnosis are met with inconsistent responses and are rarely helpful. While a number of techniques are available in the research setting to help diagnose RP (thermography, angiography, laser Doppler imaging, and direct measures of skin temperature and local blood flow), they are rarely practical in everyday clinical practice. The following criteria have been suggested as helpful for diagnosing RP[12]:

- Definite RP—Repeated episodes of biphasic or triphasic color changes upon exposure to cold
- Possible RP—Uniphasic color changes plus numbness or paresthesia upon exposure to cold
- No RP—No color changes upon exposure to cold

Once a diagnosis of RP is made, it is imperative to perform a thorough evaluation in order to distinguish PRP (Table 74-2) from definite or suspected SRP. This workup should include

- A complete history and review of systems, inquiring about symptoms concerning for an underlying connective tissue disorder (rash, skin tightening, arthralgia or joint swelling, new or severe acid reflux, shortness of breath, muscle weakness) or vascular disease (known history of cardiovascular disease, claudication).
- A review of medications (see Table 74-1 for a list of medications associated with RP).
- Thorough physical examination, with particular attention to the skin examination (looking for findings suggestive of an underlying connective tissue disease), and vascular examination (unequal, weak, or absent pulses including an abnormal Allen and/or reverse Allen test).
- Nailfold capillary microscopy can be very helpful in distinguishing PRP from SRP and in identifying those with PRP who are more likely to eventually develop a connective tissue disease.[13,14] It is accomplished by placing a drop of immersion oil or lubricating gel on the cuticle and examining the area with an ophthalmoscope (diopter set 10-40) or stereotactic microscope (Figure 74-6).
- Digital plethysmography, arterial Doppler, or ultrasound for patients with evidence of underlying vascular disease (eg, unequal blood pressures, absent pulses).
- Laboratory evaluation in suspected SRP should include
  ○ Complete blood count (CBC)
  ○ Erythrocyte sedimentation rate (ESR) and C-reactive protein (CRP)
  ○ Urinalysis
  ○ ANA by immunofluorescence (if positive, then test for disease-specific autoantibodies, including antitopoisomerase/Scl-70, anticentromere, anti-Sjögren syndrome A [anti-SSA], anti-SSB, anti-Smith, and antiribonucleoprotein [anti-RNP])

**TABLE 74-1.** Secondary Raynaud Phenomenon–Associated Conditions and Factors

| Rheumatologic |
| --- |
| Systemic sclerosis |
| Systemic lupus erythematosus |
| Dermatomyositis or polymyositis |
| Mixed connective tissue disease |
| Rheumatoid arthritis |
| Sjögren syndrome |
| Undifferentiated connective tissue disease |
| **Hematologic** |
| Cryoglobulinemia |
| Cryofibrinogenemia |
| Cold agglutinins |
| Paraproteinemia |
| Paraneoplastic syndrome |
| **Vascular** |
| Thoracic outlet syndrome |
| Thromboangiitis obliterans (Buerger disease) |
| Vasculitis |
| Atherosclerosis |
| Prinzmetal angina |
| **Endocrine** |
| Hypothyroidism |
| **Neurologic** |
| Carpal tunnel syndrome |
| **Traumatic** |
| Vibration injury |
| Frost bite |
| **Drugs or Chemicals** |
| Chemotherapeutics |
| Sympathomimetics |
| Interferons |
| Cocaine |
| Polyvinyl chloride |
| Ergots |

Adapted from Block JA, Sequiera W. *Lancet.* 2001;357:2042.

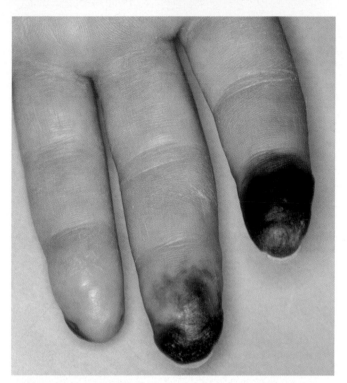

**FIGURE 74-2** Digital necrosis. Sharply demarcated necrosis of the fingertips in a patient with limited cutaneous systemic sclerosis associated with severe secondary Raynaud phenomenon (RP).

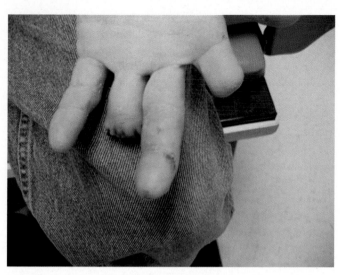

**FIGURE 74-4** Digital amputation secondary to severe Raynaud phenomenon (RP) secondary to thromboangiitis obliterans (Buerger disease). (*Photograph courtesy of Dr. Steven M. Dean.*)

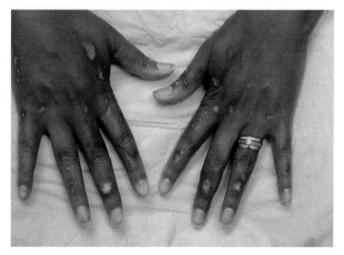

**FIGURE 74-3** Digital ulcers in a patient with scleroderma and Raynaud phenomenon (RP). This photograph also illustrates the "salt and pepper" appearance seen in some cases of scleroderma. (*Photograph courtesy of Dr. Steven M. Dean.*)

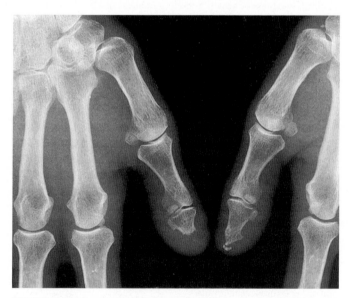

**FIGURE 74-5** Acro-osteolysis. Note dissolution of terminal phalanges in a patient with long-standing limited cutaneous systemic sclerosis and Raynaud phenomenon (RP).

## CLINICAL FEATURES

- Attacks are precipitated by cold exposure or emotional stress.

- Most often affects the hands (second to fourth digits most commonly); toes and other acral areas may also be affected.

- Triphasic color changes, with initial skin pallor (white), followed by cyanosis (blue), and then the hyperemia of rewarming (red), are classic. However, many patients only have a biphasic pattern.

- During an attack, associated symptoms may include pain, paresthesias, and clumsiness of the hands.

- Several features should heighten the concern for underlying connective tissue disease:
  - Involvement of the thumb[15]
  - Abnormal nailfold capillary microscopy
  - Presence of symptoms consistent with connective tissue disease
  - Positive ANA or disease-specific autoantibodies

## MANAGEMENT

The aims of management are symptom reduction and avoidance of critical ischemia. Patients with PRP can often be managed without medications, while those with underlying causes (especially connective tissue diseases) frequently have severe manifestations that require chronic pharmacotherapy.

### Nonpharmacologic Treatment

- Avoidance of cold temperatures and abrupt negative temperature changes.

- Wearing appropriate clothing, which includes mittens, hat, and layers to keep the whole body warm.

**TABLE 74-2.** Diagnostic Criteria for Primary Raynaud Phenomenon

Vasospastic attacks precipitated by cold or emotional stress

Symmetric attacks

No evidence of underlying connective tissue, vascular, hematologic, or other related cause

No history of critical tissue ischemia

Negative nailfold capillary microscopy

Negative ANA test and normal ESR

Adapted from LeRoy EC, Medsger TA Jr. Raynaud's phenomenon: a proposal for classification. *Clin Exp Rheumatol.* 1992;10:485.

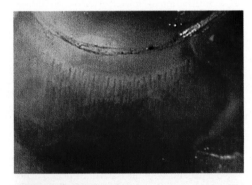
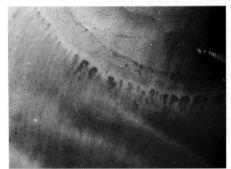
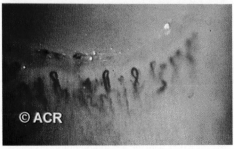
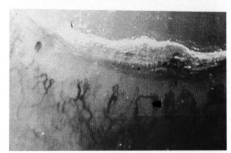

**FIGURE 74-6** Nailfold capillary microscopy. Upper left-hand panel: normal nailfold capillaries with uniform morphology and homogeneous distribution of the small capillary loops just below the cuticle. The other three panels demonstrate the abnormal findings of capillary drop out, and enlarged, dilated, tortuous capillary loops in patients with Raynaud phenomenon (RP) and underlying connective tissue disease.

- Therapies aimed at reducing emotional stress.

- Smoking cessation.

- Avoidance of sympathomimetic drugs.

- A variety of alternative or complimentary treatment strategies have been tried (eg, biofeedback, acupuncture, supplements, laser), but data supporting their efficacy is limited.[16,17]

## Pharmacologic Treatment

- Dihydropyridine calcium channel blockers (CCBs) form the cornerstone of pharmacologic treatment for RP. Several studies have demonstrated their efficacy, although effect size is modest.[16,18-20]

- Long-acting preparations are favored for chronic management. Dosing starts low and may be titrated up for maximum effectiveness, as tolerated.

- Several other medications have been investigated for chronic management of RP, but the results are inconsistent and studies are limited by small size. They include prazosin,[20,21] topical nitroglycerin,[22,23] the serotonin reuptake inhibitor fluoxetine,[20,24,25] the angiotensin II receptor antagonist losartan,[20,26,27] cilostazol,[28] the endothelin receptor antagonist bosentan,[29-31] phosphodiesterase-5 inhibitors,[20,32-36] pentoxifylline,[37,38] and HMG-CoA reductase inhibitors.[39,40] None of these agents have shown superiority over CCBs; therefore, their use is usually limited to patients who do not respond adequately or are intolerant to CCBs.

- Patients with refractory RP and severe digital ischemia have shown favorable responses to parenteral prostaglandins and prostacyclin analogues.[20,41,42] Antiplatelet therapy is often employed, and while therapeutic clinical trials are lacking, research demonstrating increased platelet activity in RP makes this a rational approach.[11] Likewise, systemic anticoagulation can be considered, but clear benefit has not been demonstrated. Chemical or surgical sympathectomy can decrease pain and may help improve blood flow and heal ulcers.[43]

## PATIENT EDUCATION

It is important for patients to know that most cases of RP are primary, will remain mild or remit, will not interfere with their daily activities, and will not require pharmacotherapy. Patients should be educated on the importance of smoking cessation, dressing warmly, and the avoidance of cold exposure.

## FOLLOW-UP

The patient presented earlier has no overt evidence for a rheumatologic condition at this time but has several features concerning for future development of a connective tissue disease (abnormal nailfold capillary microscopy, positive ANA, and family history of autoimmunity). She does not currently require pharmacotherapy directed at her RP but should be followed closely for the development of worsening symptoms and evidence of active connective tissue disease.

**PROVIDER RESOURCE**
- http://www.uptodate.com/contents/pharmacologic-and-surgi-cal-treatment-of-the-raynaudphenomenon

**PATIENT RESOURCE**
- www.raynauds.org

## REFERENCES

1. Voulgari PV, Alamanos Y, Papazisi D, et al. Prevalence of Raynaud's phenomenon in a healthy Greek population. *Ann Rheum Dis.* 2000;59(3):206.

2. Cakir N, Pamuk ON, Dönmez S, et al. Prevalence of Raynaud's phenomenon in healthy Turkish medical students and hospital personnel. *Rheum Int.* 2008;29(2):185.

3. Geographic variation in the prevalence of Raynaud's phenomenon: Charleston, SC, USA vs Tarentaise, Savoie, France. *J Rheumatol.* 1993;20(1):70.

4. Purdie G, Harrison A, Purdie D. Prevalence of Raynaud's phenomenon (RP) in the New Zealand adult population. *N Z Med J.* 2009;122(1306):55.

5. Herrick AL. Pathogenesis of Raynaud's phenomenon. *Rheumatology.* 2005;44:587.

6. Coffman JD, Cohen RA. Alpha-2-adrenergic and 5-HT2 receptor hypersensitivity in Raynaud's disease. *J Vasc Med Biol.* 1990;2:100.

7. Freedman RR, Moten M, Migály P, et al. Cold-induced potentiation of alpha 2-adrenergic vasoconstriction in primary Raynaud's disease. *Arthritis Rheum.* 1993;36:685.

8. Flavahan NA, Flavahan S, Liu Q, et al. Increased $\alpha$-2 adrenergic constriction of isolated arterioles in diffuse scleroderma. *Arthritis Rheum.* 2000;43:1886.

9. Furspan PB, Chatterjee S, Mayes MD, et al. Cooling-induced contraction and protein tyrosine kinase activity of isolated arterioles in secondary Raynaud's phenomenon. *Rheumatol.* 2005;44:488.

10. Furspan PB, Chatterjee S, Freedman RR. Increased tyrosine phosphorylation mediates the cooling-induced contraction and increased vascular reactivity of Raynaud's disease. *Arthritis Rheum.* 2004;50:1578.

11. Polidoro L, Barnabei R, Giorgini P, et al. Platelet activation in patients with the Raynaud's phenomenon. *Internal Med J.* 2012;42(5):531-535.

12. Brennan P, Silman A, Black C, et al. Validity and reliability of three methods used in the diagnosis of Raynaud's phenomenon. The UK Scleroderma Study Group. *Br J Rheumatol.* 1993;32(5):357.

13. Spencer-Green G. Outcomes in primary Raynaud phenomenon: a meta-analysis of the frequency, rates, and predictors of transition to secondary diseases. *Arch Intern Med.* 1998;158(6):595.

14. Koenig M, Joyal F, Fritzler MJ, et al. Autoantibodies and microvascular damage are independent predictive factors for the progression of Raynaud's phenomenon to systemic sclerosis: a twenty-year prospective study of 586 patients, with validation

of proposed criteria for early systemic sclerosis. *Arthritis Rheum.* 2008;58(12):3902.

15. Chikura B, Moore T, Manning J, et al. Thumb involvement in Raynaud's phenomenon as an indicator of underlying connective tissue disease. *J Rheumatol.* 2010;37(4):783.

16. Raynaud's Treatment Study Investigators. Comparison of sustained-release nifedipine and temperature biofeedback for treatment of primary Raynaud's phenomenon. Results from a randomized clinical trial with 1-year follow-up. *Arch Intern Med.* 2000;160:1101.

17. Malenfant D, Catton M, Pop JE. The efficacy of complementary and alternative medicine in the treatment of Raynaud's phenomenon: a literature review and meta-analysis. *Rheumatol.* 2009;48(7):791.

18. Thompson, AE, Shea B, Welch V, et al. Calcium-channel blockers for Raynaud's phenomenon in systemic sclerosis. *Arthritis Rheum.* 2001;44(8):1841.

19. Thompson AE, Pope JE. Calcium channel blockers for primary Raynaud's phenomenon: a meta-analysis. *Rheumatol.* 2005;44:145.

20. Henness S, Wigley, FM. Current drug therapy for scleroderma and secondary Raynaud's phenomenon: evidence-based review. *Curr Opin Rheumatol.* 2007;19(6):611.

21. Pope J, Fenlon D, Thompson A, et al. Prazosin for Raynaud's phenomenon in progressive systemic sclerosis. *Cochrane Database Syst Rev.* 2000;(2):CD000956.

22. Teh LS, Manning J, Moore, T, et al. Sustained-release transdermal glyceryl trinitrate patches as a treatment for primary and secondary Raynaud's phenomenon. *Br J Rheumatol.* 1995;34:636.

23. Chung L, Shapiro L, Fiorentino D, et al. MQX-503, a novel formulation of nitroglycerin, improves the severity of Raynaud's phenomenon: a randomized, controlled trial. *Arthritis Rheum.* 2009;60(3):870.

24. Jaffe, IA. Serotonin reuptake inhibitors in Raynaud's phenomenon. *Lancet.* 1995;345(8961):1378.

25. Coleiro B, Marshall SE, Denton, CP, et al. Treatment of Raynaud's phenomenon with the selective serotonin reuptake inhibitor fluoxetine. *Rheumatol.* 2001;40(9):1038.

26. Dziadzi M, Denton CP, Smith R, et al. Losartan therapy for Raynaud's phenomenon and scleroderma. Clinical and biochemical findings in a fifteen-week, randomized, parallel-group, controlled trial. *Arthritis Rheum.* 1999;42(12):2646.

27. Gliddon AE, Doré CJ, Black CM, et al. Prevention of vascular damage in scleroderma and autoimmune Raynaud's phenomenon. *Arthritis Rheum.* 2007;56(11):3837.

28. Rajagopalan S, Pfenninger D, Somers E, et al. Effects of cilostazol in patients with Raynaud's syndrome. *Am J Cardiol.* 2003;92:1310.

29. Korn JH, Mayes M, Matucci-Cerinic M, et al. Digital ulcers in systemic sclerosis: prevention by treatment with bosentan, an oral endothelin receptor antagonist. *Arthritis Rheum.* 2004;50(12):3985.

30. Matucci-Cerinic M, Denton CP, Furst DE, et al. Bosentan treatment of digital ulcers related to systemic sclerosis: results from the RAPIDS-2 randomized, double-blind, placebo-controlled trial. *Ann Rheum Dis.* 2011;70:32.

31. Nguyen VA, Eisendle K, Gruber I, et al. Effect of the dual endothelin receptor antagonist bosentan on Raynaud's phenomenon secondary to systemic sclerosis: a double-blind prospective, randomized, placebo-controlled pilot study. *Rheumatol.* 2010;49(3):583.

32. Shenoy PD, Kumar S, Jha LK, et al. Efficacy of tadalafil in secondary Raynaud's phenomenon resistant to vasodilator therapy: a double-blind, randomized, cross-over trial. *Rheumatol.* 2010;49:2420.

33. Schiopu E, Hsu VM, Impens AJ, et al. Randomized, placebo-controlled, crossover trial of tadalafil in Raynaud's phenomenon secondary to systemic sclerosis. *J Rheumatol.* 2009;36:2264.

34. Caglayan E, Huntgeburth M, Karasch T, et al. Phosphodiesterase type 5 inhibition is a novel therapeutic option in Raynaud's disease. *Arch Intern Med.* 2006;166:231.

35. De LaVega AJ, Derk CT. Phosphodiesterase-5 inhibitors for the treatment of Raynaud's: a novel indication. *Expert Opin Investig Drugs.* 2009;18:23.

36. HerrickAL, van den Hoogen F, Gabrielli A, et al. Modified-release sildenafil reduces Raynaud's phenomenon attack frequency in limited cutaneous systemic sclerosis. *Arthritis Rheum.* 2011;63:775.

37. Neirotti M, Longo F, Molaschi M, et al. Functional vascular disorders: treatment with pentoxifylline. *Angiology.* 1987;38(8):575.

38. Goodfield MJ, Rowell NR. Treatment of peripheral gangrene due to systemic sclerosis with intravenous pentoxifylline. *Clin Exp Dermatol.* 1989;14(2):161.

39. Kuwana M, Okazaki Y, Kaburaki J. Long-term beneficial effects of statins on vascular manifestations in patients with systemic sclerosis. *Mod Rheumatol.* 2009;19:530.

40. Abou-Raya A, Abou-Raya S, Helmii M. Statins: potentially useful in therapy of systemic sclerosis-related Raynaud's phenomenon and digital ulcers. *J Rheumatol.* 2008;35:1801.

41. Pope J, Fenlon D, Thompson A, et al. Iloprost and cisaprost for Raynaud's phenomenon in progressive systemic sclerosis. *Cochrane Database Syst Rev.* 1998;(2):CD000953.

42. Huisstede BM, Hoogvliet P, Paulis WD, et al. Effectiveness of interventions for secondary Raynaud's phenomenon: a systematic review. *Arch Phys Med Rehabil.* 2011;92:1166.

43. Polidoro L, Barnabei R, Giorgini P, et al. Platelet activation in patients with the Raynaud's phenomenon. *Intern Med J.* 2012;42(5):531-535.

# 75 LIVEDO RETICULARIS AND LIVEDO RACEMOSA

Steven M. Dean, DO, FACP, RPVI

## PATIENT STORY

A 32-year-old healthy woman with subjective cold sensitivity presents with a "fishnet" appearing rash on her thighs and calves. It has been present for at least 10 years and is symmetrical, nonpainful, and has never ulcerated (Figure 75-1). The discoloration is most pronounced when she is cold and nearly dissipates in a warm environment. Her fingers manifest the well-demarcated cold-associated pallor of Raynaud phenomenon (RP). The appearance is consistent with livedo reticularis (LR).

### EPIDEMIOLOGY

- Livedo reticularis is a common but often unrecognized vasospastic disease.[1]

- LR typically affects young to middle-aged women (20-50 years of age) who are otherwise healthy. Up to 50% of young females may be affected in cold environments.

- Relatively rare in males. When present in the male gender, a secondary cause should be suspected.

- Often coexists with RP and/or acrocyanosis.

### ETIOLOGY AND PATHOPHYSIOLOGY

- LR is most commonly a primary disorder. Less often, a variety of secondary causes can provoke LR (Table 75-1).

- Livedo racemosa is always due to a secondary disorder (Table 75-1).

- A variety of medications have been associated with LR (Table 75-2).

- LR results from physiologic or sometimes pathophysiologic changes with the cutaneous microvascular system. Livedo racemosa is always due to a pathophysiologic small vessel process.[2]

- Livedo arises from either deoxygenation or venodilatation within the conical-appearing subpapillary venous plexus. Decreased arteriolar perfusion is the predominant cause of deoxygenation within the venous plexus. Impaired arterial perfusion usually results from vasospasm, although hyperviscosity, inflammation, and/or thromboemboli can be causative as well. One or a combination of the latter three mechanisms underlies the pathophysiologic cutaneous changes of secondary LR or livedo racemosa. Increased resistance to venous outflow is a less frequent cause of deoxygenation.

- Venodilatation of the venous plexus may be caused by hypoxia or autonomic dysfunction.

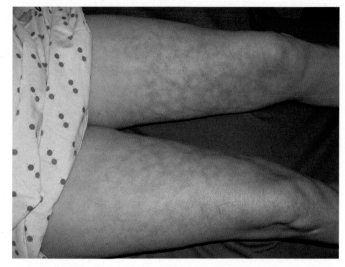

**FIGURE 75-1** Middle-aged healthy female with the characteristic ring-like mottling of livedo reticularis (LR). (*Photograph courtesy of Dr. Matt Zirwas.*)

**TABLE 75-1.** Conditions Associated With Secondary Livedo Reticularis and Livedo Racemosa

- Vasculitis (especially polyarteritis nodosa)

- Collagen vascular disease

- Myeloproliferative syndromes (polycythemia vera, essential thrombocytosis)

- Paraproteinemias

- Cryopathies (cryoglobulinemia or cryofibrinogenemia or cold agglutinin disease)

- Atheroembolic disease

- Calciphylaxis

- Hyperoxaluria

- Atrial myxoma

- Erythema ab igne

- Chronic pancreatitis

- Antiphospholipid antibody syndrome

- Sneddon syndrome

- Livedoid vasculopathy

- Infections

## DIAGNOSIS

### Clinical Features

- LR—fishnet or ring-like uniform violaceous mottling of the skin. The rings are regular and complete (Figure 75-2).

- Livedo racemosa—irregular violaceous mottling with broken rings (Figure 75-3).

- In both LR and livedo racemosa, the skin is palpably cool.

- The discoloration of livedo is provoked or exacerbated by cold exposure. Resolution or improvement occurs when exposed to heat. Primary LR is completely reversible. If the livedoid mottling fails to completely resolve in a warm environment, a secondary cause of LR should be suspected. Livedo racemosa is fixed and will not completely resolve in a warm setting.

- Leg dependency aggravates the discoloration, whereas elevation improves it.

- Usually asymptomatic, although cold-associated tingling or numbness rarely occurs.

- If concurrent purpura, nodules, macules, ulcerations, and/or atrophie blanche are noted, a secondary cause of LR or livedo racemosa exists (Figure 75-4).

- Patients with livedo racemosa have a significantly higher frequency of skin ulcerations, arthralgias, cutaneous vasculitis, and higher C-reactive protein (CRP) levels when compared to their LR counterparts.[3]

- With exception of the characteristic skin changes, the examination in primary LR is usually unremarkable with the exception of possible associated RP or acrocyanosis. Patients with secondary LR or livedo racemosa may display manifestations related to the associated disease (eg, hemiparesis in Sneddon syndrome, Gottron papules in dermatomyositis, lower extremity purpura, and ulcerations in livedoid vasculopathy).

- Livedo racemosa is a marker for arteriovenous thrombosis even in the absence of antiphospholipid antibodies.[4]

### Typical Distribution

- Most commonly involves the lower extremities, although the upper extremities can be affected (Figure 75-5).

- Frequently pronounced around the patellar and olecranon regions (Figures 75-3 and 75-6).

- Livedo racemosa tends to be more diffuse than LR and may involve the trunk, buttocks, hands, feet, and even the face (Figures 75-4, 75-7, and 75-8).

### LABORATORY STUDIES

- Not recommended in an otherwise healthy female with primary LR.

- If a secondary cause is suspected, an antiphospholipid antibody panel should always be obtained. The need for additional laboratory work should be directed by the clinical assessment (eg, vasculitis, autoimmune, or hematologic-directed serology).

**TABLE 75-2.** Medications Associated With Livedo Reticularis

- Amantadine

- Gemcitabine

- Minocycline

- Pressors (ergotamines, epinephrine or catecholamines, amphetamines, cocaine)

- Lopinavir and aripiprazole combination

- Alpha- and beta-interferons

- Quinidine

- Heparin

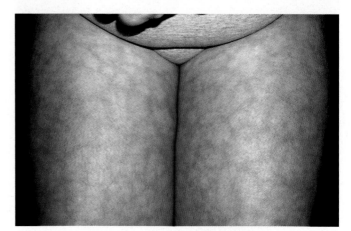

**FIGURE 75-2** Symmetric and regular erythrocyanotic livedoid pattern on the thighs of a patient with primary livedo reticularis (LR). (*Photograph courtesy of Dr. Matt Zirwas.*)

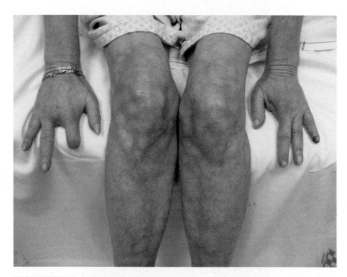

**FIGURE 75-3** Multiple broken rings of livedo racemosa along the lower extremities in a tobacco-using scleroderma patient. Note the predilection of livedo for the patellar regions. Multiple finger amputations indicate the presence of a secondary cause of vasospastic disease.

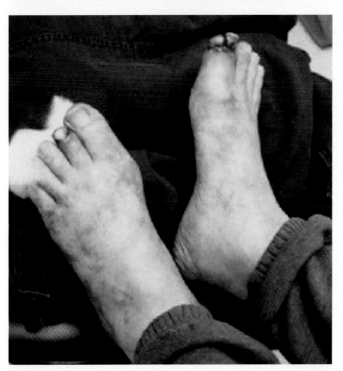

FIGURE 75-4 Highly irregular distorted rings of livedo racemosa along the dorsal feet combined with necrotic toes in the setting of rheumatoid arthritis.

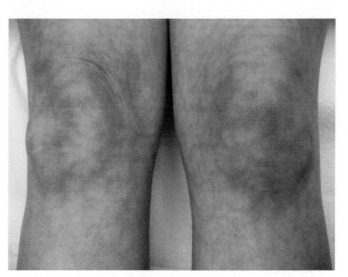

FIGURE 75-6 Fine livedo reticularis (LR) preferentially involving the patellar area in an otherwise healthy young female.

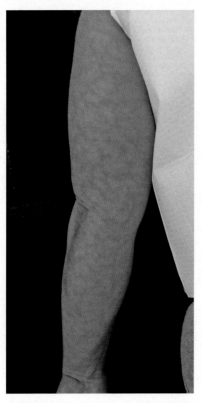

FIGURE 75-5 Although more common in the lower extremities, livedo reticularis (LR) can involve the upper extremities as well. (*Photograph courtesy of Dr. Matt Zirwas.*)

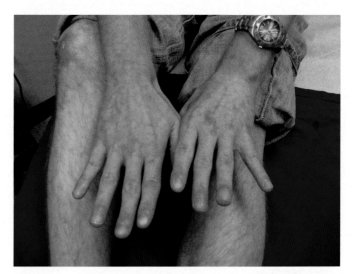

FIGURE 75-7 Irregular, broken mottling characteristic of livedo racemosa along the hands and knees of a young patient with Sneddon syndrome (multiple strokes with positive antiphospholipid antibodies).

## Skin Biopsy

- Not recommended in primary LR.
- May be helpful in elucidating the cause of secondary LR or livedo racemosa.[5]
- Several biopsies should be obtained that sample both the erythrocyanotic ring and the pallorous core.
- Biopsies of associated nodules, purpura, or ulcerations should be obtained.
- Large punch biopsies that include the medium-sized vessels within the deep reticular dermis and subcutaneous fat are ideal. If a punch biopsy is unsatisfactory, perform a wedge biopsy.
- Histologic analysis is variable and is dependent on the associated secondary etiology.

## DIFFERENTIAL DIAGNOSIS

- LR must be differentiated from its pathologic variant, livedo racemosa.
- Retiform purpura consists of branching or stellate hemorrhagic purpuric lesions caused by a complete blockage of blood flow in the dermal and subcutaneous vasculature (Figure 75-9).
- Pseudoleukoderma angiospasticum may be a variant of livedo that is characterized by a white "checkered" appearance on the soles, palms, buttocks, and flexural aspects of the forearm.
- Livedoid vasculopathy is a rare ulcerative subtype of livedo racemosa due to fibrinolytic abnormalities and microcirculatory thrombosis.

## TREATMENT

- Other than avoiding protracted cold exposure, medical treatment for primary LR is usually not needed. If necessary, a vasodilator such as a calcium channel blocker can be administered in the rare symptomatic patient or one who is publicly embarrassed by the livedoid appearance.
- Therapy of secondary LR or livedo racemosa should be focused on the causative disorder. However, even appropriate systemic therapy is unlikely to reverse both types of pathologic livedo.
- Antiphospholipid syndrome livedo racemosa with thrombosis requires anticoagulation.
- No evidence-based medicine exists to definitely guide therapy in LR or livedo racemosa.

## PATIENT EDUCATION

Admonish patients to keep their peripheral and core temperature as warm as possible. Avoid vasoconstricting medications as well as tobacco. Instruct patients to report any signs of evolving coexistent systemic disease.

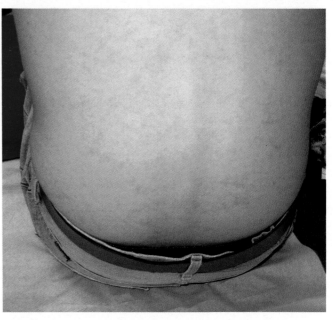

**FIGURE 75-8** When livedo is widespread and even involves the trunk, livedo racemosa should be suspected. This patient has Sneddon syndrome.

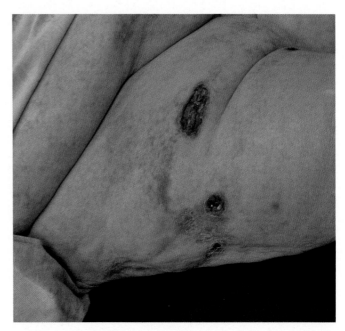

**FIGURE 75-9** Irregular purpura can be seen along the ulcerated thigh of a patient with calciphylaxis. Retiform purpura may be confused with livedo reticularis (LR) or racemosa.

## REFERENCES

1. Dean SM. Livedo reticularis and related disorders. *Curr Treat Options Cardiovasc Med.* Apr 2011;13(2):179-191.

2. Uthman IW, Khamashta MA. Livedo racemosa: a striking dermatological sign for the antiphospholipid antibody syndrome. *J Rheumatol.* 2006;33:2379-2381.

3. Kawakami T, Yamazaki M, Mizoguchk M, et al. Differences in anti-phosphatidylserine-prothrombin complex antibodies and cutaneous vasculitis between regular livedo reticularis and livedo racemosa. *Rhematology.* 2009;48:508-512.

4. Martinez-Valle F, Ordi-Ros J, Selva-O'Callaghan A, et al. Livedo racemosa as a marker of increased risk of recurrent thrombosis in patients with negative anti-phospholipid antibodies. *Med Clin (Barc).* 2009;132:785-786.

5. Herrero C, Guilabert A, Mascaro-Galy JM. Diagnosis and treatment of livedo reticularis on the legs. *Actas Dermosifiliogr.* 2008;99:598-607.

# 76 ACROCYANOSIS

Andrew K. Kurklinsky, MD, RPVI, FSVM

## PATIENT STORY

A 40-year-old woman presents with a complaint of painless blue discoloration of both hands and feet (Figure 76-1). The color changes are persistent, although their intensity seems to be greater with cold exposure. While the color improves in the summer, she experiences increased sweating of hands and feet. She has no significant medical history and takes no medications. Extensive medical workup has been unrevealing. The blue color resolves almost entirely when her hands or feet are elevated in a supine position for a few minutes. Pressing the blue skin elicits blanching; when released, the color refills in an irregular fashion from the periphery to the center.

## EPIDEMIOLOGY

- Prevalence, incidence, geographic distribution, sex, and racial characteristics are uncertain.[1,2]

- Isolated studies more commonly describe female patients in their second and third decades of life.[3,4] However, selection bias appears to be universal, and no robust epidemiologic studies exist.

- Familial presentations have been described.[3]

- May occur more frequently in areas with a cooler climate.

- Epidemiologic assessment may be confounded by prevalent factors underlying secondary cases. Such factors may be environmental or not easily identifiable, making it difficult to discern primary and secondary cases.[1,5]

- In secondary acrocyanosis, prevalence and incidence vary depending on the underlying condition.[1,6,7]

## ETIOLOGY AND PATHOPHYSIOLOGY

### Primary Acrocyanosis

- Acrocyanosis is called *primary* when no specific underlying cause can be determined. The etiology is uncertain and, given the fact that acrocyanosis is a clinical diagnosis, it is not known whether it is a unique phenomenon or different processes with similar clinical features.[3] There is a possible correlation with estrogen levels in women, and signs of acrocyanosis may resolve in some patients after menopause.

- The defect is confined to small preterminal and terminal vessels.[1] The constriction occurs within capillaries but is marked by low capillary pressures, sluggish capillary flow, and poor pressure variability.[8] Subpapillary vessels are dilated,[9] and an increased number and size of arteriovenous anastomoses with blood shunting are common.[10] There is no venous obstruction.[4]

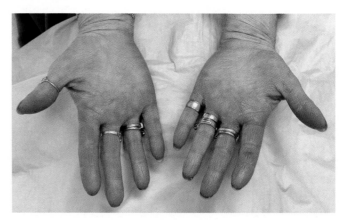

FIGURE 76-1 Acrocyanotic hands of a 40-year-old woman without causative medications or underlying diseases. (*Photograph courtesy of Dr. Steven Dean, Ohio State University, Columbus, OH.*)

## Secondary Acrocyanosis

- Associations of acrocyanosis with many other conditions have been described. When such associations are identifiable, acrocyanosis is called *secondary*. In cases of Ehlers-Danlos syndrome associated with acrocyanosis, hereditary vascular dysfunction of the pericytes in the subpapillary vascular plexus may produce abnormally twisted collagen fibrils.

- Among known associations there are many conditions that are capable of producing local tissue hypoxia and vasoconstriction. Examples include exposure to many medications and chemical substances (including environmental exposures). Other associations include congenital syndromes, infections, and solid organ and blood malignancies. Cold agglutinins, cryoglobulins, cryofibrinogens, and antiphospholipid antibodies are seen in acrocyanosis with or without malignancies.[1]

## DIAGNOSIS

The diagnosis of acrocyanosis is clinical based on persistence and typical localization of the skin color changes. It requires exclusion of other conditions characterized by blue skin color changes. The diagnosis of primary acrocyanosis should be entertained only after causes of secondary acrocyanosis have been excluded.

## Clinical Features

Primary acrocyanosis is a chronic, benign condition without tendency to progress, pain, or tissue loss. Skin changes tend to be painless and persistent and may be more pronounced in cold ambient temperatures and with dependency; skin color normalizes with elevation of the extremities (Figure 76-2A-D). Hyperhidrosis and clamminess of the hands and feet are often seen which worsens in warm temperature while skin color improves. Mild localized edema may be present.[4]

Crocq sign is classical, although nonspecific, and denotes slow and irregular return of the blood from the periphery (rather than from beneath) to the center of a blanched skin area created by local pressure (Figure 76-3A).

## Typical Distribution

Cyanotic skin changes in the distal (acral) parts of the body are seen, typically in hands and feet (Figures 76-1 to 76-4); however, nose and ears may be involved. Skin changes are diffuse and symmetric in primary acrocyanosis and are almost never proximal to the level of ankle or wrist with normal-appearing skin above that line (Figures 76-3B and 76-4).[4]

## Laboratory Studies

There are no specific laboratory tests for acrocyanosis. Hyposphygmia on plethysmography and decreased oxygen tensions with transcutaneous oximetry may be observed. Local skin temperature is low; blood flow is decreased. Various methods of capillaroscopy have been evaluated. Hemorrhages, pericapillary edema, and widened and rarified capillaries are often observed with commonly described "megacapillaries." However, there is no consensus on capillaroscopic criteria, and the method is not clinically reliable. In secondary acrocyanosis, the workup may be extensive but is focused on identifying one of the many specific causes.[1]

## DIFFERENTIAL DIAGNOSIS

### Raynaud Phenomenon

Acrocyanotic skin color changes are persistent and are not easily reversible with rewarming. There are no phasic color changes upon exposure to cold as in Raynaud phenomenon (RP). There is no or little sensory discomfort in primary acrocyanosis. These conditions may co-occur in the same patients, and some pathologic mechanisms may be shared by both conditions.[12]

### Pernio

Significant discomfort (itching, pain, burning, tenderness) is common in pernio; it is absent in acrocyanosis. Pernio cases have a clear history of damp cold exposure and may have relatively rapid onset of symptoms. Although skin changes in acrocyanosis are more pronounced, they are not a result of cold exposure. Acrocyanosis tends to persist, while pernio will see complete resolution of symptoms with warming of the weather.

### Acrorhygosis

Acrorhygosis is a purely subjective symmetrical hypothermia of the extremities. It may precede acrocyanosis. Cyanosis and hyperhydrosis are absent.[2]

### Erythromelalgia

Marked cutaneous temperature elevation with color changes that are characteristically red, so the skin may appear inflamed or scalded. It may be idiopathic or secondary to polycythemia, small fiber neuropathy, hypertension, gout, and heavy metal poisoning.[2] Significant tenderness or burning sensation is present. Heat rather than cold exposure aggravates the condition.

## MANAGEMENT

For all forms of acrocyanosis, the focus is on avoidance of cold exposure and trauma along with measures to improve local circulation. Use of calcium channel blockers is controversial. Bioflavonoids may have tonic effects on capillary-venular endothelial cells and interstitium.[13] Indoramin was shown to increase digital blood flow in acrocyanosis patients.[14] Nicotinic acid compounds were tried in clinical studies with variable success. Ketanserin induced both symptomatic and capillaroscopic improvements.[15] Cervical sympathectomy is a radical, now obsolete method. In secondary acrocyanosis, skin color may improve following treatment of the primary condition.[1]

## PATIENT EDUCATION

Primary acrocyanosis is a benign, mostly cosmetic condition without tendency to progress. In suspected secondary acrocyanosis, extensive search for the underlying process should be undertaken. Symptoms of secondary acrocyanosis may respond to treatment of the primary condition.

## FOLLOW-UP

Primary acrocyanosis does not require follow-up. Secondary acrocyanosis may require periodic follow-ups and treatment escalation if pain or tissue damage appears.

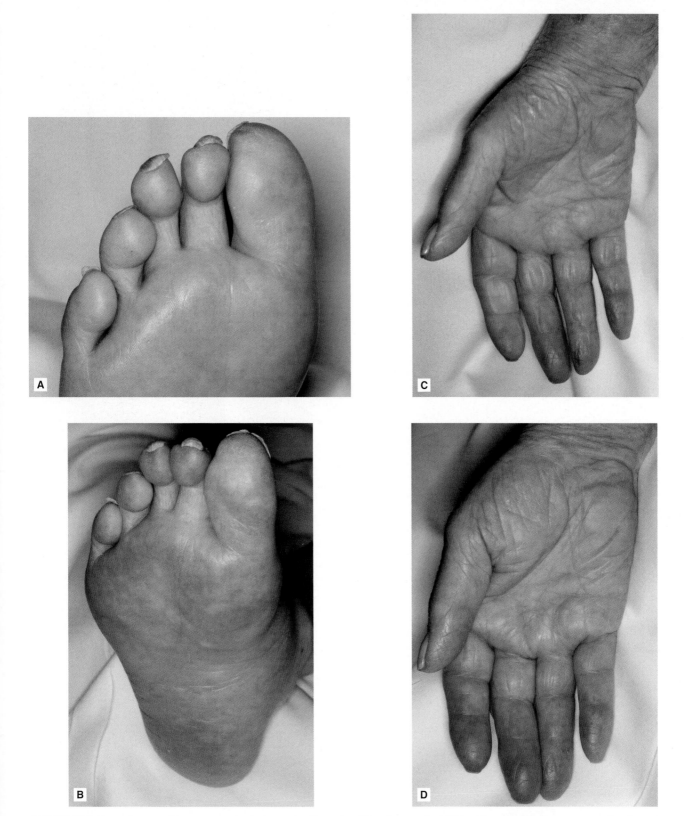

**FIGURE 76-2** Foot of a man with acrocyanosis photographed in supine (A) and dependent (B) positions. Hands of the same patient in supine (C) and (D) dependent positions.

## REFERENCES

1. Kurklinsky AK, Miller VM, Rooke TW. Acrocyanosis: the Flying Dutchman. *Vasc Med*. 2011;16(4):288-301.

2. Merlen JF. Capillary disturbances in man. *Clin Hemorheol*. 1982;2(5-6):745-751.

3. Hallam R. The relationship between erythema pernio and acrocyanosis. *Med Press Circ*. 1930;129:408-412.

4. Lewis T, Landis EM. Observations upon the vascular mechanism in acrocyanosis. *Heart*. 1929;15:229-246.

5. Borgono JM, Vicent P, Venturino H, Infante A. Arsenic in the drinking water of the city of Antofagasta: epidemiological and clinical study before and after the installation of a treatment plant. *Environ Health Perspect*. 1977;19:103-105.

6. Diógenes MJ, Diógenes PC, de Morais Carneiro RM, Neto CC, Duarte FB, Holanda RR. Cutaneous manifestations associated with antiphospholipid antibodies. *Int J Dermatol*. 2004;43(9): 632-637.

7. Naldi L, Locati F, Marchesi L, et al. Cutaneous manifestations associated with antiphospholipid antibodies in patients with suspected primary antiphospholipid syndrome: a case-control study. *Ann Rheum Dis*. 1993;52(3):219-222.

8. Boas EP. The capillaries of the extremities in acrocyanosis; blood pressure and morphology. *JAMA*. 1922;79:1404-1406.

9. Sagher F, Davis E, Sheskin J, Landau J, et al. The small blood vessels of the skin in acrocyanosis. Comparison of biomicroscopy and biopsy findings. *Br J Dermatol*. 1966;78(11):586-589.

10. Piovella C, Fratti L, Fontana S. Modification of the terminal circulation in Raynaud's disease and acrocyanosis. *Bibl Anat*. 1965;7:552-558.

11. Kobayasi T, Ullman S. Twisted collagen fibrils in acrocyanosis. *Eur J Dermatol*. 1999;9(4):285-288.

12. Cooke JP, Marshall JM. Mechanisms of Raynaud's disease. *Vasc Med*. 2005;10(4):293-307.

13. Merlen JF. Paradoxes of acrocyanosis. *Adv Microcirc*. 1982;10: 95-100.

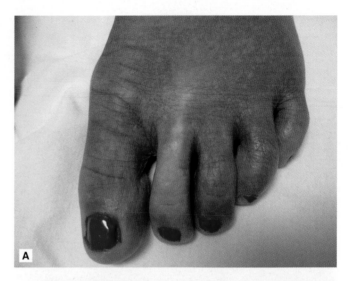

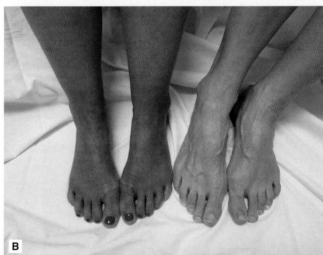

**FIGURE 76-3** (A) A 34-year-old woman with moderate positivity of immunoglobulin G (IgG) anti-beta-2 glycoprotein-1 antibodies. Purplish skin discoloration is noted in the dependent position. It improves with lifting of her feet above the head level. There are no skin changes above the ankles or in upper extremities. The blue discoloration can be pressed away, but quickly refills. (B) For comparison, feet of the patient's mother are photographed next to the patient's. (*Photograph courtesy of Dr. Stephan Moll, University of North Carolina, Chapel Hill, NC.*)

14. Clement DL. Effect of indoramin on finger blood flow in vasospastic patients. *Eur J Clin Pharmacol*. 1978;14(5):331-333.

15. Allegra C, Tonelli V. Results of a double-blind, placebo controlled study with a serotonine selective antagonist (ketanserin) in the treatment of 30 patients with acrocyanotic syndrome. *Clinica e Terapia Cardiovascolare*. 1985;4(1):39-45.

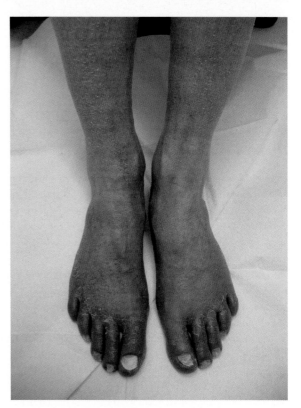

**FIGURE 76-4** A man in his 50s with a psychiatric history and significant malnourishment. He had a negative medical workup, including search for an occult malignancy. (*Photograph courtesy of Dr. Steven M. Dean, Ohio State University, Columbus, OH.*)

# 77 ANCA-NEGATIVE SMALL VESSEL VASCULITIS

Nicole C. Bundy, MD, MPH

## PATIENT STORY

A 39-year-old, previously healthy man presented to rheumatology clinic with 6 days of a progressively severe rash on his lower legs and pain in his knees and ankles. He denied recent upper respiratory or other infection. He took no medications. He was afebrile, and vital signs were normal. Physical examination revealed a rash on the feet and lower legs characterized by palpable purpura with several large areas of confluence (Figure 77-1). His knees were tender, and the ankles were tender and swollen; the remainder of the joint examination was unremarkable. The cardiopulmonary, abdominal, and neurologic examinations were normal. Laboratory values were remarkable for creatinine of 1.4 and a spot urine protein or creatinine ratio of 1.9. Chemistries, including liver functions, and a complete blood count (CBC) were normal. Antineutrophil cytoplasmic antibody (ANCA) studies were negative. A renal biopsy was performed and confirmed a diagnosis of Henoch-Schönlein purpura (HSP) (Figures 77-2 and 77-3).

## DEFINITION

The ANCA-negative small vessel vasculitis (SVV) have in common the pathogenic mechanism of immune-complex (IC) formation and deposition in and around small blood vessels, often with fixation of complement followed by varying degrees of inflammation. They also have in common almost universal cutaneous involvement that most frequently manifests clinically as palpable purpura and histologically as leukocytoclastic vasculitis. The clinical syndromes are distinguished by the nature of the immune complexes, epidemiology, and pattern of organ involvement (Table 77-1).

### Henoch-Schönlein Purpura

- Characterized by deposition of immunoglobulin A (IgA)-containing IC and complement components within the walls of affected vessels. IC deposition may also occur within the renal mesangium.

- Mainly affects the skin, joints, gastrointestinal tract, and, more rarely, kidneys.

- Frequently mild and self-limited in children, although may be complicated by severe renal disease and intussusception.

- Prognosis in adults is more guarded because of a higher incidence of progression to end-stage renal disease.

- The following classification criteria were proposed by the American College of Rheumatology (ACR) in 1990[1]:
  ○ Palpable purpura
  ○ Age 20 years or less at disease onset
  ○ Bowel angina
  ○ Granulocytes in arteriole or venule walls on biopsy

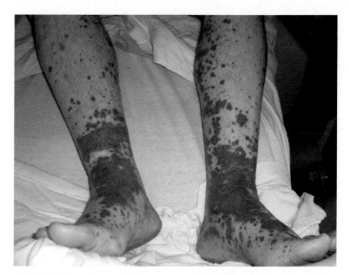

**FIGURE 77-1** A 39-year-old patient with Henoch-Schönlein purpura (HSP).

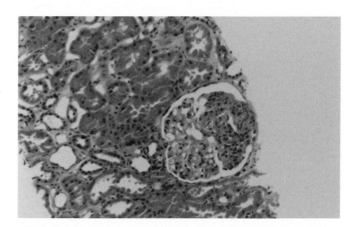

**FIGURE 77-2** Renal biopsy in Henoch-Schönlein purpura (HSP). Light microscopy reveals a glomerular tuft with mesangial expansion and hypercellularity. Note the area of adhesion to Bowman capsule.

If two or more criteria are present, the sensitivity and specificity for HSP are 87% and 88%, respectively.

## Cryoglobulinemic Vasculitis

- Cryoglobulins are ICs that precipitate from serum when exposed to cold (Figure 77-4).
- Three types are recognized:
  - Type I—isolated monoclonal IgG or IgM isotype, most often associated with Waldenström macroglobulinemia or multiple myeloma.
  - Type II—comprised of polyclonal IgG plus monoclonal IgM with rheumatoid factor (RF) activity. Represents 80% of all cryoglobulins. About 90% of cases are associated with the hepatitis C virus (HCV).
  - Type III—comprised of IgG and IgM that are both polyclonal, associated with many chronic inflammatory conditions, especially connective tissue diseases.

Type I cryoglobulinemia may cause a hyperviscosity syndrome leading to neurologic sequelae and cutaneous ischemia (Figure 77-5). Types II and III cryoglobulinemia are more likely to present with classic features of SVV: purpura, arthralgias, and glomerulonephritis. Peripheral neuropathy is common in type II; the finding of mononeuritis multiplex is highly suggestive of an SVV.

## Hypersensitivity Vasculitis

- A heterogeneous group of disorders characterized by antibody response to a foreign antigen with subsequent IC formation and deposition in small blood vessels.
- Isolated skin involvement is very common, but fever, arthralgias, and lymphadenopathy are not infrequent. Visceral organ involvement has been described but when present should prompt workup for other causes.
- Multiple inciting factors have been implicated (Table 77-2); however, a precipitating agent cannot always be identified. Antibiotics are among the most frequently implicated medications.

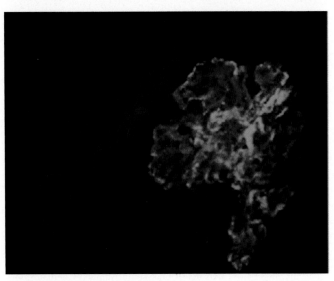

**FIGURE 77-3** Renal biopsy in Henoch-Schönlein purpura (HSP). Immunofluorescence staining positive for immunoglobulin A (IgA) deposits in the mesangium.

**TABLE 77-1.** Frequency of Organ Involvement During the Course of SVV (%)

| Disease | Skin | Musculoskeletal | Renal | GI | Pulm | Neuro | Other |
|---------|------|-----------------|-------|----|------|-------|-------|
| HSP | 100 | Up to 84 | 20 to 50 | 50 | Rare | Very rare CNS involvement | Scrotal pain and edema |
| Cryoglobulinemic vasculitis | 100 | >70 | 35 to 60 in type II; less frequent in types I and III | Liver function test (LFT) abnormalities common but related to HCV infection | 10 to 50 (may be subclinical) | 80 (almost exclusively PNS involvement) | Raynaud and sicca symptoms |
| Hypersensitivity vasculitis | 100 | Frequent | Visceral involvement may occur but is rare and should prompt workup for other causes | | | | Fever |

- The following classification criteria were proposed by the ACR in 1990[2]:
  - Age greater than 16 years
  - Use of a possible offending medication in temporal relation to the symptoms
  - Palpable purpura
  - Maculopapular rash
  - Biopsy of skin lesion showing neutrophils around an arteriole or venule

The presence of three or more criteria has a sensitivity and specificity of 71% and 84%, respectively, for the diagnosis of hypersensitivity vasculitis.

## Connective Tissue Disease–Associated Small Vessel Vasculitis

SVV is well recognized in the setting of connective tissue disease, especially rheumatoid arthritis (RA), systemic lupus erythematosus (SLE), and Sjögren disease. Clinical presentation is variable, ranging from isolated cutaneous vasculitis to severe visceral involvement.

- RA is not infrequently associated with SVV, which may remain subclinical, evolve into rheumatoid nodules, or even cause severe digital infarction (Figure 77-6).

- When RA is associated with systemic vasculitis, perinuclear ANCA (p-ANCA) is often positive.

- SVV in the setting of either SLE or Sjögren disease can cause purpura, urticaria, and skin ulceration. Pulmonary hemorrhage in SLE is a dreaded complication and thought to be secondary to SVV.

## EPIDEMIOLOGY

### Henoch-Schönlein Purpura

- Most common form of systemic vasculitis in children, with 90% of cases occurring in the pediatric age group, typically between 3 and 15 years.

- Annual incidence of 10 to 20 per 100,000 children aged less than 17 years; peak incidence of 70 per 100,000 children aged 5 to 7 years.[3]

- Much less common in adults, with an annual incidence estimated between 3.4 and 13 per million.[4]

- Male-to-female ratio of 1.2:1 to 1.8:1.[5]

- More common in whites and Asians compared with blacks.[3]

- Occurs more frequently in fall, winter, and spring with fewer cases in the summer months.

### Cryoglobulinemic Vasculitis

- Predominantly affects middle-aged to older persons (reflecting the association with malignancy, chronic infection, and long-standing connective tissue disease).

- Female-to-male ratio of 3:1.

- Prevalence varies widely from country to country and mirrors endemic presence of HCV.

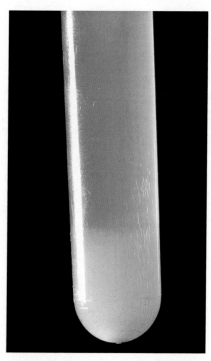

**FIGURE 77-4** Whitish cryoprecipitates, known as cryocrit, form after storing tube at 4°C for 48 to 72 hours and centrifugation.

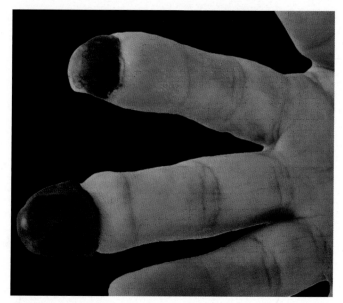

**FIGURE 77-5** Digital gangrene in a patient with type I cryoglobulinemia.

## Hypersensitivity Vasculitis

- Most common form of vasculitis.
- Reliable epidemiologic data are limited, largely because of variability and overlap in case definitions.
- In one study, the estimated annual incidence using ACR criteria[2] was 38.6 per million.[6]
- Female-to-male predominance between 1.9 and 1.[6]

## Small Vessel Vasculitis Associated With Connective Tissue Disease

- In RA patients, severe vasculitis most often occurs in those who are RF positive and have long-standing, severe disease.
- Occurrence in other connective tissue disease is difficult to predict.

## DIAGNOSIS

In the vast majority of patients with suspected vasculitis, a tissue biopsy from an involved site is mandatory to help establish the diagnosis. Cutaneous vasculitic lesions evolve rapidly; the diagnostic yield of skin biopsies is optimal when performed between 24 and 48 hours following the appearance of a specific lesion. Direct immunofluorescence is required on tissue specimens to identify immunoglobulin and complement deposition. All patients should have a urinalysis and testing for serum creatinine to look for renal involvement. A CBC with differential and platelets may be helpful: Cytopenias may imply a connective tissue disorder, while leukocytosis can point to infection. Chest x-ray should be performed in patients with pulmonary symptoms—abnormal findings should prompt consideration of the SVV more likely to affect the lung (ie, granulomatosis with polyangiitis [formerly Wegener granulomatosis], Churg-Strauss syndrome, and microscopic polyangiitis). Antinuclear antibody testing should be performed if the history or examination suggests an underlying connective tissue disease. Cultures and/or virology studies are appropriate in selected cases where infection is suspected.

## Henoch-Schönlein Purpura

- In children presenting classically (purpuric rash +/− arthralgias and abdominal pain following an upper respiratory tract infection) and with mild disease, the clinical history may be sufficient for diagnosis.
- In atypical (including adult-onset) or more severe cases, biopsy of an involved organ demonstrating marked deposition of IgA within blood vessel walls or renal parenchyma is essential to confirm the diagnosis.
- Serum IgA may be elevated.

## Cryoglobulinemic Vasculitis

In patients with suspected cryoglobulin-associated disease, the following laboratory studies can be helpful:

- Serum cryoglobulin (false negatives are common, as specimen must be kept at 37°C before processing to obtain accurate results).
- Testing for antibodies to HCV or direct measurement of HCV RNA.

**TABLE 77-2.** Selected Drugs Reported to Cause Hypersensitivity Vasculitis

Antimicrobial agents
(penicillin, sulfonamides, quinolones, tetracyclines)

Chemotherapeutic agents
(cyclophosphamide, methotrexate, tamoxifen)

NSAIDs

Cardiovascular drugs
(antiarrhythmic agents, beta-blockers, calcium channel blockers, diuretics)

Anticoagulants
(heparin, warfarin)

Anticonvulsants
(sodium valproate, phenytoin, carbamazepine)

Miscellaneous
(allopurinol, colchicine, metformin, levamisole, propylthiouracil, retinoids)

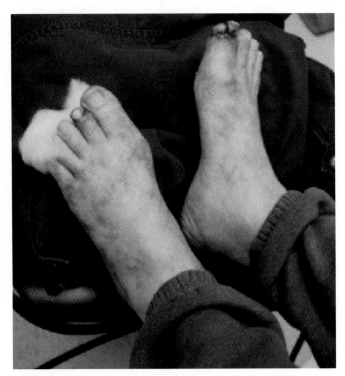

**FIGURE 77-6** Cutaneous vasculitis with digital infarction in a patient with rheumatoid arthritis (RA).

- Serum RF, which is almost universally positive in patients with type II cryoglobulins.
- Extremely low level of C4.
- ESR and C-reactive protein (CRP) may be elevated.

Biopsy of an affected organ helps to confirm the diagnosis. Skin biopsies show leukocytoclastic vasculitis with direct immunofluorescence studies revealing immunoglobulin and complement deposition (the Ig isotype will differ depending on the type of cryoglobulin). In patients with kidney involvement, renal biopsies demonstrate membranoproliferative glomerulonephritis.

## Hypersensitivity Vasculitis

- Biopsy is necessary to confirm changes consistent with SVV.
- Definitively identifying a precipitating cause may be difficult. Taking a careful history looking for antecedent infection or use of new medication in temporal relation to the disease onset is important. Drug-induced vasculitis most often occurs 7 to 10 days after the initiation of the inciting medication.[7]

## DIFFERENTIAL DIAGNOSIS

The clinician must remain astute and consider several other disease entities in the patient with suspected ANCA-negative SVV. Although uncommon, the pauci-immune ANCA-associated vasculitides can present with predominant skin involvement; therefore, ANCA testing is suggested, even in cases of vasculitis apparently limited to the skin. Noninflammatory causes of vascular disease should be considered, including embolic phenomenon and hypercoagulable disorders. Paraneoplastic syndromes, metastatic carcinoma, and several infections can mimic vasculitis and pose a diagnostic challenge.

## MANAGEMENT

The principles of management involve

- Confirming the diagnosis of vasculitis, most often by biopsy
- Defining the extent of organ involvement
- Ruling out infectious causes before instituting immunosuppressive therapy
- Weighing the risks and benefits of immunosuppressive therapies to optimize outcomes in disease with severe visceral organ involvement

## Henoch-Schönlein Purpura

- In mild cases, no specific therapy may be needed. Conservative management includes careful observation, ensuring adequate hydration, and acetaminophen or nonsteroidal anti-inflammatory drugs (NSAIDs) for analgesia (importantly, NSAIDs are contraindicated in patients with active gastrointestinal [GI] bleeding or renal disease).
- Patients with mild renal involvement do not need aggressive treatment but should be monitored closely for the development of worsening disease.
- The best treatment for severe renal disease (nephrotic range proteinuria and/or impaired renal function) remains controversial.

Biopsy is recommended. Corticosteroids are often employed, but controlled studies demonstrating their effectiveness are lacking.[8]

- Other agents that have been used, with or without steroids, include cyclophosphamide, azathioprine, and dipyridamole. Plasmapheresis[9] and intravenous immunoglobulin (IVIg)[10] have also been employed in small numbers of patients.
- Corticosteroids may hasten the resolution of abdominal pain,[11] but there is no evidence to suggest improvement in long-term outcomes or prevention of intussusception.

## Cryoglobulinemic Vasculitis

- Conservative therapy for mild disease is appropriate and may include cold avoidance, NSAIDs and other analgesics for comfort, and low-dose corticosteroids.
- More severe disease usually warrants immunosuppression and/or treatment directed at any underlying disease (eg, chemotherapy or radiation for malignancy and antiviral therapy for HCV infection).
- High-dose corticosteroids with or without cyclophosphamide are used to treat serious disease manifestations.
- Plasmapheresis is sometimes employed in life- or organ-threatening disease to quickly decrease circulating cryoglobulins.

## Hypersensitivity Vasculitis

- Identification and removal of the offending drug is the most important aspect of treatment when a medication is suspected to be the inciting factor. Most patients will recover within several days to weeks.
- If infection is thought to be responsible, appropriate antimicrobial treatment should be instituted.
- Severe or persistent disease may require the use of corticosteroids, colchicine, or dapsone.

## FOLLOW-UP

The patient presented earlier was treated with pulse corticosteroids followed by oral corticosteroids for 3 months. The rash resolved within several weeks, his urine sediment improved, and renal function returned to baseline by the end of steroid treatment. At 2 years after initial presentation, he remains well. Urinalysis and renal function continue to be checked every 6 months.

**PROVIDER RESOURCES**

- http://www.medscape.org/viewarticle/729814
- http://emedicine.medscape.com/article/1083719-overview

**PATIENT RESOURCES**

- http://www.uptodate.com/contents/vasculitis-beyond-the-basics
- http://www.rheumatology.org/Practice/Clinical/Patients/Diseases_And_Conditions/Vasculitis/

## REFERENCES

1. Mills JA, Michel BA, Bloch DA, et al. The American College of Rheumatology 1990 criteria for the classification of Henoch-Schönlein purpura. *Arthritis Rheum.* 1990;33:1114.

2. Calabrese LH, Michel BA, Bloch DA, et al. The American College of Rheumatology 1990 criteria for the classification of hypersensitivity vasculitis. *Arthritis Rheum.* 1990;33:1108.

3. Gardner-Medwin JM, Dolezalova P, Cummins C, et al. Ethnic differences in the incidence of Henoch-Schönlein purpura, Kawasaki disease and rare childhood vasculitides in children of different ethnic origins. *Lancet.* 2002;360:1197.

4. Watts RA, Jolliffe VA, Grattan CEH, et al. Cutaneous vasculitis in a defined population—clinical and epidemiological associations. *J Rheumatol.* 1998;25:920.

5. Trapani S, Micheli A, Grisolia F, et al. Henoch-Schönlein purpura in childhood: epidemiological and clinical analysis of 150 cases over a 5-year period and review of the literature. *Semin Arthritis Rheum.* 2005;35;143-153.

6. Watts RA, Jolliffe VA, Grattan CE, et al. Cutaneous vasculitis in a defined population—clinical and epidemiologic associations. *J Rheumatol.* 1998;25(5):920.

7. Carlson JA, Ng BT, Chen KR. Cutaneous vasculitis update: diagnostic criteria, classification, epidemiology, etiology, pathogenesis, evaluation and prognosis. *Am J Dermatopathol.* 2005;27:504.

8. Chartapisak W, Opastirakul S, Hodson EM, et al. Interventions for preventing and treating kidney disease in Henoch-Schönlein Purpura. *Cochrane Database Syst Rev.* Jul 8 2009;(3):CD005128.

9. Hattori M, Ito K, Konomoto T, et al. Plasmapheresis as the sole therapy for rapidly progressive Henoch-Schönlein purpura nephritis in children. *Am J Kidney Dis.* 1999;33:427.

10. Rostoker G, Desvaux-Belghiti D, Pilatte Y, et al. High-dose immunoglobulin therapy for severe IgA nephropathy and Henoch-Schönlein purpura. *Ann Intern Med.* 1994;120(6):476.

11. Rosenblum ND, Winter HS. Steroid effects on the course of abdominal pain in children with HSP. *Pediatrics.* 1987;79:1018.

# 78 GRANULOMATOSIS WITH POLYANGIITIS (WEGENER)

Tanaz A. Kermani, MD, MS
Kenneth J. Warrington, MD

## PATIENT STORY

A 32-year-old man presented with a 3-month history of fever, weight loss, sinusitis, arthralgias, and dyspnea. He had been treated with several courses of antibiotics for presumed sinusitis with no improvement. Computed tomography (CT) of the chest to evaluate his dyspnea showed multiple cavitary, pulmonary nodules (Figure 78-1). He was a lifetime nonsmoker and denied risk factors for tuberculosis. Bronchoalveolar lavage with bacterial, fungal, and mycobacterial stains and cultures were all negative. Transbronchial biopsy showed nonspecific inflammation and was negative for malignancy. Laboratory evaluation revealed anemia, elevated sedimentation rate, elevated C-reactive protein (CRP), and acute kidney injury (creatinine [1.9 mg/dL]). Urinalysis showed microscopic hematuria, red blood cell casts, and proteinuria. A renal biopsy was pursued and showed a pauci-immune, necrotizing glomerulonephritis (Figure 78-2). Antineutrophil cytoplasmic antibody (ANCA) testing was positive for a cytoplasmic staining pattern (c-ANCA) with specificity to proteinase-3 (PR3). A diagnosis of granulomatosis with polyangiitis (GPA, Wegener) was made. The patient was treated with high doses of glucocorticoids and oral cyclophosphamide with successful induction of remission. Six months later, he was transitioned to azathioprine.

## EPIDEMIOLOGY

- GPA is a necrotizing, granulomatous, systemic vasculitis affecting the small- to medium-sized blood vessels.

- Overall, estimated incidence is 8 to 10 cases per million per year. Estimated prevalence in the United States is 26 cases per million.[1]

- Males are affected slightly more frequently than females.

- Peak age at onset is between 64 and 75 years; it is uncommon in the pediatric population.[1]

## ETIOLOGY AND PATHOPHYSIOLOGY

- The causative agent in GPA is unknown.

- Human leukocyte antigen (HLA)-DPB1, HLA-DRB1, and polymorphisms in genes encoding key regulators of the immune response such as CTL4A and PTPN22 have been associated with increased risk of GPA.[1,2]

- Alpha-1-antitrypsin deficiency has been associated with GPA.[3]

- Infection with *Staphylococcus aureus* and silica exposure have also been associated with GPA.[1]

- GPA is characterized by the presence of ANCA antibodies in c-ANCA with specificity to PR3.

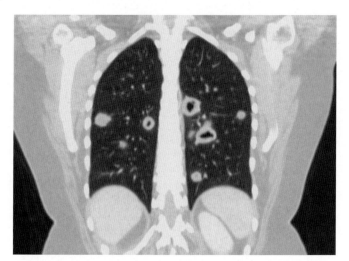

**FIGURE 78-1** Computed tomography (CT) of the chest (coronal plane) shows multiple, bilateral pulmonary nodules, some of which are cavitary, from granulomatosis with polyangiitis.

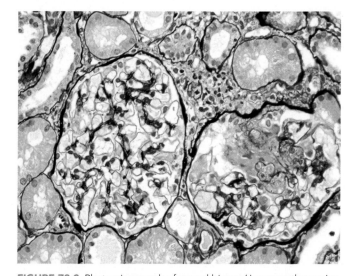

**FIGURE 78-2** Photomicrograph of a renal biopsy (Jones methenamine silver stain) demonstrates necrotizing glomerulonephritis (glomerulus on right, normal glomerulus on left for comparison) in a patient with granulomatosis with polyangiitis. (*Photograph courtesy of Dr. Lynn Cornell, Division of Anatomic Pathology, Mayo Clinic, Minnesota.*)

- In vitro studies suggest a pathogenic role for ANCA antibodies. In these studies ANCA can activate neutrophils to damage endothelial cells and induce a necrotizing vasculitis.[4]

- While the exact mechanism of vasculitis in GPA is unknown, it has been hypothesized that the ANCA antibodies interact with target antigens on primed neutrophils and monocytes, causing endothelial and tissue damage.[4]

## DIAGNOSIS

### Clinical Features

- GPA has a predilection for the upper and lower respiratory tracts, and the kidney.

- Constitutional symptoms include fever, weight loss, and fatigue. Arthralgias and myalgias are common.

- Upper airway manifestations are observed in more than 70% of patients with GPA at presentation and include sinusitis, nasal sores or crusting, septal perforation, epistaxis, saddle-nose deformity (Figure 78-3), otitis media, and conductive and/or sensorineural hearing loss.

- Symptoms of hoarseness or stridor may indicate tracheal disease that can cause subglottic or tracheal stenosis (Figure 78-4).

- Pulmonary symptoms may include cough, dyspnea, or hemoptysis.

- Renal involvement may be clinically silent and noted on testing but if present, can rapidly progress to renal failure.

- Other manifestations include scleritis, orbital masses, cutaneous vasculitis, cranial neuropathies, mononeuritis multiplex, gastrointestinal vasculitis, and central nervous system involvement with pachymeningitis, pituitary involvement, cerebral vasculitis, or thrombotic events.

### Laboratory Studies

- Nonspecific abnormalities like anemia and thrombocytosis are often present on complete blood count.

- Erythrocyte sedimentation rate (ESR) and CRP are usually elevated from systemic inflammation.

- Creatinine elevation is concerning for presence of renal disease.

- The findings of microscopic hematuria, red blood cell casts, and proteinuria on urinalysis suggest renal involvement from vasculitis.

- The presence of c-ANCA with specificity to PR3 has 90% sensitivity and 95% specificity for GPA. However, 5% to 10% patients with GPA may be ANCA negative.[5]

- A positive c-ANCA without the corresponding antibodies to PR3 (atypical ANCA) should raise suspicion for alternate conditions.

### Imaging

- Imaging of symptomatic areas can be helpful in evaluating the presence and extent of disease in patients with GPA.

- Abnormalities on plain radiographs of the sinuses include opacification or air-fluid levels. Chest radiograph may show subglottic stenosis, pulmonary nodules, masses, or alveolar opacities.

- CT or magnetic resonance (MR) imaging of the sinuses often shows opacification, air-fluid levels, or mucosal thickening indicative

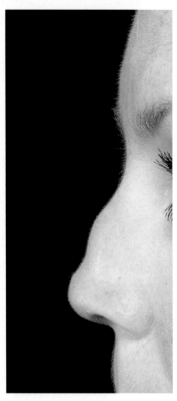

**FIGURE 78-3** Saddle nose deformity as a result of upper airway inflammation from granulomatosis with polyangiitis. (*Photograph courtesy of Dr. Steven R. Ytterberg, Division of Rheumatology, Mayo Clinic, Minnesota.*)

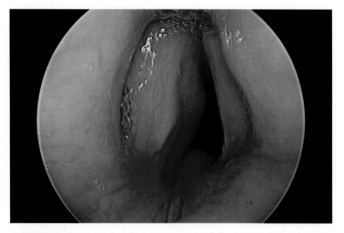

**FIGURE 78-4** Laryngoscopic examination of the upper airway shows narrowing of the trachea from a subglottic mass in a patient with granulomatosis with polyangiitis.

of chronic sinusitis. Destructive or erosive bony changes may be present.

- CT or MR imaging of the orbits in patients with proptosis is a useful modality to evaluate the extent of ocular involvement and response to therapy (Figure 78-5).

- CT imaging of the lungs is generally necessary to evaluate for pulmonary manifestations and may show pulmonary nodules (often bilateral, cavitary) or alveolar opacities (suggestive of alveolar hemorrhage).

## HISTOPATHOLOGY

- Histopathologic examination from sites of active disease is often necessary to establish the diagnosis.

- The triad of granulomatous inflammation, geographic necrosis, and small vessel vasculitis (SVV) has been established as the morphologic feature of GPA. However, in most cases, all three features may not be observed.

- Sinus or nasal biopsies are often nondiagnostic and are of limited utility due to a high frequency of false negatives.

- Cutaneous, renal, or pulmonary biopsies are helpful in establishing the diagnosis.

- Renal biopsy generally demonstrates focal segmental necrotizing glomerulonephritis that is pauci-immune (lacking immune-complex deposits).

## DIFFERENTIAL DIAGNOSIS

- The differential diagnosis of GPA is broad and includes other vasculitides, autoimmune conditions, infections, and drug-associated vasculitis.

- GPA shares clinical features with microscopic polyangiitis (MPA). However, patients with MPA do not have prominent upper airway symptoms. Granulomatous inflammation is usually absent on histopathology in MPA. Additionally, patients with MPA typically have perinuclear (p)-ANCA positivity with specificity to myeloperoxidase (MPO).

- Churg-Strauss syndrome (CSS), another form of ANCA-associated vasculitis, is characterized by the presence of eosinophilia and asthma, which is typically absent in GPA.

- Polyarteritis nodosa (PAN) is a systemic vasculitis of medium-sized muscular arteries and may present with constitutional symptoms, cutaneous manifestations, peripheral nerve involvement, and gastrointestinal (GI) and renal artery involvement. However, mesenteric and visceral angiography in PAN shows microaneurysms consistent with medium-vessel involvement. Additionally, ANCA testing is usually negative in patients with PAN, and glomerulonephritis is not a typical feature of PAN.

- Other causes of pulmonary-renal syndromes including antiglomerular basement membrane (anti-GBM) antibody disease, and connective tissue diseases (particularly systemic lupus erythematosus) are often distinguished based on clinical features and serologic testing.

- *Streptococcus* infections, endocarditis, and hepatitis C–associated cryoglobulinemia may mimic features of a systemic vasculitis but are distinguished by the presence of immune-complex deposition and absence of ANCA.

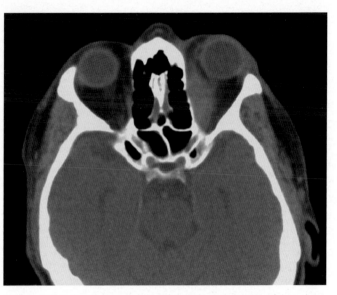

**FIGURE 78-5** Computed tomography (CT) (axial section) of the orbits in a patient with proptosis (left eye) due to an inflammatory orbital pseudotumor on the medial aspect of the orbit.

- Cocaine abuse can cause nasal destructive changes and positive ANCA, a condition called cocaine-induced midline destructive lesion (CIMDL). However, in contrast to GPA, the antigenic target of ANCA in CIMDL is human leukocyte elastase (HLE).[6]

- Adulteration of cocaine with levamisole (an antihelminthic drug) has led to reports of cases of autoimmune phenomenon including purpuric lesions from vasculopathy, which can mimic GPA and is associated with the presence of antibodies including ANCA.[7]

- Medications like propylthiouracil, methimazole, minocycline, hydralazine, and penicillamine have also been associated with drug-induced ANCA-associated vasculitis.[8]

## MANAGEMENT[9]

- Treatment of GPA involves induction of remission and maintenance of remission.

- The choice of induction therapy depends on the severity of organ manifestations and includes high doses of glucocorticoids along with cyclophosphamide (oral or intravenous for 3-6 months) or rituximab. In cases of limited disease, methotrexate at doses of 20 to 25 mg weekly may be used.

- Plasma exchange may be helpful in cases of severe renal impairment or pulmonary hemorrhage with respiratory failure.

- For maintenance of remission, medications such as methotrexate, azathioprine, or mycophenolate mofetil are used. Patients treated with rituximab for induction of remission may be retreated with repeat courses of rituximab to maintain remission, but the optimal frequency and dosing schedule have not been well studied.

- Relapses are common and often require increase or change in immunosuppression.

- Treatment-associated morbidity, particularly infections, is significant.

- Patients should receive prophylaxis against *Pneumocystis jiroveci* pneumonia, and measures to prevent steroid-induced bone loss should also be implemented.

- Patients with exposure to cyclophosphamide need follow-up for long-term complications including bladder and hematologic malignancies.

## PATIENT EDUCATION

Given the rarity of this condition, patients should be encouraged to seek information from reliable sources about their diagnosis, treatment, and potential complications. Patients with GPA need to recognize the need and importance of frequent and close monitoring of their health status even after the symptoms improve. Patients should partner with their physicians and inform them of any changes in symptoms so that relapses or complications of treatment like infections can be diagnosed and treated promptly.

## FOLLOW-UP

- Patients with GPA should be managed by specialists with expertise in vasculitis.

- Patients should be followed closely for symptoms or signs of disease relapse and treatment-related complications.

- Clinic visits may be required monthly initially and then at 3-month intervals depending on clinical course.

- Long-term follow-up is necessary as delayed complications may develop.

- Laboratory studies including markers of inflammation, urinalysis, and assessment of renal function should be checked at every visit.

### PATIENT AND PROVIDER RESOURCES

- http://www.rheumatology.org/practice/clinical/patients/ diseases_and_conditions/wegeners.asp

- http://www.vasculitisfoundation.org

- http://www.mayoclinic.com/

- www.hopkinsvasculitis.org

- www.clevelandclinic.org/arthritis/vasculitis

- http://rarediseasesnetwork.epi.usf.edu/vcrc/

## REFERENCES

1. Ntatsaki E, Watts RA, Scott DG. Epidemiology of ANCA-associated vasculitis. *Rheum Dis Clin North Am*. 2010;36:447-461.

2. Chung SA, Xie G, Roshandel D, et al. Meta-analysis in granulomatosis with polyangiitis reveals shared susceptibility loci with rheumatoid arthritis. *Arthritis Rheum*. Oct 2012;64(10): 3463-3471.

3. Mahr AD, Edberg JC, Stone JH, et al. Alpha(1)-antitrypsin deficiency-related alleles Z and S and the risk of Wegener's granulomatosis. *Arthritis Rheum*. 2010;62:3760-3767.

4. Kallenberg CG. Pathogenesis of ANCA-associated vasculitides. *Ann Rheum Dis*. 2011;70(suppl 1):i59-i63.

5. Berden A, Goceroglu A, Jayne D, et al. Diagnosis and management of ANCA associated vasculitis. *BMJ*. 2012;344:e26.

6. Trimarchi M, Bussi M, Sinico RA, Meroni P, Specks U. Cocaine-induced midline destructive lesions—an autoimmune disease? *Autoimmun Rev*. Feb 2013;12(4):496-500.

7. Espinoza LR, Perez Alamino R. Cocaine-induced vasculitis: clinical and immunological spectrum. *Curr Rheumatol Rep*. Dec 2012;14(6):532-538.

8. Merkel PA. Drug-induced vasculitis. *Rheum Dis Clin North Am*. 2001;27:849-862.

9. Chen M, Kallenberg CG. ANCA-associated vasculitides—advances in pathogenesis and treatment. *Nat Rev Rheumatol*. 2010;6:653-664.

# 79 MICROSCOPIC POLYANGIITIS

Ashima Makol, MD
Kenneth J. Warrington, MD

## PATIENT STORY

A 68-year-old woman was hospitalized for evaluation of progressive dyspnea, cough, and hemoptysis. She had a 2-month history of malaise, anorexia, arthralgias, and a 30-lb weight loss. Symptoms did not improve with outpatient antibiotic therapy. Laboratory studies were significant for profound anemia, elevated erythrocyte sedimentation rate (ESR), C-reactive protein (CRP), and decreased renal function. Perinuclear-pattern antineutrophil cytoplasmic antibody (p-ANCA) and myeloperoxidase (MPO) antibody were positive. Urinalysis showed microscopic hematuria with granular and red blood cell casts. Chest radiograph revealed bilateral alveolar infiltrates (Figure 79-1). Bronchoscopy with bronchoalveolar lavage was consistent with alveolar hemorrhage, and transbronchial lung biopsy showed changes of pulmonary capillaritis (Figure 79-2). An extensive infectious workup was negative. A diagnosis of microscopic polyangiitis (MPA) was made. The patient was treated with high-dose corticosteroids and oral cyclophosphamide, resulting in gradual clinical improvement. She was subsequently switched to azathioprine for maintenance of remission.

## EPIDEMIOLOGY

- MPA is a rare, multisystem autoimmune disorder.
- It is characterized by inflammation of small blood vessels such as arterioles, venules, and capillaries.
- It most commonly occurs in the 65- to 74-year age group.
- Males are affected slightly more frequently than females.
- Incidence of MPA is 3 to 6 per million per year; prevalence is about 60 per million population.[1,2]

## ETIOLOGY AND PATHOPHYSIOLOGY

- The exact etiology of MPA remains unknown.
- Genetic and environmental factors, including infections, are thought to play a role in disease pathogenesis.
- Antineutrophil cytoplasmic antibodies (ANCAs) are present in most patients with MPA and are specific for MPO, an antigen in neutrophil granules and monocyte lysosomes.
- In vitro and experimental animal observations suggest that ANCAs have an important pathogenic role in the pathogenesis of MPA. However, other proinflammatory stimuli are required for the development of clinical disease.
- Antiendothelial cell antibodies (AECAs) may also play a role in pathogenesis.
- Histologically, MPA is characterized by necrotizing small vessel vasculitis (SVV) without evidence of granulomatous inflammation.[2,3]

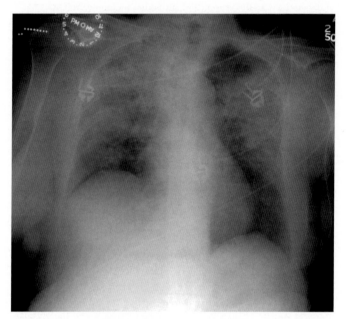

**FIGURE 79-1** Chest radiograph showing bilateral alveolar infiltrates due to pulmonary hemorrhage.

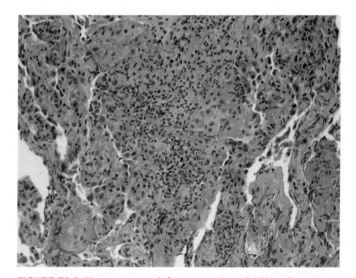

**FIGURE 79-2** Photomicrograph from a transbronchial lung biopsy specimen demonstrates pulmonary capillaritis with acute and organizing intra-alveolar hemorrhage. Neutrophilic infiltrate and hemosiderin-laden macrophages are seen.

## DIAGNOSIS

### Clinical Features

- MPA mainly involves the kidney along with the upper and lower respiratory tract.

- Symptoms are variable and related to pattern of involvement of the internal organs.

- Constitutional symptoms including fever and weight loss are common.

- Almost all patients have renal involvement, characterized by rapidly progressive glomerulonephritis, which may progress to end-stage kidney disease.

- Pulmonary manifestations occur in about 50% of patients. Pulmonary capillaritis from MPA causes alveolar hemorrhage with hemoptysis, dyspnea, cough, and pleuritic chest pain. Other pulmonary features may include pulmonary nodules, infiltrates, or pleural effusion.

- Skin involvement occurs in 30% to 60% of patients and typically presents with palpable purpura (Figure 79-3), livedo reticularis, nodules, or ulcerations.

- Upper respiratory involvement may present as sinusitis (Figure 79-4) and/or otitis media and occurs in about a third of cases.

- Other manifestations of MPA may include ocular inflammation such as scleritis or episcleritis (Figure 79-5) or retinal vasculitis, peripheral neuropathy or mononeuritis multiplex, arthritis, and gastrointestinal vasculitis.[2-4]

### Laboratory Studies

- Nonspecific tests reflect the systemic inflammation associated with MPA. These include elevated ESR, CRP, platelet count, and low hemoglobin (normocytic normochromic anemia).

- Elevated serum creatinine, microscopic hematuria, and proteinuria reflect renal disease.

- About 75% of patients with MPA are p-ANCA MPO positive. A subset of patients with MPA are ANCA negative. Serial measurements of ANCA over time do not correlate well with disease activity or risk of relapse.[4]

### Imaging

- Patients should undergo chest imaging for assessment of pulmonary involvement.

- Chest CT scan may show pulmonary nodules, alveolar infiltrates, or fibrosis in the lung bases.

### Histopathology

- Histopathologic examination of involved tissue, such as kidney, lung, skin, or nerve, is often necessary to document SSV.

- Lung biopsy in a patient with alveolar hemorrhage typically shows intra-alveolar and interstitial red blood cells, hemorrhagic necrotizing alveolar capillaritis, neutrophilic infiltration resulting in fibrinoid necrosis of vessel walls, and intra-alveolar hemosiderosis.[4]

- Kidney biopsy generally demonstrates focal segmental necrotizing glomerulonephritis, often with glomerular crescents.

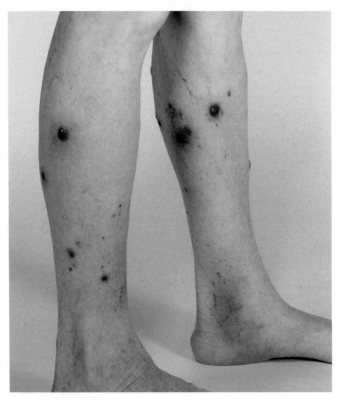

**FIGURE 79-3** Vasculitic skin eruption in a patient with microscopic polyangiitis (MPA). Lesions of palpable purpura and hemorrhagic bullae are present.

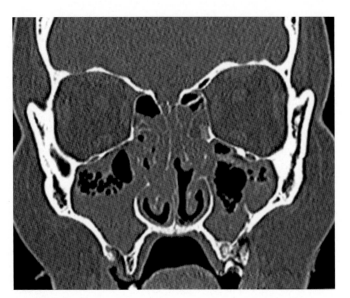

**FIGURE 79-4** Extensive sinus inflammation seen on computed tomography (CT) scan of the sinuses in a patient with microscopic polyangiitis (MPA).

Immunofluorescence studies show few or no immune deposits (pauci-immune).[3]

- Nasal biopsy is often nonspecific and of limited utility.

- Organ- and life-threatening damage from vasculitis can progress rapidly. Therefore, prompt diagnosis is essential.

## DIFFERENTIAL DIAGNOSIS

- Granulomatosis with polyangiitis (GPA, formerly Wegener granulomatosis), can be difficult to distinguish from MPA as the clinical characteristics are very similar. Histologically, MPA can be distinguished from GPA by the absence of granuloma formation. Patients with MPA are typically p-ANCA or MPO positive, while most patients with GPA have a positive c-ANCA or proteinase-3 (PR3) antibody.

- Churg-Strauss syndrome (CSS) is also a form of SVV. However, eosinophilia and asthma are typical of CSS and are not usually seen in MPA.

- Classic polyarteritis nodosa (PAN) is a vasculitis of medium-sized muscular arteries that causes renal infarcts, renal vasculitis, and visceral microaneurysms. ANCAs are not detected in patients with PAN. Glomerulonephritis is seen in MPA but not classic PAN.

- Antiglomerular basement membrane (anti-GBM) antibody disease (Goodpasture syndrome) can present with glomerulonephritis and pulmonary hemorrhage. The diagnosis is made by serologic testing for anti-GBM antibodies and by renal biopsy.

## MANAGEMENT

Treatment of MPA can be divided into three phases: induction of remission, maintenance of remission, and treatment of relapses.

- Induction therapy: For severe forms of MPA, treatment consists of high-dose corticosteroids with either cyclophosphamide (oral or intravenous pulses for 3-6 months) or rituximab (by intravenous infusion, once weekly for 4 weeks).[5]

- Remission maintenance: Azathioprine or methotrexate (contraindicated in patients with renal insufficiency) is generally given for 12 to 18 months.[6] Mycophenolate mofetil is sometimes used, but may be less effective. Patients treated with rituximab for remission induction can be treated with repeated courses of rituximab to maintain remission. However, the optimal frequency and dosing schedule have not been studied to date.

- Plasma exchange can increase the rate of renal recovery in patients with acute renal failure secondary to MPA.

- Morbidity associated with therapy is significant. Preventive measures to minimize treatment-related complications, particularly infections, are essential. Patients should receive prophylaxis against *Pneumocystis jiroveci* pneumonia with trimethoprim or sulfamethoxazole. Measures to prevent steroid-induced bone loss should also be implemented.

- In patients with nonsevere forms of MPA, methotrexate in combination with prednisone can be used as remission-induction therapy.[7]

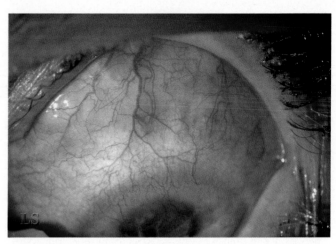

**FIGURE 79-5** Photograph of the right eye (slit-lamp examination) in a patient with scleritis due to microscopic polyangiitis (MPA).

## PATIENT EDUCATION

Patients should learn as much as possible about their disease and its treatment. That way, patients can participate in their health care, and disease flares can be diagnosed and treated promptly. Patients should also understand the possible side effects of medications so that treatment changes can be made when necessary. Patients who have a good understanding of their illness are more likely to have better outcomes.

## FOLLOW-UP

- Patients with MPA should be managed at, or in collaboration with, centers of expertise in vasculitis.
- Patients should be followed closely for symptoms or signs of disease flare and for treatment-related complications.
- Clinic visits may be required monthly initially and then at 3-month intervals depending on clinical progress. Long-term follow-up is necessary as delayed complications may develop.
- Laboratory studies including markers of inflammation, urinalysis, and assessment of renal function should be checked at every visit.

### PATIENT AND PROVIDER RESOURCES

- http://www.vasculitisfoundation.org/microscopicpolyangiitis
- http://www.mayoclinic.com/health/vasculitis/DS00513
- http://rarediseasesnetwork.epi.usf.edu/vcrc/

## REFERENCES

1. Watts RA, Mooney J, Skinner J, Scott DG, Macgregor AJ. The contrasting epidemiology of granulomatosis with polyangiitis (Wegener's) and microscopic polyangiitis. *Rheumatology (Oxford)*. 2012;51:926-931.

2. Ntatsaki E, Watts RA, Scott DG. Epidemiology of ANCA-associated vasculitis. *Rheum Dis Clin North Am*. 2010;36:447-461.

3. Guillevin L, Pagnoux C, Teixeira L. Microscopic polyangiitis. In: Ball GV, Bridges SL, eds. *Vasculitis*. 2nd ed. Oxford, UK: Oxford University Press; 2008:355-364.

4. Chung SA, Seo P. Microscopic polyangiitis. *Rheum Dis Clin North Am*. 2010;36:545-558.

5. Stone JH, Merkel PA, Spiera R, et al. Rituximab versus cyclophosphamide for ANCA-associated vasculitis. *N Engl J Med*. 2010;363:221-232.

6. Jayne D, Rasmussen N, Andrassy K, et al. A randomized trial of maintenance therapy for vasculitis associated with antineutrophil cytoplasmic autoantibodies. *N Engl J Med*. 2003;349:36-44.

7. Mukhtyar C, Guillevin L, Cid MC, et al. EULAR recommendations for the management of primary small and medium vessel vasculitis. *Ann Rheum Dis*. 2009;68:310-317.

# 80 CHURG-STRAUSS SYNDROME (EOSINOPHILIC GRANULOMATOSIS WITH POLYANGIITIS)

Ashima Makol, MD
Kenneth J. Warrington, MD

## PATIENT STORY

A 58-year-old man with recurrent rhinosinusitis and nasal polyps developed new-onset asthma poorly responsive to inhaled bronchodilators. He responded well to oral corticosteroids but developed exacerbations each time steroids were tapered. Two years later, he developed weakness and paraesthesias in his right arm and leg that progressed to right wrist and foot drop. Electromyography confirmed mononeuritis multiplex. Laboratory studies were pertinent for leucocytosis with predominant eosinophilia (48%), elevated erythrocyte sedimentation rate (ESR) and C-reactive protein (CRP), a positive myeloperoxidase (MPO) antibody, and perinuclear antineutrophil cytoplasmic antibody (p-ANCA) pattern (Figure 80-1) on immunofluorescence study. A purpuric rash (Figure 80-2) over the left ankle revealed leukocytoclastic vasculitis (Figure 80-3) with eosinophils on histopathology. A diagnosis of Churg-Strauss syndrome (CSS) was made. He was treated with high-dose steroids and oral cyclophosphamide with resolution of eosinophilia and remarkable clinical improvement by 6 months. He was subsequently switched to azathioprine for maintenance of remission.

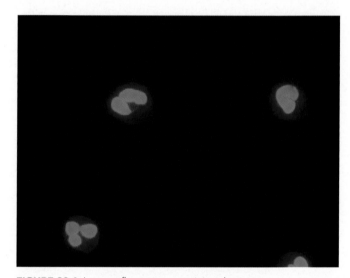

**FIGURE 80-1** Immunofluorescence staining demonstrates a perinuclear antineutrophil cytoplasmic antibody (p-ANCA) pattern in a patient with Churg-Strauss syndrome (CSS). (*Photograph courtesy of Melissa Snyder, PhD, and Brian E. Peters, BS.*)

## EPIDEMIOLOGY

- Rare, multisystem, autoimmune disorder
- First described by Churg and Strauss in 1951
- Classified as a vasculitis and characterized by inflammation of small- to medium-sized arteries, arterioles, and venules in association with allergic syndromes like asthma, rhinitis, and sinusitis
- Mean age at onset 38 to 54 years[1]
- Rare, but more severe in children and adolescents
- Slight male predominance[1]
- Prevalence: 10.7 to 14 per 1 million adults; incidence: 0.11 to 2.66 per 1 million adults per year[1]

## ETIOLOGY AND PATHOPHYSIOLOGY

- Exact pathogenesis is not well understood.
- Autoimmunity is suggested by the presence of hypergammaglobulinemia, increased levels of immunoglobulin E (IgE), ANCA, and rheumatoid factor (RF) in some patients.[1]
- Human leukocyte antigen (HLA)-DRB4 is the main genetic risk factor and may increase the risk of developing vasculitic manifestations.[1]

- Polymorphisms in interleukin (IL)-10 gene have been associated with CSS.[2]

- CD4+ CD25+ T-regulatory cells (Tregs) that produce IL-10 are diminished in CSS patients with asthma or eosinophilia but not in CSS patients in remission.[2]

- The prominence of allergic features suggests a heightened T helper 2 (Th2) immunity, and pulmonary angiocentric granulomatosis suggests heightened Th1 immunity.[2]

- Abnormal eosinophil function is likely as a result of increased eosinophil recruitment by Th2 cytokines (IL-4 and 5) and decreased eosinophil apoptosis.[2]

- Association of CSS with use of leukotriene receptor antagonists (eg, montelukast) in steroid-dependent asthma has been reported but causality has not been proven.[2,3]

- Rare reports of cases associated with cocaine and omalizumab (anti-IgE monoclonal antibody) use.[1,2]

## DIAGNOSIS

### Clinical Features

CSS is characterized by three phases[4]:

- Prodromal phase—second or third decades of life, atopic disease, allergic rhinitis, and asthma (>95%).

- Eosinophilic phase—peripheral blood eosinophilia, eosinophilic infiltration of multiple organs, especially the lung and gastrointestinal tract.

- Vasculitic phase—fourth or fifth decades of life, a life-threatening systemic vasculitis of the small-medium vessels, often associated with vascular and extravascular granulomatosis. Heralded by nonspecific constitutional symptoms, especially fever, fatigue, weight loss, and malaise.

- American College of Rheumatology (ACR) criteria for classification of CSS[5] in a patient with documented vasculitis have a sensitivity of 85% and a specificity of 99.7% for CSS if four of six criteria are met:
    1. Asthma (a history of wheezing or the finding of diffuse high-pitched wheezes on expiration)
    2. Greater than 10% eosinophils on the differential leukocyte count
    3. Mononeuropathy (including mononeuritis multiplex) or polyneuropathy
    4. Migratory or transient pulmonary opacities detected radiographically
    5. Paranasal sinus abnormality
    6. Biopsy containing a blood vessel showing the accumulation of eosinophils in extravascular areas

- Skin is the most common site of vasculitis[4] with lesions ranging from palpable purpura to tender subcutaneous nodules. Vasculitic neuropathy is common. Skin and sural nerve biopsy can be helpful in confirming vasculitis.

- Gastrointestinal involvement leads to eosinophilic gastroenteritis with abdominal pain and bleeding.[4]

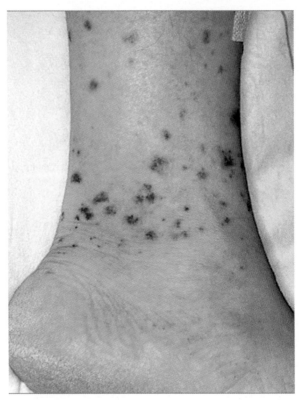

FIGURE 80-2 Palpable purpura on the left ankle of a 58-year-old man with Churg-Strauss syndrome (CSS).

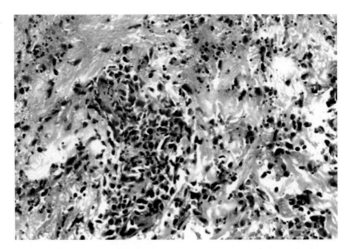

FIGURE 80-3 Skin biopsy from a patient with Churg-Strauss syndrome (CSS) demonstrating leukocytoclastic vasculitis. Vascular necrosis with nuclear dust, perivascular lymphocytes, and eosinophils. Many polymorphonuclear leucocytes are fragmented. Dermal edema is noted.

- Cardiac involvement (Figure 80-4) is the most serious and accounts for 50% of deaths from CSS. Myocarditis, congestive heart failure, and arrhythmias are seen.[4]

- Renal involvement is seen in up to 27% patients and is characterized by hematuria and proteinuria. Necrotizing glomerulonephritis is seen on kidney biopsy.[2]

## Laboratory Studies

- There are no diagnostic tests specific for CSS.

- A complete blood count commonly demonstrates peripheral blood eosinophilia (>10% of total leucocyte count or >1500/µL). This may normalize rapidly if steroids are initiated, but tissue eosinophilia persists.

- Elevated IgE level is common.

- 40% of cases have ANCA, directed against MPO, with the majority having a perinuclear pattern on immunofluorescence staining (MPO-pANCA).[1,3]

- Other nonspecific markers include normocytic normochromic anemia, elevated ESR or CRP, hypergammaglobulinemia, and low titer RF.

## Imaging

- Chest x-ray should be obtained in all patients. Transient, patchy, nodular or interstitial opacities without lobar or segmental distribution are seen in 75% of patients. Pleural effusions are seen in 30% (exudative, eosinophilic). Hilar adenopathy is uncommon. Pulmonary hemorrhage is evident as widespread alveolar infiltrates.

- Patients with dyspnea or abnormal lung function tests should have a high-resolution computer tomography (HRCT). Typical findings for CSS include peribronchial and/or septal thickening and scattered nodular or patchy indistinct opacities (Figure 80-5).

## Histopathology

One or more of these may be seen on tissue biopsy depending on the phase of disease:

- Eosinophilic infiltration

- Prominent, sometimes extensive areas of necrosis

- An eosinophilic, giant cell vasculitis, especially of the small arteries and veins

- Interstitial and perivascular necrotizing granulomas

## DIFFERENTIAL DIAGNOSIS

- Eosinophilic pneumonia (acute or chronic)—Presents with asthma, progressive dyspnea, fever, cough, night sweats, and weight loss. Respiratory failure in acute cases. Characterized by abnormal accumulation of eosinophils in the lung without granulomas or vasculitis on biopsy. Bilateral peripheral or pleural-based opacities described as the "photographic negative" of pulmonary edema is virtually pathognomonic. Organs other than the lung are not involved.

- Allergic bronchopulmonary aspergillosis—This is a complex hypersensitivity reaction to bronchial colonization with *Aspergillus* in patients with asthma or cystic fibrosis. Eosinophilia is milder than in CSS. Central bronchiectasis is noted on HRCT and

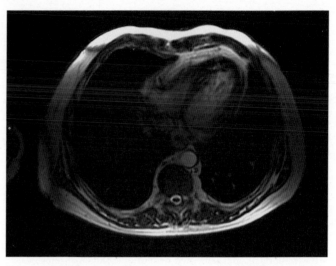

FIGURE 80-4 Cardiac magnetic resonance imaging (MRI) in a patient with Churg-Strauss syndrome (CSS). A rim of circumferential subendocardial delayed enhancement is noted along the inferior wall, most prominent at the base of the heart, suggestive of subendocardial inflammation. Functional imaging showed global hypokinesis and severely reduced systolic function with an ejection fraction of 36%.

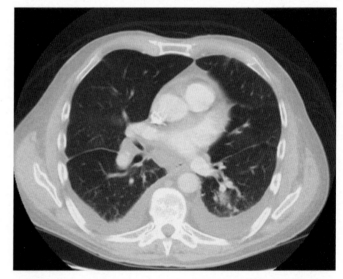

FIGURE 80-5 Computed tomography (CT) of the chest in a patient with Churg-Strauss syndrome (CSS). Large bilateral pleural effusions and scattered patchy, reticulonodular opacities along the bronchovascular bundles in the lung bases.

bronchocentric granulomatosis on histopathology. Extrapulmonary organs other than the nose and sinuses are not affected.

- Hypereosinophilic syndrome (HES)—A rare condition characterized by persistent blood and bone marrow eosinophilia lasting longer than 6 months associated with evidence of tissue infiltration by eosinophils. Heart, skin, nervous system, lungs, gastrointestinal tract, liver, and spleen are frequently involved. Some patients may have a cough, a minority has pulmonary infiltrates, and asthma is rare. Molecular testing for the FIP1L1/PDGFR alpha mutation may be helpful as this is suggestive of HES.

- Aspirin-exacerbated respiratory disease (AERD)—This is a combination of asthma, chronic rhinosinusitis with nasal polyposis, and reactions to aspirin and other cyclo-oxygenase-1 (COX-1) inhibiting nonsteroidal anti-inflammatory drugs (NSAIDs) characterized by bronchoconstriction, nasal congestion, and rhinorrhea. Eosinophilia may be present, but these patients do not have eosinophilic pneumonia or the other organ system involvement seen in CSS. In few cases, AERD may evolve into CSS.

- Other vasculitides—Granulomatosis with polyangiitis (Wegener), microscopic polyangiitis (MPA), and CSS can all affect the lung, although the degree of eosinophilia and presence of asthma are typical of CSS and not usually seen in the other two. The type of ANCA seen in CSS is more typically anti-MPO, whereas in granulomatosis with polyangiitis it is more likely antiproteinase-3 (anti-PR3).

## MANAGEMENT

- The primary therapy for CSS is high-dose oral corticosteroids.[3,4]
- Major life-threatening organ involvement may require treatment with pulse doses of intravenous corticosteroids and other cytotoxic agents.[3,4]
- Cyclophosphamide is typically given for 3 to 6 months, after which patients are switched to either oral methotrexate or azathioprine as maintenance therapy for at least 18 months.[3,4]
- Asthma is treated according to standard guidelines.
- Rituximab, intravenous immunoglobulin (IVIg), or anti–IL-5 (mepolizumab) may be used in refractory cases not responding to conventional treatment.[1,4]

## PATIENT EDUCATION

Patients with CSS can experience relapse of their disease. The likelihood of experiencing a severe relapse can be minimized by prompt reporting of any new symptoms to the doctor, regular follow-up, and ongoing monitoring with laboratory tests and imaging.

## FOLLOW-UP

- Patients should be reassessed at 3-month intervals or more frequently if needed to monitor responsiveness to treatment, drug side effects, and development of recurrences by following symptoms, eosinophil count, previously abnormal laboratory markers, and spirometry.

- Urinalysis and serum creatinine must be checked at every visit to assess for renal involvement.

### PATIENT AND PROVIDER RESOURCES

- http://www.vasculitisfoundation.org/churgstraussresources
- http://www.cssassociation.org/
- http://www.uptodate.com

## REFERENCES

1. Abril A. Churg-Strauss syndrome: an update. *Curr Rheumatol Rep.* Dec 2011;13(6):489-495.

2. http://uptodate.com/ topic- Epidemiology, pathogenesis, and pathology of Churg-Strauss syndrome (allergic granulomatosis and angiitis)

3. Pagnoux C. Churg-Strauss syndrome: evolving concepts. *Discov Med.* Mar 2010; 9(46):243-252.

4. Baldini C, Talarico R, Della Rossa A, Bombardieri S. Clinical manifestations and treatment of Churg-Strauss syndrome. *Rheum Dis Clin North Am.* 2010;36(3):527-543.

5. Masi AT, Hunder GG, Lie JT, et al. The American College of Rheumatology 1990 criteria for the classification of Churg-Strauss syndrome (allergic granulomatosis and angiitis). *Arthritis Rheum.* Aug 1990;33(8):1094-1100.

# 81 POLYARTERITIS NODOSA

Shalene Badhan, MD
Sheryl Mascarenhas, MD
Stacy P. Ardoin, MD, MS

## PATIENT STORY

A 48-year-old man presented with a 2-week history of left-foot drop and diffuse muscle pain. He also reported 3 months of progressive, postprandial abdominal pain, fever, and 15-lb weight loss. His past medical history was notable only for mild hypertension, and his only medication was amlodipine. Physical examination was remarkable for hypertension (175/85 mm Hg), fever (39.8°C), livedo reticularis on his thighs, tenderness with palpation of quadricep muscles, and tenderness with palpation of abdomen without audible bruits, guarding, rebound, or palpable masses. Neurologic examination confirmed a left-foot drop.

Complete blood count (CBC) displayed leukocytosis (white blood cell count 15,500/mm$^3$), normocytic anemia (hematocrit 30%), and thrombocytosis (platelet count 670,000/mm$^3$). Blood urea nitrogen (BUN) (44 mg/dL), serum creatinine (2.1 mg/dL), and urinalysis showed only trace proteinuria. Creatine kinase was elevated at 650 U/L. Erythrocyte sedimentation rate (ESR) (87 mm/h) and C-reactive protein (CRP) (46 mg/L) were also elevated.

A mesenteric arteriogram revealed several areas of aneurysmal dilation in the mesenteric arteries. A biopsy of the left sural nerve identified transmural arterial inflammation with infiltration of polymorphonuclear lymphocytes. Subsequently, a diagnosis of polyarteritis nodosa was made. Testing for hepatitis B infection was negative. He was treated with high-dose oral glucocorticoids and oral cyclophosphamide and gradually improved.

## EPIDEMIOLOGY

Polyarteritis nodosa (PAN) is a rare disease that can present at any age and has no racial or ethnic predilection. PAN affects males slightly more frequently than females (1:1.17 male-to-female ratio). The incidence of PAN is higher in populations with a high burden of hepatitis B virus infection, and the frequency of hepatitis B–related PAN has decreased with the increasing availability of the hepatitis B vaccination.[1,2]

## ETIOLOGY AND PATHOPHYSIOLOGY

PAN is a vasculitis primarily of medium-sized arteries, particularly in the kidney, gastrointestinal tract, peripheral nervous system, skin, and central nervous system. Other potential targets of the disease include joints, muscles, liver, spleen, heart, gonads, and eyes. PAN may involve nearly any medium-sized artery, although the pulmonary arteries are usually spared.[1,3,4]

In PAN, biopsies of affected arteries show patchy, transmural inflammation sparing capillaries, larger arteries, and the venous system. Fibrinoid necrosis and pleomorphic cellular infiltrate without granulomatous inflammation are characteristically seen in the affected vessel walls. Aneurysmal dilation and stenosis occur as a result of disruption of the vessel walls' elastic laminae.[1,2,4]

## DIAGNOSIS

PAN is challenging to diagnose as patients often present with nonspecific symptoms including fever, malaise, arthralgias, and weight loss. Postprandial abdominal pain is often present when the mesenteric arteries are involved. Gonadal involvement may mimic testicular or ovarian torsion. Physical examination may reveal hypertension, livedo reticularis (Figure 81-1), purpuric skin lesions (Figures 81-2 and 81-3), digital ulcerations, skin ulcers (Figure 81-3), arthritis, myositis, or signs of neuropathy (typically mononeuritis multiplex). The pulmonary vasculature is typically spared.[1,2,4-6]

The laboratory findings in PAN are nonspecific, nondiagnostic, and may include leukocytosis, anemia, and elevated inflammatory markers (ESR or CRP). Urinalysis is typically bland as the pathology is arterial insufficiency rather than glomerulonephritis. Autoantibody tests are not useful except to exclude other disorders. Testing for hepatitis B infection should always be performed when PAN is suspected.[1,4]

The diagnosis of PAN hinges on demonstration of characteristic histologic changes on biopsy (discussed earlier) or radiographic findings in affected arteries. Angiography reveals dilation and stenosis of affected arteries as a result of fibrinoid necrosis, leading to the classic "beads on a string" appearance often seen on mesenteric or renal angiography (Figure 81-4). While computed tomography (CT) and magnetic resonance imaging (MRI) angiography are less invasive and can be diagnostic, these modalities lack sensitivity in detecting smaller vessel involvement. As a result, conventional angiography remains the imaging gold standard in suspected PAN.[1] The PAN classification criteria developed by the American College of Rheumatology (ACR) are highlighted in Table 81-1.[7]

### Common Clinical Features

- Cutaneous involvement: livedo reticularis (Figures 81-1 and 81-5), palpable purpura (Figures 81-2 and 81-3), digital ulcerations (Figure 81-6), nodules, ulcers (Figures 81-3 and 81-5)

- Musculoskeletal involvement: arthralgia, arthritis, myositis

- Nervous system involvement: mononeuritis multiplex, other peripheral neuropathy, central nervous system (CNS) arterial involvement

- Renal: hypertension, renal insufficiency, non-nephrotic proteinuria (glomerulonephritis is not present)

- Genitourinary system: orchitis or oophoritis

### Laboratory Studies

- Nonspecific laboratory abnormalities are typical in PAN including leukocytosis, anemia, thrombocytosis, and elevated inflammatory markers (ESR and CRP).

- If the renal arteries are affected, elevated BUN and serum creatinine may be seen along with non-nephrotic range proteinuria and

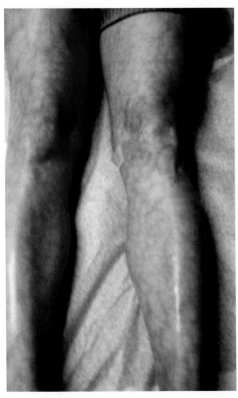

FIGURE 81-1 Livedo reticularis characteristic of polyarteritis nodosa (PAN).

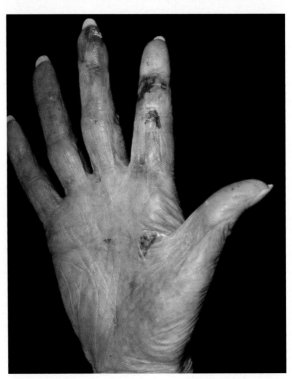

FIGURE 81-3 Purpuric lesions and ulcers on index finger and palm in a patient with polyarteritis nodosa (PAN). (*Photograph courtesy of Dr. Nancy Bates Allen.*)

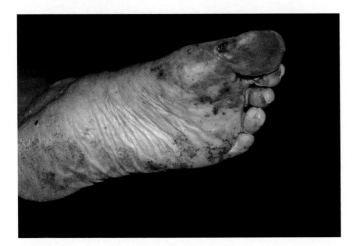

FIGURE 81-2 Extensive purpuric lesions involving the foot in a patient with polyarteritis nodosa (PAN). (*Photograph courtesy of Dr. Nancy Bates Allen.*)

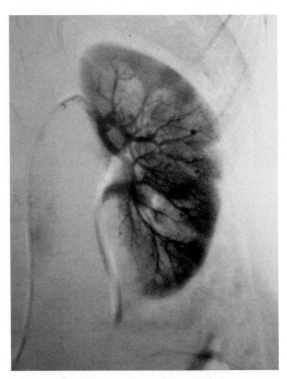

FIGURE 81-4 Microaneurysms in the renal arteries detected by conventional subtraction angiography in a patient with polyarteritis nodosa (PAN). (*Photograph courtesy of Dr. Nancy Bates Allen.*)

**TABLE 81-1.** The American College of Rheumatology Criteria for the Classification of PAN[a]

1. Weight loss ≥10 kg

2. Livedo reticularis

3. Testicular pain or tenderness

4. Myalgias, weakness, or leg tenderness

5. Mononeuropathy or polyneuropathy

6. Diastolic blood pressure of >90 mm Hg

7. Elevated serum nitrogen urea (>40 mg/dL) or creatinine (>1.5 mg/dL)

8. Hepatitis B virus infection

9. Arteriographic abnormality

10. Biopsy of small- or medium-sized artery with intramural polymorphonuclear neutrophils

[a]These criteria were developed for use in clinical studies and not for diagnosing individual patients. A patient is classified as having PAN if three or more criteria are present. These criteria have a reported sensitivity of 82.2% and a specificity of 86.6% for the classification of polyarteritis nodosa (PAN) compared with other vasculitides.[7]

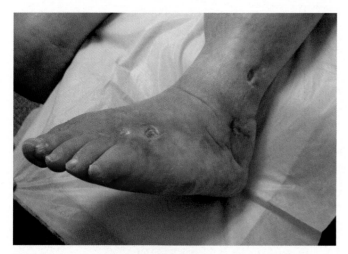

**FIGURE 81-5** Cutaneous ulcerations, retiform purpura, and livedo reticularis in a patient with cutaneous polyarteritis nodosa (PAN). (*Photograph courtesy of Dr. Steven M. Dean, Ohio State University, Columbus, OH.*)

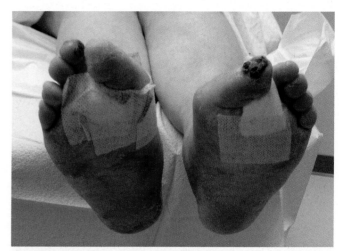

**FIGURE 81-6** Digital ischemia and ulcerations in a patient with cutaneous polyarteritis nodosa (PAN). Retiform purpura is present on the soles. (*Photograph courtesy of Dr. Steven M. Dean, Ohio State University, Columbus, OH.*)

mild hematuria. Glomerular findings such as white and red cell casts and acanthocytes are usually absent.

- Muscle enzymes (creatine kinase and aldolase) may be elevated if myositis is present.

- Except to exclude other disorders, autoantibody tests are not helpful in diagnosing PAN.

- Testing for hepatitis B infection is indicated if PAN is suspected.

- Electromyography and nerve conduction velocity studies can confirm and localize muscle and nerve involvement.[1,4,5]

## Imaging

- Imaging of the arterial vasculature can establish the presence of vasculitis. Classically, arteriography (often of the renal and mesenteric arteries) reveals strictures and aneurysms (Figure 81-3), resulting in the classic "beads on a string" appearance characteristic of PAN.

## Biopsy

- Biopsy of affected tissue is recommended if feasible. Common biopsy sites in PAN include skin, muscle, and peripheral nerve.[2] A full-thickness skin biopsy that includes subcutaneous fat from the center of a nodule or edge of a vasculitis ulcer is recommended.[2] Peripheral nerve biopsy (often of sural nerve) as well as muscle biopsy (often of gastrocnemius muscle) may be diagnostic.[2,4]

## DIFFERENTIAL DIAGNOSIS

- ANCA-associated vasculitides: Respiratory tract involvement and ANCAs directed against antiproteinase-3 (anti-PR3) or myeloperoxidase (MPO) are distinctive features of a majority of the cases of granulomatosis with polyangiitis (GPA, previously known as Wegener granulomatosis), microscopic polyangiitis, and Churg-Strauss syndrome (CSS). In contrast to the ANCA-associated vasculitides, in PAN, ANCA and enzyme immunoassays for PR3 and MPO-ANCA are usually negative, and the respiratory tract and renal capillaries are not affected.

- Immune-complex–mediated vasculitides
  - Cryoglobulinemia—Mixed essential cryoglobulinemia may induce a small vessel vasculitis (SVV) characterized by fever, arthralgias, and purpuric rash. In contrast to PAN, serum cryoglobulins, rheumatoid factor, and hypocomplementemia are usually present. In addition, cryoglobulinemia often causes glomerulonephritis, whereas PAN does not.[2] While PAN is often associated with hepatitis B infection, mixed essential cryoglobulinemia is associated with hepatitis C infection.
  - Henoch-Schönlein purpura—HSP is an SVV that is more common in children than adults. HSP classically presents with purpuric rash, arthritis, and abdominal pain due to inflammation of the small vessels of the gut. Glomerulonephritis is a common complication of HSP, while orchitis and CNS involvement occur less frequently. In contrast to PAN, HSP is an SVV, and biopsy of affected tissue shows immunoglobulin A (IgA) deposition within blood vessels.[2]
  - Hypersensitivity vasculitis—Hypersensitivity vasculitis may present with fever, systemic symptoms, rash, and arthralgias and often is induced by infections or medications. Histologically, hypersensitivity vasculitis is characterized by nonspecific

immune-complex deposition in small vessels including capillaries, postcapillary venules, and arterioles.[2]

- PAN mimics—Vasculitis mimics include viral hepatitis, subacute bacterial endocarditis, and other chronic infections or embolic diseases.[2] Autoimmune diseases such as systemic lupus erythematosus, rheumatoid arthritis, or systemic sclerosis may also present with secondary small- and medium-vessel vasculitis.[2]

## MANAGEMENT

The mortality of untreated PAN was high (13% 5-year survival) prior to introduction of glucocorticoid therapy, but with aggressive immunosuppressive therapy, the 5-year survival has improved to more than 80%.[8,9] The treatment of PAN depends on the severity of disease and whether hepatitis B infection is present. Overall, the risk of relapse is approximately 20% at 1 year and greater than 50% at 5 years. The risk of relapse is lowest in PAN associated with hepatitis B infection.[9]

- PAN associated with hepatitis B infection—Initial treatment involves high-dose prednisone (1 mg/kg/d) followed by rapid taper to suppress the inflammation. Antiviral therapy is critical to treat the hepatitis B infection. Plasma exchange may be considered in severe disease.[1,10-12]

- Cutaneous PAN—In a subset of patients, PAN is limited to the skin. In these patients, nonsteroidal anti-inflammatory drugs (NSAIDs), dapsone, or glucocorticoid therapy can be effective. However, if the disease persists or recurs, steroid-sparing therapy with agents such as methotrexate or azathioprine may be needed. Patients with cutaneous PAN must be monitored closely for the development of systemic PAN.[1,13]

- Idiopathic PAN—The approach to treatment involves high-dose steroids (either oral prednisone at 1 mg/kg/d or intravenous methylprednisolone in doses up to 1 g per day) followed by a gradual taper. With severe disease, oral cyclophosphamide (1-2 mg/kg/d) is often used. Alternate steroid-sparing, immunosuppressive agents that may be used to treat less severe PAN include azathioprine and methotrexate. In rapidly progressive or life- or organ-threatening PAN, plasma exchange is an option.[11,12] After remission is induced with high-dose steroids and cyclophosphamide, a less toxic maintenance agent such as azathioprine or methotrexate can be used. Even after immunosuppression is gradually discontinued, surveillance for recurrence is needed.[1,2,11]

- Prevention—Calcium, vitamin D, and bisphosphonate therapy should be considered for patients on high-dose steroids. Patients taking cyclophosphamide require prophylaxis against *Pneumocystis jiroveci* pneumonia and need to be monitored closely for cytopenias, signs of bladder toxicity, gonadal failure, and secondary malignancies.

## PATIENT EDUCATION

Patients on immunosuppressive therapy should be educated about treatment-related risks of glucocorticoids, cyclophosphamide, and other immunosuppressive agents.

## FOLLOW-UP

Once remission has been achieved, patients need to be monitored for recurrence and long-term medication toxicity.[2]

## REFERENCES

1. Stone JH. Polyarteritis nodosa. *JAMA*. 2002;288:1632-1639.

2. Weiss PF. Pediatric vasculitis. *Pediatr Clin North Am*. 2012;59:
407-423.

3. Ebert EC, Hagspiel KD, Nagar M, Schlesinger N. Gastrointestinal involvement in polyarteritis nodosa. *Clin Gastroenterol Hepatol*.
2008;6:960-966.

4. Pagnoux C, Seror R, Henegar C, et al. Clinical features and
outcomes in 348 patients with polyarteritis nodosa: a systematic
retrospective study of patients diagnosed between 1963 and 2005
and entered into the French Vasculitis Study Group Database.
*Arthritis Rheum*. 2010;62:616-626.

5. Rothschild PR, Pagnoux C, Seror R, Brezin AP, Delair E,
Guillevin L. Ophthalmologic manifestations of systemic necrotizing
vasculitides at diagnosis: a retrospective study of 1286 patients and
review of the literature. *Semin Arthritis Rheum*. 2013;42:507-514.

6. Levine SM, Hellmann DB, Stone JH. Gastrointestinal involvement in polyarteritis nodosa (1986-2000): presentation and
outcomes in 24 patients. *Am J Med*. 2002;112:386-391.

7. Lightfoot RW Jr, Michel BA, Bloch DA, et al. The American
College of Rheumatology 1990 criteria for the classification of
polyarteritis nodosa. *Arthritis Rheum*. 1990;33:1088-1093.

8. Mohammad AJ, Jacobsson LT, Westman KW, Sturfelt G,
Segelmark M. Incidence and survival rates in Wegener's
granulomatosis, microscopic polyangiitis, Churg-Strauss
syndrome and polyarteritis nodosa. *Rheumatology (Oxford)*.
2009;48:1560-1565.

9. Pagnoux C, Seror R, Henegar C, et al. Clinical features and
outcomes in 348 patients with polyarteritis nodosa: a systematic
retrospective study of patients diagnosed between 1963 and 2005
and entered into the French Vasculitis Study Group Database.
*Arthritis Rheum*. 2010;62:616-626.

10. Ribi C, Cohen P, Pagnoux C, et al. Treatment of polyarteritis
nodosa and microscopic polyangiitis without poor-prognosis
factors: a prospective randomized study of one hundred
twenty-four patients. *Arthritis Rheum*. 2010;62:1186-1197.

11. de Menthon M, Mahr A. Treating polyarteritis nodosa: current
state of the art. *Clin Exp Rheumatol*. 2011;29:S110-S116.

12. Pons-Estel GJ, Salerni GE, Serrano RM, et al. Therapeutic
plasma exchange for the management of refractory systemic
autoimmune diseases: report of 31 cases and review of the
literature. *Autoimmun Rev*. 2011;10:679-684.

13. Morgan AJ, Schwartz RA. Cutaneous polyarteritis nodosa: a
comprehensive review. *Int J Dermatol*. 2010;49:750-756.

# 82 THROMBOANGIITIS OBLITERANS (BUERGER DISEASE)

Ari J. Mintz, DO
Bruce D. Mintz, DO

## PATIENT STORY

A 38-year-old male smoker presented with a 1-year history of left-calf discomfort during ambulation and a 3-month history of progressive bluish discoloration of the toes. He had previously been seen by a vascular surgeon and diagnosed with a 'near' occlusion of the tibioperoneal trunk. Physical examination revealed diminished radial artery pulses bilaterally, and the Allen test was positive bilaterally. Tender subcutaneous nodules on the medial aspect of the left calf and a mottled appearance of the skin on the bilateral lower extremities were noted. Computed tomographic (CT) angiography displayed stenosis within the tibioperoneal trunk as well as the infrageniculate arteries bilaterally. Additionally, characteristic "corkscrewing" of distal tibioperoneal and digital arteries was identified. Duplex ultrasonography documented segmental thrombosis of the left great saphenous vein.

## EPIDEMIOLOGY

- Initially described by von Winiwarter in 1879, although the eponym was given to Leo Buerger who published extensive pathologic findings from the amputated limbs of afflicted patients in 1908.[1,2]

- Segmental, nonatherosclerotic inflammatory disease of the small- and medium-sized arteries, veins, and nerves most commonly affecting the hands and feet.[1,2]

- Typically occurs in young adults (20-45 years old) with a higher incidence in men over women (2:1 ratio).[3]

- There is a high association with current or recent tobacco smokers. There are cases in which thromboangiitis obliterans (TAO) has been associated with chewing tobacco as well as marijuana.[3,4]

- Prevalence has diminished over the past 5 years on account of decreased smoking as well as adherence to more stringent diagnostic criteria.

- Highest incidence occurs in Israeli Jews of Ashkenazi descent and natives of Indian, Korean, and Japanese descent. It is less frequent in subjects of northern European descent.

- Death from TAO is unusual, but morbidity is substantial. When affected patients continue to smoke, 43% require one or more amputations in 7.6 years.

## ETIOLOGY AND PATHOPHYSIOLOGY

- The definitive etiology of TAO is not known, yet tobacco exposure is required for both disease initiation and progression.

- The mechanism of disease remains cryptic but may involve immunologic dysfunction and tobacco hypersensitivity that is associated with enhanced cellular sensitivity to type I and III collagen, impaired endothelium-dependent vasorelaxation, and increased antiendothelial cell antibody titers.

- A genetic link may exist as affected subjects have an increased prevalence of human leukocyte antigen (HLA)-A9, HLA-B5, and HLA-54.

## DIAGNOSIS

- TAO should be suspected in young (<45 year old) smokers with a compatible history and symptoms of arterial insufficiency with concurrent superficial venous thrombosis.

- Peripheral artery disease (PAD) can mimic TAO and many times presents with similar manifestations and risk factors. Affected populations are typically older than 50 years and may have concurrent coronary artery disease and/or cerebrovascular disease.[5] However, the combination of arterial insufficiency with superficial venous thrombosis suggests a diagnosis of TAO. In addition, involvement of both upper and lower extremities favors a diagnosis of TAO over atherosclerosis.

### Clinical Features

- Patients with TAO typically present with ischemic signs and symptoms in the distribution of the distal arteries of the upper or lower extremities.[3]

- Manifestations may include claudication (arch of the foot as well as the calf); Raynaud phenomenon (40%) or livedo reticularis; rest pain in hands, feet, and digits; ischemic ulcerations; and/or gangrene (Figures 82-1 to 82-3).[6]

- Foot or arch claudication is often erroneously diagnosed as a musculoskeletal problem.

- Although symptoms of TAO commonly begin in the distal extremities, the disease typically progresses to involve more proximal vessels.

- Allen and reverse Allen tests may reveal ulnar or radial artery obstruction, respectively.

- Superficial thrombophlebitis complicates almost half of all cases of TAO (Figure 82-4).

- Due to associated neurologic involvement, paresthesias of the acral portions of the upper and lower extremities are often described.

### Laboratory Studies

- No specific laboratory tests are available that confirm the diagnosis of TAO.

- Comprehensive serology should be completed to rule out other causes for ischemic digits including thrombophilic states, diabetes, and autoimmune diseases.

- Some studies show that the level of anticardiolipin antibody may be a predictor of age of onset of disease as well as risk of amputation.

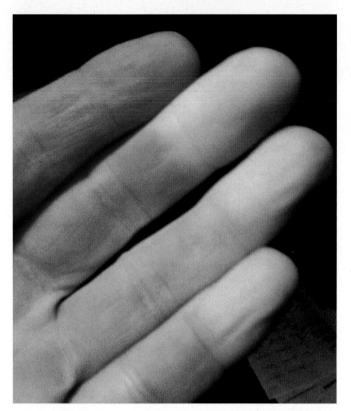

FIGURE 82-1 Preulcerative phase of thromboangiitis obliterans (TAO) with classic well-demarcated digital pallor of Raynaud phenomenon. (*Photograph courtesy of Dr. Steven M. Dean.*)

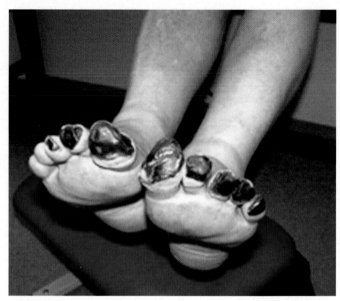

FIGURE 82-3 Diffuse necrotic toes due to thromboangiitis obliterans (TAO).

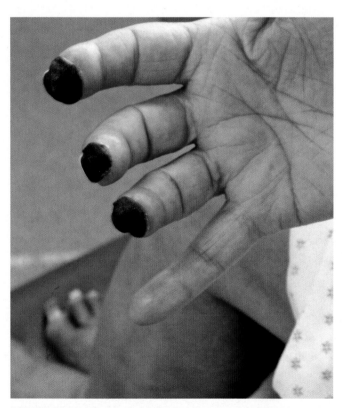

FIGURE 82-2 Multiple necrotic fingers in association with thromboangiitis obliterans (TAO).

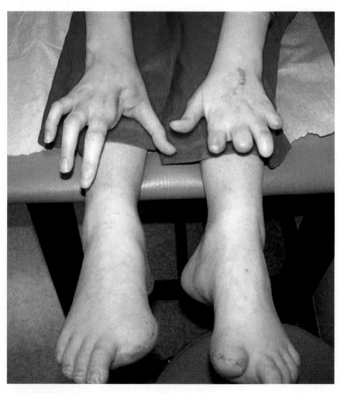

FIGURE 82-4 An inveterate smoker with thromboangiitis obliterans (TAO) who has undergone multiple toe and finger amputations. Note the erythematous cord along the dorsum of the left hand (medial to the cicatrix) due to superficial venous thrombosis.

## Radiographic Studies

- Classic arteriographic findings include nonatherosclerotic segmental occlusions of the small- and medium-sized arteries (eg, tibioperoneal, radioulnar, palmoplantar, and digital arteries). Arteriography may show the characteristic "pigtailing" or "corkscrewing" of the arteries representing small collateral arteries around associated occlusions. However, corkscrew arteries are not specific for TAO.

- Echocardiography should be obtained in order to exclude a proximal source of emboli.

## Histology

A biopsy is usually reserved for unusual cases complicated by significant proximal large artery involvement or when a patient is older than 45 years.

- Acute phase: Initial inflammatory response leads to neutrophil infiltration and granulomatous formation resulting in vessel occlusion by inflammatory thrombus with relative sparing of the vessel wall.

- Subacute phase: After the initial inflammation the thrombus organizes with continuing platelet adherence.

- Chronic phase: Inflammatory mediators are no longer present and the vessel is occluded by organized thrombus and vascular fibrosis. The chronic phase may resemble atherosclerotic disease as well as other vasculitides; however, TAO may be distinguished through the maintenance of the internal elastic lamina.

## DIFFERENTIAL DIAGNOSIS

- PAD
- Peripheral arterial embolism
- Antiphospholipid syndrome
- Frostbite
- Giant cell arteritis or Takayasu arteritis
- Gout
- Polyarteritis nodosa (PAN)
- Raynaud phenomenon
- Reflex sympathetic dystrophy
- Autoimmune disease (scleroderma, systemic lupus erythematosus [SLE])
- Thoracic outlet syndrome

## MANAGEMENT

- Although there is no cure for TAO, the cornerstone of management is smoking cessation. Even smoking one or two cigarettes per day can perpetuate the disease.

- Symptomatic management with calcium channel blockers or other vasodilators can be implemented, especially if there is concurrent Raynaud phenomenon.

- Prostaglandin analogs such as intravenous iloprost can be used to treat the pain and ischemic complications.

- Intramuscular vascular endothelial growth factor (**VEGF**) has been used experimentally.

- Lumbar and/or cervical sympathectomy or spinal cord stimulators have been sporadically utilized.

## PATIENT EDUCATION

- Complete smoking cessation is the cornerstone of management.

## FOLLOW-UP

TAO patients should be carefully assessed at appropriate intervals to monitor disease activity and progression.

### PROVIDER RESOURCES

- http://emedicine.medscape.com/article/460027-overview
- http://www.uptodate.com/contents/thromboangiitis-obliterans-buergers-disease

### PATIENT RESOURCES

- http://health.nytimes.com/health/guides/disease/thromboangiitis-obliterans/overview.html
- http://www.patient.co.uk/health/Buerger''s-Disease.htm

## REFERENCES

1. Buerger L. Landmark publication from the *American Journal of the Medical Sciences*, "Thromboangiitis obliterans: a study of the vascular lesions leading to presenile spontaneous gangrene." 1908. *Am J Med Sci*. 2009;337:274.

2. Piazza G, Creager MA. Thromboangiitis obliterans. *Circulation*. 2010;121:1858.

3. Olin JW. Thromboangiitis obliterans (Buerger's disease). *N Engl J Med*. 2000;343:864.

4. Salimi J, Tavakkoli H, Salimzadeh A, et al. Clinical characteristics of Buerger's disease in Iran. *J Coll Physicians Surg Pak*. 2008;18:502.

5. Shammas NW. Epidemiology, classification, and modifiable risk factors of peripheral arterial disease. *Vasc Health Risk Manag*. 2007;3(2):229-234.

6. Combemale P, Consort T, Denis-Thelis L, et al. Cannabis arteritis. *Br J Dermatol*. 2005;152:166.

# 83 GIANT CELL AND TAKAYASU ARTERITIS

Irving L. Rosenberg, MD
Wael N. Jarjour, MD, FACP

## PATIENT STORY

A 68-year-old woman presented to the hospital with a 2-day history of left-eye blindness and a discolored lower lip and tongue. One week prior she presented to her dentist complaining her dentures were not fitting correctly and was treated for thrush. She was previously in good health and never had visual or oral complaints. Figures 83-1 and 83-2 demonstrate how giant cell arteritis (GCA) can present with nonspecific findings yet cause significant ischemia and organ damage. Below is a comparison demonstrating how GCA and Takayasu arteritis (TA) are points on a continuum of an inflammatory clinical process differing by age of onset, pathogenic mechanism, and the vascular beds commonly affected.

## EPIDEMIOLOGY

### Giant Cell Arteritis

- Increasing frequency with age and average age of diagnosis 72 years.[1]

- Women are more likely affected than men.[2]

- Prevalence up to 1 in 500 among individuals older than 50 years.[2]

- Northern European ancestry living in the United States or Europe.[3]

- History of smoking and atheromatous disease increase risk in women.[4]

- Human leukocyte antigen (HLA)-DR4 positivity.[4]

### Takayasu Arteritis

- 80% to 90% of cases are in women between the ages of 10 and 40.

- Greatest prevalence in Asia. Japan reports 150 new cases per year compared to one to three new cases per million people in the United States and Europe.[5]

- Additional risk factors: HLA-B52, HLA-B39 positivity.

## ETIOLOGY AND PATHOPHYSIOLOGY

### Giant Cell Arteritis

- The pathogenic mechanism of GCA is unknown. However, current understanding implicates a foreign antigen in a cascade of events that understanding results in arterial inflammation.
  - An antigenic stimulant activates dendritic cells, which in turn activate CD4 T lymphocytes that produce interferon-gamma (INF-γ), which has significant effects on macrophage activation and function.
  - This leads to further cytokine and chemokine production, especially interleukin 1 (IL-1), IL-6, transforming growth factor, and monocyte chemoattractant protein 1 (MCP-1).

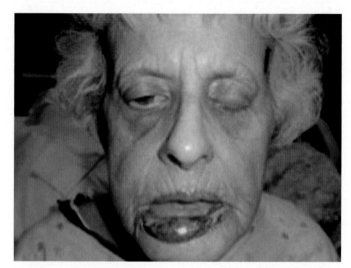

FIGURE 83-1 Giant cell arteritis (GCA) presenting with blindness and ptosis of the left eye. Note the swollen, discolored lower lip and left temporal necrotic tissue.

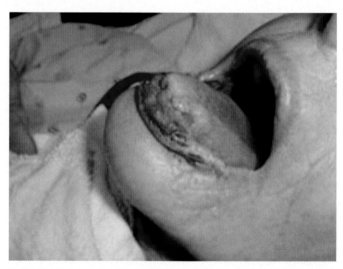

FIGURE 83-2 Giant cell arteritis (GCA) patient with a necrotic lower lip and left side of the tongue.

○ These processes cause immune activation in the adventitia, which ultimately leads to inflammatory changes including granuloma formation, multinucleated giant cells, growth factors, and reactive oxygen intermediates.

○ This entire process subsequently leads to remodeling of the luminal wall caused by matrix digestion, smooth muscle loss, proliferation of myofibroblast, and intimal hyperplasia.

○ All of the above processes contribute to luminal occlusion.

## Takayasu Arteritis

• The etiology and pathogenesis of TA remains unknown, but like GCA is thought to be antigen driven. Several differentiating observations separate TA from GCA that includes the role of gamma delta (γδ) T cells and CD8 T cells in TA.

○ HLA class I molecules, in particular HLA-B52, are more prevalent in TA patients.[6] This is of interest since HLA class I molecules bound to antigens are required for CD8 T-cell recognition.

○ Pathology in TA reveals granulomas and multinucleated giant cells in the media of the blood vessels. There is also proliferation of fibroblasts in the smooth muscle layer.

○ The release of perforin and granzyme B by CD8 T cells in the smooth muscle layer is thought to lead to smooth muscle cell destruction.[7] The fibrotic deposition in this layer leads to vessel wall dilation and aneurysm formation.

○ Intimal thickening can lead to luminal narrowing and vessel occlusion.

## DIAGNOSIS

### Giant Cell Arteritis

• American College of Rheumatology (ACR) classification criteria, which is not used in diagnosis but is useful as a research tool to separate GCA from other vasculitides include age greater than 50, new-onset localized headaches, tenderness or decreased pulse of the temporal artery, erythrocyte sedimentation rate (ESR) greater than 50 mm/h, or biopsy demonstrating multinucleated giant cells in a granulomatous process or a necrotizing arteritis with predominance of mononuclear cells.[8] Patients are said to have GCA if they have three out of five of the above criteria.

### Takayasu Arteritis

• ACR criteria: age less than 40, claudication of the extremities, decreased pulsation of one or both brachial arteries, difference of at least 10 mm Hg in systolic blood pressure between the arms, bruit over one or both subclavian arteries or the abdominal aorta, or arteriographic narrowing or occlusion of the entire aorta, its primary branches or large arteries in the proximal upper or lower extremities, not due to arteriosclerosis, fibromuscular dysplasia, or other causes. Three of the six are required to make the diagnosis.[5]

## CLINICAL FEATURES

### Giant Cell Arteritis

• Systemic symptoms such as fever, weight loss, malaise, and fatigue. A significant number of patients with GCA have polymyalgia-type symptoms characterized by morning stiffness, gelling (stiffness that occurs after being stationary), and proximal muscle pain.

• Cranial arteritis

○ Often presents with a sudden-onset throbbing, sharp or dull headache, mostly localized to the temporal region but it can affect other areas. Patients also often complain of scalp tenderness. One of the most serious complications of GCA is permanent vision loss, which is sudden and painless. Occasionally patients complain of preceding transient vision blurring (amaurosis fugax) or diplopia.

○ Additional neurologic complaints include visual hallucinations depending on the degree and the location of central nervous system (CNS) involvement.

○ Jaw claudication or pain in the masseter and temporalis muscles with prolonged use is reported in half of GCA patients. Claudication of the tongue as well as tongue infarctions have been reported as well (Figures 83-1 and 83-2).

○ Physical examination may reveal firm nodularity or tenderness over the temporal arteries, with or without decreased pulse. GCA patients may have a carotid bruit and/or murmur of aortic insufficiency.

• Large vessel arteritis: Up to 15% of GCA patients have involvement of larger vessels in addition to cranial vessels. The most commonly affected vessels are the carotid, subclavian, and axillary arteries. Consequently, patients will often complain of claudication, numbness, or tingling of extremities. This may make the clinical presentation difficult to differentiate from TA.

### Takayasu Arteritis

• The patient may be asymptomatic; however, the initial presentation often reflects systemic inflammation that manifests as fevers, night sweats, weight loss, and muscle aches.

• The clinical manifestations reflect the vascular bed affected.

○ Visual symptoms, dizziness, headache, syncope, carotidynia, or stroke may be seen in patients with carotid and vertebral artery disease.

○ Inflammation of the subclavian and brachiocephalic arteries may lead to ischemia and claudication.

○ Patients may develop congestive heart failure, arrhythmias, myocardial infarction, or aortic insufficiency.

○ Other effects include severe renovascular hypertension from renal artery stenosis or suprarenal abdominal coarctation.

○ Patients can present with the manifestations of chronic mesenteric ischemia typically in association with severe superior mesenteric artery stenosis.

○ Pulmonary hypertension from pulmonary artery stenosis may occur.

○ Aneurysmal rupture has been reported mostly in patients from Japanese descent.

## LABORATORY STUDIES

### Giant Cell Arteritis

• No specific single test can rule out GCA, and the interpretation of laboratory tests should always be considered in the context of the clinical presentation.

• Complete blood count often reveals an elevated platelet count and anemia of chronic disease.

- ESR is often elevated, but up to 25% of biopsy-positive patients have a normal ESR.[9]

- C-reactive protein (CRP) is elevated but varies more from patient to patient than other tests, decreasing its reliability.[10]

- IL-6 inflammatory marker is often elevated, which correlates with severity and expression of systemic symptoms. Systemic steroids can suppress levels of IL-6, yielding an improvement of symptoms.[11]

- Liver function may demonstrate elevated alkaline phosphatase in 25% to 30% of GCA patients.[10]

- Biopsy of large segments of the temporal arteries bilaterally is a useful tool when positive to establish a tissue diagnosis of GCA (Figure 83-3). However, a negative biopsy does not exclude the diagnosis.

## Takayasu Arteritis

- Similar to GCA, no single test can rule out TA.

- Acute phase reactants such as ESR and CRP are often elevated.

- Hypoalbuminemia may be present.

- Complete blood count may reveal an elevated platelet count and normocytic anemia of chronic inflammation.

## IMAGING

### Giant Cell Arteritis

There is no specific preferred imaging modality for the diagnosis, but the radiographic choice is often based on specific clinical complaints.

Angiography/CTA/MRA: Dramatic findings on angiography, magnetic resonance angiography (MRA), and computed tomography angiography (CTA) may include long segments of smooth stenosis and occlusions within the aorta and/or subclavian, axillary, and/or brachial arteries (Figure 83-4). Thoracoabdominal aortic dissections and aneurysms may occur, and even intracranial aneurysms have been reported (Figure 83-5).

- MRA is often the preferred modality due to the minimal invasiveness and comparatively high sensitivity.[12]

- MRI: Delayed gadolinium-enhanced magnetic resonance imaging (MRI) can be a useful tool to detect inflammation in the vessel wall.

- Ultrasonography of the temporal arteries can reveal hypoechoic ring around arteries (halo sign) when these arteries are inflamed (Figure 83-6). This study has a good positive predictive value when compared with temporal artery biopsy.[13]

### Takayasu Arteritis

- Plain films: May reveal widened mediastinum, dilation of the thoracic aorta, and prominence of the great vessels with aneurysmal dilation.

- CT/MRA/MRI: Classically shows smooth narrowing or blockage of the affected vessel lumen, surrounded by a thickened vessel wall (Figure 83-7). As discussed earlier, delayed gadolinium-enhanced MRI is one of the most advanced techniques available to detect inflammation in the blood vessel wall. These modalities are useful for aneurysm detection as well (Figure 83-8).

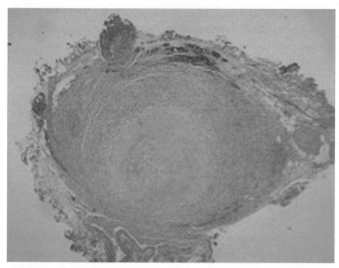

**FIGURE 83-3** Temporal artery biopsy in giant cell arteritis (GCA). The whole artery is infiltrated with mononuclear inflammatory cells (lymphocytes and histiocytes), mostly in the media and adventitia.

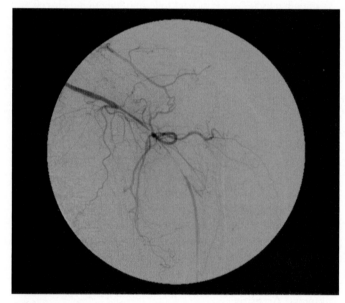

**FIGURE 83-4** Arteriographic evidence of long, segmental, smooth narrowing in the left axillary and brachial arteries in a 64-year-old woman with GCA who presented with arm claudication. (*Photograph courtesy of Dr. Steven M. Dean.*)

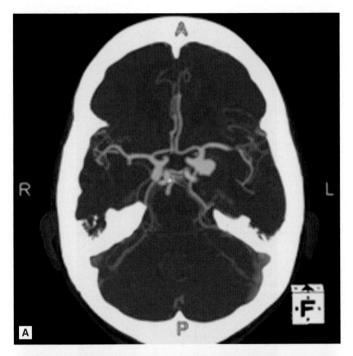

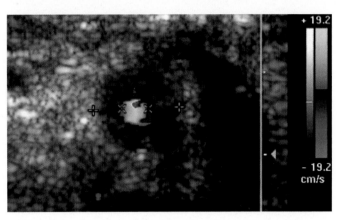

FIGURE 83-6 The classic ultrasonographic "halo sign" illustrating inflammation within the common carotid artery of an elderly patient with headaches associated with giant cell arteritis (GCA). (*Photograph courtesy of Dennis Kiser, RVT.*)

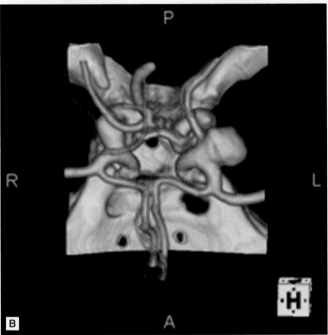

FIGURE 83-5 (A and B) Giant cell arteritis (GCA)–associated large aneurysm arising from the left supraclinoid internal carotid artery on computed tomography angiography (CTA). The posterior cerebral artery is incorporated into the aneurysm (A). Note magnified three-dimensional (3D) reconstruction of the aneurysm (B).

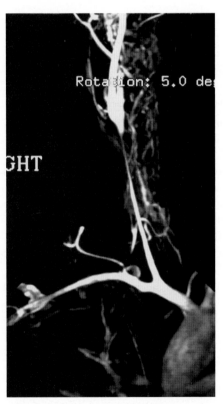

FIGURE 83-7 Long, segmental, smooth narrowing within the right internal carotid artery of a 21-year-old patient with Takayasu arteritis (TA). (*Photograph courtsey of Dr. Michael Jaff.*)

- Angiography: Can show smooth-walled arteries that taper to a long stenotic area (Figures 83-9 and 83-10). Some areas of dilation or aneurysm may be present as well.

- Positron emission tomography (PET): [18]F-fluorodeoxyglucose can be used to image the aorta and its branches to determine the degree of stenosis. Areas of increased uptake correlate with abnormal areas on MRI and likely represent areas of inflammation.[14]

- Ultrasonography: Can be used to detect inflammation in accessible arteries (Figure 83-11).

## DIFFERENTIAL DIAGNOSIS

- Large vessel vasculitis of the aorta and major proximal blood vessels is predominantly due to TA, GCA, and tertiary syphilis. Rare causes for large vessel vasculitis include Behçet syndrome, ankylosing spondylitis, Cogan syndrome, Kawasaki disease, lupus, sarcoidosis, and granulomatosis with polyangiitis (formerly Wegener granulomatosis).

- Other conditions in the differential for large vessel vasculitis include

1. Fibromuscular dysplasia (FMD): Characterized by headache, neck pain, and difficult-to-control hypertension. Patients with FMD develop ischemia related to stenosis, spontaneous dissection with occlusion of arteries, and embolization of thrombi. As opposed to chronic inflammatory states, FMD lacks the chronic anemia, elevated CRP, ESR, or other acute phase reactants.

2. Congenital coarctation of the aorta: Manifests as narrowing of the thoracic aorta with asymmetry of upper versus lower extremity pulses (radiofemoral delay). Less often, asymmetry of the upper extremity pulses and brachial pressure may occur when the coarctation is proximal to the left subclavian artery. It may lead to arterial hypertension, aortic dissection, intermittent claudication, and an increased rate of CNS aneurysms. This condition lacks the elevated inflammatory markers or acute phase reactants. "Rib notching" in association with collateral arterial flow is suggestive of coarctation.

3. Connective tissue disorders: Ehlers-Danlos syndrome, for example, predisposes patients to aneurysms and rupture. Patients generally lack elevated inflammatory markers but demonstrate joint hypermobility and have musculoskeletal complaints.

## MANAGEMENT

### Giant Cell Arteritis

- Glucocorticoids should be given as soon as possible, even before a definitive diagnosis, if there is high clinical and laboratory suspicion in order to avoid the most concerning complication—permanent vision loss. The workup is not affected adversely for at least several weeks after starting steroids. A typical starting dose is prednisone 60 mg. High-dose steroids should be continued for up to 4 weeks or until symptoms improve and then slowly tapered over the course of 9 to 12 months. Close clinical and laboratory monitoring is essential to evaluate for disease flares and reactivation of the inflammatory state.

- Antiplatelet therapy: Although the mechanism is not well defined, patients on aspirin therapy have significantly decreased incidence of

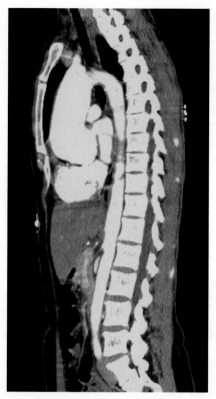

**FIGURE 83-8** Ascending thoracic aortic aneurysm in a patient with Takayasu arteritis (TA).

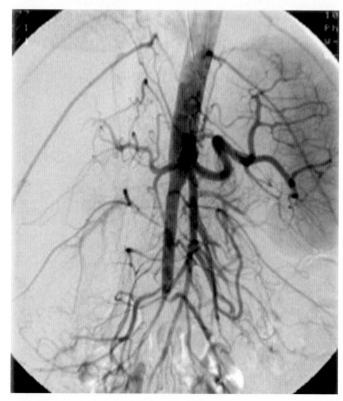

**FIGURE 83-9** Long segment narrowing within the infrarenal aorta and bilateral common iliac artery occlusions displayed via arteriography in a young woman with Takayasu arteritis (TA). (*Photograph courtsey of John Angle.*)

visual loss and cerebral vascular events.[15] This effect is thought to be due to aspirin's inhibitory effect on IFN-γ, a key mediator in the inflammatory cascade in GCA.[16]

- Antitumor necrosis factor-alpha (anti–TNF-α) therapy appears to be very promising in refractory cases.

## Takayasu Arteritis

- Glucocorticoids are usually administered at a dose ranging from 30 to 60 mg of prednisone daily when there is evidence of an active inflammatory disease process. Response to treatment is assessed by decreasing ESR and CRP, as well as decreasing vessel wall thickening and edema. Prednisone should be tapered slowly at a rate of a 10% decrease in the total daily dose per week. TA patients may need chronic low-dose glucocorticoid daily therapy.

- Up to 50% of TA patients have resistance to glucocorticoids and chronic inflammation requiring adjuvant therapy. Agents that have been shown to have benefit are methotrexate, azathioprine, and anti-TNF agents.

## PATIENT EDUCATION

Response to therapy varies among individuals. For example, treatment can result in cessation of symptoms immediately for some, while others may require lifelong treatment. It is important for the patient to understand that despite treatment the disease may progress, and that side effects from the medication may be equally concerning.

## FOLLOW-UP

Depending on the severity of disease at the time of presentation, management may range from immediate hospitalization to outpatient follow-up. In all cases, patients need close monitoring to evaluate treatment response and to dictate future treatment.

### PROVIDER RESOURCE

- http://emedicine.medscape.com/article/332378-overview

### PATIENT RESOURCES

- http://www.uptodate.com/contents/vasculitis-beyond-the-basics
- http://www.uptodate.com/contents/vasculitis-beyond-the-basics#H4

## REFERENCES

1. Smetana GW, Shmerling RH. Does this patient have temporal arteritis? *JAMA.* 2002;287:92.

2. Lawrence RC, Helmick CG, Arnett FC, et al. Estimates of the prevalence of arthritis and selected musculoskeletal disorders in the United States. *Arthritis Rheum.* 1998;41:778.

3. Salvarani C, Gabriel SE, O'Fallon WM, Hunder GG. The incidence of giant cell arteritis in Olmsted County, Minnesota: apparent fluctuations in a cyclic pattern. *Ann Intern Med.* 1995;123:192.

4. Weyand CM, Hicok KC, Hunder GG, Goronzy JJ. The HLA-DRB1 locus as a genetic component in giant cell arteritis.

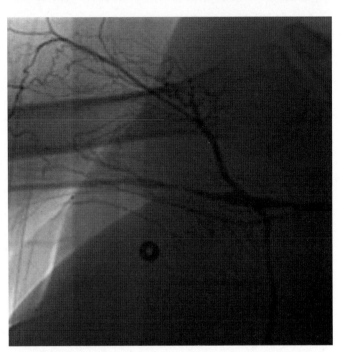

**FIGURE 83-10** Right upper extremity arteriogram demonstrating a segment of severe smooth stenosis within the proximal brachial artery characteristic of Takayasu arteritis (TA). Several collateral branches are seen bridging this segment. The patient presented with arm claudication.

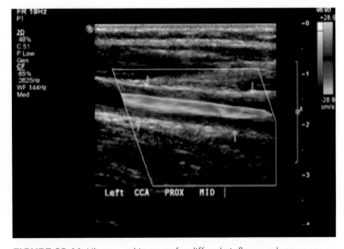

**FIGURE 83-11** Ultrasound image of a diffusely inflamed common carotid artery in a young woman with Takayasu arteritis (TA). (*Photograph courtsey of Dr. Teresa Carmen.*)

Mapping of a disease-linked sequence motif to the antigen binding site of the HLA-DR molecule. *J Clin Invest*. 1992;90:2355.

5. Arend WP, Michel BA, Bloch DA, et al. The American College of Rheumatology 1990 criteria for the classification of Takayasu arteritis. *Arthritis Rheum*. 1990;33:1129.

6. Kimura A, Kitamura H, Date Y, et al. Comprehensive analysis of HLA genes in Takayasu arteritis in Japan. *Int J Cardiol*. 1996;54(suppl):S61-S69.

7. Seko Y. Takayasu's arteritis: insights into immunopathology. *Jpn Heart J*. 2000;411:15-26.

8. Hunder GG, Bloch DA, Michel BA, et al. The American College of Rheumatology 1990 criteria for the classification of giant cell arteritis. *Arthritis Rheum*. 1990;33:1122.

9. Salvarani C, Hunder GG. Giant cell arteritis with low erythrocyte sedimentation rate: frequency of occurrence in a population-based study. *Arthritis Rheum*. 2001;45:140.

10. Hazleman B. Laboratory investigations useful in the evaluation of polymyalgia rheumatica (PMR) and giant cell arteritis (GCA). *Clin Exp Rheumatol*. 2000;18:S29.

11. Roche NE, Fulbright JW, Wagner AD, et al. Correlation of interleukin-6 production and disease activity in polymyalgia rheumatica and giant cell arteritis. *Arthritis Rheum*. 1993; 36:1286.

12. Bley TA, Wieben O, Uhl M, et al. High-resolution MRI in giant cell arteritis: imaging of the wall of the superficial temporal artery. *AJR Am J Roentgenol*. 2005;184:283.

13. Pipitone, N. Role of imaging studies in the diagnosis and follow-up of large-vessel vasculitis: an update. *Rheumatology*. 2008;47(4):403-408.

14. Meller J, Strutz F, Siefker U, et al. Early diagnosis and follow-up of aortitis with [(18)F] FDG PET and MRI. *Eur J Nucl Med Mol Imaging*. 2003;30:730.

15. Nesher G, Berkun Y, Mates M, et al. Low-dose aspirin and prevention of cranial ischemic complications in giant cell arteritis. *Arthritis Rheum*. 2004;50:1332.

16. Weyand CM, Kaiser M, Yang H, et al. Therapeutic effects of acetylsalicylic acid in giant cell arteritis. *Arthritis Rheum*. 2002; 46:457.

# 84 BEHÇET SYNDROME

Ali Mehdi, MD
Rula A. Hajj-Ali, MD

## PATIENT STORY

A 38-year-old Middle Eastern man presented to the emergency department complaining of sudden onset of chest pain associated with hemoptysis. Physical examination was notable for swelling in his right lower extremity. A provisional diagnosis of right leg DVT and secondary pulmonary embolism was suspected, and the patient underwent a computed tomography (CT) scan of the chest that revealed a 3-cm arterial aneurysm involving the right pulmonary artery (Figure 84-1). Further questioning revealed the patient had been suffering from recurrent painful oral aphthous ulcers for the past 5 years. He reported that the ulcers recurred around 6 times yearly. He also complained of two scrotal ulcers in the past 2 years. Moreover, the patient reported recurrent bilateral eye redness and pain over the past couple of years that were treated as conjunctivitis; no evaluation by an ophthalmologist was performed. This constellation of clinical symptoms, venous thrombosis, as well as the pulmonary aneurysms lead to the diagnosis of Behçet syndrome (BS)—a relapsing systemic vasculitis syndrome that can be as benign as isolated mucocutaneous lesions or be associated with significant morbidity and mortality as in this case.

## INTRODUCTION

- BS is a systemic inflammatory vasculitis characterized by recurrent oral aphthous ulcerations, genital ulcers, and skin and ocular lesions.[1]

- It is a heterogeneous disease with systemic involvement of cardiovascular, gastrointestinal, renal, and nervous systems.

- BS is also known as the "Old Silk Route" disease, as the first description of the disease is attributed to Hippocrates in the fifth century BC in the *Third Book of Endemic Diseases* where he describes a disease characterized by aphthous ulcers endemic in Asia Minor.

- Hulusi Behçet, a Turkish dermatologist, identified the major manifestations of oral aphthous ulcers, genital ulcers, and recurrent hypopyon uveitis (Figure 84-2) and clumped them into a clinical entity that he called the "triple symptom complex" in 1937.

## EPIDEMIOLOGY

- BS is most commonly encountered in Mediterranean countries and countries of the far east along the old "Silk Route"—an ancient commercial line stretching between the Mediterranean, Middle East, and the Far East.

- Prevalence is between 20 and 421 per 100,000 adults in Turkey; Japan follows with reported prevalence between 13.5 and 20 cases per 100,000 adults. Prevalence is much lower in Western countries ranging from 0.12 to 0.64 cases per 100,000 adults.

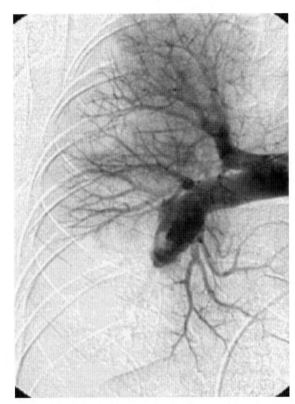

**FIGURE 84-1** Computed tomography (CT) scan of the chest of a Behçet syndrome (BS) patient demonstrating an aneurysm of the right pulmonary artery. (*Reproduced with permission of Informa HealthCare—Books.*)

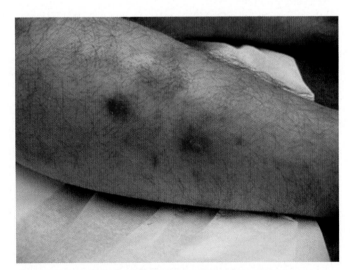

**FIGURE 84-2** Resolving erythema nodosum in a patient with Behçet syndrome (BS).

- A recent epidemiologic study revealed an 18-fold increase in the prevalence of this syndrome in the United States. The causes of this increase are not exactly known, but it is in part due to migration of population but could also be due to better recognition and awareness of this disorder.

- Environmental components influence the prevalence of BS. Migrant studies suggest that immigration might be associated with an alteration of BS risk.

- Typical age of onset is the third or fourth decade of life.

- BS has a more aggressive and severe course in young male adults in Eastern Mediterranean cohorts, Turkey, the Middle and Far East, and Japan than in Western populations.

## ETIOLOGY AND PATHOPHYSIOLOGY

### Genetics

- Genetics of BS are mostly uncertain; however, it is a polygenic disorder.

- Genetic factors are suggested by the fact that immigrants of endemic areas to areas of low prevalence show higher disease prevalence than the general population of the area.

- Human leukocyte antigen (HLA)-B51 allele expression signifies an increased risk of developing BS. HLA-B51 phenotype appears to be more prevalent in the familial cases of BS, and its contribution is actually limited to 20% of BS cases.

- Other non-HLA genes have also been reported in the pathogenicity of the disease including intracellular adhesion molecule (ICAM)-1 gene, interleukin (IL)-1 gene, endothelin nitric oxide synthase (eNOS) gene, vascular endothelial growth factor (VEGF) gene, manganese superoxide dismutase gene, and cytochrome P450. Mutations in the Mediterranean fever gene (MEFV) encoding the protein pyrin have been implicated as well.

### Infectious Factors or Molecular Mimicry

- Many studies point to a possible role for an infectious process in the pathogenicity of BS.

- It is theorized that bacterial or viral antigens share some homology in terms of sequences and thus cross-react with the heat shock family of proteins (HSP), resulting in a cell-mediated and humoral immune response.

- Specific pathogens studied include *Streptococcus* species, *Helicobacter pylori*, herpes simplex virus, and parvovirus B19.

### Cellular Immunity and Cytokines[2]

- Immune system dysfunction is the hallmark of BS; this includes both the innate as well as the acquired immune systems, both the cell-mediated and the humoral components.

- As noted earlier, HSP and bacterial or viral antigens lead to stimulation of T lymphocytes and oligoclonal expansion; these autoreactive T cells appear to have a critical role in the pathogenic cascade of the disease.

- T helper 1 (Th1) polarization of the immune response occurs in BS; this seems to be integral to the mechanistic cascade that leads to the inflammatory state of BS. These TH1-primed cells overproduce

IL-2,-6,-8, -12, and -18; tumor necrosis factor-alpha (TNF-$\alpha$); and interferon-gamma (IFN-$\gamma$).

- Neutrophils in BS patients also demonstrate an activated phenotype with increased chemotaxis, phagocytosis, superoxide production, and myeloperoxidase expression.

### Humoral Immunity and Autoantibodies

- Higher numbers of circulating B lymphocytes have been reported in BS patients.

- Many autoantibodies have been reported in BS patients. The pathogenicity and the clinical significance of these antibodies are yet to be determined. Targets include oral mucosal antigens, endothelial cells, T-cell costimulatory molecule, cytotoxic T lymphocyte antigen-4 (CTLA-4), and oxidized low-density lipoprotein, among others.

- Anti-*Saccharomyces cerevisiae* antibodies have also been reported in BS patients, particularly in patients with intestinal involvement.

### Endothelial Dysfunction and Coagulation Abnormalities

- Endothelial dysfunction is a hallmark of BS with reduced flow-mediated dilation. This promotes vascular inflammation and provides a prothrombotic milieu in BS.

- Nitric oxide (NO) evokes endothelial dysfunction, with increased NO concentrations reported in the serum of BS patients as well as their synovium and aqueous humor.

- Thrombotic events can occur in up to 25% of BS patients; although some evidence exists for defects in the hemostasis or coagulation or fibrinolysis cascade, it is currently believed that the thrombotic manifestations of BS are secondary to vascular damage resulting from inflammation and endothelial dysfunction rather than a generalized hypercoagulable state.

- Table 84-1 summarizes the major disturbances in the immune or hemostatic or coagulation and fibrinolytic systems in BS patients.

## DIAGNOSIS

- The diagnosis of BS remains a challenge given the protean manifestations, and the multiple diseases, which mimic this syndrome as well as the lack of specific diagnostic tests.

- The diagnosis of BS should be based on collective information from the pattern of clinical involvement, laboratory findings, tissue histology, and imaging.

## CLINICAL MANIFESTATIONS[3]

### Mucocutaneous Manifestations

- Recurrent oral ulcers: Present in almost all BS patients. This is the earliest sign of disease and may precede other symptoms by years; most common sites are the gingival and buccal mucosa, tongues, and lips.

- Genital ulcers: Occur in 57% to 93% of patients, commonly heal with scarring.

- Most common site is the scrotum in males; vulvar, vaginal, and cervical lesions occur in females.

- Cutaneous lesions: Occur in 38% to 90% of patients.

- Papulopustular lesions (acne-like) are the most common and occur in usual sites of acne (face, upper chest, and back) as well as in atypical sites like the legs and arms.
- Nodular lesions in the form of erythema nodosum (Figure 84-2) usually affect the lower extremities.
- The pathergy reaction: Hyper-reactivity of skin in response to trauma, defined as an erythematous papular or pustular lesion that appears 48 hours after skin prick by a 20-gauge needle.
- Cutaneous ulcers, similar to the orogenital ulcers, are much less frequent and occur in 3% of patients and usually heal with scarring.

## Ocular Manifestations[4]

- Occurs in 30% to 70% of patients within 3 years of disease onset; associated with significant morbidity as 25% of patients with ocular involvement become blind despite treatment.
- More frequent and more severe in males from the endemic countries.
- Clinical symptoms include photophobia, lacrimation, blurred vision, hyperemia, and pain.
- Typically, it is a bilateral chronic relapsing nongranulomatous uveitis that could affect the anterior segment, posterior segment, or both.
- In about a third of affected patients, inflammatory exudates form a layer in the anterior chamber, yielding the classic hypopyon (Figure 84-3).
- In addition to uveitis, retinal occlusive vasculitis occurs and involves the arteries and the veins.
- Recurrent inflammatory attacks eventually lead to the formation of synechiae, iris atrophy, cataract, glaucoma, chorioretinal scars, atrophic retina, and optic atrophy; all these complications eventually lead to loss of vision.
- Other less frequent ocular manifestations include conjunctivitis, keratitis, iridocyclitis, scleritis, and episcleritis.

## Musculoskeletal Manifestations

- Affects between 45% and 60% of patients.
- Most frequently presents with nonerosive, nondeforming oligoarthritis involving the knees, ankles, and wrists.

## Vascular Manifestations

- BS is a peculiar systemic vasculitis that affects both the arterial and venous system.
- Cardiovascular involvement occurs in 7% to 49% of patients 3 to 16 years after disease onset; more common in males.[5]
- Veins more commonly affected with deep or superficial venous thrombosis; rarely thrombosis of the superior or inferior vena cava can occur; thrombosis can also involve hepatic veins leading to Budd-Chiari syndrome or involve the dural sinuses.
- Arterial disease (manifested as aneurysms or occlusions) is less common but is associated with significant morbidity; arteries involved include the pulmonary arteries, abdominal aorta, carotid, femoral, popliteal, and rarely the coronaries.

**TABLE 84-1.** Summary of Disturbances in the Immune and Hemostatic Systems in BS Patients

Low serum levels of mannose-binding lectin

Increased toll-like receptor 2 and 4 activity by monocytes

Increased gamma delta (γδ) T cells

Elevated TH1 activity

Divergence in cytokine production profile with elevated IL-2, -6, -8, -12, and -18; TNF-α; IFN-γ

Antigen-presenting cell activation

Increased neutrophil activity (increased serum soluble selectin and ICAM-1; increased ROS and MMPs)

Elevated number of circulating B cells

Elevation in various autoantibodies (mucosal antigens, endothelial cells, CTLA-4, LDL, kinectin, ASCA)

Endothelial dysfunction with proinflammatory phenotype activation (elevated NO concentrations; increased VEGF; increased leptin)

Increased oxidative stress (reduced glutathione/oxidized glutathione; reduced SOD; elevated catalase)

Increased thrombin formation with decreased fibrinolysis (decreased activated protein C, thrombomodulin, and tPA)

Increased platelet activation

ASCA, anti-*Saccharomyces cerevisiae* antibodies; BS, Behçet syndrome; CTLA, cytotoxic T lymphocyte antigen; ICAM, intracellular adhesion molecules; IFN, interferon; IL, interleukin; LDL, low-density lipoprotein; MMP, matrix-metalloproteinase; NO, nitric oxide; ROS, reactive oxygen species; SOD, superoxide dismutase; Th1, T helper 1; TNF, tumor necrosis factor; tPA, tissue plasminogen activator; VEGF, vascular endothelial growth factor.

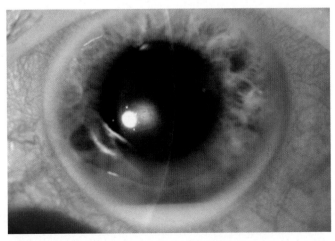

**FIGURE 84-3** Hypopyon uveitis in a patient with Behçet syndrome (BS).

- Pulmonary artery aneurysm (Figure 84-1)[6] occurs in around 1% of patients. Misdiagnosis with pulmonary emboli is common given the similar clinical presentation and the association with venous thrombosis.

## Neurologic Manifestations

- Is the most serious manifestation of BS carrying high mortality and morbidity.
- Occur in 5% to 10% of patients within 5 years of disease onset, more frequent in males.
- Parenchymal disease is the most common form of neuro-Behçet, affecting mainly the brain stem and manifesting as recurrent meningoencephalitis; symptoms include pyramidal signs, cerebellar signs, behavioral changes, sphincter disturbances, headaches, and cranial nerve palsies.
- Cerebral venous thrombosis is a common nonparenchymal neurologic disease; symptoms mainly include severe headaches.
- Peripheral neuropathy is uncommon in BS as opposed to other vasculitis syndromes.

## Gastrointestinal Manifestations

- Quite common among the Japanese BS population (up to 30%); less common in the Middle East.
- Symptomatology includes anorexia, vomiting, diarrhea, dyspepsia, and abdominal pain.
- Mucosal ulceration can occur throughout the gastrointestinal (GI) tract, most commonly in the ileum.

## Renal Manifestations

- Renal involvement in BS is less frequent and less severe than in other forms of vasculitis.
- Renal involvement could manifest as AA amyloidosis, glomerulonephritis, vascular disease, and interstitial nephritis.

## LABORATORY STUDIES

- No specific laboratory findings for BS are available.
- An increase in the inflammatory markers such as C-reactive protein (CRP), erythrocyte sedimentation rate (ESR), leukocytes, and platelets may be found during the active phase of the disease.

## Classification Criteria

- Different classification criteria have been developed in BS. These criteria were developed for research purposes and should not be used as diagnostic criteria. The mostly used criteria are the International Study Group (ISG) criteria[7] detailed in Table 84-2.

## DIFFERENTIAL DIAGNOSIS

- The differential diagnosis varies based on the presentation of the patient suspected of having BS.
- Table 84-3 lists the most common diseases that mimic BS.

**TABLE 84-2.** International Study Group Criteria for Classification of Behçet Syndrome

| | |
|---|---|
| Recurrent oral ulcerations | Minor aphthous, major aphthous, or herpetiform ulcers observed by the physician, recurring at least three times over a 12-month period |
| **Plus Two of the Following** | |
| Recurrent genital ulcers | Aphthous ulceration or scarring observed by physician or patient |
| Eye lesions | Anterior uveitis, posterior uveitis, or cells in the vitreous on slit lamp examination, or retinal vasculitis detected by an ophthalmologist |
| Skin lesions | Erythema nodosum, pseudofolliculitis, or papulopustular lesions, or acneiform nodules observed by the physician |
| Positive pathergy test | Interpreted as positive by the physician at 24 to 48 hours |

**TABLE 84-3.** Differential Diagnosis of Behçet Syndrome Symptomatology

Reactive arthritis

Inflammatory arthropathies

Celiac disease

Sarcoidosis

Stevens-Johnson syndrome

Systemic infections

Familial Mediterranean fever

Seronegative arthropathies

Inflammatory bowel disease

Multiple sclerosis

Systemic vasculitis

Venereal diseases

Malignancies

Bullous skin disorders

## PROGNOSIS[8]

- BS has a variable course with relapses and remissions.
- It is more severe in young males of Middle Eastern or Far Eastern descent.
- Mortality rate is highest in Turkey (9.8%), mostly due to large vessel vasculitis.
- The greatest morbidity and mortality is related to the neurologic, ocular, and vascular involvement.
- Disease activity generally decreases with time in terms of mucocutaneous and articular manifestations; total disease burden, however, increases due to accumulating vascular, ocular, and neurologic insults.
- There has been improvement in the ocular prognosis over the years, which is probably attributed to earlier recognition and aggressive treatment strategies.

## MANAGEMENT

- Few randomized controlled trials have been performed in BS (Table 84-4).
- Treatment of BS is based on the clinical presentation and affected site, in addition to the severity of disease.

### Articular Disease

- Colchicine has been shown in a controlled trial to be effective for arthritis in both males and females. Anti-inflammatory medications can be added.
- Unresponsive cases might warrant low-dose steroid therapy. Although widely used and thought to be effective, no solid data exists to support the clinical experience.
- Patients receiving azathioprine therapy had fewer trends to develop arthritis than those who did not.
- Favorable response has been reported with anti–TNF-α agents.
- Methotrexate is sometimes used but efficacy data is very limited.

### Mucocutaneous Disease

- Topical corticosteroids are frequently used for oral and genital ulcers during the early active phase of the disease. Other symptomatic treatments include lidocaine and chlorhexidine.
- Major oral or genital ulcers can be treated with intralesional steroids.
- Colchicine is widely used for mucocutaneous lesions; its efficacy was shown only in genital ulcers and erythema nodosum in female patients.
- When oral and genital ulcerations are resistant to topical measures and colchicine, systemic glucocorticoids are utilized; a randomized controlled trial using low-dose depot steroid was found to be helpful in controlling erythema nodosum in females.
- Dapsone is effective for mucocutaneous manifestations.
- Methotrexate has been reported to be effective.
- Resistant cases might warrant immunosuppressive therapy with azathioprine, cyclosporine A, IFN-α, and TNF-blocking agents.

**TABLE 84-4.** Summary of Double-Blind Randomized, Controlled Systemic Drug Trials in Behçet Syndrome[10,a]

| Study Limbs | Result |
| --- | --- |
| Methylprednisolone IM 40 mg/3 weekly vs placebo | Effective for erythema nodosum in females |
| Etanercept SC 25 mg 2 × weekly vs placebo | Effective for oral ulcers, nodular, and papulopustular lesions |
| IFN-α-2a 6 MU 3 × weekly vs placebo | Effective for oral ulcers, genital ulcers, and papulopustular lesions |
| Dapsone 100 mg daily vs placebo | Effective for mucocutaneous lesions |
| Thalidomide 100 to 300 mg daily vs placebo | Effective for oral ulcers, genital ulcers, and follicular lesions |
| Cyclosporine 10 mg/kg/d vs colchicine 1 mg daily | Cyclosporine found to be more effective for ocular disease and mucocutaneous lesions |
| Azathioprine 2.5 mg/kg/d vs placebo | Effective for ocular disease, arthritis, and mucocutaneous lesions |
| Colchicine 1 to 2 mg daily vs placebo | Effective for genital ulcers, erythema nodosum, and arthritis in the female population; only for arthritis in males |

[a]Table adapted from Yurdakul S, Yazici H. Behçet syndrome. *Best Pract Res Clin Rheumatol.* 2008;22(5):793-809. IM, intramuscular; SC, subcutaneous.

## Ocular Disease

- Topical corticosteroid may be used in the management of mild anterior uveitis.

- Patients who are not adequately controlled with topical treatment warrant a short course of glucocorticoid therapy.

- Posterior uveitis patients require a more aggressive management approach including high-dose glucocorticoid therapy in addition to another immunosuppressive agent.
  - High-dose intravenous pulse methylprednisolone therapy has been reported to be effective.
  - Azathioprine was shown, in a randomized controlled study, to decrease the recurrence risk and severity of ocular disease in BS.
  - Alternatively, cyclosporine can be used, as it was shown in a controlled trial to reduce the frequency of ocular exacerbations and improve visual acuity.
  - Many large, prospective case series demonstrated that anti-TNF therapy is effective in controlling resistant ocular disease in BS. Although randomized controlled trails are lacking, data suggest that TNF blockade represents an important advancement in the treatment of ocular manifestations in BS.
  - Recently, mycophenolate mofetil (MMF) was shown to be safe and effective in controlling macular edema and uveitis relapses.

## Gastrointestinal Disease

- Corticosteroids, sulfasalazine, and azathioprine are the mainstay of treatment.

- Successful treatment of GI manifestations of the disease has been reported with infliximab.

## Neurologic Disease

- Aggressive treatment with combination therapy is warranted.

- High-dose corticosteroid therapy is universally recommended; positive reports have been described with cyclophosphamide, azathioprine, methotrexate, IFN-$\alpha$, and anti-TNF therapy.

## Vascular Disease

- Little data is available to direct the treatment of vascular disease in BS.

- A combined medical and surgical approach is needed in large arterial disease. High-dose glucocorticoid therapy in addition to cyclophosphamide improves prognosis. Lower complication rates occur when surgical interventions are performed when the disease is inactive.

- There is a lack of consensus on the treatment of venous thrombosis in BS. The use of immunosuppressive therapy and/or anticoagulation is used in many centers.

  Table 84-5 summarizes the European League Against Rheumatism (EULAR)[9] recommendations for the management of BS.

## FOLLOW-UP

- BS patients are at a risk for serious complications of the disease process. Close follow-up with an experienced rheumatologist is required to identify early signs of disease activity and initiate the appropriate therapeutic strategy in order to prevent the dreaded complications of this disease.

**TABLE 84-5.** The European League Against Rheumatism (EULAR) Recommendations for the Management of BS

| | |
|---|---|
| Mucocutaneous disease | • Topical measures |
| | • Erythema nodosum: colchicine |
| | • Resistant cases: azathioprine, IFN-$\alpha$, or anti-TNF agents |
| Articular disease | • Colchicine is the first choice |
| | • Resistant cases: azathioprine, IFN-$\alpha$, or anti-TNF agents |
| Ocular disease | • Azathioprine and local and systemic corticosteroids |
| | • Refractory cases: cyclosporine A or infliximab in combination with azathioprine and corticosteroids, or IFN-$\alpha$ alone or with corticosteroids |
| Gastrointestinal disease | • Sulfasalazine, corticosteroids, azathioprine, anti-TNF agents |
| | • Surgery for perforation or intractable bleeding |
| Major vessel disease | • Acute deep vein thrombosis: corticosteroids, azathioprine, cyclophosphamide, or cyclosporine A |
| | • Thrombosis of the vena cava and Budd-Chiari: cyclophosphamide |
| | • Arterial aneurysm: corticosteroids and cyclophosphamide, surgery |
| Neurologic disease | • Parenchymal disease: corticosteroids, IFN-$\alpha$, azathioprine, cyclophosphamide, methotrexate, or anti-TNF agents |
| | • Dural sinus thrombosis: corticosteroids |

BS, Behçet syndrome; IFN, interferon; TNF, tumor necrosis factor.

## REFERENCES

1. Sakane T, Takeno M, Suzuki N, Inaba G. Behcet's disease. *N Engl J Med*. 1999;341(17):1284-1291.

2. Pay S, Şimşek I, Erdem H, Dinç A. Immunopathogenesis of Behcet's disease with special emphasis on the possible role of antigen presenting cells. *Rheumatol Int*. 2007;27(5):417-424.

3. Tursen U, Gurler A, Boyvat A. Evaluation of clinical findings according to sex in 2313 Turkish patients with Behcet's disease. *Int J Dermatol*. 2003;42(5):346-351.

4. Kitaichi N, Miyazaki A, Iwata D, Ohno S, Stanford MR, Chams H. Ocular features of Behcet's disease: an international collaborative study. *Br J Ophthalmol*. 2007;91(12):1579-1582.

5. Atzeni F, Sarzi-Puttini P, Doria A, Boiardi L, Pipitone N, Salvarani C. Behcet's disease and cardiovascular involvement. *Lupus*. 2005;14(9):723-726.

6. Hamuryudan V, Er T, Seyahi E, et al. Pulmonary artery aneurysms in Behcet syndrome. *Am J Med*. 2004;117(11):867-870.

7. International Study Group for Behcet's Disease. Criteria for diagnosis of Behcet's disease. *Lancet*. 1990;335(8697):1078-1080.

8. Kural-Seyahi E, Fresko I, Seyahi N, et al. The long-term mortality and morbidity of Behcet syndrome: a 2-decade outcome survey of 387 patients followed at a dedicated center. *Medicine (Baltimore)*. 2003;82(1):60-76.

9. Hatemi G, Silman A, Bang D, et al. EULAR recommendations for the management of Behcet disease. *Ann Rheum Dis*. 2008;67(12):1656-1662.

10. Yurdakul S, Yazici H. Behcet's syndrome. *Best Pract Res Clin Rheumatol*. 2008;22(5):793-809.

# 85 NEPHROGENIC SYSTEMIC FIBROSIS

Jason Prosek, MD

## PATIENT STORY

A dialysis-dependent 48-year-old white man with polycystic kidney disease was admitted to the hospital for a living-related renal transplantation. In the immediate post-op course he was evaluated for arrhythmias via cardiac magnetic resonance imaging (MRI) with gadolinium contrast. Three weeks post-op he underwent a renal biopsy for an elevated serum creatinine, which showed acute tubular necrosis (ATN). At that time he developed a painful, erythematous sclerotic plaque with a small erosion in the center of his abdominal wall. Skin biopsies were consistent with nephrogenic systemic fibrosis (NSF).

## EPIDEMIOLOGY[1,2]

- Rare systemic fibrosing disorder presenting as symmetrical, thickened, fibrotic skin leading to flexion contractures and immobility.
- Skin involvement is the predominant feature, leading to its former description as nephrogenic fibrosing dermopathy (NFD). However, increased understanding of this disorder as a systemic process with systemic manifestations has necessitated changing the nomenclature to NSF.
- 95% of cases occur in patients with advanced stages of renal dysfunction.
  - This represents mostly hemodialysis, but also includes peritoneal dialysis, reduced transplant allograft function, and acute kidney injury (AKI) not requiring dialysis.
- Rate of incidence is estimated between 1% and 5% of dialysis-dependent patients.
  - Risk is higher in peritoneal dialysis versus hemodialysis.
  - Gadolinium dose-response relationship has been suggested in a study comparing double dose versus single dose. Odds ratio comparing the two doses was found to be 22.3 for the double dose versus single dose.
- First published case series chronicled patients from 1997 to 2002.

## ETIOLOGY[3-6]

- Gadolinium-based contrast agents
  - Gadolinium is a cationic contrast agent used in MRI. Free gadolinium is relatively water insoluble and toxic to tissue. Thus it is chelated for use in humans. There are various molecular structures used to accomplish this with varying degrees of binding strength. Ionic and cyclical compounds are more stable, compared to nonionic, linear structures.
  - Chelates are excreted unchanged through the kidney, thus diminished renal function significantly prolongs the half-life of gadolinium, from 1.5 to 2 hours with normal renal function, to greater than 30 hours in renal failure.

- One US/FDA registry of 75 cases revealed an exposure to gadolinium 2 days to 18 months prior to diagnosis of NSF. An international registry noted more than 95% of cases reported fell within 2 to 3 months of exposure.
  - The acidosis, hyperphosphatemia, and abnormal iron metabolism associated with renal failure may contribute to destabilization of the gadolinium-chelate complex causing the release of free gadolinium into circulation.
- Erythropoietin therapy
  - Postulated because of its fibrogenic properties, bone marrow stimulation, and iron mobilization.
  - An association has been described, suggesting that high and escalated doses of erythropoietin are an additional risk factor for NSF.
- Infection
  - One single center, retrospective study found that the presence of infection at the time of gadolinium administration markedly increased the risk of NSF in dialysis patients (odds ratio [OR] 25, 95% confidence interval [CI] 3.9-264).

## PATHOLOGY[7]

- Light microscopy
  - Early disease is characterized by subtle proliferation of dermal fibrocytes.
  - Late disease is characterized by marked thickening of the dermis with florid proliferation of fibrocytes with long dendritic processes.
  - Thick collagen bundles with surrounding clefts are prominent, while there is a variable increase in dermal mucin and elastic fibers.
- Immunohistochemical staining
  - Abundance of CD34+ dermal cells typically associated with tissue injury and wound healing.
  - Dendritic processes align with elastic fibers and around collagen bundles in dense networks.
  - Special stainings may reveal gadolinium in tissue; however, at this time chelated versus nonchelated gadolinium cannot be distinguished.

## PATHOGENESIS[6,7]

- Two proposed mechanisms involve activated transforming growth factor beta 1 (TGF-$\beta$1) pathway and increased circulating fibrocytes:
  - TGF-$\beta$1
    - Upregulated messenger ribonucleic acid (mRNA) levels discovered in skin and fascia of affected tissue.
    - TGF-$\beta$1 produced by local CD68+/factor IIIa+ dendritic cells on activation by noxious stimuli.

- TGF-β1 in turn regulates dendritic cell maturation and antigen presentation, leading to a vicious cycle responsible for generating tissue fibrosis.
  - Increased circulating fibrocytes
    - Toxin directly stimulates bone marrow to produce CD34+ fibrocytes.
    - Accumulate in affected tissue and produce collagen.
- Superimposed on these two postulates are the roles of proinflammatory cytokines and gadolinium itself:
  - Proinflammatory/profibrotic cytokines
    - NSF tissue found to have accumulation of macrophages, fibroblasts, TGF-β expression.
    - In vitro studies of human peripheral blood monocytes (PBMCs) exposed to gadolinium chelates showed marked expression of interleukin (IL)-13, IL-4, IL-6, IL-13, TGF-β, and vascular endothelial growth factor (VEGF).
  - Free gadolinium
    - Believed to be the initial toxin/stimuli that initiates the above mechanisms.
    - In vivo studies have demonstrated precipitation in tissue, disruption of calcium movement through nerve and muscle cells, and displacement of endogenous metals thus interfering with intracellular enzymes and cell membranes.

## CLINICAL MANIFESTATIONS[7]

- Skin manifestations
  - Typically present as symmetrical, bilateral fibrotic lesions (Figure 85-1).
  - Manifest as indurated plaques, papules, or subcutaneous nodules (Figures 85-2 and 85-3). The skin may be erythematous, suggestive of cellulitis. The erythema eventually resolves, leaving behind thickened skin with cobblestoning, woody, or peau d'orange features (Figure 85-4).
  - Lesions typically first develop distally (ankles, lower legs, feet, hands) and progress proximally (thighs, forearms, occasionally trunk and buttocks).
  - The head is spared, pruritic and neuropathic pain may develop, and progressive fibrosis over joints can lead to loss of flexibility, hairlessness, hyperpigmentation, and epidermal atrophy.
- Systemic manifestations
  - Muscle induration without loss of strength can be seen early in disease course. This can progress to joint contractures later in the disease.[8]
  - Pulmonary involvement includes alveolar fibrosis (decreased diffusion capacity of carbon monoxide [CO]) and diaphragm (respiratory failure).
  - Cardiac involvement includes myocardium and pericardium.

## DIAGNOSIS[9]

Histopathologic examination of an involved site is required to make a definitive diagnosis. Deep incisional or punch biopsy is recommended since the lesion can extend deep into subcutaneous tissue. Laboratory testing can show elevated erythrocyte sedimentation rate, C-related peptide, ferritin, and decreased albumin—all consistent with a chronic inflammatory state, but these are nonspecific findings.

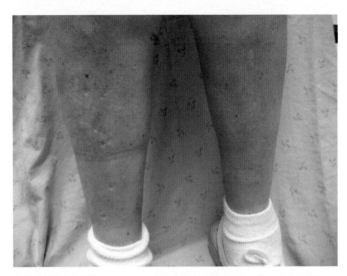

FIGURE 85-1 Bilateral lower extremity involvement of nephrogenic systemic fibrosis (NSF) with mildly hyperpigmented thickened and indurated skin. Superimposed bilateral hypopigmented plaques (right worse than left) as well as a faint peau d'orange appearance along the proximal right anterior calf are evident. (*Photograph courtesy of Dr. Steven M. Dean.*)

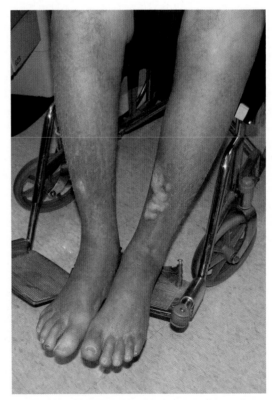

FIGURE 85-2 Typical thickened, indurated skin extending from the patient's knees into his feet. Notice the loss of hair distally, the large nodules on the anterior surface, as well as a bronzed, cobblestoned discoloration throughout. (*Photograph courtesy of Dr. Michael Jaff.*)

When clinically warranted, a surface echocardiogram can demonstrate cardiomyopathy, while pulmonary function tests can document diminished diffusion capacity and lung volumes.

## DIFFERENTIAL DIAGNOSIS

- Scleroderma—absence of Raynaud phenomenon, anticentromere, and anti-Scl-70 antibodies all argue against systemic sclerosis.
- Scleromyxedema—the skin lesions may be similar, but head involvement and immunoglobulin G (IgG)-$\lambda$ paraprotein are more suggestive of scleromyxedema.
- Eosinophilic fasciitis—the skin lesions are similar, but hands and feet are typically spared. Blood will reveal an eosinophilia, while tissue will reveal eosinophilic infiltration.
- Calciphylaxis—appearance may be similar in early stages, and patient population (chronic kidney disease) overlaps considerably. Tissue biopsy can typically differentiate the two.

## DISEASE COURSE

- Typical presentation follows 2 to 4 weeks after gadolinium exposure, but the reported range is 2 days to 18 months.
- Course is typically chronic and unremitting. More rapid disease progression is associated with poor outcomes and death.
- A fulminant form has been described in 5% of patients involving contractures, loss of mobility, and significant morbidity. It is postulated that these cases represent repeated gadolinium exposures.

## PREVENTION[5]

- Avoidance of gadolinium in cases of advanced kidney dysfunction is the major preventative strategy recommended to prevent NSF.
  - The Food and Drug Administration (FDA) defines at-risk patients as those with estimated glomerular filtration rate (eGFR) less than 30 mL/min or those with AKI.
  - Only two cases of NSF have occurred in patients with GFRs in the 30 to 60 mL/min range, but both happened in the setting of AKI, rendering true GFR measurements unreliable.
  - Recommendation is to consider MR without contrast or computed tomography (CT) with or without contrast as an alternative.
- Role of hemodialysis[10]
  - No study has confirmed that the risk of NSF is reduced by hemodialysis.
  - When initiated immediately following gadolinium exposure, hemodialysis removes 78%, 96%, and 99% of the total gadolinium exposure after the first, second, and third treatments, respectively.
  - For chronic hemodialysis patients, imaging studies should be arranged as close to the scheduled dialysis treatment as possible.
  - For peritoneal dialysis patients, it is recommended to initiate at least one treatment of hemodialysis following the exposure to maximize clearance.
  - For chronic kidney disease patients not on dialysis but with GFR less than 30, hemodialysis is recommended, but must be weighed versus the risks of temporary access placement and dialysis itself.

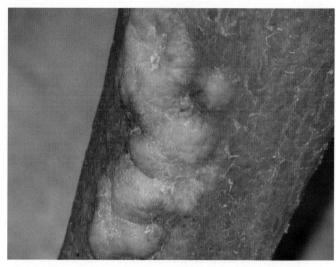

**FIGURE 85-3** Magnified image of the subcutaneous tumor-like nodules on the lower extremity with surrounding hyperpigmentation. (*Photograph courtesy of Dr. Michael Jaff.*)

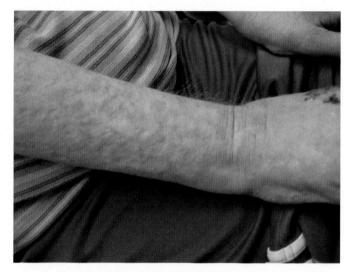

**FIGURE 85-4** Characteristic peau d'orange appearance on a nephrogenic systemic fibrosis (NSF) patient's forearm. In addition the skin is thickened, tight, and woody. (*Photograph courtesy of Dr. Steven M. Dean.*)

## TREATMENT[2]

In general, only recovery of kidney function via resolution of AKI or renal transplantation offers the possibility of reversing NSF. Notably, NSF does not currently impact transplant wait time. Intensive physical therapy is recommended to prevent further disability related to joint contractures. Several other treatment modalities have been studied:

- Extracorporeal photopheresis (ECP)
  - Exposure of PBMCs to photoactivated 8-methoxypsoralen, then reinfused.
  - This induces monocyte-derived tumor necrosis factor-alpha (TNF-$\alpha$), which suppresses collagen synthesis and enhances collagenase production.
  - Current studies are small in scale, but have been favorable.
- Ultraviolet A phototherapy
  - Inhibits procollagen synthesis in human skin.
  - Debated whether this wavelength actually penetrates to the dermis.
  - Results have been inconsistent, but the safety of this procedure makes it an often-used modality alone or in conjunction with other therapies.

### PROVIDER RESOURCES

- http://www.icnfdr.org/
- http://emedicine.medscape.com/article/1097889-overview
- http://www.uptodate.com/contents/nephrogenic-systemic-fibrosis-nephrogenic-fibrosing-dermopathy-in-advanced-renal-failure

### PATIENT RESOURCE

- http://www.ismrm.org/special/QNA.pdf

## REFERENCES

1. Cowper SE, Robin HS, Steinberg SM, et al. Scleromyxedema-like cutaneous diseases in renal-dialysis patients. *Lancet*. 2000;356:1000-1001.

2. Swartz RD, Crofford LJ, Phan SH, Ike RW, Su LD. Nephrogenic fibrosing dermopathy: a novel cutaneous fibrosing disorder in patients with renal failure. *Am J Med*. 2003;114(7):563.

3. Marckmann P, Skov L, Rossen K, et al. Nephrogenic systemic fibrosis: suspected causative role of gadodiamide used for contrast-enhanced magnetic resonance imaging. *J Am SocNephrol*. 2006;17(9):2359.

4. Sadowski EA, Bennet LK, Chan MR, et al. Nephrogenic systemic fibrosis: risk factors and incidence estimation. *Radiology*. 2007;243:148.

5. Swaminathan S, Ahmed I, McCarthy JT, et al. Nephrogenic fibrosing dermopathy and high-dose erythropoietin therapy. *Ann Intern Med*. 2006;145:234.

6. Swaminathan S, Horn TD, Pellowski D, et al. Nephrogenic systemic fibrosis, gadolinium, and iron mobilization. *N Engl J Med*. 2007;357(7):720.

7. Cowper SE, Su LD, Bhawan J, Robin HS, LeBoit PE. Nephrogenic fibrosing dermopathy. *Am J Dermatopathol*. 2001;23(5):383.

8. Levine JM, Taylor RA, Elman LB, et al. Involvement of skeletal muscle in dialysis-associated systemic fibrosis (nephrogenic fibrosing dermopathy). *Muscle Nerve*. 2004;30:569.

9. Cowper SE. Nephrogenic fibrosing dermopathy: the first 6 years. *Curr Opin Rheumatol*. 2003;15:785.

10. Okada S, Katagiri K, Kumazaki T, et al. Safety of gadolinium contrast agent in hemodialysis patients. *Acta Radiol*. 2001;42:339.

## PART 10

# ENVIRONMENTAL DISEASES

# 86 FROSTBITE

Ari J. Mintz, DO
Bruce Mintz, DO, FSVM

## PATIENT STORY

A 48-year-old homeless man presented to the emergency department with bilateral black toes on a subzero temperature morning in January. He states that initially he felt a tingling sensation followed by clumsiness, which led to a total loss of sensation of both feet. The patient's history included tobacco smoking as well as poorly controlled diabetes mellitus. Examination revealed bilateral segments of profound, dark distal eschar, along with bullous erythema of the toes. A dusky area of mid foot tissue demarcation was apparent with segmental dark ischemic borders. Immediate amputation of the left leg was undertaken and the right foot was given a chance to demarcate over the ensuing days.

## EPIDEMIOLOGY

- The prevalence of frostbite in the United States is unknown since no specific system for reporting cases exists.

- Rare in North America with the exception of Canada, Alaska, and other northern states.

- Proclivity for males aged 30 to 49 years, which probably reflects increased outdoor activity as opposed to genetic predisposition.

- Young children are at greater risk of frostbite due to impaired behavioral modification.

- Increased risk in the black population.

- The highest-risk groups are participants in extreme sports (ie, mountaineers) and the military population.

- The most affected areas are the hands, feet, face, lips, and ears.[1,2]

## ETIOLOGY AND PATHOPHYSIOLOGY

- Frostbite injury is due to the absolute temperature as well as duration of exposure. Of these two factors, the exposure duration has the greater impact on the level of injury and severity of tissue damage. The wind chill factor also influences susceptibility to and severity of frostbite.

- Risk factors: malnutrition, substance abuse, mental illness, homelessness, moisture, previous cold injury, and vasoconstrictive medications.

- Predisposing medical conditions: peripheral artery disease (PAD), stroke, Raynaud phenomenon, diabetes, and peripheral neuropathy.

- Frostbite involves three pathophysiologic components—extracellular and intracellular ice crystallization, intracellular dehydration, and ischemia.
  - Extracellular ice crystal formation results in damage to the cellular membrane. Further exposure causes a shift of intracellular fluid into the extracellular matrix, resulting in intracellular dehydration and eventual intracellular ice crystal formation. Damage caused by the expansion of the ice crystals is irreversible.
  - Alternating vasoconstriction and vasodilation ("the hunting reaction") causes rewarming of peripheral tissues with warm core blood. Throughout this cycling, cellular mediators are released including prostaglandins and thromboxane A2, augmenting platelet aggregation, thrombosis, and vasoconstriction.
  - Continued exposure to colder temperatures slows the hunting reaction and eventually stops the vasodilation phase, resulting in unopposed vasoconstriction. This ultimately leads to tissue hypoxia, acidosis, venular and arteriolar thrombosis, and ischemic necrosis.

## DIAGNOSIS

### Clinical Features

- Common symptoms include paresthesias, throbbing, numbness, anesthesia, joint pain, and loss of muscle dexterity.

- First degree: superficial distribution with a central pallor and surrounding edema. The surrounding skin often experiences sensory changes.

- Second degree: characterized by blister formation within 48 hours of tissue exposure. At this stage there is no tissue loss. Eschar may form and slough, revealing healthy granulation tissue.

- Third degree: more extensive blistering occurs expanding past the superficial layer of skin. Blisters may at this point be hemorrhagic, and skin may form eschar within weeks.

- Fourth degree: further extension into the deep layers occurs including muscle, muscle tendon, and bone. This stage is characterized by tissue necrosis and irreversible tissue loss.

Many authorities now use a more simplistic scheme that classifies frostbite injury as superficial (first and second degree, see Figure 86-1) or deep (third and fourth degree, see Figure 86-2). This yields a better correlation between tissue injury and outcome.

### Typical Distribution

Commonly affected areas include the distal digits (ie, fingers and toes) as well as areas of exposure such as cheeks, nose, and ears, although frostbite of the cornea has been described.[3,4]

### Laboratory Studies

- In the absence of concurrent comorbidities, routine blood work does not typically provide useful clinical information.

- A workup to exclude other potential causes of ischemic digits should be considered; however, frostbite is largely a clinical diagnosis based on appearance and exposure history.

- Radiologic studies such as technetium-99 ($^{99}$Tc) scintigraphy or magnetic resonance imaging (MRI) may be useful to establish the degree of involvement and to determine long-term tissue viability.[5] However, neither of these techniques has shown definitive superiority to 3 to 4 weeks of observation for demarcation.

## DIFFERENTIAL DIAGNOSIS

- Thermal burns.
- Severe PAD.
- Frostnip.
  - Localized paresthesias due to superficial cooling of skin and subcutaneous tissues.
  - Occurs without permanent cellular damage.
  - Resolves upon rewarming.
- Pernio (chilblain).
  - Superficial inflammatory ulcerations typically occurring on the digits after repeated exposure to damp, nonfreezing temperatures.
  - Typically occurs during the fall or spring months.
  - Reddish-purple plaques and nodules, vesicles, or bullae are characteristic that are often intensely pruritic or painful.
- Immersion foot (trench foot).
  - Neurovascular damage of the feet.
  - Due to repeated and prolonged exposure to damp nonfreezing temperatures.
  - Tissue loss may occur.

## MANAGEMENT

### Prehospital Treatment

- Removal from cold exposure.
- Avoid use of affected areas.
- Do not rewarm frostbitten tissue if refreezing is a possibility. This may cause further tissue damage.
- Do not use fire heat to rewarm, as sensory loss may result in burns.

### Hospital Treatment

- Rapid rewarming is essential.
- Rewarming is most effective through immersion of the affected tissue into water heated to 40 to 42°C for 15 to 30 mintutes.[6]
- Debridement of white or clear blisters; apply aloe vera every 6 hours.
- Leave hemorrhagic blisters intact and apply topical aloe vera every 6 hours.
- Elevation of the affected parts.
- Antitetanus prophylaxis (toxoid of immunoglobulin [Ig]).
- Analgesia as needed.
- Benzyl penicillin 600 mg every 6 hours for 48 to 72 hours.
- Daily hydrotherapy for 30 to 45 minutes at 40°C.

Due to its potential association with vascular thrombosis, intravenous or intra-arterial tissue plasminogen activator (tPA) along with intravenous heparin has been shown to improve outcome.[7]

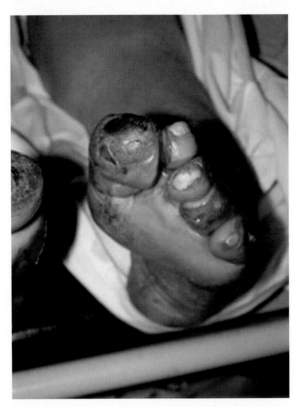

**FIGURE 86-1** Digital ischemic lesions without necrotic tissue suggestive of superficial frostbite within all of the toes.

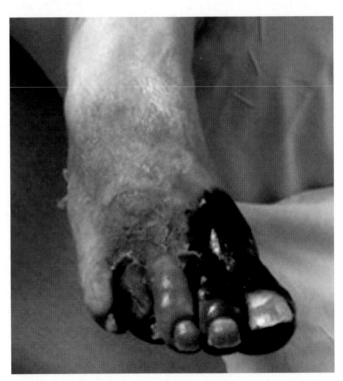

**FIGURE 86-2** Ischemic eschar with well-demarcated border and dusky margins on first and second toes, along with a hemorrhagic bulla on the second digit and a clear bulla on the third digit with surrounding erythema. The fourth toe is necrotic. This is consistent with deep frostbite.

Initial surgical therapies, such as debridement and amputation, should be avoided within the first 3 to 4 weeks in order to prevent the removal of potentially viable tissue. Once complete demarcation and separation of gangrenous tissue occurs, then surgery can be undertaken if needed. Early amputation may be required in the setting of frostbite-associated wet gangrene or infection (Figure 86-3).

## PATIENT EDUCATION

Minimizing exposure risk is primary to the prevention of frostbite. Patients should be warned that they are at increased risk of developing frostbite in the future with exposure and that permanent sensory loss and hyperhidrosis often ensue.

For further information please visit http://emedicine.medscape.com/article/194957-overview or http://www.emedicinehealth.com/script/main/art.asp?articlekey=124962.

## FOLLOW-UP

- Follow-up is critical to avoid intercurrent tissue trauma. Clinicians should maintain a high index of suspicion for compartment syndrome, and the affected extremity should be examined regularly.

- Weekly follow-up is suggested until wounds are stable.

### PROVIDER RESOURCES

- http://emedicine.medscape.com/article/926249-overview
- http://www.uptodate.com/contents/frostbite

### PATIENT RESOURCES

- http://www.patient.co.uk/health/Frostbite.htm
- http://firstaid.webmd.com/frostbite-treatment

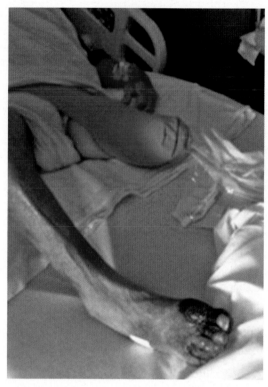

FIGURE 86-3 A recent contralateral amputation was required from the same deep frostbite injury shown in Figure 86-2.

## REFERENCES

1. Legmuskallio E, Lindholm H, Koskenvuo K, et al. Frostbite of the face and ears: epidemiological study of risk factors in Finnish conscripts. *BMJ*. 1995;311:1661.

2. Ervasti O, Juopperi K, Kettunen P, et al. The occurrence of frostbite and its risk factors in young men. *Int J Circumpolar Health*. 2004;63:71.

3. Long WB 3rd, Edlich RF, Winters KL, Britt LD. Cold injuries. *J Long Term Eff Med Implants*. 2005;15:67.

4. Cauchy E, Chetaille E, Marchand V, Marsigny B. Retrospective study of 70 cases of severe frostbite lesions: a proposed new classification scheme. *Wilderness Environ Med*. 2001;12:248.

5. McIntosh SE, Hamonko M, Freer L, et al. Wilderness Medical Society practice guidelines for the prevention and treatment of frostbite. *Wilderness Environ Med*. Jun 2011;22(2):156-166.

6. Aygit AC, Sarikaya A. Imaging of frostbite injury by technetium-99m-sestamibi scintigraphy: a case report. *Foot Ankle Int*. Jan 2002;23(1):56-59.

7. Bruen KJ, Ballard JR, Morris SE, Cochran A, Edelman LS, Saffle JR. Reduction of the incidence of amputation in frostbite injury with thrombolytic therapy. *Arch Surg*. Jun 2007;142(6): 546-551.

# 87 PERNIO

Andrew K. Kurklinsky, MD, RPVI

## PATIENT STORY

A 68-year-old woman from Idaho presented in February with complaints of burning, painful reddish-blue skin changes in four of her right and three of her left toes. These changes have recurred for the past 3 years appearing in the fall and resolving in the spring; specifically, skin changes are absent during the warmer seasons. Blistering and superficial ulcerations were described in the first year yet they were subsequently preventable by wearing well-insulated shoes and warm socks. She has no peripheral arterial disease (PAD) and underwent extensive workup, which was unrevealing. Her serologies were negative for rheumatic diseases, and the nail fold capillaries pattern was normal. She had marked improvement after a week of nifedipine treatment. A diagnosis of pernio was ultimately made.

## EPIDEMIOLOGY

- More common in geographic areas with moist cold conditions.[1]
- Occurs more frequently among women than men.[1-3]
- More common in young and middle age, although patients of any age and race may be affected.
- Low body mass is common.

## ETIOLOGY AND PATHOPHYSIOLOGY

- Intermittent or prolonged cold exposure with local hypoxemia and localized inflammation.[4]
- Typically an essential process affecting susceptible individuals, but some cases are seen in association with connective tissue disorders where pernio may be their early or the only sign.[3,5,6]
- PAD and/or vasospastic disease is a risk factor.

## DIAGNOSIS

The diagnosis is clinical, and laboratory studies and biopsies are not helpful (unless alternative diagnoses have to be ruled out). The key historic factor to establishing the diagnosis is cold exposure. It precedes skin changes by less than 1 day to several decades. The skin lesions are persistent and recur during the cold season or with repeat cold exposure; they disappear in warm climate or with stable warm weather.[1,7]

### Clinical Features

- Acute or repeat cold exposure history is identifiable.[1] The cold is typically nonfreezing and moist, rather than dry.[7,8]
- The onset and spontaneous disappearance of the lesions are noted in relation to prevailing ambient temperature. Many patients go through multiple cycles.[1]
- The lesions are typically macules, less frequently nodules, papules, or plaques, with color changes ranging from blue to erythematous

with doughy subcutaneous swelling. Occasionally they may ulcerate, form vesicles, or hemorrhage with variable stages of resolution present at the same time[1,2,7] (Figures 87-1 to 87-3).

- Symptoms often include local itching, burning, or pain.[7]
- Digital paresthesia may be present.[1]
- Capillary refill time ranges from normal to prolonged.[8]
- Multiple clinical variants and synonymous terms are known.[9]
- More commonly an isolated benign condition but may be observed with connective tissue diseases and then is marked by greater persistence beyond the cold season.[3]

### Typical Distribution

- Acral distribution, usually toes and fingers, but sometimes feet, lower legs, ears[1,3,10] (Figure 87-1).
- May involve a single toe, but lesions are typically bilateral and often symmetrical[1] (Figures 87-1 to 87-3).

### Laboratory Studies

- Low digital pulse volumes and reduced toe temperatures may be confirmed.[1]
- Most patients exhibit vasospastic responses.[1] Nail fold capillaries are normal, unless there is a concurrent connective tissue disease.[8]
- Cold agglutinins, cryoglobulins, rheumatoid factor, lupus anticoagulant, anticardiolipin, and other antiphospholipid antibodies may be positive but are not used to confirm or rule out the diagnosis.[10,11]

### Histologic Findings

- Nonspecific changes of mild perivascular inflammation with endothelial swelling without evidence of epidermal injury.[10,12]
- The infiltrates are predominantly T cells in the papillary and deep layers with perieccrine reinforcement, associated with dermal edema and necrotic keratinocytes.[13]
- Immunohistochemistry is not helpful in differentiating idiopathic cases from lupus erythematosus–associated ones.[13]
- Infiltration of the vessel wall with lymphocytes may be a distinctive feature in some cases.[2]
- Histologic patterns may vary depending on the depth and type of the lesion.[14]

## DIFFERENTIAL DIAGNOSIS

### Raynaud Phenomenon

Pernio lesions do not have the characteristic white-blue-red phasicity and are markedly more lasting compared to Raynaud manifestations (days to weeks rather than minutes to hours). Unlike pernio, in Raynaud phenomenon color changes are induced and reversed rather quickly (in a matter of minutes) with cold exposure and local rewarming, respectively.

## Acrocyanosis

Acrocyanosis does not have the clearly identifiable cold antecedent, although the color changes are aggravated by cold exposure. Acrocyanosis skin changes are more diffuse, while pernio may affect some toes, and the symmetry of its lesions, if present, is not perfect. Pernio lesions and associated symptoms will completely resolve in stable warm temperature, while in acrocyanosis the color changes may only improve or be replaced with prominent hyperhydrosis.

## Frostbite

Frostbite results from complete freezing of the skin, rather than subfreezing cooling as in pernio. This results in subsequent exudative inflammation with blistering, marked pain, and tissue necrosis. Frostbite reactions are more severe and will progress more rapidly, while pernio changes, although less dramatic, may persist for weeks and eventually become chronic-recurrent.

## Erythema Nodosum

Erythema nodosum is an acute, usually self-limited syndrome without identifiable cold antecedent. It usually occurs in the legs, but not in the characteristically acral locations like pernio. Systemic symptoms (fever, arthralgias, malaise) often accompany erythema nodosum, and there is a frequent association with a systemic illness (eg, sarcoidosis) or drug exposures (sulfas, oral contraceptives).

## Erythema Induratum (Bazin Disease)

Erythema induratum was long considered a cutaneous form of tuberculosis, but other etiologies are possible. Histologically, granulomatous tuberculous lesions may be seen with panniculitis and vasculitis. Skin probes are positive for tuberculosis in most patients. Like pernio, it is more common in women and located more typically on the calves with possible exacerbation by cold weather.

## MANAGEMENT

- Tobacco cessation for smokers.
- Prevention of cold exposure is the most important and usually sufficient intervention.[1,10]
- Prazosin,[1] nifedipine,[8] and capsaicin[15] have been shown effective in treatment and prevention.
- In cases associated with lupus erythematosus, mycophenolate mofetil has been effective.[5]

## PATIENT EDUCATION

Prognosis is excellent. The condition is typically benign and nonprogressing. Reduction of cold exposure with appropriate changes to footwear and clothing usually are sufficient.

## FOLLOW-UP

Follow-up is not required unless there is no response to prophylactic measures. If weatherproofing efforts are not sufficient, and significant or recurring tissue damage is noted, connective tissue workup may be justified.

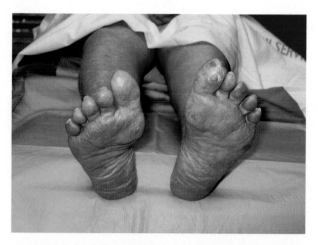

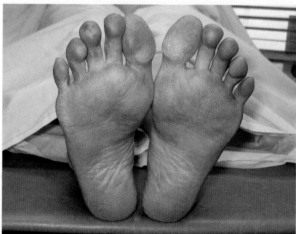

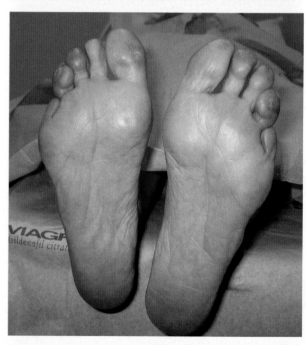

**FIGURES 87-1 TO 87-3** Bilateral toe lesions of pernio vary in color intensity from erythematous red to purple. Different hues may be seen on the same toe. Occasional superficial ulcerations and hemorrhages are present. The distal portions of the toes display a swollen, bulbous appearance. (*Images are courtesy of Dr. Steven Dean, Ohio State University, Columbus, OH.*)

## REFERENCES

1. Spittell J, Spittell P. Chronic pernio: another cause of blue toes. *Int Angiol.* 1992;11(1):46-50.

2. Herman EW, Kezis JS, Silvers DN. A distinctive variant of pernio. Clinical and histopathologic study of nine cases. *Arch Dermatol.* 1981;117(1):26-28.

3. Viguier M, Pinquier L, Cavelier-Balloy B, et al. Clinical and histopathologic features and immunologic variables in patients with severe chilblains. A study of the relationship to lupus erythematosus. *Medicine.* 2001;80(3):180-188.

4. Goette D. Chilblains (perniosis). *J Am Acad Dermatol.* 1990; 23(2 pt 1):257-262.

5. Hedrich CM, Fiebig B, Hauck FH, et al. Chilblain lupus erythematosus—a review of literature. *Clin Rheumatol.* 2008;27(8):949-954.

6. Franceschini F, Calzavara-Pinton P, Quinzanini M, et al. Chilblain lupus erythematosus is associated with antibodies to SSA/Ro. *Lupus.* 1999;8(3):215-219.

7. Lewis T. Observations on some normal and injurious effects of cold upon the skin and underlying tissues: II. Chilblains and allied conditions. *Br Med J.* 1941;2(4223):837-839.

8. Simon T, Soep J, Hollister J. Pernio in pediatrics. *Pediatrics.* 2005;116(3):e472-e475.

9. Al Mahameed A, Olin JW. Pernio (chilblains). In: Creager MA, Dzau VJ, Loscalzo J, eds. *Vascular Medicine: A Companion to Braunwald's Heart Disease.* Philadelphia, PA: Saunders Elsevier; 2006.

10. Weston WL, Morelli JG. Childhood pernio and cryoproteins. *Pediatr Dermatol.* 2000;17(2):97-99.

11. Olson JC, Esterly NB. Painful digital vesicles and acrocyanosis in a toddler. *Pediatr Dermatol.* 1992;9(1):77-79.

12. Coskey R, Mehregan A. Shoe boot pernio. *Arch Dermatol.* 1974;109(1):56-57.

13. Cribier B, Djeridi N, Peltre B, Grosshans E. A histologic and immunohistochemical study of chilblains. *J Am Acad Dermatol.* 2001;45(6):924-929.

14. Wall LM, Smith NP. Perniosis: a histopathological review. *Clin Exp Dermatol.* 1981;6(3):263-271.

15. Cappugi P, Zippi P, Isolani D, et al. Topical capsaicin as useful therapy in the treatment of chilblains. *Pain Clinic.* 1995;8(4): 347-351.

# 88 IMMERSION FOOT SYNDROME

Adil Sattar, MD
Raghu Kolluri, MD, FACP, FSVM

## PATIENT STORY

A 43-year-old woman presented with severe pain, burning, and swelling of the feet. Her symptoms began 2 days prior after returning from a 7-day camping and hiking trip. She reported that her boots were soaked during this period. Examination revealed that both feet were swollen, acrocyanotic, and cold with decreased capillary refill in all 10 toes; pedal pulses were palpable bilaterally. There were dried up blisters in the bilateral feet and ankles (Figure 88-1). Arterial duplex documented normal posterior tibial and dorsalis pedis arteries. A diagnosis of bilateral immersion foot was made. She was initially treated with bed rest, intravenous antibiotics, elevation, and hydration. Her swelling improved over the next few weeks, but she continued to have symptoms of pain and discomfort which were treated with gabapentin therapy. There was no tissue or limb loss due to early detection and treatment.

## INTRODUCTION

- Immersion foot syndrome (IFS) is a clinical syndrome that results from damage to peripheral tissues in the extremities exposed to cold in a wet environment for prolonged periods at temperatures just above their freezing point (0-15°C).

- It has also been referred to as nonfreezing cold injury (NFCI) to differentiate clinically and pathologically from frostbite, which is a freezing cold injury.[1]

- It is not uncommon to have both freezing and nonfreezing injuries in the same individual when exposed to harsh conditions for a prolonged period.

- IFS, besides trench foot, also includes less recognized conditions like warm water immersion foot, shelter limb, and paddy foot (tropical immersion foot). Trench foot is considered a serious military problem for soldiers exposed to cold and wet conditions during battle time,[2] but due to infrequent reporting in civilian personnel, it has remained rather obscure as a civilian medical problem.

## EPIDEMIOLOGY

- Trench foot was described in World War 1 when trench warfare was employed and soldiers wore wet boots and socks for prolonged periods under cold conditions. Cold injuries have been described as early as the Crimean War of 1853 in the men stuck in trenches filled with mud.

- During the Second World War, American forces sustained 11,000 cases of trench foot, and the German army performed more than 15,000 amputations for cold-related injuries.[3]

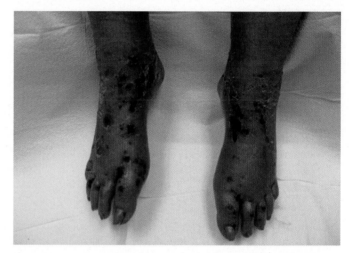

**FIGURE 88-1** The early hyperemic phase of trench foot with edema, cyanosis, and hemorrhagic crusts. (*Photograph courtesy of Steven M. Dean, DO.*)

- African Americans are more susceptible to cold weather injury as observed in the American Civil War and also during the cold winter conflict of Ardennes in 1944.

- Hikers exposed to cold and wet conditions for prolonged periods are at risk if they do not take appropriate care of wet boots and socks. Civilian cases of IFS have also been reported in homeless, older adults, and alcoholics where environmental factors and decreased alertness can lead to injury. Injury to mountaineers has also been reported in the context of inappropriate clothing, incorrect equipment, and lack of knowledge of cold injuries.[4]

## PATHOPHYSIOLOGY

### Normal Skin Physiology

- Skin is a major thermoregulatory organ and functions to either conserve or dissipate heat according to the individual's body temperature.

- The vascular anastomosis of the skin is under dual neural control.
  - Under cold conditions the increased central sympathetic tone causes vasoconstriction.
  - Direct local control of the vasculature causes vasoconstriction in cold and dilation in warm conditions.[5]

- An important protective mechanism of the skin is cold-induced vasodilation (CIVD), where the vasoconstrictive response in cold conditions is interrupted by periods of vasodilation and increased heat flow. Maximal vasoconstriction and minimal cutaneous blood flow occurs when skin is cooled to 15°C or below. If, however, cooling continues to lower temperatures, CIVD is observed in 5- to 10-minute cycles. CIVD results from a cessation of vasoconstrictor transmitter release from adrenergic nerve endings and also as a direct cold-induced relaxation of vascular smooth muscle. The thermoprotective nature of CIVD is evidenced by the fact that Eskimos and Nordics have a very strong CIVD response occurring at much shorter intervals than others.

### Pathophysiology of IFS

- Vasoconstriction—Prolonged vasoconstriction leads to vasospasm of the vessels that supply blood to nerve and muscle cells. Exposure to cold stimulates the release of norepinephrine in the peripheral circulation, which acts on the alpha-2 adrenergic receptors, causing constriction of vascular smooth muscle.[6]

- Increased sympathetic drive—The degree and severity of cold injury depends on duration of cold exposure. Pain and fear can activate the sympathetic nervous system, leading to vasoconstriction.

- Cold-induced ischemia—Leads to injury to the endothelium, resulting in platelet and leukocyte accumulation leading to tissue hypoxia.

- Reperfusion injury—Results in free radical generation, which leads to further endothelial damage and eventually edema.[7]

- CIVD—Absence of CIVD with prolonged cold exposure is an additional factor contributing to IFS.

- Nerve injury—Ischemia of the nerves causes hypoxia and results in primary nervous system injury. Thick, large, myelinated fibers (C fibers) are most susceptible to injury after prolonged cold exposure. However, the full extent of nerve fiber involvement depends on the actual duration and severity of the cold exposure. Cold exposure also results in nerve conduction blockade and associated cessation of axoplasmic transport.[6]

## DIAGNOSIS AND CLINICAL STAGES

Ungley has described four clinical stages of trench foot[8]:

- Prehyperemic: Initial stage of IFS occurs during the period of exposure to cold. This stage is marked by intense vasoconstriction, which causes the affected limb to be blanched, pale, or mottled in appearance. Loss of proprioception occurs, causing gait disturbances. Sluggish capillary refill is noted. Peripheral pulses are generally not palpable, and are often only demonstrable by Doppler.

- Cyanotic phase: Occurs during or immediately following removal from cold environment and onset of rewarming. Peripheral arteries are often not palpable.

- Hyperemic phase: Develops when rewarming of the affected extremities leads to increased blood flow and is marked by erythema and warmth of the skin. The onset is abrupt and this stage may last from days to months. Pulses can be palpated during this phase. Delayed capillary refill continues. Characterized by throbbing pain, hypesthesia, and edema of the extremities. In severe cases, blister formation with serous or bloody fluid is also seen (Figure 88-2). Anhydrosis is often present in addition to a loss of neuromuscular function and generalized muscle weakness.

- Posthyperemic phase: This phase can last from weeks to months and is characterized by hyperhidrosis. The affected limbs demonstrate increased sensitivity to cold stimuli with pain, which can be permanent. There is often a lack of obvious physical signs during this stage. There is increased risk of fungal infections due to increased sweating.

## DIAGNOSIS

- IFS is a clinical syndrome and there are no pathognomonic physical signs or laboratory investigations that can diagnose trench foot.

- Diagnosis should include a careful history about the timing and type of cold exposure and history of rewarming-related signs and symptoms.

- Infrared thermography has been used in experimental studies to confirm the diagnosis of trench foot, assess the severity of damage, and monitor response to treatment.

## DIFFERENTIAL DIAGNOSIS

- Frostbite—Frostbite is a severe, localized cold-induced injury characterized by the following (Figures 88-3A and B):
  - Pain and numbness.
  - Skin appears hard, pale, cold, and waxy.
  - Swelling, burning sensation, and blister formation that may last for weeks.
  - Development of black scabs that develop after several weeks.

- Frostnip—Frostnip refers to cold-induced, localized paresthesias that resolve with rewarming. There is no permanent tissue damage.

- Pernio or chilblain—Localized inflammatory lesions result from acute or repetitive exposure to damp cold above the freezing point.

Lesions are edematous, often reddish or purple, and may be very painful or pruritic (Figures 88-4A and B).

## MANAGEMENT

- Initial supportive care—Once diagnosed, rewarming of trench foot limb must be undertaken gradually as the increases in the metabolic demands of tissues cannot be met by vessels damaged by cold injury. The affected extremities should be kept cool by exposure to steady air from a fan while the core body temperature is slowly raised.
  - IFS can also be seen in association with core body hypothermia, which warrants careful management of both. This is a complex situation where the trench foot requires a very gradual rewarming, while core hypothermia may require rewarming of body as quickly as possible.
  - Individuals suffering from cold injuries will also often be dehydrated as a consequence of cold diuresis. Rehydration with warm liquids should be initiated.[9]
- Pain management: Due to the neuropathic nature of the pain, medications such as amitriptyline, gabapentin, or pregabalin should be considered. Pain specialists should be involved early in the management.
- Pressure offload and physical rehab: Custom shoes and orthotics must be used appropriately, which help improve functional outcome. Physical therapy can be beneficial when initiated early and helps with adequate joint articulation.
- Vasodilation: Alpha-adrenergic blockers provide no benefit to patients suffering from trench foot. Sympathectomy may give short-term improvement with local pain and with increased sensitivity to the cold, but these symptoms eventually return by 6 months with a greater severity.[9]

## PREVENTION AND PATIENT EDUCATION

- High-risk individuals should avoid protracted exposure to cold and wet environments. Sometimes hostile conditions may not be avoidable, such as in battle conditions, in which case soldiers should be instructed to keep the feet dry by periodic changing of wet socks, rotating personnel to prevent prolonged exposures, and limiting sweat accumulation.[9]
- Thermal protective clothing is necessary.
- Air drying of feet for at least 8 hours a day is recommended.[10] Footwear should be appropriately sized so as not to constrict blood flow to the feet.

In summary, IFS is a clinical entity that is best treated by timely diagnosis and supportive care.

### PROVIDER RESOURCE

- http://emedicine.medscape.com/article/1278523-overview#a1

### PATIENT RESOURCES

- www.emedicinehealth.com/cold_hands_and_feet/article_em.htm
- http://www.adventurenetwork.com/2010/first-aid-for-trenchfoot-prevention-and-treatment-tips/

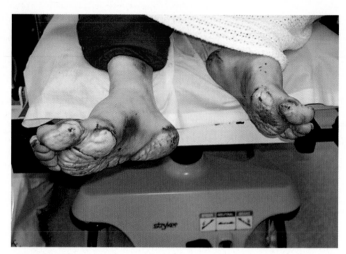

FIGURE 88-2 Severe case of trench foot in hyperemic phase with plantar blisters.

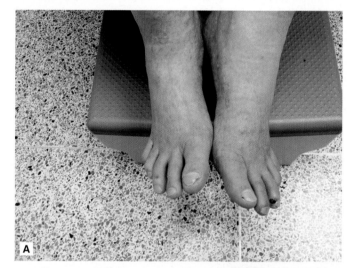

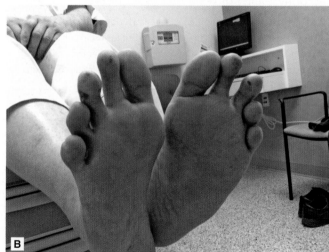

FIGURE 88-3 This is a 38-year-old male electrician who presented with severe painful ulceration and discomfort of the feet after spending 4 hours outdoors in a sleet storm. Note the generalized cyanosis, ulceration on the dorsum (A), and waxy-appearing lesions on the plantar surface characteristic of frostbite (B).

## REFERENCES

1. Francis TJ, Golden FS. Non-freezing cold injury: the pathogenesis. *J R Nav Med Serv*. 1985;71(1):3-8.

2. Francis TJ. Nonfreezing cold injury: a historical review. *J R Nav Med Serv*. 1984;70(3):134-139.

3. Atenstaedt RL. Trench foot: the medical response in the first World War 1914-1918. *Wilderness Environ Med*. 2006;17(4): 282-289.

4. Harirchi I, Arvin A, Vash J, Zafarmand V, Conway G. Frostbite: incidence and predisposing factors in mountaineers. *Br J Sports Med*. 2005;39(12):898-901; discussion 901.

5. Imray CH, Richards P, Greeves J, Castellani JW. Nonfreezing cold-induced injuries. *J R Army Med Corps*. 2011;157(1):79-84.

6. Irwin MS. Nature and mechanism of peripheral nerve damage in an experimental model of non-freezing cold injury. *Ann R Coll Surg Engl*. 1996;78(4):372-379.

7. Mohr WJ, Jenabzadeh K, Ahrenholz DH. Cold injury. *Hand Clin*. 2009;25(4):481-496.

8. Ungley CC, Channell GD, Richards RL. The immersion foot syndrome. 1946. *Wilderness Environ Med*. 2003;14(2):135-141; discussion 134.

9. Hallam MJ, Cubison T, Dheansa B, et al. Managing frostbite. *BMJ*. 2010;341:c5864.

10. Wrenn K. Immersion foot. A problem of the homeless in the 1990s. *Arch Intern Med*. 1991;151(4):785-788.

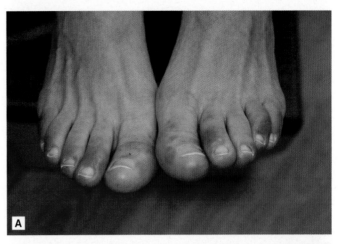

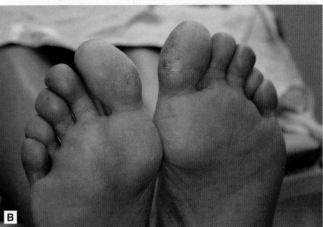

**FIGURE 88-4** A 52-year-old woman presented with edematous, reddish purple, and painful, pruritic lesions that developed in fall and early winter. She had similar lesions in the preceding two winters with resolution of symptoms in summer. This is characteristic of pernio.

# 89 ERYTHROMELALGIA

W. David Arnold, MD
Miriam L. Freimer, MD

A 52-year-old woman with controlled hypothyroidism presented for symptoms of painful burning and discolored feet. She reported 1 to 2 years of progressive disabling lower limb burning pain and numbness associated with fluctuating skin discoloration. Her symptoms were worsened with lower limb dependency, warmth, and exertion. Examination was notable for erythema of the distal legs and feet associated with slightly increased palpable warmth. There was distal pain and temperature sensation loss with relative preservation of vibration and position sense. Distal pulses were normal as were strength and muscle stretch reflexes. Her workup included electromyography and nerve conduction studies that confirmed a length-dependent, predominantly axonal neuropathy. Skin biopsy showed severely diminished intraepidural nerve fiber density consistent with small fiber neuropathy. Laboratory evaluation demonstrated an elevated hemoglobin A1c of 9%, but otherwise no additional contributing factors were identified. She was diagnosed with small fiber predominant neuropathy related to diabetic mellitus and secondary erythromelalgia (EM). Management of her diabetes and symptomatic treatment with gabapentin resulted in partial pain relief.

## INTRODUCTION

EM describes a complex group of distinct disorders associated with overlapping, nonspecific symptoms of distal limb (melos) burning pain (algos) and redness (erythos). This largely unrecognized and infrequently diagnosed syndrome was originally described and named by S. Weir Mitchell in 1878.[1] Later the modified term, erythermalgia, was suggested due to the presence of exacerbation with heat, but this term is infrequently used today.[2]

EM is usually broadly categorized as either primary or secondary. Primary forms are usually idiopathic in nature, but a very small fraction of patients have a hereditary or familial form. Secondary cases occur with other medical conditions or as a side effect related to certain medications.

## EPIDEMIOLOGY

- Rare painful condition with an incidence of 1.3 per 100,000 people per year.[3]

- Primary EM is significantly more common, accounting for approximately 85% of all cases.

- Most cases of primary EM are idiopathic, but exceedingly rare cases have been described in association with a mutation in the voltage-gated sodium channel alpha-subunit gene (SCN9A) on chromosome 2.[4]

- Secondary EM may be seen in association with various myeloproliferative disorders.[5] Over 50% of patients with polycythemia vera may develop EM. The symptoms of EM may precede diagnosis of the underlying myeloproliferative disorder by over 2 years.[5,6]

## ETIOLOGY AND PATHOPHYSIOLOGY

- The etiology of most cases of EM remains obscure.

- Retrospective studies have demonstrated high prevalence of small fiber predominant neuropathy suggesting the possibility of neurogenic disruption of vascular tone.[7,8]

- The discovery of a gain-of-function mutation in the voltage-gated SCN9A gene on chromosome 2 in patients with familial EM prompted significant progress in the understanding of idiopathic EM.[4,9] The mutation in the SCN9A gene results in a lower threshold for action potential generation in the dorsal root ganglia and sympathetic ganglia causing vascular changes and severe pain that is poorly responsive to treatment. The pattern of inheritance is usually autosomal dominant, but sporadic cases have been described.[10]

- Processes of abnormal platelet activation have been attributed to secondary EM associated with thrombocythemia.[11,12]

- Other conditions or exposures reported in association with EM include but are not limited to toxins associated with certain species of mushrooms, diabetes mellitus, lupus, rheumatoid arthritis, lichen sclerosis, gout, spinal cord disorders, multiple sclerosis, and some drugs (pergolide, nifedipine, verapamil, diltiazem, bromocriptine).[6,13-15]

## DIAGNOSIS

### Clinical Features

In isolation, each of the cardinal features of EM is nonspecific. However, when clustered in a single patient the symptoms are quite characteristic. Thompson reported criteria that are helpful in excluding other disorders with overlapping symptoms.[16] Typically patients present with erythema and burning of the distal limbs, especially the hands and feet (Figures 89-1 and 89-2). Usually the lower limbs are more severely affected. Asymmetric symptoms are unusual in primary EM but common in secondary forms.

Thompson EM Criteria[16]:

1. Burning extremity pain
2. Pain aggravated by warming
3. Pain relieved by cooling
4. Erythema of affected skin
5. Increased temperature of affected skin

### Laboratory Features

- There are no specific diagnostic laboratory findings for most forms of EM. The diagnosis is established on a clinical basis.

- The evaluation may include electromyography and nerve conduction studies, autonomic and small fiber nerve testing, vascular studies, and laboratory testing to exclude mimicking or coexistent conditions.

- The quantitative sudomotor axon reflex test (QSART) is the most sensitive diagnostic assessment for small fiber neuropathy. During a QSART acetylcholine is applied to the skin using iontophoresis in order to activate sympathetic C-fibers of the sweat glands (Figure 89-3). The evoked sweat response is quantified. A normal response suggests intact small fiber function, and absent or reduced response is indicative of small fiber nerve dysfunction (Figure 89-4).

- Skin biopsy is another tool frequently used to assess for underlying small fiber neuropathy. Reduced intraepidermal nerve fiber density is indicative of small fiber neuropathy (Figure 89-5).

- Patients should have a complete blood count to investigate for thrombocythemia or other features of an underlying myeloproliferative disorder.

- Genetic testing is available to identify exceedingly rare patients with SCN9A-related familial EM. (See http://www.ncbi.nlm.nih.gov/sites/GeneTests/.)

## DIFFERENTIAL DIAGNOSIS

- The differential includes other disorders that may lead to similar signs and symptoms overlapping with that of EM. Most, if not all, mimicking conditions may be eliminated clinically due to the distinct nature of EM.

- The most common mimicking conditions include those associated with distal limb burning pain and skin temperature or color changes.

- Raynaud phenomenon is easily distinguished on the basis of worsening symptoms with cold exposure rather than worsening with warmth. Interestingly, patients with EM and coexistent Raynaud phenomenon have been rarely reported.[17]

- Peripheral artery disease may present with distal burning pain and skin changes, but examination features of diminished pulses and distal limb coolness help eliminate this disorder.

- Complex regional pain syndrome may most closely mimic the features of EM, but the lack of bilateral involvement helps to exclude these cases.

## MANAGEMENT

- Treatment strategies depend on the underlying pathophysiology and whether the process is primary or secondary. Symptomatic management is often less than satisfactory.

- Management may include antiepileptic medications such as gabapentin or pregabalin or antidepressants including the tricyclic antidepressants and serotonin-norepinephrine reuptake inhibitors.

- In many cases patients resort to cooling the affected limbs and lifestyle modifications to avoid overheating. These strategies may be effective, but chronic immersion into cold water frequently leads to skin maceration and even immersion foot syndrome.

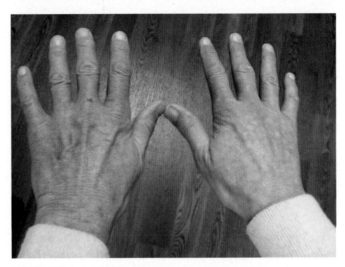

FIGURE 89-1 Subtle hand erythema in a 64-year-old man with erythromelalgia (EM) and associated distal limb numbness and burning pain.

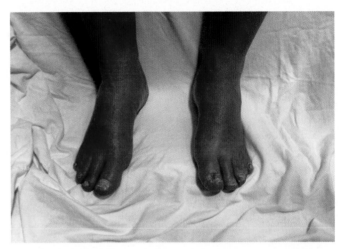

FIGURE 89-2 Prominent erythema and warmth associated with severe burning pain in a 57-year-old man with erythromelalgia (EM) in the setting of nifedipine treatment.

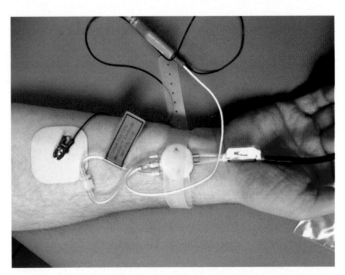

FIGURE 89-3 Apparatus used during the quantitative sudomotor axon reflex test (QSART) for acetylcholine iontophoresis and sweat output measurement.

- A proportion of patients, usually with thrombocythemia-associated EM, will respond dramatically to low-dose aspirin therapy.

## PATIENT EDUCATION

The Erythromelalgia Association is an international patient organization founded in 1999 communicating with physicians and EM sufferers. (The Erythromelalgia Association; 200 Old Castle Lane; Wallingford, PA 19086 USA; telephone: 610-566-0797; e-mail: memberservices@burningfeet.org; website: http://www.erythromelalgia.org/)

## FOLLOW-UP

- Follow-up for ongoing symptomatic management is appropriate.
- For patients with secondary EM, treatment and follow-up for underlying primary process should occur as needed.

### PROVIDER RESOURCE

- http://emedicine.medscape.com/article/200071-overview

## REFERENCES

1. Mitchell SW. On a rare vaso-motor neurosis of the extremities, and on the maladies with which it may be confounded. *Am J Med Sci*. 1878;76:2-36.

2. Smith LA, Allen EV. Erythermalgia (erythromelalgia) of the extremities: a syndrome characterized by redness, heat, and pain. *Am Heart J*. 1938;16:175-188.

3. Reed KB, Davis MD. Incidence of erythromelalgia: a population-based study in Olmsted County, Minnesota. *J Eur Acad Dermatol Venereol*. 2009;23(1):13-15.

4. Waxman SG, Dib-Hajj SD. Erythromelalgia: a hereditary pain syndrome enters the molecular era. *Ann Neurol*. 2005;57(6):785-788.

5. Drenth JP, Michiels JJ. Three types of erythromelalgia. *BMJ*. 1990;301(6750):454-455.

6. Kurzrock R, Cohen PR. Erythromelalgia and myeloproliferative disorders. *Arch Intern Med*. 1989;149(1):105-109.

7. Davis MD, Sandroni P, Rooke TW, Low PA. Erythromelalgia: vasculopathy, neuropathy, or both? A prospective study of vascular and neurophysiologic studies in erythromelalgia. *Arch Dermatol*. 1337;139(10):1337-1343.

8. Davis MD, Genebriera J, Sandroni P, Fealey RD. Thermoregulatory sweat testing in patients with erythromelalgia. *Arch Dermatol*. 1583;142(12):1583-1588.

9. Han C, Dib-Hajj SD, Lin Z, et al. Early- and late-onset inherited erythromelalgia: genotype-phenotype correlation. *Brain*. 1711;132(pt 7):1711-1722.

10. Han C, Rush AM, Dib-Hajj SD, et al. Sporadic onset of erythermalgia: a gain-of-function mutation in Nav1.7. *Ann Neurol*. 2006;59(3):553-558.

11. Michiels JJ, Abels J, Steketee J, van Vliet HH, Vuzevski VD. Erythromelalgia caused by platelet-mediated arteriolar

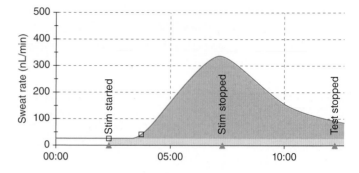

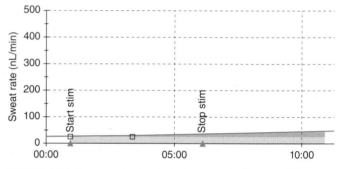

**FIGURE 89-4** Two quantitative sudomotor axon reflex test (QSART) tracings: a normal QSART response in an individual without neuropathy (upper tracing) and an abnormal QSART response consistent with small fiber neuropathy (lower tracing).

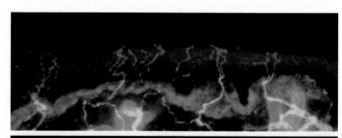

**FIGURE 89-5** An abnormal skin biopsy demonstrating reduced intraepidermal nerve fiber density consistent with small fiber neuropathy (lower image) and a normal skin biopsy (upper image).

inflammation and thrombosis in thrombocythemia. *Ann Intern Med*. 1985;102(4):466-471.

12. van Genderen PJ, Lucas IS, van Strik R, et al. Erythromelalgia in essential thrombocythemia is characterized by platelet activation and endothelial cell damage but not by thrombin generation. *Thromb Haemost*. 1996;76(3):333-338.

13. Saviuc PF, Danel VC, Moreau PA, et al. Erythromelalgia and mushroom poisoning. *J Toxicol Clin Toxicol*. 2001;39(4):403-407.

14. Babb RR, Alarcon-Segovia D, Fairbairn JF 2nd. Erythermalgia. Review of 51 cases. *Circulation*. 1964;29:136-141.

15. Ioulios P, Charalampos M, Efrossini T. The spectrum of cutaneous reactions associated with calcium antagonists: a review of the literature and the possible etiopathogenic mechanisms. *Dermatol Online J*. 2003;9(5):6.

16. Thompson GH, Hahn G, Rang M. Erythromelalgia. *Clin Orthop Relat Res*. 1979;144:249-254.

17. Berlin AL, Pehr K. Coexistence of erythromelalgia and Raynaud's phenomenon. *J Am Acad Dermatol*. 2004;50(3):456-460.

# 90 ERYTHEMA AB IGNE

Steven M. Dean, DO, FACP, RPVI

## PATIENT STORY

A 47-year-old woman with chronic low back pain presents with a chief complaint of a persistent rash along her posterior trunk. The discoloration has slowly progressed over the last year and does not fluctuate in response to hot or cold temperatures. She has no history of vasospastic disease. On examination an irregular reticular fixed brownish discoloration overlies her entire back. She admits to sleeping on a heating pad for the last 3 years due to her unremitting back pain. A diagnosis of erythema ab igne (EAI) or "toasted skin syndrome" is rendered (Figure 90-1).

## EPIDEMIOLOGY

- Due to infrequency of EAI, limited epidemiologic data exists.

- Although previously a disorder associated with protracted exposure to stoves and open fires, the majority of cases are now linked to laptops and heating pads or blankets.

- Slight female predominance but no overt racial predilection.

- While EIA was formerly primarily identified in middle-aged subjects, in a recent review, affected women averaged 25 years and men averaged 20 years of age.[1]

## ETIOLOGY AND PATHOPHYSIOLOGY

- Table 90-1 lists various causes of EAI.

- Occupations at risk include cooks, bakers, foundry workers, silversmiths, and glass blowers.

- Patients with chronic pain are at risk due to heating pad or hot water bottle application to various body sites.

- Modern day cases are increasingly linked to laptop use on the thighs.

- EIA results from prolonged and repeated exposure to thermal radiation. The heat exposure is not intense enough to burn the skin, yet it is severe enough to evoke injury and subsequent discoloration.

- Causative temperatures typically range from 43 to 47°C (109-117°F)

- The definitive pathomechanism that leads to EIA is unclear, yet appears to involve heat injury to the epidermis and superficial vascular plexus that ultimately leads to dilation and hemosiderin deposition in a reticulate pattern.[2]

- The length of recurrent thermal exposure required to elicit EIA typically ranges from months to several years. Rarely, the discoloration has been reported as early as 1 to 2 weeks after contact with a heat source. The exposure risk is cumulative.

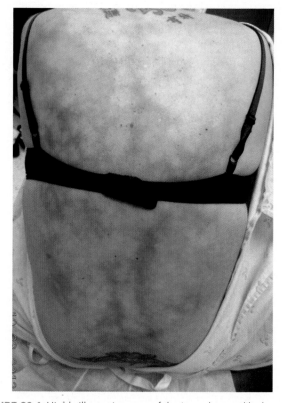

**FIGURE 90-1** Highly illustrative case of the irregular, net-like hyper-pigmentation of erythema ab igne (EIA) along the entire back of a patient with chronic back pain. She admitted to sleeping on a heating pad for the last 3 years.

**TABLE 90-1.** Causes of Erythema Ab Igne

Laptop computers

Heating pads

Hot water bottles

Open fires

Stoves

Electric space heaters

Electric blankets

Car heaters

Infrared lamps

Heated car seats

## DIAGNOSIS

### Clinical Features

- EAI is a clinical diagnosis.

- Initial or early heat exposure provokes a mild reversible net-like blanching erythema (Figures 90-2 and 90-3). When thermal contact persists, the reticular hyperpigmentation becomes fixed or nonblanching and darker (Figure 90-4). Chronic cases can manifest associated hyperkeratosis, telangiectasias, bullae, scaling, and ulcerations. In severely affected patients, a large area of nonreticulate atrophic and pigmented skin evolves surrounded by a peripheral stereotypical reticular pattern.[3]

- Commonly affected areas include the anterior calves (fires), anterior thighs (laptops), and back or peripheral joints (heating pads or bottles). Less frequent sites include the face and arms or palms of cooks. Abdominopelvic involvement in patients with visceral malignancies, peptic ulcer disease, and chronic pancreatitis has been reported (Figure 90-5).

- Usually asymptomatic, yet pruritus and a burning sensation can occur.

- If long-standing EAI becomes complicated by nodules, chronic ulcerations, and/or unusual pain, degeneration into a squamous cell or Merkel cell carcinoma should be suspected. Squamous cell transformation is the most common heat-associated cancer. Although most cases of squamous cell carcinoma are low to intermediate grade, around 30% are aggressive and metastatic.[4] Merkel cell carcinoma is virulent with up to 30% mortality.[5]

### Laboratory Studies and Imaging

- There is no laboratory or imaging study that confirms or refutes the diagnosis of EAI.

### Histology

- Although a biopsy is typically not required, it should be completed if signs of malignant transformation exist (eg, nodules or ulceration).

- Histology of EAI resembles actinic keratosis with squamous cell atypia within the epidermis. Abnormal dermal elastic tissue, epidermal and dermal atrophy, hyperkeratosis or dyskeratosis as well as melanin and hemosiderin deposition are present.[6]

- Histology of carcinomatous evolution is consistent with either squamous cell or neuroendocrine carcinoma (Merkel cell carcinoma).

## DIFFERENTIAL DIAGNOSIS

- Livedo reticularis—more diffuse reticular discoloration that is aggravated by cold, usually reversible with warming, and most often found in otherwise healthy females.

- Livedo racemosa—more closely resembles EIA than livedo reticularis as the irregular net-like discoloration is fixed. However, in contrast to EIA the discoloration is much more diffuse and an associated systemic disease exists.

- Poikiloderma atrophicans vasculare—rare variant of early mycosis fungoides with generalized hyperkeratotic scaly macules

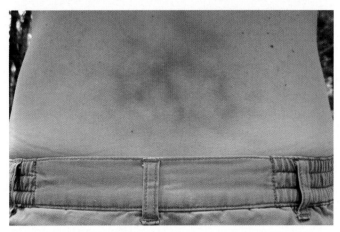

FIGURE 90-2 Mild focal case of erythema ab igne (EIA) in a patient with lumbar pain. The discoloration completely resolved with heating pad discontinuance. (*Photograph courtesy of Dr. Michael Jaff.*)

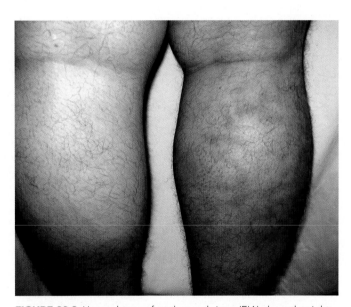

FIGURE 90-3 Unusual case of erythema ab igne (EIA) along the right posterior calf in a patient with superficial venous thrombosis of the small saphenous vein. A heating pad had been applied for the preceding 3 months. The discoloration fully resolved, although 7 months were required.

and papules in a retiform or reticular distribution. Typically found on the trunk and flexural regions.

## MANAGEMENT

- Mainstay of therapy is immediate removal of the infrared radiation source. When the heat exposure has been of short duration, EAI is typically reversible. Resolution usually occurs within several months.

- In more protracted and severe cases associated with marked hyperpigmentation, topical tretinoin or hydroquinone can be prescribed. Laser therapy (Nd:YAG, alexandrite, ruby) may reduce the discoloration as well.

- Epithelial atypia can be treated with 5-fluorouracil.[7]

## PATIENT EDUCATION

Patients must be fully cognizant of the relationship between excessive thermal radiation and EAI. Further exposure to heat must cease. The potential for carcinomatous evolution should be explained and documented.

## FOLLOW-UP

Periodic follow-up examinations are recommended to assess for malignant conversion.

### PROVIDER RESOURCES

- http://dermnetnz.org/vascular/erythema-ab-igne.html
- http://emedicine.medscape.com/article/1087535-overview

### PATIENT RESOURCES

- http://en.wikipedia.org/wiki/Erythema_ab_igne
- http://www.dermapics.com/erythema%20ab%20igne.html

## REFERENCES

1. Riahi RR, Cohen PR. Laptop-induced erythema ab igne: report and review of literature. *Dermatol Online J.* 2012;18(6):5.

2. Botten D, Langley RG, Webb A. Academic branding: erythema ab igne and use of laptop computers. *CMAJ.* 2010;182(18):E857.

3. Kennedy CTC. Reactions to mechanical and thermal injury. In: Champion RH, Burton JL, Ebling FJG, eds. *Textbook of Dermatology.* 5th ed. Oxford: Blackwell Scientific Publications; 1992:777-832.

4. Page EH, Shear NH. Temperature-dependent skin disorders. *J Am Acad Dermatol.* 1988;18:1003-1009.

5. Sahl WJ, Taira JW. Erythema ab igne: treatment with 5-fluorouracil cream. *J Am Acad Dermatol.* 1992;27:109-110.

6. Kaplan RP. Cancer complicating chronic ulcerative and scarifying mucocutaneous disorders. *Adv Dermatol.* 1987;2:19-46.

7. Sibley RK, Dehmer LP, Rosai J. Primary neuroendocrine (Merkel cell?) carcinoma of the skin. A clinicopathologic and ultrastructural study of 43 cases. *Am J Surg Pathol.* 1985;9:95-108.

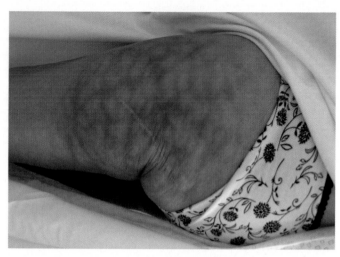

**FIGURE 90-4** Deeply pigmented discoloration along the left lateral thigh of a patient with chronic hip pain and 2-year history of frequent heating pad application. Despite discontinuance of heat for 9 months, the discoloration has only lightened and not resolved.

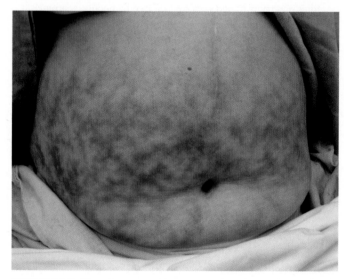

**FIGURE 90-5** Chronic pancreatitis-associated erythema ab igne (EIA) of the abdomen.

## PART 11

# LIMB ULCERATIONS

# 91 VENOUS STASIS ULCERATION

Kevin P. Cohoon, DO, MSc
Thom W. Rooke, MD, FSVM
David H. Pfizenmaier II, MD, DPM

## PATIENT STORY

A 60-year-old woman presents with a 3-month history of painful ulceration of her lower left leg. She has a history of congestive heart failure, diabetes, and has varicosities on the lower limbs.

Her physical examination is unremarkable except for the presence of a 6-cm$^2$ ulcer over her left medial malleolus. The ulcer is shallow, with a yellowish base and scattered islands of granulation tissue. There is a scaly brown-reddish hyperpigmentation surrounding the ulcer's borders without signs of infection. The patient's extremities are cool, with the presence of varicosities and edema of the left extremity making palpation of the dorsalis pedis pulses difficult. Figures 91-1 and 91-2 demonstrate a typical case of venous ulceration that may be misdiagnosed as cellulitis in its earliest stage prior to ulceration. Figures 91-3 and 91-4 illustrate an atypical location of a stasis ulceration that can be located on the lateral or posterior calf.

### EPIDEMIOLOGY

- Venous ulcers affect 500,000 to 600,000 people in the United States every year and account for 80% to 90% of all leg ulcers.[1]

- Venous stasis ulcers are common in patients who have a history of leg swelling, varicose veins, or a history of blood clots in either the superficial or the deep veins of the legs.

- Peak incidence occurs in women aged 40 to 49 years and in men aged 70 to 79 years.

### ETIOLOGY AND PATHOPHYSIOLOGY

- Venous ulcers are chronic nonhealing ulcers that occur in the lower extremities of patients with venous obstruction or valvular incompetence (often caused by a previous venous thrombosis).

- Venous ulcers classically develop in regions of dependent swelling and edema.

- Comorbidities that aggravate edema (such as heart failure, renal failure, hepatic failure, the use of medications such as calcium channel blockers, nonsteroidal anti-inflammatory drugs, and cyclo-oxygenase 2 inhibitors, and many others) may contribute to the formation of ulcers.

- Patients with venous incompetency typically present with unilateral edema or bilateral edema that is worse in one leg.

- Dilatation of the capillaries and leakage of plasma proteins and red blood cells are a direct result of venous hypertension and may lead to fibrin deposition and impaired oxygen transport, producing ischemia and hypoxia that results in cell death and ulcerations.[2]

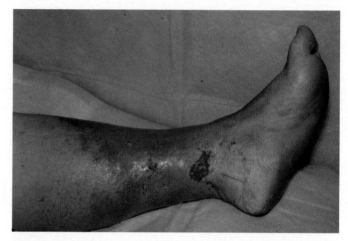

FIGURE 91-1 Classic venous ulceration near the medial malleolus of a 60-year-old woman. Other characteristic features include an irregular margin, moist red base, and surrounding stasis hyperpigmentation. (*Photograph courtesy of Thom Rooke, MD.*)

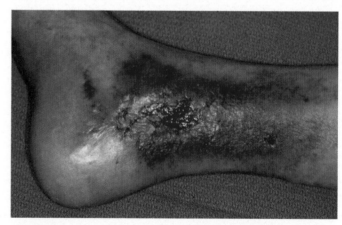

FIGURE 91-2 Another stereotypical venous stasis ulceration and surrounding hyperpigmentation within the distal medial gaiter distribution. (*Photograph courtesy of Thom Rooke, MD.*)

## DIAGNOSIS

Patients with severe venous stasis typically have edema of the legs, hyperpigmentation, and red and scaly areas (stasis dermatitis). The initial assessment of clinical severity is made by simple observation and specialized testing is not required. Venous disease can be characterized using the CEAP classification system.

**CEAP classification:**

**C**linical severity

**E**tiology or cause

**A**natomy

**P**athophysiology

Grade description (based on clinical severity):

C0—No evidence of venous disease

C1—Superficial spider veins (reticular veins) only

C2—Simple varicose veins only

C3—Ankle edema of venous origin (not foot edema)

C4—Skin pigmentation in the gaiter area (lipodermatosclerosis)

C5—A healed venous ulcer

C6—An open venous ulcer

## CLINICAL FEATURES

Venous ulcers develop in regions of dependent swelling and edema. They often appear as an irregularly shaped moist wound along the medial aspect of the lower leg or ankle. Dermatologic signs of venous stasis include pigmentation changes in the legs. The surrounding skin is often discolored and swollen. The skin may appear shiny and tight, depending on the amount of edema. The ulcers can be painful; however, they usually are not as painful as ischemic ulcers. Maceration and excess exudate generally occur.

## TYPICAL DISTRIBUTION

Although most commonly found along the medial aspect of the leg, the ulcer may occur around the medial or lateral malleolus. Ulcers may affect one or both legs.

## LABORATORY STUDIES

Duplex ultrasonography is helpful to evaluate for venous obstruction or venous incompetence. The superficial veins evaluated for venous incompetence should include the great saphenous vein (GSV) and small saphenous vein (SSV). Special attention should be given to the great saphenous vein near its confluence with the common femoral vein, mid saphenous vein, and distally on the leg as well as the small saphenous vein near its confluence with the popliteal vein. Incompetence of the superficial and/or perforating veins is determined by spectral Doppler waveform and/or color Doppler imaging. Incompetence documented with color Doppler is considered to be present when the appearance of retrograde color flow on release of compression is observed. Absence of retrograde color on release of the compression indicates competent valves. Spectral Doppler waveform analysis can confirm the presence of venous incompetence and is considered to be present if the duration of the reverse flow is greater than 0.5 seconds.

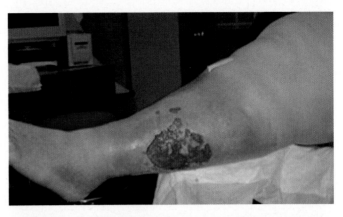

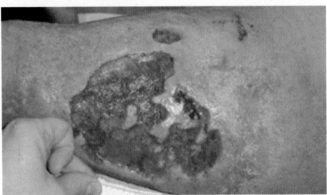

**FIGURES 91-3 AND 91-4** Less often, stasis ulcerations may affect the lateral portion of the calf. This distribution suggests incompetence within the small saphenous vein with associated tributaries and lateral based perforating veins. (*Photograph courtesy of Thom Rooke, MD.*)

## DIFFERENTIAL DIAGNOSIS

- Arterial insufficiency (arterial ulcer)
- Bacterial pyoderma (eg, infected wound or bite)
- Trauma
- Diabetic ulcer
- Pressure ulcer
- Vasculitis
- Pyoderma gangrenosum
- Skin cancer
- Infection (eg, mycobacterial, fungal, tertiary syphilis, leishmaniasis, amebiasis)
- Sickle cell anemia
- Embolic disease (including cholesterol emboli)
- Cryoglobulinemia
- Calciphylaxis

## MANAGEMENT

- The primary objective of treatment is to reduce or eliminate venous (blood) pooling and edema. This initially involves treatment of any causative chronic medical problem, including cardiac disease and liver or renal failure.
- Reducing or eliminating lower extremity edema can be accomplished with compression treatment and elevation of the legs. Patients should elevate their legs to reduce gravity-induced edema.
- Compression treatments (including compression stockings, multilayer compression wraps, or wrapping an ACE bandage or dressing from the toes or foot to the area below the knee) are essential for effective healing of venous ulcers. Patients who receive adequate compression heal faster than those who do not receive compression.
- There are two primary methods of wrap compression: (1) a single-layer compression method with stretch or nonstretch wraps and (2) a multilayer method, with one layer placed on a second layer. Multilayer methods are better than single-layer methods; however, the single-layer method is superior to no compression.
- Compression wraps should be applied several times a day to continue reduction of swelling. Often a "figure 8" pattern is used.
- Application of a foam pad around the medial or lateral malleolus can provide local compression to reduce edema.
- Dressings may be required to maintain a healthy wound environment with proper moisture and debridement.
- Types of dressings include
  - Moist dressings
  - Hydrogels or hydrocolloids
  - Alginate dressings
  - Collagen wound dressings
  - Debriding agents
  - Antimicrobial dressings
  - Composite dressings
  - Synthetic skin substitutes
- Treatment of underlying cellulitis and infection is important for chronic venous ulcers.

- Preventing recurrent stasis ulcerations involves aggressive treatment to control edema (typically using compression hosiery if the chronic ulcer has healed).
- 20 to 30 mm Hg compression hosiery up to the knee can reduce and improve peripheral edema in the lower legs. Stronger or weaker compression can be used, depending on the need for compression and the comfort level of the patient.
- Healing times for venous stasis ulcer is unpredictable (delayed healing may occur because delivery of oxygen and other nutrients are impaired by edema and fibrin deposition).[3]
- Endovenous thermal ablation is the recommended treatment of an incompetent GSV and has replaced the classic high ligation and inversion stripping of the saphenous vein to the level of the knee.[4]
- The Effect of Surgery and Compression on Healing and Recurrence (ESCHAR) study of 500 randomized patients illustrated that compression therapy alone was as effective as compression and surgery (saphenous vein ablation with high ligation and stripping) in healing venous ulcerations; however, 12-month ulcer recurrence rates were significantly decreased in the surgery with compression cohort when compared to isolated compression.[4]
- Pentoxifylline should be considered to accelerate healing of stasis ulcerations. If available, other pharmacologic considerations to expedite tissue healing include micronized purified flavonoid fraction, diosmin, hesperidin, horse chestnut seed extract, rutosides, and sulodexide.[4]

## PATIENT EDUCATION

Proper education and educational reinforcement are crucial for the successful treatment and prevention of venous ulcers.

## FOLLOW-UP

Prevention of recurrent venous ulcers is often more important than treatment and involves continued aggressive control of edema.

### PATIENT AND PROVIDER RESOURCES

- http://www.woundsource.com/blog/causes-and-treatment-venous-stasis-ulcers
- http://my.clevelandclinic.org/heart/disorders/vascular/leg-footulcer.aspx
- http://www.patient.co.uk/doctor/Venous-Leg-Ulcer.htm
- http://www.uptodate.com/contents/chronic-venous-disease-beyond-the-basics

## REFERENCES

1. Phillips TJ, Dover JS. Continuing medical education: leg ulcers. *J Am Acad Dermatol*. 1991;25:965-987.

2. Browse NL, Buenard KG. The cause of venous ulceration. *Lancet*. 1982;ii:243-245.

3. Falanga V. Venous ulceration. *Chronic Would Care Previews*. 1996;8:101-108.

4. Gloviczki P, Comerota AJ, Dalsing MC, et al. The care of patient with varicose veins and associated chronic venous diseases: clinical practice guidelines of the Society for Vascular Surgery and the American Venous Forum. *J Vasc Surg*. 2011;53:S2-S48.

# 92 ARTERIAL ULCERATIONS

John H. Fish III, MD, FSVM, RPVI

## PATIENT STORY

An 82-year-old man with peripheral artery disease (PAD) was evaluated for a painful right foot. Over the past 3 weeks the patient began to have constant dull aching in his foot that improved when standing or walking. His pain was particularly intense at night, and he found that sleeping in a chair helped the disomfort. Three weeks prior to this presentation, small sores on the dorsal surface of the foot evolved and subsequently coalesced with dry gangrene in the small toe (Figure 92-1). The right foot was found to be tender, pulseless, cool, and ruborous with mild edema and elevation pallor.

Debridement of the wounds was subsequently performed (Figure 92-2) and aspirin and cilostazol were started. The ankle pressure on the right was 48 mm Hg with an ankle-brachial index (ABI) of 0.29. Infrainguinal arterial duplex ultrasound revealed diffusely monophasic waveforms with an occlusion of the distal superficial femoral artery. An angiogram further delineated an occlusion of the right external iliac artery that was treated with percutaneous atherectomy, angioplasty, and stent placement. The patient required a small-digit amputation that healed within 6 weeks after revascularization (Figure 92-3).

## EPIDEMIOLOGY

- Lower extremity ulcers caused by ischemia from arterial disease are becoming more frequent in aging populations in Western countries.

- In addition to age, risk factors include smoking, diabetes, hypertension, and dyslipidemia.

- Chronic critical limb ischemia (CLI) is defined as ulcers and tissue loss or rest pain for more than 2 weeks without open lesions due to a lack of nutritive blood flow.

- The 2007 TransAtlantic Inter-Society Consensus (TASC II) further defined CLI as an absolute ankle pressure of less than 50 mm Hg or a toe pressure of less than 30 mm Hg.

- The incidence and prevalence of CLI has been difficult to calculate, but based on the assumption that 25% of patients with CLI will require amputation and that roughly 5% of claudicants will progress to CLI, one can estimate anywhere from 300 to 1000 affected patients per million per year.[1]

- Arteriosclerosis occurs at a much younger age in diabetics with its hallmark involvement of the tibioperoneal arteries and relative sparing of the pedal vessels. Amputation is 10 times more frequent in diabetics with PAD and 45% of major amputees are diabetic.[1]

- Purely ischemic ulcers without a neuropathic component only account for around 15% of ulcers in diabetics.[2]

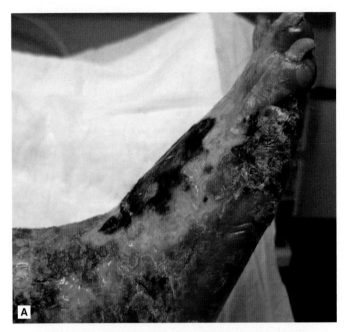

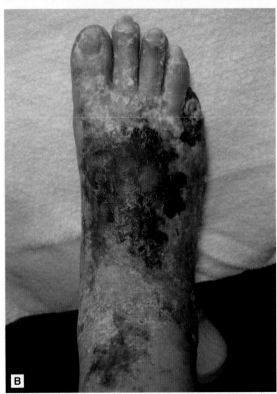

**FIGURE 92-1** An 82-year-old man with ischemic rest pain, extensive necrosis and dry gangrene of the 5th toe. Additionally, photograph A displays a bullous lesion along the lateral portion of the 3rd toe. Photograph B illustrates dependent rubor within the distal forefoot and distal cyanosis involving the 3rd toe.

## PATHOPHYSIOLOGY AND DIAGNOSIS

### Etiology

- A lack of nutritive perfusion to the periphery leads to decreased tissue resilience and tissue death.
- At ankle pressures less than 50 mm Hg and digital perfusion of less than 30 mm Hg, dermal ischemia impairs normal repair mechanisms of cell regeneration, especially over areas of mechanical pressure that lack sufficient cushioning.
- The amount of oxygen-rich blood supply needed for healing of damaged and ulcerated dermis and subdermal tissue is much higher than that to maintain tissue integrity.
- Chronic ischemic wounds are not able to adequately enter the initial inflammatory phase of healing where vasodilation and increased vascular permeability occur along with platelet and neutrophil infiltration, fibrin deposition, and mucopolysaccharide production to produce a natural protective barrier.

## CLINICAL FEATURES

- A chronically ischemic leg will usually exhibit thin, dry, shiny skin that is hairless and hypohidrotic.
- Ischemic ulcers are extremely painful and typically involve the dorsum of the foot, the toes, or the lateral aspects of the foot (first and first metatarsal heads) and ankle where friction and pressure will lead to devitalization of skin.
- Purely ischemic ulcers are rarely on the plantar surface of the foot, although areas of the heel may become involved with prolonged bed rest (Table 92-1). Other examples of ischemic ulcerations are shown in Figures 92-4 and 92-5.

## VASCULAR EXAMINATION AND LABORATORY STUDIES

- The patient should be examined supine with a thorough pulse examination beginning in the groin.
- The leg should be elevated to evaluate for color change and the time to pallor onset (<15 seconds in severe disease). With dependency of the affected leg, the amount of time it takes to return to its usual color is also a useful marker of severity (normally <20 seconds).
- With prolonged dependency, there is often rubor, and the foot will remain cold to the touch and often edema will manifest.
- The ulcer may be quite tender but should be gently probed for sinus tracts or exposed bone.
- Bedside handheld Doppler for ABI determination has been shown to be predictive for tissue loss when the index is below 0.5 and ankle pressure is less than 50 mm Hg.
- Studies utilizing transcutaneous oxygen tension measurement suggest that values of less than 20 mm Hg predict poor healing, while a tension of greater than 40 mm Hg measured on the skin surrounding an ulcer will be predictive for healing.[3]
- The use of laser Doppler to determine skin perfusion pressures can also provide information about capillary and arteriolar flow and has been employed to predict the healing potential of chronic ischemic lesions.

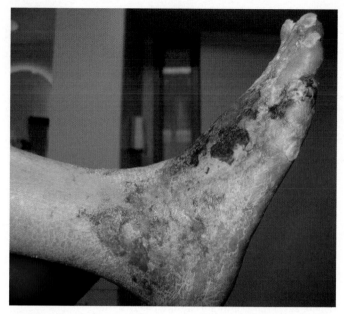

**FIGURE 92-2** Patient from Figure 92-1 following debridement.

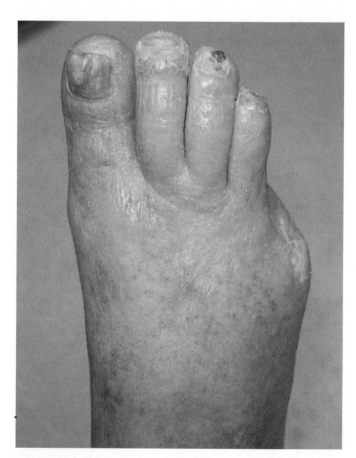

**FIGURE 92-3** The patient from Figure 92-1 following revascularization and fifth digit amputation.

**TABLE 92-1.** Summary of Classic Characteristics of Vascular Ulcers

| | Arterial | Venous | Mixed (Arterial/Venous) | Neurotrophic (Diabetic) |
|---|---|---|---|---|
| Localization | Toes, dorsal foot, pressure points, and bony prominences | Medial lower leg and ankle | Medial and lateral lower leg and ankle | Medial and lateral forefoot, plantar foot, and metatarsal heads |
| Ulcer base | Variable color or necrotic, usually dry and bloodless | Weeping with fibrinous discharge and red granulation | Variable, fibrotic with smooth base | Pink to red granulation, often deep and tracking |
| Ulcer border | Punched-out, sharp, smooth, round | Irregular shape, surrounding skin discoloration | Variable | Punched-out, surrounding callous, undermined |
| Skin color | Dependent rubor, elevation pallor | Hyperpigmented | Hyperpigmented | Normal or pale |
| Skin temperature | ↓↓ | ↑ | ↓ | Normal |
| Sensory | Normal to ↓, sensitive, very painful ulcer | Normal | ↓ | ↓↓ |
| Reflexes | Normal to ↓ | Normal | Normal to ↓ | ↓↓ |

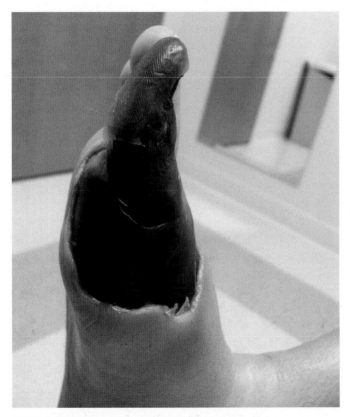

**FIGURE 92-4** Dry gangrene of the forefoot. Notice the dry mummified appearance with a discreet, punched-out demarcation border. (*Photograph courtesy of Steven Dean, DO.*)

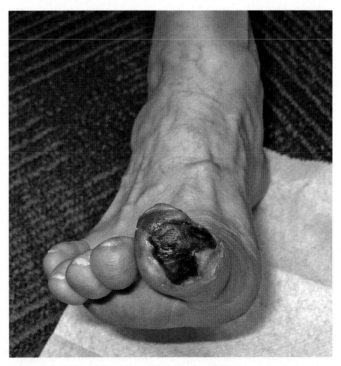

**FIGURE 92-5** Ischemic ulceration of the distal hallux. This example displays the typical punched-out or "cookie cutter" appearance along with surrounding dependent rubor. (*Photograph courtesy of Steven Dean, DO.*)

- Noninvasive imaging techniques utilizing ultrasound, magnetic resonance angiography (MRA), and/or computed tomographic angiography (CTA) should be considered to evaluate the macrovasculature, while digital subtraction angiography still remains the gold standard for complete imaging of the macro- and microvasculature of the extremities.

## DIFFERENTIAL DIAGNOSIS

- Lower extremity ulcerations may be due to a long list of potential causative factors. Various etiologies are listed in Table 92-2.

- Classic characteristics of the four most common varieties of vascular lesions in the lower extremities (arterial, venous, mixed, and neurotrophic) are outlined in Table 92-1.

- An example of a chronic venous stasis ulceration is displayed in Figure 92-6, and a diabetic neurotrophic ulceration is illustrated in Figure 92-7.

## MANAGEMENT

- First and foremost, re-establishment of adequate perfusion to the ulcer bed must be the initial goal of therapy.

- Wounds need to be off-loaded, and elastic or inelastic compressive bandages may need to be avoided.

- Wounds with a mixed mild arterial and venous etiology may benefit from inelastic compression; an increase in periwound laser Doppler flow was recently shown in patients with an ankle pressure greater than 60 mm Hg when up to 40 mm Hg of pressure was applied.[4]

- Edema control is important in cases of chronic ulcerations of any type, although the avoidance of chronic dependency in CLI may be difficult to achieve due to pain. Specialized sequential compression pumps have been designed to augment venular emptying and, subsequently, downstream arteriolar filling via the Venturi effect.

- Mechanical debridement and careful removal of devitalized tissue is the next integral step.

- Infection and contamination should be avoided and aggressively treated if suspected.

- Local wound therapies and specialized dressings should be used judiciously; randomized studies have not shown any product to be superior to standard saline wet to damp or dry sterile gauze dressings in ischemic wounds.[2]

- Medical treatment of ischemic ulcers can be considered with antiplatelet agents (aspirin, ticlopidine, and clopidogrel), xanthine derivatives (pentoxifylline), phosphodiesterase inhibitors (cilostazol), or even potent vasodilators such as prostaglandin infusions (indication in Europe).

- Newer modalities such as human growth factors and bioengineered skin substitutes hold promise in treating ischemic wounds.

- Hyperbaric oxygen therapy has taken on a role in the United States in treating ischemic wounds in diabetics.

- Patients who are not candidates for revascularization and have poor skin microcirculation may be best served with amputation rather than aggressive local therapy.[5]

**TABLE 92-2.** Lower Extremity Ulcer Etiologies

- Vascular
  - Venous stasis
  - Arteriosclerosis
  - Diabetic or neurotrophic
  - Lymphedema
  - Thromboangiitis obliterans
- Vasculitis
  - Leukocytoclastic
  - Autoimmune related
  - Polyarteritis nodosa
  - Granulomatosis with polyangiitis
- Neoplastic
  - Malignant conversion (Margolin ulcer)
  - Leukemia cutis
  - Lymphoma (mycosis fungoides)
  - Kaposi sarcoma
  - Primary neoplasms
- Traumatic
  - Thermal
  - Blunt trauma and factitious ulcers
- Infectious
  - Bacterial
    - Staph or strep
    - Nocardiosis
    - Ecthyma gangrenosum
    - Anthrax
    - Spirochete infections
    - Atypical mycobacteria
  - Viral
    - HIV
    - Herpetic
  - Fungal and parasitic causes
- Hematologic or rheologic
  - Antiphospholipid antibodies
  - Cryoglobulinemia
- Primary or secondary vasospasm
  - Raynaud phenomenon
  - Chronic pernio (chilblains)
  - Acrocyanosis
- Chemical or drug induced
  - Insect or spider venom
  - Stevens-Johnson syndrome
  - Ergotamine toxicity
  - Hydroxyurea induced
- Other
  - Calciphylaxis
  - Distal embolization
  - Pyoderma gangrenosum
  - Radiotherapy induced
  - Hypertensive ulcer

## FOLLOW-UP

- Close surveillance of arterial ulcerations along with the perfusion status must follow any revascularization attempt, usually with scheduled interval arterial Doppler and ultrasound scanning to detect signs of early restenosis or stent or graft failure.

- Conservative management may dictate even closer follow-up intervals with frequent dressing changes.

- All-cause mortality among patients with CLI is high, with estimates of a threefold increase in rates of myocardial infarction over patients with intermittent claudication; death within 1 year has been estimated at 20% in multiple studies[1] and 40% to 70% at 5 years.[6]

## REFERENCES

1. Tzoulaki I, Fowkes FGR. Epidemiology of peripheral arterial disease. In: Mohler ER, Jaff MR, eds. *Peripheral Arterial Disease.* Philadelphia, PA: American College of Physicians; 2008:6.

2. Sumpio BE, Paszkowiak J, Aruny J, Blume P. Lower extremity ulceration. In: Creager MA, Dzau VJ, Loscalzo J, eds. *Vascular Medicine.* Philadelphia, PA: Saunders; 2006:880-893.

3. Ruangsetakit C, Chisakchai K, Mahawongkajit P, Wongwanit C, Mutirangura P. Transcutaneous oxygen tension: a useful predictor of ulcer healing in critical limb ischemia. *J Wound Care.* 2010;19(5):202-206.

4. Mosti G, Iabichella ML, Partsch H. Compression therapy in mixed ulcers increases venous output and arterial perfusion. *J Vasc Surg.* 2012;55(1):122-128.

5. Slovut DP, Sullivan TM. Critical limb ischemia: medical and surgical management. *Vasc Med.* 2008;13:281-291.

6. Dormandy J, Heeck L, Vig S. The fate of patients with critical limb ischemia. *Semin Vasc Surg.* 1999;12:142-147.

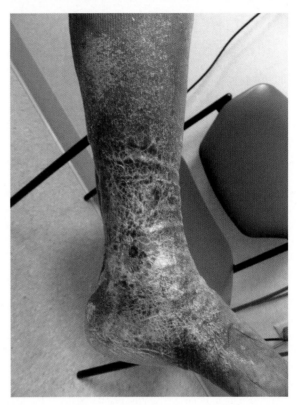

**FIGURE 92-6** Venous stasis ulceration.

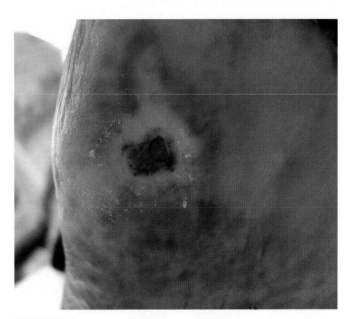

**FIGURE 92-7** Neurotrophic first metatarsophalangeal plantar ulcer with surrounding callous in a diabetic Charcot foot.

# 93 NEUROPATHIC ULCERATION

Travis Hubbuch, DPM
Michael Maier, DPM

## PATIENT STORY

A 58-year-old overweight diabetic man presented with bloody drainage from a callous on the plantar aspect of the right first metatarsophalangeal joint (MPJ) for approximately 1 week (Figure 93-1). He has a history of bilateral plantar first MPJ ulcers that healed with conservative treatment. He is a truck driver and wears custom-molded accommodative orthotics that are approximately 1-year old within work boots (Figure 93-2).

On physical examination, pedal pulses are palpable. The feet are warm and of equal temperature. Protective sensation is plantarly absent on testing with a 10-g monofilament. He has a planus (flat) foot type with limited first MPJ range of motion and mallet toe deformity (flexion contracture of the hallux interphalangeal joint) (Figure 93-3). Following debridement of hyperkeratotic tissue and cutaneous sanguinous drainage from the plantar aspect of the right first MPJ, a small surface area, full-thickness skin ulceration is identified (Figure 93-4). The wound base is granular and healthy with no signs of active infection. Treatment includes topical use of a hydrogel with silver (to address surface contaminants and facilitate moist wound healing) and a prescription for new orthotic devices. Due to the recurrent callous despite use of the orthotics, routine visits are recommended every 10 to 12 weeks for callous debridement and diabetic foot care. He is not interested in surgical correction of the abnormal mechanics in the forefoot (hallux malleus correction).

### EPIDEMIOLOGY

- The incidence of diabetic ulcers in the United States is approximately 1.5 million[1] and this is expected to increase as diabetes increases.

- There are currently nearly 800,000 new cases of diabetes diagnosed every year, affecting approximately 6% of the population.[1]

- Approximately 60% of all nontraumatic lower extremity amputations occur in diabetics.[2]

- Approximately 85% of diabetic lower extremity amputations are preceded by a foot ulcer.[2]

- Within 5 years of amputation, 28% to 51% of diabetic amputees undergo contralateral leg amputation.[2]

- 5-year mortality following bilateral amputation: 39% to 68%.[2]

- The direct cost of treating noninfected diabetic foot ulcers is more than $6 billion annually.[3]

### ETIOLOGY AND PATHOPHYSIOLOGY

- Neuropathic ulceration is typically the result of repetitive, moderate soft tissue trauma in the setting of peripheral sensory neuropathy and abnormal foot mechanics.

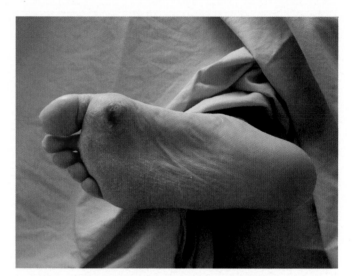

**FIGURE 93-1** Bleeding callous on plantar aspect of first metatarsophalangeal joint (MPJ).

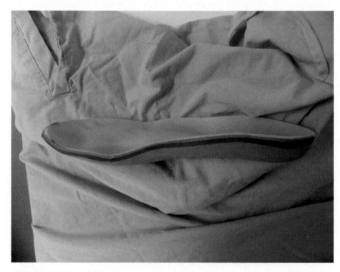

**FIGURE 93-2** Multilaminate custom-molded accommodative foot orthotic.

- The most common causes of peripheral neuropathy include
  - Diabetes
  - Alcoholism
  - Nutritional deficiencies
  - Guillain-Barré syndrome
  - Toxicities (heavy metals)
  - Hereditary
  - Endocrine
  - Rheumatologic (SLE)
  - Amyloidosis
  - Pressure neuropathy
  - Idiopathic
  - Sarcoidosis
  - Hypothyroidism

- Diabetes mellitus is the most common cause of neuropathic ulceration.

- Diabetic peripheral neuropathy often occurs in a stocking or glove and "dying back" (distal to proximal) distribution. It includes sensory, motor, and autonomic components. Sensory neuropathy is the most common component[4] and is defined as the absence of protective sensation (inability to distinguish a 10-g monofilament). Motor neuropathy results in mechanical imbalance between opposing muscle groups (flexors or extensors) and can affect both large muscle groups as well as the intrinsic musculature of the foot. This can lead to foot deformities such as foot drop, equinus, hammertoes, and prominent metatarsal heads.[5] Autonomic neuropathy often results in dry, cracked skin creating potential portals of entry for infection. Sympathetic denervation, arteriovenous shunting, and microvascular dysfunction impair tissue perfusion and normal response to injury. These autonomic dysfunctions combined with motor and sensory components are implicated in the pathogenesis of ulceration.[6]

- Trauma to the neuropathic foot plays a key role in the development of ulceration. Beyond overt trauma such as that of puncture wounds or blunt trauma, moderate repetitive stress associated with walking and day-to-day activity is most commonly associated with ulceration. Further, variability in activity level or periodic bursts of increased activity can precipitate ulceration.[7,8]

- It is widely accepted that there is a strong association between neuropathic foot ulceration and increased plantar pressures.[9] Glycosylation of collagen (as a result of long-standing diabetes) may lead to stiffening of capsular and ligamentous structures.[10] Subsequently, limited ranges of motion at the ankle, subtalar, and MPJs lead to increased plantar pressures.[11] These abnormal plantar pressures often manifest clinically as calluses, corns, blisters, or skin fissures. The locations are specific to the underlying structural deformities. In the absence of adequate off-loading mechanisms, neuropathic ulceration may occur.[4]

- Other factors frequently associated with increased risk for neuropathic ulceration include poor glycemic control, duration of diabetes, peripheral arterial disease, nephropathy, visual impairment, advanced age, and prior foot surgery.[12]

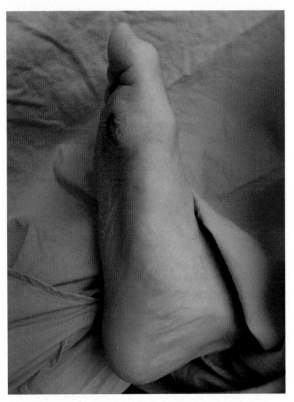

FIGURE 93-3 Lateral view of foot demonstrates severe flatfoot deformity with plantar callous and digital contracture.

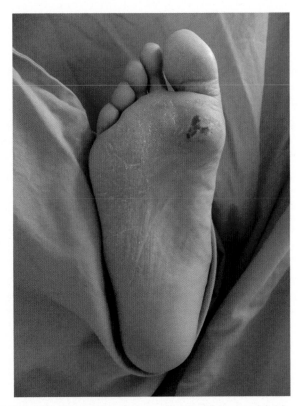

FIGURE 93-4 Neuropathic ulceration identified following debridement of all hyperkeratotic tissue and sanguinous drainage.

## DIAGNOSIS

- Neuropathic ulceration is primarily a clinical diagnosis. Typically, these wounds are accompanied by hyperkeratotic tissue at increased pressure points on the foot.

- Patients may be unaware of such wounds due to the presence of callous tissue in the setting of peripheral sensory neuropathy.

- All hyperkeratotic debris must be debrided to assess the full extent of ulceration including depth.

- Most neuropathic ulcers occur on the plantar surface of the foot; however, ulcers on the dorsal, medial, and lateral aspects can also occur in the setting of poorly fitting shoe gear.

  Comprehensive assessment should include the following.

### Foot Specific History

- Daily activity or work activity
- Neuropathic symptoms
- Claudication or rest pain
- Previous infections or ulcers or amputations

### Wound History

- Inciting event or trauma
- Current wound care
- Footwear or off-loading technique
- Patient compliance

## CLINICAL FEATURES

- Most patients with neuropathic ulceration demonstrate some degree of orthopedic foot deformity. These range in terms of severity and distribution on the foot (digits, mid foot, hindfoot, and ankle). Based on individual patient characteristics, these deformities may be treated conservatively with off-loading modalities or with surgical correction or a combination of the two.

- Patients with Charcot arthropathy may have overt mid foot collapse with ulceration and present some of the most challenging management problems.

- In addition to structural deformities, musculoskeletal evaluation should include muscle strength testing, joint range of motion assessment, and gait analysis to identify any functional deformities.

- Patients with neuropathic ulceration may also have concomitant peripheral arterial disease, and assessment should include comprehensive vascular evaluation.

- Typically, neuropathic ulcers are well circumscribed over bony prominences or pressure points on the foot. The quality of tissue in the wound base as well as the characteristics and volume of drainage are dependent on multiple factors including perfusion and the presence or absence of infection.

- Imaging studies (radiographs, magnetic resonance imaging [MRI], bone scan) are useful to assess bone architecture as well as the extent of wound involvement and infection.[13]

## MANAGEMENT

- The hallmark of therapy for neuropathic ulceration is off-loading pressure from the wound itself. Wound location, patient activity level, and body habitus are all considerations for device choice.

- If patient compliance is in question, total contact casting forces nonweightbearing and is very effective for off-loading the plantar foot.[12]

- Orthotics are of multilaminate design and custom molded to the patient's foot. Shoe design is equally important, and patients with severely contracted digits or dorsal ulceration may require shoes with expandable or heat-moldable uppers (Figure 93-5). Depending on the severity of deformity, shoe modifications may be necessary as well to further reduce pressure and shear forces on the plantar foot (Figure 93-6).

- Finally, for patients with severe deformity such as those with Charcot arthropathy or partial foot amputation, advanced custom bracing is necessary (Figures 93-7 and 93-8).

- Orthopedic surgery is required in some patients if the deformity cannot be accommodated in conservative fashion.

## PATIENT EDUCATION

- Patients should be educated on the need for daily foot inspection and counseled against any *unprotected weightbearing* (walking without the prescribed offloading device).

## FOLLOW-UP

- Initially, patients with neuropathic ulceration may need to be seen often for wound debridement. Once healed, periodic follow-up is indicated for debridement of any residual hyperkeratotic tissue and regular foot examination.

- Finally, patients should wear any prescribed off-loading devices daily and replace these regularly (usually once annually).

### PROVIDER RESOURCES

- http://emedicine.medscape.com/article/460282-overview
- http://www.woundsource.com/blog/neuropathic-ulcers-and-wound-care-symptoms-causes-and-treatments

### PATIENT RESOURCES

- http://www.patient.co.uk/health/Diabetes,-Foot-Care-and-Foot-Ulcers.htm
- http://www.nlm.nih.gov/medlineplus/ency/patientinstructions/000077.htm

## REFERENCES

1. Advanced Medical Technology Association. Advanced wound management: healing and restoring lives. Jun 2006;7-8.

2. Diabetes in America. 2nd ed. National Diabetes Data Group, National Institutes of Health, National Institute of Diabetes and

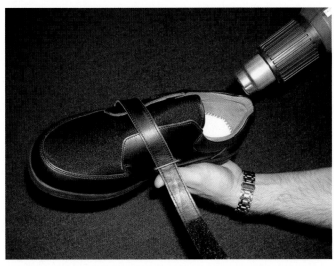

FIGURE 93-5 Extra-depth shoe with heat moldable, neoprene upper used to accommodate digital deformities.

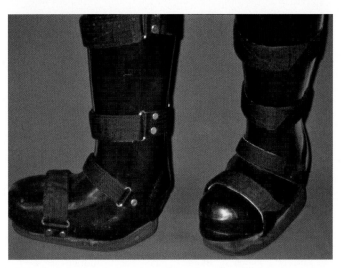

FIGURE 93-7 Charcot restraint orthopedic walker (CROW devices) used for patients with Charcot arthropathy and associated mid foot bony collapse.

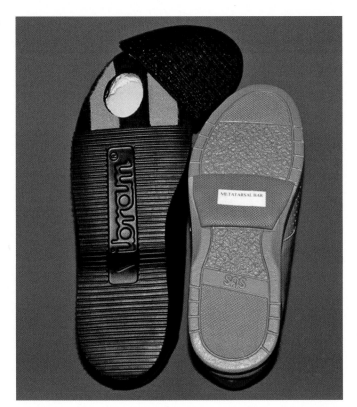

FIGURE 93-6 Shoe modification with drill-n-fill and metatarsal bar to reduce pressure in central aspect of plantar forefoot.

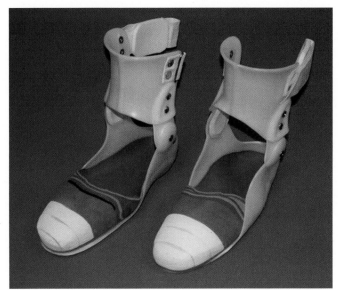

FIGURE 93-8 Short-leg articulated ankle-foot orthoses with accommodative inlays and forefoot fillers used for patients with transmetatarsal amputations and ankle instability.

Digestive and Kidney Diseases. NIH Publication No. 95-1468, 1995. 2. *Diabetes Atlas*. 3rd ed. International Diabetes Federation, 2006.

3. Gordois A, Scuffham P, Shearer A, Oglesby A, Tobian JA. The health care costs of diabetic peripheral neuropathy in the US. *Diabetes Care*. Jun 2003;26(6):1790-1795.

4. Reiber GE, Vileikyte L, Boyko EJ, et al. Causal pathways for incident lower-extremity ulcers in patients with diabetes from two settings. *Diabetes Care*. 1999;22:157-162.

5. Frykberg RG. Diabetic foot ulcers: pathogenesis and management. *Am Fam Physician*. 2002;66:1655-1662.

6. Flynn MD, Tooke JE. Aetiology of diabetic foot ulcerations: a role for the microcirculation. *Diabetic Med*. 1992;8: 320-329.

7. Knox RC, Dutch W, Blume P, et al. Diabetic foot disease. *Int J Angiography*. 2000;9:1-6.

8. Armstrong DG, Lavery LA, Holtz-Neiderer K, et al. Variability in activity may precede diabetic foot ulceration. *Diabetes Care*. 2004;27:1980-1984.

9. Brownlee M. Glycosylation products and the pathogenesis of diabetic complications. *Diabetes Care*. 1991;14:8-11.

10. Delbridge L, Perry P, Marr S, et al. Limited joint mobility in the diabetic foot: relationship to neuropathic ulceration. *Diabetic Med*. 1988;5:333-337.

11. Boulton AJ, Kirsner GE, Vileikyte L. Clinical practice. Neuro-pathic diabetic foot ulcers. *New Engl J Med*. 2004;351:48-55.

12. Veves A, Murray HJ, Young MJ, et al. The risk of foot ulceration in diabetic patients with high foot pressure: a prospective study. *Diabetologia*. 2002;35:660-663.

13. Frykberg RG, Zgonis T, Armstrong DG, et al. Diabetic foot disorders: a clinical practice guideline. *J Foot and Ankle Surg*. 2006;45(8):S10-S12, S14.

# 94 PYODERMA GANGRENOSUM

Stephanie Jacks, MD
Steven M. Dean, DO, FACP, RPVI

## PATIENT STORY

A 35-year-old woman with no significant medical history presented with a painful ulcer on the right pretibial area. It started as a small pustule that subsequently evolved into a rapidly enlarging ulcer over the course of several weeks. She may have injured the area after falling from her bicycle just prior to the onset of the lesion. A comprehensive review of systems is notable for intermittent crampy abdominal pain and diarrhea for the past year, which had been attributed to irritable bowel syndrome. Laboratory evaluation shows only a mild anemia, but biopsy samples from the terminal ileum are consistent with Crohn disease. A skin biopsy from the edge of the ulcer itself is nondiagnostic. The ulcer improves after initiation of therapy with infliximab for her Crohn disease. Pyoderma gangrenosum is suspected.

## EPIDEMIOLOGY

- The incidence of the disease is 1 patient in 100,000 people per year.[1]

- While pyoderma gangrenosum (PG) can occur at any age, it is most common in women aged 20 to 50 years old, and children represent only about 4% of cases.[2,3]

- In about half of patients, PG is idiopathic.[2]

- Roughly half of patients have an underlying disease association, most commonly inflammatory bowel disease, followed by inflammatory arthritis and hematologic disorders, such as acute myelogenous leukemia, chronic myelogenous leukemia, or myelodysplasia.[2]

- Other less common disease associations include human immunodeficiency virus (HIV), hepatitis C, systemic lupus erythematosus, and Takayasu arteritis.[4,5]

- The condition may occur in several syndromes, including pyogenic arthritis, pyoderma gangrenosum, acne (PAPA) syndrome; synovitis, acne, pustulosis, hyperostosis, osteitis (SAPHO) syndrome; and chronic recurrent multifocal osteomyelitis.[3]

## ETIOLOGY AND PATHOPHYSIOLOGY

- An alteration in neutrophil chemotaxis is most likely involved, but the pathophysiology is not well characterized.[1]

- Defects in cell-mediated immunity, humoral immunity, and monocyte function have also been reported; however, no consistent association has been determined.[4]

- Cutaneous lesions are initiated and aggravated by trauma (eg, needle sticks or other minor injuries), a phenomenon known as pathergy (Figure 94-1).[4]

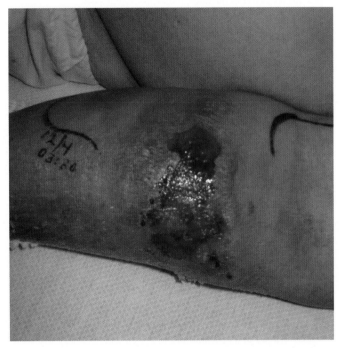

**FIGURE 94-1** Pyoderma gangrenosum (PG), illustrating the phenomenon of pathergy. This lesion occurred at the site of intravenous (IV) placement on the antecubital fossa. (*Photograph courtesy of Benjamin Kaffenberger, MD, The Ohio State University.*)

## DIAGNOSIS

### Clinical Features

- The classic presentation is a painful ulcer with a purulent base and irregular edges (Figures 94-2 through 94-9).[1,2]
- The border of the ulcer classically appears undermined with a gunmetal gray color.[2]
- Lesions may start as pustules, bullae, or nodules that subsequently undergo necrosis leading to the classic ulcerated appearance.[2]
- Ulcers often expand rapidly and coalesce with one another but may present with a more chronic, slowly enlarging course.[2]
- Particularly in peristomal lesions, crater-like holes representing the openings of fistulous tracts that may drain pus can be seen.[6]
- After healing, the lesions leave atrophic, cribriform, hyperpigmented scars (Figures 94-10 and 94-11).[2,6]

### Clinical Variants

- Vesiculobullous eruption—This variant presents with bullous lesions on the face and arms, and is more commonly seen in patients with hematologic disorders. These more superficial lesions may overlap with bullous Sweet syndrome, another cutaneous neutrophilic disorder.[2]
- Sterile pustular eruption—This subtype presents with multiple small, diffuse pustules that may not progress to ulcerations, and is most often seen in patients with inflammatory bowel disease.[2]
- Pyostomatitis vegetans—This variant displays chronic vegetative lesions in a perioral distribution and is seen with increased frequency in patients with inflammatory bowel disease.[2]

### Distribution

- Ulcers most frequently appear on the lower extremities, in particular the pretibial areas, but may occur anywhere.[2]
- Peristomal ulcers also are characteristic of PG.[6]
- In cases that are associated with medications or hematologic disorders, patients often develop widespread, rapidly necrotic ulcers in association with systemic symptoms such as fever.[2]
- Lesions on the face and dorsal hands are more commonly seen in association with hematologic disorders.[2]
- In children, the head, genital, and perianal areas are more frequently involved.[2]
- Sterile neutrophilic infiltrates may involve multiple organs, including the bones, lungs, and liver.[2]

### Laboratory Studies and Further Workup

- PG represents a diagnosis of exclusion, as there are no specific laboratory or histologic findings for the disease.
- Laboratory findings may include nonspecific evidence of inflammation, such as leukocytosis or an elevated erythrocyte sedimentation rate and C-reactive protein.[2]
- 15% of patients will have a monoclonal gammopathy, usually immunoglobulin A (IgA).[2]

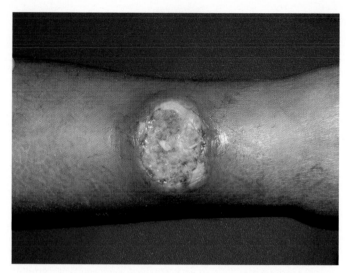

**FIGURE 94-2** Classic appearance of pyoderma gangrenosum (PG), showing an ulcer with undermined, gunmetal gray borders and a purulent base. The patient had Crohn disease. (*Photograph courtesy of Matthew Zirwas, MD, The Ohio State University.*)

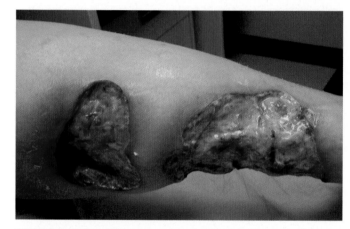

**FIGURE 94-3** Pyoderma gangrenosum (PG). Note the markedly fibropurulent ulceration base with associated necrosis. A violaceous-appearing periulcerative discoloration exists as well. (*Photograph courtesy of Dr. Michael Jaff, Harvard Medical School.*)

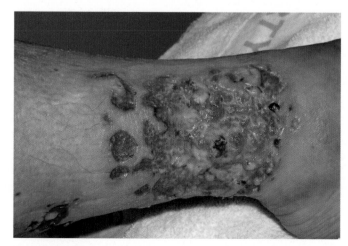

**FIGURE 94-4** Pyoderma gangrenosum (PG). (*Photograph courtesy of Matthew Zirwas, MD, The Ohio State University.*)

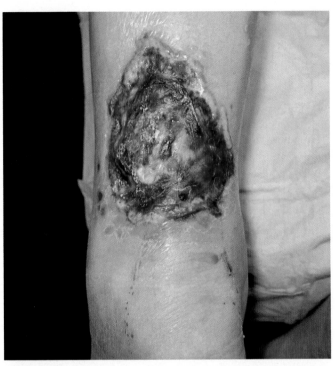

FIGURE 94-5 Pyoderma gangrenosum (PG). A painful fibronecrotic base exists with an inflammatory appearing border. The patient had long-standing hepatitis C with early cirrhosis. (*Photograph courtesy of Steven M. Dean, DO, The Ohio State University.*)

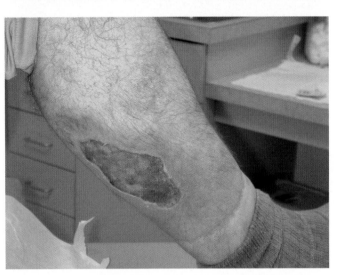

FIGURE 94-7 Pyoderma gangrenosum (PG). Large PG ulceration along the posterolateral calf of a 45-year-old man with seronegative arthritis. Note the mildly rolled border and periulcerative erythema. (*Photograph courtesy of Steven M. Dean, DO, The Ohio State University.*)

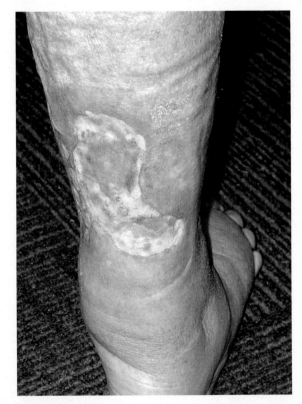

FIGURE 94-6 Pyoderma gangrenosum (PG). A large fibrous PG ulceration in an unusual location (posterior calf) in a 59-year-old woman with CREST syndrome. Early granulation tissue and ulceration contraction evolved after cyclosporine was started 6 weeks prior. (*Photograph courtesy of Steven M. Dean, DO, The Ohio State University.*)

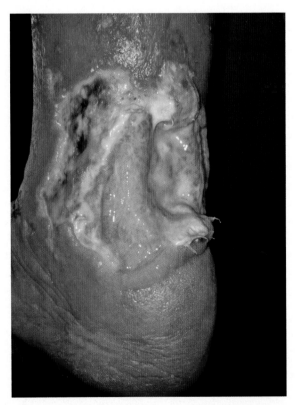

FIGURE 94-8 Pyoderma gangrenosum (PG) of the posterior ankle. (*Photograph courtesy of Seth Bendo, MD, The Ohio State University.*)

- A search for any undiagnosed underlying systemic disease, as well as a thorough history and physical examination, is warranted in all patients.
- Further studies should be dictated by symptoms and examination findings, but may include
  - Skin biopsy and tissue cultures (including bacterial, fungal, viral, and mycobacterial cultures)
  - Gastrointestinal workup—stool ova and parasites, colonoscopy, radiographic imaging, liver function tests, hepatitis serologies.
  - Hematologic workup—complete blood count, platelet count, peripheral blood smear, bone marrow biopsy
  - Serologic studies—serum protein electrophoresis, immunofixation electrophoresis, antinuclear antibodies, antiphospholipid antibodies, antineutrophil cytoplasmic antibodies, and syphilis serologies.
  - Chest x-ray
  - Urinalysis[2]
- Histopathologic findings are nonspecific, but untreated early lesions may show a neutrophilic infiltrate, and more chronic lesions may show tissue necrosis at the center and fibrosing inflammation at the edge of the ulcer.[2]

## DIFFERENTIAL DIAGNOSIS

- Infectious—Bacterial infections, such as folliculitis, cellulitis, streptococcal synergistic gangrene, and ecthyma gangrenosum, as well as deep mycotic, parasitic, syphilitic, and atypical or typical mycobacterial infections
- Malignant—Cutaneous T-cell and B-cell lymphomas, squamous cell carcinoma, and basal cell carcinomas
- Vascular—Venous hypertension (stasis ulceration) or severe arterial insufficiency
- Vasculitic—Polyarteritis nodosa, microscopic polyangiitis, granulomatosis with polyangiitis (Wegener disease), Churg-Strauss disease, Behçet disease, and other autoimmune disorders, such as systemic lupus erythematosus and rheumatoid arthritis
- Miscellaneous—Brown recluse spider bites, panniculitides, factitious ulcers, pustular drug eruptions[2]

## MANAGEMENT

- There is no specific treatment for PG, but the goals of treatment are to promote healing, minimize pain, control the underlying disease process (if present), and minimize the risk of adverse effects.[2]
- As the disease is rare, a gold standard for therapy based on large-scale clinical trials is lacking, and current treatment recommendations are based on case studies or case series.
- Standard treatment involves local or systemic corticosteroids or topical immunomodulators, either alone or in combination with adjunctive systemic immunosuppressants.[2]
- For patients with mild disease, superpotent topical or intralesional corticosteroids or topical tacrolimus represent the first line of treatment.[2]
- These may be combined with oral antibiotics (such as minocycline), colchicine, dapsone, or potassium iodide.[2]

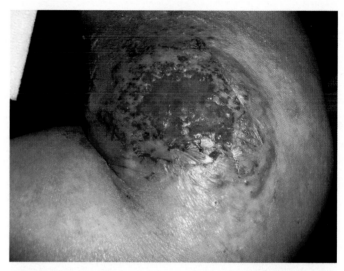

**FIGURE 94-9** Pyoderma gangrenosum (PG). (*Photograph courtesy of Shane Clark, MD, The Ohio State University.*)

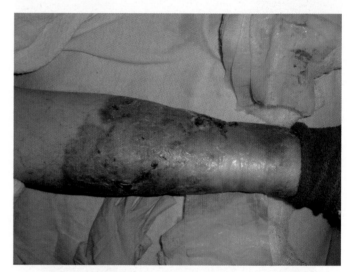

**FIGURE 94-10** Pyoderma gangrenosum (PG), healing. Note the atrophy and hyperpigmentation of the healing areas. (*Photograph courtesy of Stephanie Jacks, MD, The Ohio State University.*)

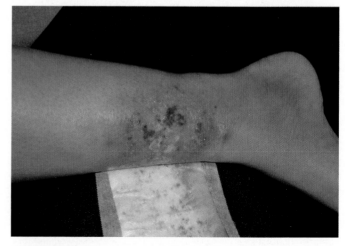

**FIGURE 94-11** Pyoderma gangrenosum (PG), healing. Note the cribriform pattern of healing, with atrophy and hyperpigmentation. (*Photograph courtesy of Matthew Zirwas, MD, The Ohio State University.*)

- For patients with more severe disease, oral systemic corticosteroids (standard starting dose of prednisone is 60-120 mg by mouth daily) or intravenous pulse steroids (methylprednisolone at a dose of 1 g daily for 3-5 days) are often necessary.[2]

- For patients requiring protracted courses of systemic corticosteroids to control the disease, or for those with contraindications to systemic corticosteroids, other therapeutic options include cyclosporine, thalidomide, cyclophosphamide, and azathioprine, although many other systemic immunosuppressants have been used with some success.[2,5]

- For patients with inflammatory bowel disease, infliximab or other tumor necrosis factor-alpha (TNF-α) inhibitors may be particularly helpful, and improvement in cutaneous lesions may accompany improvement in gastrointestinal pathology.[2,5]

- Surgical excision of the ulcers should be avoided due to pathergy, as the ulceration may enlarge at the site of surgical manipulation.[1]

## PATIENT EDUCATION

- Patients should be informed that a thorough workup is crucial in suspected cases of PG, both to exclude other causes of ulcers as well as to search for any underlying associated diseases.

- Realistic expectations regarding treatment outcomes must also be set, as there is no specific treatment for the condition, and response to therapy varies widely.

## FOLLOW-UP

- The disease course and response to therapy are unpredictable.

- A recent case series of 103 patients reported a mortality rate of 16%, although mortality rates of up to 30% have been reported elsewhere.[1,7]

- Ongoing management should be tailored to the individual, taking into consideration the severity of the disease and the chosen treatment course (eg, need for laboratory monitoring with many of the immunosuppressants).

### PROVIDER RESOURCE

- http://emedicine.medscape.com/article/1123821-overview

### PATIENT RESOURCES

- http://www.mayoclinic.com/health/pyoderma-gangrenosum/DS00723

- http://www.bad.org.uk/site/1396/default.aspx

## REFERENCES

1. Binus AM, Qureshi AA, Li VW, Winterfield LS. Pyoderma gangrenosum: a retrospective review of patient characteristics, comorbidities and therapy in 103 patients. *Br J Dermatol.* 2011;165(6):1244-1250.

2. Bolognia JL, Jorizzo JL, Rapini RP, et al. *Dermatology.* 2nd ed. Philadelphia, PA: Mosby Elsevier; 2008.

3. Hadi A, Lebwohl M. Clinical features of pyoderma gangrenosum and current diagnostic trends. *J Am Acad Dermatol.* 2011;64(5): 950-954.

4. Jackson MJ. Pyoderma gangrenosum. eMedicine. Available at: http://emedicine.medscape.com/article/1123821-overview. Accessed January 7, 2012.

5. James WD, Berger T, Elston D. *Andrews' Diseases of the Skin: Clinical Dermatology.* 10th ed. Philadelphia, PA: Saunders; 2006.

6. Paller AS, Mancini AJ. *Hurwitz Clinical Pediatric Dermatology: A Textbook of Skin Disorders of Childhood and Adolescence.* 3rd ed. Philadelphia, PA: Saunders; 2005.

7. Ruocco E, Sanguiliano S, Gravina AG, Miranda A, Nicoletti G. Pyoderma gangrenosum: an updated review. *J Eur Acad Dermatol Venereol.* 2009;23(9):1008-1017.

# 95 NECROBIOSIS LIPOIDICA AND DIABETIC DERMOPATHY

Katya L. Harfmann, MD

## PATIENT STORY

A 40-year-old woman with a history of diabetes presents with red plaques on her shins (Figures 95-1 and 95-2). They are asymptomatic, though continue to increase in size. A biopsy was previously taken and revealed necrobiosis lipoidica. She had been working closely with her primary care physician to better control her glucose, but the lesions continued to progress. She has been applying topical corticosteroids with minimal improvement. This story demonstrates a typical case of necrobiosis lipoidica refractory to treatment in spite of well-controlled diabetes.

## EPIDEMIOLOGY

### Necrobiosis Lipoidica

- Strongly associated with diabetes mellitus (usually type 1), though rarely may occur in patients who are not diabetic.[1]

- Percentage of patients with diabetes at the time of presentation ranges from 11% to 65%.[1]

- Patients without diabetes on presentation may have impaired glucose tolerance, develop diabetes at a later date, or have positive family histories of diabetes.[1]

- May occur at any age, though tends to develop at an earlier age in patients with pre-existing diabetes.[2]

- Women are affected three times as often as men.[1]

### Diabetic Dermopathy

- Most common cutaneous finding in patients with diabetes mellitus, occurring in 9% to 55% of diabetics.[3]

- Incidence increased in diabetics with other microangiopathic complications of diabetes (retinal, neuropathic, and/or nephrogenic).[3]

- Occurs in both insulin-dependent and noninsulin-dependent diabetics.[2]

- Incidence increases with age, typically seen in patients older than 50 years.[3]

- Men are affected more often than women.[4]

## ETIOLOGY AND PATHOPHYSIOLOGY

### Necrobiosis Lipoidica

- Disorder of collagen degeneration with granuloma formation and fat deposition.[1]

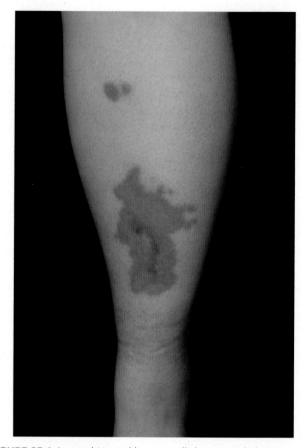

**FIGURE 95-1** Large shiny, red-brown, well-demarcated plaque characteristic of necrobiosis lipoidica. A few satellite papules exist as well. (*Photograph courtesy of Dr. Matthew Zirwas.*)

- Etiology remains unknown; however, it may be related to immunologically mediated vascular disease, diabetic microangiopathy, or defective collagen.[1]

## Diabetic Dermopathy

- Etiology largely unknown; however, trauma may be a causative factor.[3]

- Previously thought to be related to ischemia, though lesions are now recognized to have more blood flow than surrounding skin.[5]

## DIAGNOSIS

- Necrobiosis lipoidica—A biopsy is typically performed for diagnosis. No further laboratory workup is helpful in making a diagnosis.[1]

- Diabetic dermopathy—This is a clinical diagnosis with no laboratory workup or biopsy necessary.[3]

## Clinical Features

- Necrobiosis lipoidica—characterized by asymptomatic shiny, red-brown, telangiectatic papules, patches, plaques, or nodules (Figures 95-1 and 95-2).[1] Koebnerization may be involved in new lesion formation. Over time, the lesions enlarge and coalesce, often becoming waxy and atrophic centrally (Figure 95-3). Painful ulcers occur at sites of trauma in 35% of lesions (Figures 95-3 and 95-4).[1]

- Diabetic dermopathy—characterized by asymptomatic reddish-brown macules, patches, and papules (Figures 95-5, 95-6, 95-7). They are usually oval, round, or linear in shape, clearly demarcated from surrounding skin. Older lesions may be covered with a thin scale and may appear atrophic and hyperpigmented. Individual lesions may resolve completely over a period of 18 to 24 months; however, new lesions continuously form.[3]

## Typical Distribution

- Necrobiosis lipoidica—most commonly seen in the pretibial area, as well as the dorsal hands, and forearms.[6] Less commonly, the ankles, calves, thighs, feet, face, scalp, and trunk are involved. Typically lesions are bilaterally symmetric.[1]

- Diabetic dermopathy—like necrobiosis lipoidica, lesions are most commonly seen in the pretibial area, though are classically asymmetric. Less frequently, the upper extremities, thighs, trunk, and lower abdomen are involved.[3]

## Pathology

- Necrobiosis lipoidica—The epidermis is usually normal or atrophic, with occasional ulceration. Necrobiotic collagen is seen in the dermis with palisading granulomas, often in tiers oriented parallel to the epidermis. There is a dermal interstitial infiltrate of histiocytes, multinucleated giant cells, lymphocytes, and plasma cells.[7]

- Diabetic dermopathy—Though rarely biopsied, the skin lesions demonstrate dermal hemosiderin, perivascular lymphocytes, and an increase in papillary dermal blood vessels.[8]

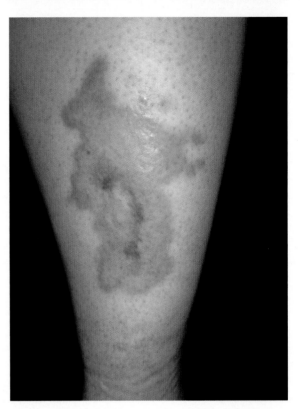

**FIGURE 95-2** Close up of the previous photograph. A waxy appearance to the plaque is evident. (*Photograph courtesy of Dr. Matthew Zirwas.*)

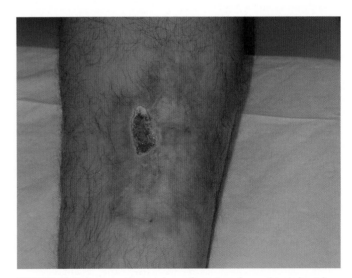

**FIGURE 95-3** A more advanced manifestation of necrobiosis lipoidica with an associated ulceration. Note the periulcerative yellow-orange atrophic features of the plaque. (*Photograph courtesy of Dr. Steven M. Dean.*)

## DIFFERENTIAL DIAGNOSIS

- Granuloma annulare—Typically on the distal extremities, rather than the pretibial area. Often does not have the same degree of atrophy, telangiectasias, and yellow-brown color as necrobiosis lipoidica. Histopathologically, inflammation is more patchy with deposition of mucin within granulomatous inflammation.[1]

- Necrobiotic xanthogranuloma—Lesions typically yellow, indurated plaques occurring periorbitally. Associated with a paraproteinemia.[1]

- Sarcoidosis—May coexist with necrobiosis lipoidica. Like granuloma annulare, sarcoidosis does not demonstrate the same degree of atrophy, telangiectasias, and yellow-brown color as necrobiosis lipoidica. If clinical suspicion for sarcoidosis is high, a chest radiograph to look for bilateral hilar lymphadenopathy may be helpful.[1]

- Stasis dermatitis—Though also on the pretibial area, differs clinically with the presence of an eczematous rash in addition to other signs of vascular insufficiency such as varicose veins, edema, hyperpigmentation, lipodermatosclerosis, and occasional ulcers.[1]

- Panniculitis, such as erythema nodosum—Usually appears as erythematous nodules on the lower legs of young women. Usually painful rather than asymptomatic. No epidermal atrophy or ulceration.[1]

- Granulomatous infections—Infections such as syphilis, leprosy, and dimorphic fungal infections are often distinguished clinically.[1]

- Sclerosing lipogranuloma—May be indurated plaques with ulcerations. Developing after injection of substances such as paraffin, cottonseed oil, sesame oil, or beeswax, these lesions rarely occur on the legs.[1]

- Pigmented purpuric dermatoses—Several of these disorders may occur on the lower extremities, including Schamberg disease, purpura annularis telangiectodes of Majocchi, and pigmented purpuric lichenoid dermatitis of Gougerot-Blum. Schamberg disease has the classic "cayenne pepper" spots within the patches of orange or brown pigmentation. The others are primarily purpuric, rather than hyperpigmented.[3]

## MANAGEMENT

### Necrobiosis Lipoidica

- No treatment has proven to be effective in large, placebo-controlled studies.[1]

- Topical corticosteroids—both intralesional triamcinolone and 0.1% betamethasone under occlusion. Active or established lesions benefit most from injections into the active border, as histologic changes extend into normal skin surrounding lesions (Figures 95-1 and 95-3).[1]

- Antiplatelet agents—aspirin and dipyridamole.[6]

- Systemic corticosteroids—short courses tapered over 5 weeks. Need to monitor blood glucose given association of conditions with glucose intolerance or diabetes.[1]

- Single case reports of pentoxifylline, topical tacrolimus, infliximab, PUVA, tretinoin, ticlopidine, mycophenolate mofetil, nicotinamide, clofazimine, perilesional heparin injections.[9]

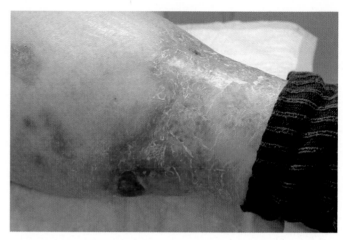

**FIGURE 95-4** Scattered atrophic-appearing red-brown patches and plaques as well as an ulceration in necrobiosis lipoidica. (*Photograph courtesy of Dr. Steven M. Dean.*)

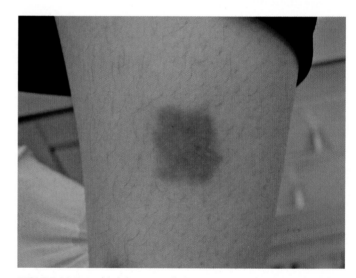

**FIGURE 95-5** Reddish-brown well-demarcated oval patch exemplifying diabetic dermopathy.

- Pulsed dye laser to treat prominent telangiectasias.[9]

- Cyclosporine 2.5 mg/kg/d and granulocyte-macrophage colony-stimulating factor (GM-CSF) have healed a few cases of ulcerated necrobiosis lipoidica.[1]

- Surgical excision with split-thickness skin grafting for recalcitrant ulcers.[1]

- Upregulation of gli-1 oncogene in necrobiosis lipoidica may guide future therapeutic investigations with gli-1 oncogene inhibitors (tacrolimus and sirolimus).[10]

## Diabetic Dermopathy

- Nonspecific treatment, because lesions are asymptomatic and treatments are generally ineffective.[3]

- Blood sugar control will not affect present lesions, but is essential to prevent future lesions.[3]

## FOLLOW-UP

- In patients with a new diagnosis of necrobiosis lipoidica without diabetes, periodic glucose tolerance tests should be performed. Existing lesions should also be examined for squamous cell carcinoma.[1]

### PROVIDER RESOURCES

- http://emedicine.medscape.com/article/1103467-overview
- http://www.patient.co.uk/doctor/Necrobiosis-Lipoidica.htm

### PATIENT RESOURCES

- http://www.dlife.com/diabetes/complications/skin/necrobiosis-lipoidica
- http://www.diabetescare.net/content_detail.asp?id=815

### REFERENCES

1. Howard A, White CR Jr. Non-infectious granulomas. In: Bolognia J, Jorizzo JL, Rapini RP, eds. *Dermatology.* 2nd ed. St. Louis, MO: Mosby/Elsevier; 2008:1429-1431.

2. Romano G, Moretti G, Di Benedetto A, et al. Skin lesions in diabetes mellitus: prevalence and clinical correlations. *Diabetes Res Clin Pract.* Feb 1998;39(2):101-106.

3. Morgan AJ, Schwartz RA. Diabetic dermopathy: a subtle sign with grave implications. *J Am Acad Dermatol.* Mar 2008;58(3):447-451.

4. Ahmed I, Goldstein B. Diabetes mellitus. *Clin Dermatol.* Jul-Aug 2006;24(4):237-246.

5. Wigington G, Ngo B, Rendell M. Skin blood flow in diabetic dermopathy. *Arch Dermatol.* Oct 2004;140(10):1248-1250.

6. Körber A, Dissemond J. Necrobiosis lipoidica diabeticorum. *CMAJ.* Dec 4 2007;177(12):1498.

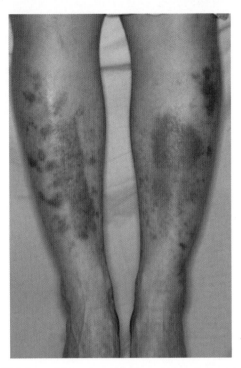

FIGURE 95-6 Large bilateral pretibial hyperpigmented patches consistent with diabetic dermopathy. (*Photograph courtesy of Dr. Mark Davis, Department of Dermatology, Mayo Clinic.*)

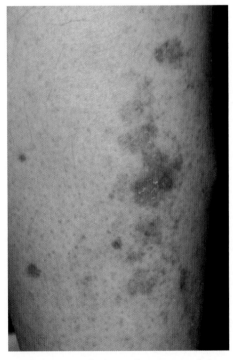

FIGURE 95-7 Close up pretibial view illustrating well demarcated brownish patches, macules, and papules of diabetic dermopathy. (*Photograph courtesy of Dr. Mark Davis, Department of Dermatology, Mayo Clinic.*)

7. Rapini RP. Noninfectious granulomas. In: Rapini RP, ed. *Practical Dermatopathology*. St. Louis, MO: Mosby/Elsevier; 2005:100-101.

8. Rapini RP. Other Non-neoplastic diseases. In: Rapini RP, ed. *Practical Dermatopathology*. St. Louis, MO: Mosby/Elsevier; 2005:230.

9. Moreno-Arias GA, Camps-Fresneda A. Necrobiosis lipoidica diabeticorum treated with the pulsed dye laser. *J Cosmet Laser Ther*. Sep 2001;3(3):143-146.

10. Macaron NC, Cohen C, Chen SC, Arbiser JL. gli-1 Oncogene is highly expressed in granulomatous skin disorders, including sarcoidosis, granuloma annulare, and necrobiosis lipoidica diabeticorum. *Arch Dermatol*. Feb 2005;141(2):259-262.

# 96 CALCIPHYLAXIS

Jason Prosek, MD
Christopher Valentine, MD

## PATIENT STORY

A 55-year-old woman with end-stage renal disease (ESRD), dependent on dialysis for 14 years, presented with multiple highly painful plaques on her abdomen and flank over the last month (Figure 96-1). The lesions ulcerated over that period of time. Her intact parathyroid hormone level was 1514 pg/mL at the time of presentation. This patient underwent parathyroidectomy for tertiary hyperparathyroidism and sodium thiosulfate treatments with dialysis but continued to have chronic pain related to the skin manifestations of calciphylaxis.

## EPIDEMIOLOGY

- Calciphylaxis is most likely to occur in ESRD, with reported prevalence of 4.1% in dialysis patients.

- Primary hyperparathyroidism is the second most commonly associated disorder.[1]

- Clinical risk factors in dialysis patients are obesity, female gender, Caucasian race, diabetes mellitus, hyperphosphatemia, malnutrition, and hypercoagulable state (protein S or C deficiency).[2]

- Associated medications include warfarin, steroids, calcium-containing phosphate binders, vitamin D analogues, and calcineurin inhibitors.

- Prospective data for 36 cases demonstrated 33% mortality at 6 months for plaque lesions and 80% mortality at 6 months for ulcerative lesions.[3]

- Retrospective data from 64 patients revealed overall 1-year survival of 45.8%.[4] Patients who had surgical debridement did better, with 61% 1-year survival. Sepsis from infected ulcers is a common cause of death.

- There are reports of calciphylaxis associated with acute kidney injury, alcoholic cirrhosis, systemic lupus erythematosus, rheumatoid arthritis, endometrial carcinoma, and Hodgkin lymphoma all in the absence of ESRD.

## ETIOLOGY AND PATHOGENESIS

- Pathogenesis is complex and only partially understood.

- Vascular smooth muscle cells (VSMCs) differentiate into chondrocyte- or osteoblast-like cells.

- Uremic toxins, hyperphosphatemia, and reactive oxygen species have been implicated in the change in phenotype of the VSMC.

- Decrease in vascular calcification inhibitory proteins including fetuin-A and matrix Gla protein.

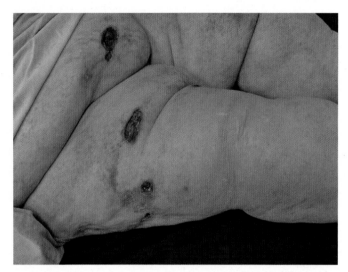

**FIGURE 96-1** Proximally located, highly painful ulcerative plaques and eschar characteristically involving the fatty portions of the extremities and lower abdomen. Note the associated livedo racemosa and retiform purpura indicative of ischemia caused by medial arteriolar calcification. (*Photograph courtesy of Steven M. Dean, DO.*)

- Fetuin-A is a glycoprotein made in the liver. It binds calcium and phosphorous in the circulation, and is a systemic inhibitor of vascular calcification. Fetuin-A levels are diminished in dialysis patients, and are also lower in chronic inflammation.

- Matrix Gla protein is made by VSMC and chondrocytes. It binds calcium and prevents calcification of arteries. Activity is vitamin K dependent, which may explain the association of calciphylaxis with warfarin use.

- Systemic medial calcification of arterioles is the first step and leads to epidermal ischemia, tissue infarction, and ulceration.[4]

- Hyperphosphatemia and elevated parathyroid hormone level have been implicated, but calciphylaxis may occur with normal serum levels of calcium, phosphorous, and parathyroid hormone (PTH).

- Administration of PTH induces ischemic skin necrosis in animals, and some patients have clinical improvement after parathyroidectomy.

- Hypercoagulability may play a role in the pathogenesis, either due to a thrombotic disorder or procoagulant effects of warfarin.[5]

- Wilmer and Magro proposed a two-stage concept in which stage one is development of the vascular lesion, and stage two is development of end-organ ischemia due to expanding calcific vascular lesions, obliterative endovascular thrombosis, and/or vascular thrombosis.[2]

## DIAGNOSIS

### Clinical Features

- Painful lesions in adipose areas including abdomen, buttocks, thighs.

- Early lesions are painful purpuric plaques, livedo racemosa, and subcutaneous nodules (Figure 96-2).

- At later stages the lesions become ischemic and necrotic (Figure 96-3).

- Infection of necrotic lesions may lead to bacteremia or sepsis.

- A painful proximal myopathy may be present even without skin lesions.

- An optic neuropathy related to calciphylaxis has been described.

### Typical Distribution

- May occur on the distal extremities (Figures 96-3 to 96-5).

- Typically involves area with greatest amount of adipose tissue—abdomen, buttocks, and thighs (Figures 96-1, 96-2, 96-6).

- Penile calciphylaxis has been reported in patients with ESRD, and 76% of cases are in diabetic patients. Overall mortality was 69% at 6 months. Survival rate was 28% with local debridement or penectomy, but improved to 75% in those who had parathyroidectomy.

### Laboratory Studies

- There is no diagnostic laboratory test.

- Elevated PTH is common, but most patients with a high PTH will not develop calciphylaxis.

- Calcium × phosphorous product greater than 70 is a risk factor for calciphylaxis.

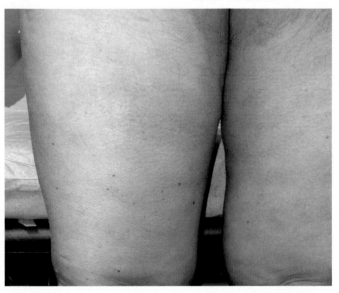

FIGURE 96-2 Early preulcerative calciphylaxis of the proximal fatty lower extremities. Tender irregular erythematous patches along the anteromedial thighs suggestive of livedo racemosa are evident.

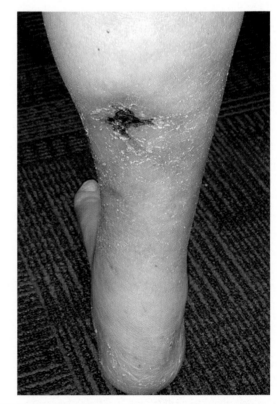

FIGURE 96-3 Stereotypical painful necrotic ulcer with small eschar on the posterior surface of right lower extremity with surrounding purpuric ischemic discoloration. (*Photograph courtesy of Steven M. Dean, DO.*)

- Plain radiographs, computed tomographic (CT) scans, and mammography may all be used to detect soft tissue calcification. Mammography is superior to plain films and CT scans, but use is limited by the pain caused by the technique.
- Bone scan may show vascular and subcutaneous calcification.
- Skin biopsy for diagnosis of calciphylaxis is controversial. The risks of skin ulceration, poor wound healing, and infection must be weighed against the benefit of a definitive diagnosis.
- Pathology: Skin biopsy demonstrates arteriolar medial calcification, intimal hyperplasia, endovascular fibrosis, subcutaneous or dermal vascular thrombosis, and chronic calcifying panniculitis.

## DIFFERENTIAL DIAGNOSIS

- Nephrogenic fibrosing dermopathy
- Warfarin skin necrosis
- Antiphospholipid syndrome
- Atheroemboli
- Vasculitis
- Cryoglobulinemia
- Severe peripheral vascular disease
- Hypercoagulable states—protein C or S deficiency, antithrombin III deficiency
- Pyoderma gangrenosum
- Necrotizing fasciitis

## MANAGEMENT

- Increase frequency of dialysis in ESRD patients to five to six times weekly with low calcium dialysate.[6]
- Avoid use of calcium-containing phosphate binders.
- Avoid or minimize use of vitamin D analogues.
- Strict control of serum phosphorous to less than 6 mg/dL by dietary restriction and use of noncalcium-based binders.[7]
- Goal for calcium × phosphorous product in stage 3-5 chronic kidney disease (CKD) is less than 55 mg$^2$/dL$^2$.
- Use of cinacalcet, a calcimimetic agent that increases the sensitivity of the calcium-sensing receptor on the parathyroid gland. Evidence supporting its use is only in case reports.[8]
- Surgical parathyroidectomy—indications include calciphylaxis, PTH level greater than 800 pg/mL associated with hypercalcemia, and/or hyperphosphatemia despite medical therapy.
- Intravenous sodium thiosulfate (12.5-25 g three times a week) to enhance calcium solubility and removal during dialysis.
- Topical 25% sodium thiosulfate was effective in two patients.
- Bisphosphonates—proposed mechanism is inhibition of macrophages and proinflammatory cytokines as well as binding to calcified VSMCs.[8]
- Hyperbaric oxygen has been effective in small series.
- Avoid injections in involved areas.
- Optimize anemia management.

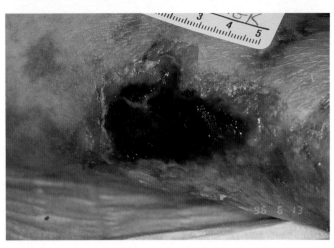

FIGURE 96-4 Large, painful necrotic ulcer with eschar of the left medial calf. Note the violaceous lesions and erythema surrounding the necrotic area. (*Photograph courtesy of Steven M. Dean, DO.*)

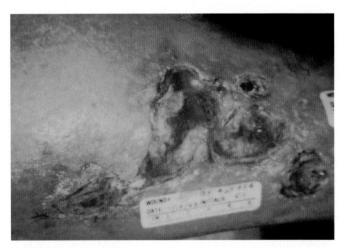

FIGURE 96-5 Multiple necrotic lesions with black eschar of the right lateral calf with periulcerative violaceous patches. (*Photograph courtesy of Steven M. Dean, DO.*)

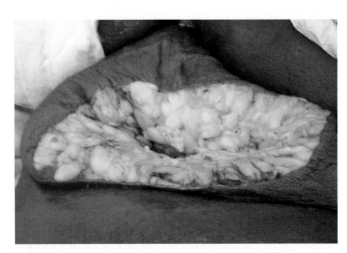

FIGURE 96-6 Postdebridement photograph of a large calciphylaxis ulceration illustrating the predilection for the fatty region of the thigh.

• For acral lesions, evaluate for peripheral arterial disease that may be amenable to angioplasty or stenting.

## PATIENT EDUCATION

• In ESRD patients obesity and elevated phosphorous are the potentially modifiable risk factors.
• Dietary phosphorous restriction and compliance with phosphorous binders must be emphasized.
• Weight loss programs based on carbohydrate restriction and exercise should be encouraged unless there are medical contraindications.

## FOLLOW-UP

• Frequent physical examination to verify response to therapy and monitor for signs of infection.

### PATIENT AND PROVIDER RESOURCES

• There is a calciphylaxis registry at the University of Kansas. www2.kumc.edu/calciphylaxisregistry/
• Moorthi RN, Moe SM. CKD—mineral and bone disorder: core curriculum 2011. *Am J Kidney Dis*. Dec 2011;58(6):1022-1036.

## REFERENCES

1. Nigwekar SU, Wolf M, Sterns RH, et al. Calciphylaxis from nonuremic causes: a systematic review. *Clin J Am Soc Nephrol*. 2008;3:1139.
2. Wilmer WA, Magro CM. Calciphylaxis: emerging concepts in prevention, diagnosis, and treatment. *Semin Dial*. May-Jun 2002;15(3):172-186.
3. Fine A, Zacharias J. Calciphylaxis is usually non-ulcerating: risk factors, outcome and therapy. *Kidney Int*. 2002 Jun;61:2210-2217.
4. Weenig RH. Pathogenesis of calciphylaxis: Hans Selye to nuclear factor kappa-B. *J Am Acad Dermatol*. 2008;58:458.
5. Ross EA. Evolution of treatment strategies for calciphylaxis. *Am J Nephrol*. 2011;34(5):460-467.
6. Baldwin C, Farah M, Leung M, et al. Multi-intervention management of calciphylaxis: a report of 7 cases. *Am J Kidney Dis*. Dec 2011;58(6):988-991.
7. Block GA. Control of serum phosphorous: implications for coronary artery calcification and calcific uremic arteriolopathy (calciphylaxis). *Curr Opin Nephrol Hypertens*. Nov 2001;10(6): 741-747.
8. Raymond CB, Wazny LD. Sodium thiosulfate, bisphosphonates, and cinacalcet for treatment of calciphylaxis. *Am J Health Syst Pharm*. Aug 1 2008;65(15):1419-1429.

# APPENDIX

# LOWER EXTREMITY: ARTERIOVENOUS FISTULA

A. George Akingba, MD, PhD
Gary W. Lemmon, MD

## PATIENT STORY

A 58-year-old healthy man initially presented to the emergency room with gunshot wound (GSW) birdshot injuries to the back of his left leg that occurred on a hunting trip. His initial examination showed normal pulses without any localized neurologic deficits. He was reevaluated in the clinic 1 month later with a thrill in the popliteal fossa and diminished pedal pulses. A duplex ultrasound study confirmed an arteriovenous fistula (AVF) at the level of the proximal posterior tibial artery (PTA) or distal popliteal artery. An endovascular intervention resulted in successful coverage of the AVF and improvement of distal limb perfusion (Figure 1).

### ETIOLOGICAL DEFINITION AND CLASSIFICATION

- An AVF is an abnormal connection between an artery and vein with a persistent endothelialized tract. They are often classified as either congenital or acquired.

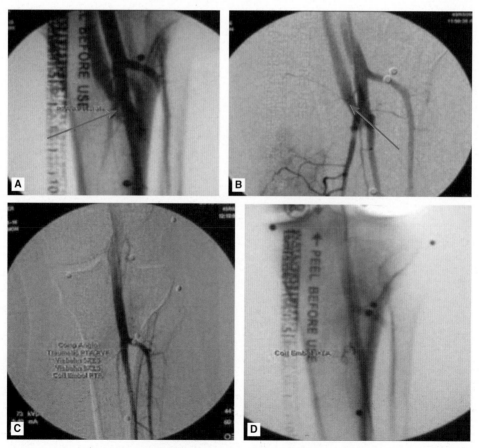

**FIGURE 1** An angiogram of an AVF between the PTA and contiguous vein after a GSW with birdshot injuries, showing (A) the site of the fistula, (B) venous filling through the fistula, and (C) and (D) postendovascular intervention angiogram showing resolution of AVF.

- Congenital AVFs are rare and often secondary to persistent embryonic vessels that fail to distinctively differentiate into an artery or vein.
- Acquired AVFs are more common and often secondary to the following causes: traumatic, iatrogenic, therapeutic, and degenerative aneurysmal changes.

## ETIOPATHOLOGY OF ACQUIRED AVFs

1. Traumatic injury most commonly following stab wounds (63%), GSW (26%), or blunt trauma (1%).[1,2]

2. Iatrogenic injury most commonly occurs after percutaneous vascular interventions. The common femoral artery (CFA) is the most common site of iatrogenic AVFs.[3,4]

3. Therapeutic procedures performed for complex hemodialysis vascular access in patients with inadequate access at more conventional sites (eg, femoral vein transposition).

4. Degenerative aneurysmal changes resulting in rupture of an arterial aneurysm into a contiguous vein (Figure 2A and B).[5-8]

## PATHOPHYSIOLOGY OF ACQUIRED AVFs

- The natural history of an AVF is often determined by the size and adequacy of the inflow and outflow vessels, as well as the size and location of fistula tract.
- Some AVFs spontaneously close, but most continue to enlarge.
- In chronic AVFs the proximal artery and proximal vein enlarge with an associated increase in flow through the respective vessels. These vessels also undergo tortuous changes as they enlarge. If the fistula outflow resistance is very low, it can result in a distal arterial steal phenomenon that can manifest as tissue ischemia.
- Over time, the proximal arterial wall can undergo thinning and aneurysmal dilation while the proximal vein wall often thickens. Also, the high venous pressure in the distal veins can result in valvular incompetence that can manifest as varicose veins, hyperpigmentation, and stasis ulcers.
- Systemically, in chronic AVFs the increase in venous return results in compensatory increase in stroke volume and cardiac output, which leads to cardiomegaly that can manifest as high-output congestive heart failure (CHF).

## CLINICAL PRESENTATION

- Small AVFs may be asymptomatic, only being discovered incidentally.
- Larger AVFs can present acutely or chronically.
- Acute presentations of AVFs are more commonly associated with traumatic AVFs and degenerative aneurysms that rupture into a contiguous vein.
- Chronic presentations are associated with missed iatrogenic or traumatic injury.
- The most common presentation is a thrill (or bruit) or a pulsatile mass.[9,10] Other modes of presentation include limb swelling/heaviness, varicose veins, hyperpigmentation, stasis ulcers, painful ischemia, neurologic deficits (from a pulsatile mass compression effect), and cardiac manifestations associated with high-output CHF.

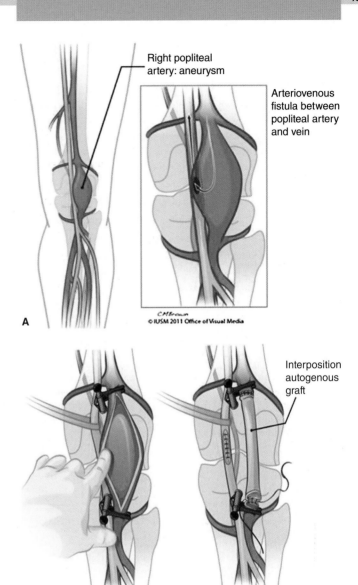

**FIGURE 2** A schematic drawing showing (A) a popliteal artery aneurysm rupture into a contiguous vein and (B) open surgical repair of the AVF and popliteal artery aneurysm.

## DIAGNOSIS

- A plain x-ray of the chest or local area can be useful in identifying evidence of CHF or previous penetrating trauma (missiles).

- Ankle brachial indices (ABIs) and lower extremity arterial duplex ultrasound scanning can be useful for screening when AVFs are suspected. They can also be useful in objectively determining the severity of the arterial component of the AVF while lower extremity venous duplex scanning does the same for the venous component.

- Additional noninvasive imaging techniques include computed tomography (CT), contrast angiography, and magnetic resonance (MR) angiography.

- A commonly used minimally invasive diagnostic technique is digital subtraction angiography (DSA). This modality also provides the opportunity for therapeutic intervention.

## TREATMENT OPTIONS

- Small asymptomatic AVFs do not require treatment as they usually spontaneously involute.

- The technical principles for treating AVFs are varied and can be based on the following:
  - Durability of repair
  - Comorbidities of the patient
  - Anatomical dimensions of fistula tract

- Conservative management with ultrasound-guided compression has been found to be useful in a small number of AVFs with a long communication tract between the artery and vein.[11-15] Success rates are relatively poor and even more unlikely if the AVF tract has a short length, large diameter, or occurs at a bifurcation.

- Endovascular therapies have increased with the technological improvement associated with this option. It is becoming the treatment of choice for stable patients with suitable anatomy, in poor-risk surgical candidates, and in patients with poorly accessible lesions in the abdomen and extremities.

- Some of these endovascular techniques involve embolization and stent grafting of the lesion. Embolization involves accurately delivering an appropriate caliber occlusive device to the AVF. Its major risk involves embolization of the occlusive device to the lungs or distal arterial circulation. Stent grafting involves delivering a fabric-covered stent that occludes the arterial orifice of the AVF while maintaining flow to the distal arterial circulation. Its major risk involves endoleaks that can predispose to a recurrent AVF.

- For the most part endovascular interventions have been promising with good success rates and relatively low complication rates.

- Finally, an open surgical approach is indicated for patients with acute AVFs associated with hemodynamic decompensation or ischemia, as well as with chronic AVFs that are not amenable to other approaches. The surgical option is also often the preferred treatment of choice when procedural durability in young patients is essential or in some cases where patient follow-up is not anticipated.

## COMPLICATIONS OF TREATMENT

- Embolization of the occlusive device to the lungs or distal arterial circulation
- Bleeding
- Infection
- Nonresolution of AVF
- Recurrence
- Injury to surrounding structures
- Progression of disease

## FOLLOW-UP

- Surveillance clinical and duplex evaluations may be typically performed at 1, 3, 6, and 12 months postintervention.

- Recurrent AVFs usually result from incomplete treatment and can present similar to the primary presentation (ie, acutely or chronically). They can also be worked-up in a similar fashion as the initial presentation.

**PROVIDER RESOURCES**

- Yu PT, Rice-Townsend S, Naheedy J, Almodavar H, Mooney DP. Delayed presentation of traumatic infrapopliteal arteriovenous fistula and pseudoaneursym in a 10-year-old boy managed by coil embolization. *J Pediatr Surg*. 2012 Feb;47(2):e7-e10.

- http://emedicine.medscape.com/article/459842-clinical.

**PATIENT RESOURCES**

- http://www.vascularweb.org/vascularhealth/pages/vascular-conditions-,-tests-,-treatments.aspx.

- http://emedicine.medscape.com/article/459842-clinical.

## REFERENCES

1. Robbs JV, Carrim AA, Kadwa AM, Mars M. Traumatic arteriovenous fistula: experience with 202 patients. *Br J Surg*. 1994;81:1296-1299.

2. Johnston W, Jack L. Cronenwett JL. *Rutherford's Vascular Surgery*, 2-volume set e-book.

3. Kelm M, Perings SM, Jax T, et al. Incidence and clinical outcome of iatrogenic femoral arteriovenous fistulas. *J Am Coll Cardiol*. 2002;40:291-297.

4. Kent KC, McArdle CR, Kennedy B, et al. A prospective study of the clinical outcome of femoral pseudoaneurysms and arteriovenous fistulas induced by arterial puncture. *J Vasc Surg*. 1993;17:125-133.

5. Syme J. Case of spontaneous varicose aneurysms. *Edin Med J*. 1831;36:104-105.

6. Brewster DG, Cambria RP, Moncirol A, et al. Aortocaval and iliac arteriovenous fistulas: recognition and treatment. *J Vasc Surg*. 1991;13:258-265.

7. Scher LA, Veith F. Arteriovenous fistulas of the aorto-iliac territory. In: Bergan JJ, Yao JST, eds. *Aneurysms: Diagnosis and Treatment*. New York, NY: Grune & Stratton; 1982:599-610.

8. Davis PM, Gloviczki P, Cherry KJ Jr, et al. Aorta-caval and ilio-iliac arteriovenous fistulae. *Am J Surg*. 1998;176:115-118.

9. Rich NM, Hobson RW, Collins GJ. Traumatic arteriovenous fistulas and false aneurysms: a review of 558 lesions. *Surgery*. 1975;78:817-828.

10. Khoury G, Sfeir R, Nabbout G, et al. Traumatic arteriovenous fistulae: "the Lebanese war experience." *Eur J Vasc Surg*. 1994;8:171-173.

11. Ruebben A, Tettoni S, Muratore P, et al. Arteriovenous fistulas induced by femoral arterial catheterization: percutaneous treatment. *Radiology*. 1998;209:729-734.

12. Thalhammer C, Kircherr AS, Uhlich F, et al. Postcatheterization pseudoaneurysms and arteriovenous fistulas: repair with percutaneous implantation of endovascular covered stents. *Radiology*. 2000;2:127-131.

13. Fellmeth BD, Roberts AC, Bookstein JJ, et al. Postangiographic femoral artery injuries: nonsurgical repair with ultrasound guided compression. *Radiology*. 1991;178:671-675.

14. Schaub F, Theiss W, Heinz M, et al. New aspects in ultrasound-guided compression repair of post catheterization femoral artery injuries. *Circulation*. 1994;90:1861-1865.

15. Feld R, Patton GM, Carabasi RA, et al. Treatment of iatrogenic femoral artery injuries with ultrasound guided compression. *J Vasc Surg*. 1992;16:832-840.

Page numbers followed by f and t refer to figures and tables, respectively.

**A**

Abdominal aorta bifurcation, 43f
Abdominal aortic aneurysms
  clinical findings of, 118
  diagnosis of, 118
  endovascular repair of, 118-120
    angiography after, 120f
    complications associated with, 120
    devices, 120, 120f
    endoleak after, 120
    follow-up after, 120, 123
    patient selection for, 119
    ruptured AAA, 123
    technique, 119
  epidemiology of, 118
  etiology of, 118
  imaging of, 118
  laboratory tests for, 118
  management of, 118-119
  open repair of, 118-119
  pathophysiology of, 118
  patient education about, 123-124
  ruptured
    clinical presentation of, 123
    endograft for, 124f
    endovascular repair of, 123
    epidemiology of, 122-123
    open surgical repair of, 123
Abdominal aortogram, 14f
Above-knee amputations, 23
Acral ischemia, 51f
Acroangiodermatitis
  clinical features of, 279f-280f, 280
  definition of, 276, 279
  diagnosis of, 280
  differential diagnosis of, 281
  epidemiology of, 279
  etiology of, 279-280
  histopathologic features of, 281
  imaging of, 281
  laboratory studies, 280
  management of, 281
  pathogenesis of, 279-280
  patient education about, 281
  physical examination of, 280
  stasis dermatitis versus, 281
Acrocyanosis, 260
  clinical features of, 353f, 354, 355f-356f
  diagnosis of, 354
  differential diagnosis of, 354
  distribution of, 354
  epidemiology of, 353
  etiology of, 353
  follow-up for, 354
  laboratory studies of, 354
  patient education about, 354
  pernio versus, 408
  primary, 353-354
  secondary, 354
Acro-osteolysis, 342, 344f
Acrorhygosis, 354
Acute compartment syndrome, 51
Acute lipodermatosclerosis, 309
Acute mesenteric ischemia
  clinical presentation of, 194
  diagnosis of, 194-195
  duplex ultrasound of, 195
  endovascular therapy for, 198
  epidemiology of, 193
  mesenteric angiogram for, 195, 195f
  nonocclusive, 194, 198
  pathophysiology of, 193-194
  patient education about, 198
  prognosis for, 198
  signs and symptoms of, 194
  treatment of, 195-198
Acute pancreatitis, 216
Acute right brachial deep venous thrombosis, 255f
Adson test, 55, 59
Adventitial fibromuscular dysplasia, 187
Allen test, 79-81, 80f
Allergic bronchopulmonary aspergillosis, 374-375
Allergic contact dermatitis, 276-277, 277f
Alpha-1 antitrypsin deficiency, 269-273, 364
Alpha-adrenergic blockers, 412
Amaurosis fugax, 89, 92
Ambulatory venous hypertension, 243, 289
American College of Rheumatology
  Churg-Strauss syndrome criteria, 373
  giant cell arteritis criteria, 385
  Henoch-Schönlein purpura criteria, 358
  polyarteritis nodosa criteria, 376, 378t
  Takayasu arteritis criteria, 385
Amputation
  digit, 426f
  limb, 22-24
Anastomotic pseudoaneurysms, 5
ANCA-negative small vessel vasculitis
  cryoglobulinemic vasculitis, 359, 359t, 360f
  definition of, 358
  diagnosis of, 361-362
  differential diagnosis of, 362
  follow-up for, 362
  Henoch-Schönlein purpura, 358f, 358-362, 379
  hypersensitivity vasculitis, 359, 359t, 361t, 361-362, 379
  management of, 362
  polyarteritis nodosa versus, 379

Aneurysms. *See also* Pseudoaneurysms
  abdominal aortic. *See* Abdominal aortic aneurysms
  aortic. *See* Aortic aneurysms
  brachial artery, 51
  carotid artery, 108f-110f, 108-110
  fusiform, 126
  popliteal artery, 133f
  radial artery, 51
  subclavian artery, 55f
Angiography
  aortoiliac occlusive disease evaluations, 7f
  carotid artery traumatic injury evaluations, 113
  celiac axis compression syndrome evaluations, 200
  chronic mesenteric ischemia evaluations, 202-203
  computed tomography. *See* Computed tomography
      angiography
  endovascular aneurysm repair, 120f
  fibromuscular dysplasia evaluations, 189
  iliac artery endofibrosis evaluations, 165f
  superficial femoral artery occlusion evaluations, 11f-12f
  thoracic outlet syndrome evaluations, 55
Angiojet device, 245f
Angioplasty, 64
  atherosclerotic arch vessel disease treated with, 39-40
  femoral popliteal disease treated with, 14-16
  fibromuscular dysplasia treated with, 191
Angiotensin-converting enzyme inhibitors, 127
Ankle-brachial index, 291
  in aortoiliac occlusive disease, 6f, 9f
  in iliac artery endofibrosis, 163f-164f
  in peripheral arterial disease, 13
  in tibioperoneal occlusive disease, 20
Ankle-foot orthoses, 433f
Anterior tibial artery
  disease of, 19f
  pseudoaneurysm of, 144f
Anticoagulation
  calf vein thrombosis treated with, 233
  complications of, 241
  deep venous thrombosis treated with, 240-241
  guidelines for, 241
  hemorrhage caused by, 241
  for May-Thurner syndrome, 253
  for percutaneous endovenous intervention for femoropopliteal
      deep venous thrombosis, 246
  superficial venous thrombosis treated with, 228
Antiglomerular basement membrane antibody disease,
      370
Antihypertensive agents, 127
Antineutrophil cytoplasmic antibodies, 364, 368
Antinuclear antibodies, 343
Antiplatelet agents
  atheroemboli and, 31
  atherosclerotic arch vessel disease treated with, 39
  blunt carotid artery injuries treated with, 114
  giant cell arteritis treated with, 388-389
Antitumor necrosis factor-alpha therapy, 389

Aorta
  coarctation of, 388
  dissection of. *See* Aortic dissection
  occlusion of, 10
  shaggy, 30, 30f
Aorta-to-iliofemoral bypass, 27
Aortic aneurysms
  abdominal, 118
  infrarenal, 147f
  thoracic. *See* Thoracic aortic aneurysms
  thoracoabdominal. *See* Thoracoabdominal aortic aneurysms
Aortic arch
  angiography of, 46f-47f
  atherosclerosis of. *See* Atherosclerotic arch vessel disease
  computed tomographic angiography of, 37, 39f
  steepness of, 93f
Aortic dissection
  DeBakey classification of, 42, 43f
  malperfusion with, 198
  in Marfan syndrome, 150, 152f
  pathology of, 42
  Stanford classification of, 43, 45f
  superior mesenteric artery extension of, 194f
  thoracic. *See* Thoracic aortic dissection
Aortic root dilatation
  in Loeys Dietz syndrome, 155f
  prophylactic surgical repair of, 152
Aortobifemoral grafting
  ankle-brachial index after, 10
  aortoiliac occlusive disease treated with, 4, 10
Aortoceliac bypass, 207f
Aortoenteric fistula, 5
Aortofemoral bypass, 25
Aortoiliac occlusive disease
  aggressive form of, 2
  angiogram of, 7f
  ankle-brachial index in, 6f, 9f
  atherosclerosis as cause of, 8
  blood pressure measurements in, 3
  case study of, 2, 6
  claudication associated with, 8
  clinical features of, 8
  collateralization, 2f, 2-3
  complications of, 4-5, 10
  computed tomography of, 3
  diagnosis of, 3, 8
  differential diagnosis of, 8
  duplex ultrasound of, 3
  epidemiology of, 2, 8
  etiology of, 2-3, 8
  follow-up, 5, 10
  imaging of, 2f, 3, 7f
  infrainguinal disease and, 3
  magnetic resonance angiography of, 3
  morbidity rates for, 4
  pathology of, 2-3, 8
  patient education about, 10

risk factors for, 7
symptoms of, 8
TASC II classification system for, 7t, 10
treatment of
    aortobifemoral grafting, 4, 10
    complications of, 4-5, 10
    early complications of, 4
    endovascular, 10
    end-to-end anastomosis, 4
    end-to-side anastomosis, 4, 4f
    late complications of, 4-5
    open repair, 3-4, 4f
    results of, 4
    stents, 9f
Aortomesenteric plaque, 209f
Arachnodactyly, 149
Arc of Riolan, 3, 196f, 206f
Arch vessel disease. *See* Atherosclerotic arch vessel disease
Arterial tortuosity syndrome, 156
Arterial ulceration, 425-429, 427t-428t
Arteriography
    atherosclerotic renal artery stenosis, 184f
    giant cell arteritis, 386f
    popliteal artery entrapment syndrome, 162f
    thoracic outlet syndrome evaluations, 59
    vascular Ehlers-Danlos syndrome and, 147
Arteriovenous fistula, 74, 85
Arteriovenous malformation
    acroangiodermatitis associated with, 280
    angiography of, 173f
    computed tomography of, 173f, 175f
    endovascular therapy for, 178
    epidemiology of, 172
    ethanol sclerotherapy for, 178
    etiology of, 174
    extratruncular, 174, 176
    hemodynamics of, 174
    management of, 177t, 177-178
    multidisciplinary approach to, 177t, 177-178
    patient education about, 178
    recurrence of, 177-178
    surgical resection of, 174f
    truncular, 176
Aspirin, 246
Aspirin-exacerbated respiratory disease, 375
Asteatotic eczema, 276
Atheroembolism. *See also* Blue toe syndrome
    acutely ischemic limb from, 134
    diagnosis of, 30
    follow-up for, 31
Atheromatous emboli, 30
Atherosclerosis
    aortoiliac occlusive disease caused by, 8
    carotid occlusive disease caused by. *See* Carotid artery occlusive disease
    fibromuscular dysplasia versus, 189
    risk factors for, 88, 92, 184
    tibioperoneal occlusive disease and, 19

Atherosclerotic arch vessel disease
    angioplasty for, 39-40
    clinical presentation of, 34
    color duplex ultrasonography of, 36-37
    computed tomographic angiography of, 35f, 37
    diagnosis of, 34, 36-38
    endovascular management of, 39-40
    epidemiology of, 34
    etiology of, 34
    laboratory evaluation, 36-37, 37f
    management of, 39-40
    medical management of, 39
    pathophysiology of, 34
    physical examination of, 34, 36
    radiographic evaluation of, 37, 38f
    risk factors for, 34
    stent placement for, 40
    surgical management of, 39
Atherosclerotic renal artery stenosis
    angiographic features of, 184, 184f
    arteriography of, 184f
    clinical features of, 183
    computed tomography angiography of, 183
    diagnosis of, 183-184
    differential diagnosis of, 184
    duplex ultrasound of, 182f, 183t
    epidemiology of, 182
    follow-up for, 185-186
    hypertension in, 182-183
    magnetic resonance angiography of, 183
    management of, 184-185
    natural history of, 185-186
    pathophysiology of, 182
    patient education about, 185
    stents for, 186
Atopic dermatitis, 277
Autologous vein conduits, 12
Autonomic neuropathy, 431
Axillary artery, 83f
Axillofemoral bypass, 26, 26f
Axillosubclavian vein deep venous thrombosis, 255f, 257f
Azathioprine, 370, 395t, 396

**B**
Baker cyst, 232, 314
Balloon angioplasty, for renal artery fibromuscular dysplasia, 103, 191
Balloon venoplasty and stenting, for femoropopliteal deep venous thrombosis, 246-247, 248f
BASIL trial, 21
Bazin disease, 408
Beals syndrome, 152
Behçet syndrome
    arterial disease associated with, 393
    articular disease, 395, 396t
    autoantibodies in, 392
    cellular immunity and, 392

Behçet syndrome (*Cont.*):
  classification criteria for, 394, 394t
  clinical manifestations of, 392-394
  coagulation abnormalities associated with, 392
  computed tomography of, 391f
  corticosteroids for, 395-396
  definition of, 391
  diagnosis of, 392
  differential diagnosis of, 394, 394t
  endothelial dysfunction associated with, 392
  epidemiology of, 391-392
  erythema nodosum associated with, 391f
  etiology of, 392
  follow-up for, 396
  gastrointestinal manifestations of, 394, 396, 396t
  genetics of, 392
  hemostasis dysfunctions in, 393t
  humoral immunity and, 392
  immune dysfunctions in, 393t
  infectious factors, 392
  laboratory studies, 394
  management of, 395-396
  mucocutaneous manifestations of, 392-393, 395, 396t
  musculoskeletal manifestations of, 393
  neurologic manifestations of, 394, 396, 396t
  ocular manifestations of, 393, 393f, 396, 396t
  parenchymal disease versus, 394
  pathophysiology of, 392
  prognosis for, 395
  renal manifestations of, 394
  systemic drug trials in, 395t
  vascular manifestations of, 393-394, 396
Below-knee amputations, 23
Benign acute blue finger, 259f-260f, 259-261, 261t
Beta-blockers, 127
Bicuspid aortic valve disease, 152
Bioflavonoids, 354
Bisphosphonates, 447
Blood pressure, in aortoiliac occlusive disease, 3
Blue toe syndrome
  diagnosis of, 30
  differential diagnosis of, 31
  endovascular therapy for, 31
  epidemiology of, 29
  etiology of, 29-30
  follow-up for, 31
  illustration of, 29f-30f
  imaging modalities for, 30
  laboratory tests, 30
  management of, 31
  medical therapy for, 31
  pathophysiology of, 29-30
  surgical therapy for, 31
Blunt carotid artery injuries
  antiplatelet therapy for, 114
  endovascular treatment for, 115
  epidemiology of, 111-113
  grading of, 113-114
  mechanisms of, 111-112
  medical treatment for, 114
  mortality rate for, 112
  screening criteria for, 112-113
  surgical treatment of, 115-116
Brachial artery
  anatomy of, 83f
  occlusion of, 52, 60
  pseudoaneurysm of, 49f-50f, 51
  true aneurysm of, 51, 52f
Brachial artery access
  complications of
    diagnosis of, 51
    epidemiology of, 49
    etiology of, 49-50
    follow-up, 52
    imaging of, 51
    management of, 51-52
    occlusion, 52
    pathophysiology of, 49-50
    patient education about, 52
    thrombosis, 50-51
    types of, 50
  declining use of, 49
Brachiocephalic arteries
  aneurysms of, 47
  imaging of, 82f
  peripheral arterial disease of, 47
Budd-Chiari syndrome, 212-214
Buerger disease. *See* Thromboangiitis obliterans

**C**
Calciphylaxis
  clinical features of, 445f, 446, 446f-447f
  diagnosis of, 446-447
  in dialysis patients, 445
  differential diagnosis of, 400, 447
  distribution of, 446, 446f-447f
  epidemiology of, 445
  etiology of, 445
  laboratory studies, 446-447
  management of, 447-448
  pathogenesis of, 445-446
  penile, 446
Calf hematoma, 313
Calf muscle rupture, 312-315
Calf swelling, 313
Calf vein thrombosis
  anticoagulation for, 233
  diagnosis of, 231-232
  differential diagnosis of, 232-233
  distal, 230
  duplex ultrasound of, 231-232, 232f
  epidemiology of, 230

etiology of, 230
follow-up for, 234
heparin for, 233
magnetic resonance venography of, 232
management of, 233
pathophysiology of, 230
patient education about, 233
superficial venous thrombosis as cause of, 232
Wells score, 231, 231t
Capillary hemangioma, 72
Capillary malformations
    description of, 75, 75f
    in Klippel-Trenaunay syndrome, 169f, 169-170
Carotid artery. *See also* Common carotid artery; External carotid
        artery occlusion; Internal carotid artery
    aneurysm of, 108f-110f, 108-110
    cervical. *See* Cervical carotid artery
    dissection of, 105-107, 111f
    duplex imaging of, for fibromuscular dysplasia, 103
Carotid artery occlusive disease
    carotid artery stenting for, 92-94, 94f-95f
    carotid endarterectomy for, 88f-89f, 88-90, 92, 100
    clinical features of, 89
    diagnosis of, 88-89
    epidemiology of, 88
    etiology of, 88
    management of, 92-94, 94f-95f
    occlusion, 99f-101f, 99-101
    pathophysiology of, 88
    ulceration, 97-98
Carotid artery shunt, 109f
Carotid artery stenting
    age of patient and, 93
    carotid artery occlusive disease treated with, 92-94,
        94f-95f
    illustration of, 95f
    surveillance after, 94
Carotid artery traumatic injuries
    angiography for, 113
    blunt
        antiplatelet therapy for, 114
        endovascular treatment for, 115
        epidemiology of, 111-113
        grading of, 113-114
        mechanisms of, 111-112
        medical treatment for, 114
        mortality rate for, 112
        screening criteria for, 112-113
        surgical treatment of, 115-116
    computed tomographic angiography for, 113
    diagnosis of, 112-113
    duplex ultrasound of, 113
    epidemiology of, 111-112
    follow-up for, 116
    imaging of, 113-114
    management of, 114-116

penetrating
    epidemiology of, 111
    management of, 114, 114f
    screening criteria for, 112
    pseudoaneurysm formation secondary to, 115f, 116
    sequelae of, 112
Carotid endarterectomy
    carotid artery occlusive disease treated with, 88f-89f, 88-90,
        92, 100
    high-risk patients, 90, 93
    recurrent stenosis after, 90
Catheter-based angiography, 55
Catheter-directed thrombolytic therapy, 198, 214, 257, 266
Cavernous hemangioma, 72
Celiac artery
    anatomy of, 193f
    computed tomographic angiography of, 126f
    ostial calcification of, 204f
    stenosis of, 210f
    in thoracic endovascular aneurysm repair, 126f, 131
Celiac axis compression syndrome, 199-201
Cellulitis
    factitial edema versus, 338
    infectious
        follow-up for, 305
        in lymphedema, 302, 305, 305f
        patient education about, 305
        prevention of, 305
        treatment of, 305
    lower extremity
        clinical features of, 307f, 308
        computed tomography of, 309
        diagnosis of, 308-309
        differential diagnosis of, 309-310
        epidemiology of, 307
        etiology of, 307-308
        imaging of, 309
        laboratory studies, 308
        magnetic resonance imaging of, 309
        management of, 310-311
        nonpurulent, 310
        pathogens that cause, 307-308
        pathophysiology of, 308
        predisposing factors, 308, 308f-309f
        purulent, 310
        recurrent, 308f
    stasis dermatitis and, 277, 278f
Center for Medicare and Medicaid Services, 93
Cephalic vein, 85f
Cerebral venous disease, 394
Cervical carotid artery
    dissection of, 105
    ulcerative disease of, 97-98
Cervical carotid stroke, 88, 92
Cervical rib, 54, 54f, 56, 58, 60f
Charcot arthropathy, 432

Charcot restraint orthopedic walker, 433f
Chest radiographs
    cervical ribs, 54f
    Churg-Strauss syndrome, 374
    thoracic outlet syndrome evaluations, 55
Chilblains, 260-261, 405, 411. *See also* Pernio
Cholesterol crystal emboli, 30
Chronic ischemia
    in diabetic patients, 20
    symptoms of, 134
Chronic mesenteric ischemia
    angiography of, 202-203
    antegrade bypass for, 203, 205, 207f
    clinical presentation of, 202
    computed tomography of, 204f
    description of, 194
    diagnosis of, 202-203
    duplex ultrasound of, 202, 203f
    endovascular revascularization for, 208, 209f
    epidemiology of, 202
    follow-up for, 211
    mesenteric bypass for, 203
    pathophysiology of, 202
    patient education about, 208
    prognosis for, 208
    retrograde bypass for, 205, 208f
    signs and symptoms of, 202
    transaortic mesenteric endarterectomy for, 205, 208, 209f
    treatment of, 203-208, 205f-210f
Chronic thromboembolic pulmonary hypertension, 239, 241
Chronic total occlusion device, 11
Chronic venous disease
    CEAP classification, 288, 290t
    clinical features of, 288, 288f-289f, 304
    compression therapy for, 291
    diagnosis of, 289-291
    duplex ultrasound of, 289
    epidemiology of, 288-289
    risk factors for, 288-289
    signs of, 297
    treatment of, 291
    varicose veins. *See* Varicose veins
    venous reflux as cause of, 289, 291
Chronic venous insufficiency
    acroangiodermatitis associated with, 279-280
    cutaneous manifestations of, 338
    description of, 232
    duplex ultrasound of, 334-335
    epidemiology of, 333
    etiology of, 333-334
    pathophysiology of, 333-334
    phlebolymphedema caused by, 333-336
    risk factors for, 289
    signs of, 334
Churg-Strauss syndrome, 366, 370, 372-375, 373f-374f

Cilostazol, 10
Cinacalcet, 447
Claudication
    in aortoiliac occlusive disease, 8
    critical limb ischemia versus, 15
    diagnostic studies for, 8
    in iliac artery endofibrosis, 164-165
    in tibioperoneal occlusive disease, 20
Coarctation of the aorta, 388
Cocaine abuse, 367
Coil embolization, 140f
Coil embolotherapy, 178
Colchicine, 395
Cold-induced vasodilation, 411
Collateralization, 2f, 2-3
Common carotid artery. *See also* Carotid artery
    lesions of, 40
    occlusion of, 100f
    stenosis of, 36, 37f
Common femoral artery, 235f
Common iliac deep venous thrombosis, 251f
Compartment syndrome, acute, 51
Complex regional pain syndrome, 415
Compression maneuvers, for thoracic outlet syndrome
        diagnosis, 55
Compression therapy, 291, 424
Computed tomography
    aortoiliac occlusive disease evaluations, 3
    arteriovenous malformation evaluations, 173f, 175f
    Behçet syndrome evaluations, 391f
    chronic mesenteric ischemia evaluations, 204f
    Churg-Strauss syndrome evaluations, 374f
    granulomatosis with polyangiitis evaluations, 364f, 366, 366f
    iliac artery endofibrosis evaluations, 165
    liver imaging uses of, 213
    lymphedema evaluations, 304
    microscopic polyangiitis evaluations, 369f
    retroperitoneal hematoma evaluations, 122f
    splenic vein thrombosis evaluations, 215f, 217
    thoracic outlet syndrome evaluations, 55
Computed tomography angiography
    aortic arch evaluations, 37, 39f
    atherosclerotic arch vessel disease evaluations, 35f, 37
    atherosclerotic renal artery stenosis evaluations, 183
    carotid artery traumatic injury evaluations, 113
    celiac axis compression syndrome evaluations, 199f, 200
    disadvantages of, 183
    femoropopliteal aneurysm evaluations, 134f
    fibromuscular dysplasia evaluations, 103
    giant cell arteritis evaluations, 387f
    median arcuate ligament syndrome evaluations, 199f
    peripheral arterial disease evaluations, 12, 15
    renal artery stenosis evaluations, 183, 189, 190f
    subclavian steal syndrome evaluations, 62f, 64
    thoracic aortic aneurysm evaluations, 130, 131f

thoracic outlet syndrome evaluations, 59
thoracoabdominal aortic aneurysm evaluations, 125-126
tibioperoneal occlusive disease evaluations, 20
Computed tomography venography, 252
Conduits, for femoropopliteal bypass, 12
Congenital lymphedema, 302
Congenital vascular anomalies
  definition of, 71
  hemangiomas. *See* Hemangiomas
  vascular malformations. *See* Congenital vascular malformations
Congenital vascular malformations
  arteriovenous malformation. *See* Arteriovenous malformation
  classification of, 73, 73f
  clinical presentation of, 74-76
  coil embolotherapy for, 178
  definition of, 73
  diagnosis of, 76, 176
  duplex ultrasonography of, 176
  epidemiology of, 73, 172
  ethanol sclerotherapy for, 77, 178
  etiology of, 74, 174
  fast-flow, 74f
  follow-up for, 178
  glue embolotherapy for, 178
  Hamburg classification of, 175t
  hemangiomas. *See* Hemangiomas
  high-flow, 73-75, 74f, 77
  imaging of, 176
  low-flow, 73, 75
  magnetic resonance imaging of, 176
  management of, 76-77, 177t, 177-178
  multidisciplinary approach to, 177t, 177-178
  pathogenesis of, 74
  pathophysiology of, 174
  patient education about, 77, 178
  sclerotherapy for, 76-77, 77f
  transarterial lung perfusion scintigraphy of, 176
Connective tissue diseases
  differential diagnosis of, 388
  small vessel vasculitis associated with, 360-361
Contact dermatitis, 276-277
Coronary artery bypass grafting, 50
Coronary subclavian steal syndrome
  clinical features of, 68-69
  diagnosis of, 69
  differential diagnosis of, 34, 69
  follow-up for, 70
  management of, 69, 69f
  pathophysiology of, 67-68
  patient education about, 69-70
  subclavian artery stenosis as cause of, 67-68
Corticosteroids
  atheromatous embolization and, 31
  Behçet syndrome treated with, 395-396
  microscopic polyangiitis treated with, 370

necrobiosis lipoidica treated with, 442
pyoderma gangrenosum treated with, 439
Cranial arteritis, 385
Critical limb ischemia
  definition of, 425
  description of, 15-16
  epidemiology of, 425
  mortality rates, 429
  treatment of, 22
Crocq sign, 354
Cryoglobulinemia, 379
Cryoglobulinemic vasculitis, 359, 359t, 360f, 362
Cryoglobulins, 359, 361
Cullen sign, 123
Cyclophosphamide, 375, 379
Cyclosporine, 395t, 443
Cytokines, 392, 399

**D**
Dapsone, 395t
D-Dimer, 231, 237
DeBakey classification, of aortic dissection, 42, 43f
Deep venous thrombosis
  acute, 237, 241, 244f
  acute right brachial, 255f
  anticoagulation for, 240
  axillosubclavian vein, 255f
  chronic venous disease caused by, 289
  complications of, 237-238
  description of, 23
  after endovenous laser ablation, 298
  epidemiology of, 236t
  etiology of, 236
  factitial edema versus, 338
  femoropopliteal. *See* Femoropopliteal deep venous thrombosis
  heparin for, 240
  iliofemoral, 252f
  long-term management of, 241
  lower extremity cellulitis versus, 310
  low-molecular-weight heparin for, 240-241
  management of, 239-241
  in May-Thurner syndrome, 251, 251f, 251-254, 253f-254f
  pathophysiology of, 237
  percutaneous endovenous intervention for, 243-249
  pharmacomechanical therapy for, 241
  in phlegmasia cerulea dolens, 264
  recurrence of, 237
  risk factors for, 236, 236t
  superficial venous thrombosis, 226-227
  ultrasound of, 238f
  unfractionated heparin for, 240-241
  warfarin for, 241
Dermatitis
  acroangiodermatitis. *See* Acroangiodermatitis
  allergic contact, 276-277, 277f

Dermatitis (*Cont.*):
  atopic, 277
  stasis. *See* Stasis dermatitis
Diabetes mellitus
  foot ulcers associated with, 18f
  neuropathic ulcerations associated with, 430
Diabetic Charcot foot, 429f
Diabetic dermopathy
  clinical features of, 441, 443f
  diagnosis of, 441
  differential diagnosis of, 442
  distribution of, 441
  epidemiology of, 440
  etiology of, 441
  follow-up for, 443
  management of, 443
  pathology of, 441
  pathophysiology of, 441
Diabetic peripheral neuropathy, 431
Digital gangrene, 360f
Digital necrosis, 344f
Digital plethysmography, 79, 80f
Dihydropyridine calcium channel blockers, 346
Distal anastomosis, for aortoiliac occlusive disease, 4, 4f
Distal aortic false aneurysm, 141f-142f
Dorsal pedal hump, 302, 303f
DREAM trial, 119
Drug-eluting stents, 16
Duplex ultrasound/ultrasonography
  acute mesenteric ischemia evaluations, 195
  aortoiliac occlusive disease evaluations, 3
  atherosclerotic renal artery stenosis evaluations, 183t
  calf vein thrombosis evaluations, 231-232, 232f
  carotid artery dissection evaluations, 105, 106f
  carotid artery traumatic injury evaluations, 113
  celiac axis compression syndrome evaluations, 200, 200f
  chronic mesenteric ischemia evaluations, 202, 203f
  chronic venous disease evaluations, 289
  chronic venous insufficiency evaluations, 334-335
  congenital vascular malformations evaluations, 176
  coronary subclavian steal syndrome evaluations, 69
  femoropopliteal deep venous thrombosis evaluations, 237, 238f
  giant cell arteritis evaluations, 386, 387f
  leg swelling evaluations, 313-314
  May-Thurner syndrome evaluations, 252
  mesenteric vein thrombosis evaluations, 221, 222f-223f
  muscle rupture evaluations, 313-314
  peripheral arterial disease evaluations, 15
  popliteal artery entrapment syndrome evaluations, 160, 161f-162f
  radial artery evaluations, 79
  renal artery stenosis evaluations, 182f, 187
  stasis dermatitis evaluations, 275
  subclavian artery peripheral arterial disease evaluations, 47
  subclavian steal syndrome evaluations, 63f

  Takayasu arteritis evaluations, 389f
  thoracic outlet syndrome evaluations, 55, 59
  tibioperoneal occlusive disease evaluations, 20
  venous stasis ulceration evaluations, 423
  vertebral artery evaluations, 67f

**E**
Echocardiography, 43
Ectopia lentis, 149, 151f
Edema
  in chronic ulcerations, 428
  factitial, 337-339, 338f
  lipedema. *See* Lipedema
  lipolymphedema. *See* Lipolymphedema
  lymphedema. *See* Lymphedema
  management of, 304
  muscle rupture as cause of, 312-315
  systemic causes of, 304
Ehlers-Danlos syndrome
  acrocyanosis associated with, 354
  clinical manifestations of, 145
  epidemiology of, 144
  forms of, 145
  genetic counseling, 147
  medical therapy for, 146-147
  obturator artery aneurysm associated with, 145f
  pathophysiology of, 144-145
  surgical considerations for, 147-148
  vascular, 145-147
Elephantiasis nostras verrucosa, 304f, 316-317
Embosclerosants, 178
Endarterectomy
  carotid artery occlusive disease treated with, 88f-89f, 88-90, 92, 100
    high-risk patients, 90, 93
    recurrent stenosis after, 90
  transaortic mesenteric, for chronic mesenteric ischemia, 205, 208, 209f
Endograft
  aortic, for false aneurysm, 142f
  ruptured abdominal aortic aneurysm treated with, 124f, 131f
Endoleak, after endovascular aneurysm repair, 120, 131
Endoscopic ultrasound, 217
Endovascular treatment
  abdominal aortic aneurysm. *See* Abdominal aortic aneurysms, endovascular repair of
  acute mesenteric ischemia, 198
  aortoiliac occlusive disease, 10
  arteriovenous malformations, 178
  blunt carotid artery injuries, 115
  chronic mesenteric ischemia, 208, 209f
  femoral popliteal disease, 15
  iliac artery endofibrosis, 165-166
  mesenteric vein thrombosis, 223
  popliteal artery entrapment syndrome, 161

subclavian steal syndrome, 64
   thoracic aortic aneurysms, 130-132, 131f-132f
   thoracic aortic dissection, 44
Endovenous laser ablation, 291, 296-299, 298f-299f
End-stage renal disease, 445, 448
End-to-end anastomosis, 4
End-to-side anastomosis, 4, 4f
Eosinophilic fasciitis, 400
Eosinophilic granulomatosis with polyangiitis. *See* Churg-Strauss
   syndrome
Eosinophilic pneumonia, 374
Erythema ab igne, 418f-420f, 418-420
Erythema induratum, 408
Erythema nodosum, 269, 269f, 270t, 271-273, 391f, 408, 442
Erythromelalgia
   acrocyanosis versus, 354
   clinical features of, 414, 415f
   definition of, 414
   diagnosis of, 414-415
   differential diagnosis of, 415
   epidemiology of, 414
   etiology of, 414
   laboratory features of, 414-415
   management of, 415-416
   pathophysiology of, 414
   patient education about, 416
   quantitative sudomotor axon reflex test for, 415, 415f
Erythropoietin, 398
Etanercept, 395t
Ethanol sclerotherapy, 77, 178
European League Against Rheumatism, 396, 396t
EVAR 1 trial, 119
External carotid artery occlusion, 100. *See also* Carotid artery
Extra-anatomic bypass grafts
   aorta-to-iliofemoral bypass, 27
   aortofemoral bypass, 25
   axillofemoral bypass, 26, 26f
   complications of, 27
   contraindications for, 26
   femorofemoral bypass, 25f-26f, 27
   follow-up for, 27
   general concepts regarding, 25-26
   indications for, 26
   obturator bypass, 27, 27f
   patient education about, 27
   subclavian steal syndrome treated with, 64
   supraceliac aorta-to-iliofemoral bypass, 27
   surgical options for, 26-27
   thoracofemoral aorta-to-iliofemoral bypass, 27
   types of, 25
Extracorporeal photopheresis, 401

**F**
Factitial edema, 337-339, 338f
Factitial panniculitis, 269-273

Fast-flow vascular malformations, 74f
*FBN1* mutations, 151
Femoral artery pseudoaneurysm, 137f
Femoral popliteal disease
   bypass for, 11-13
   case study of, 14
   endovascular treatment of, 15
   percutaneous transluminal angioplasty for, 14-16
   stenting for, 14-16
Femorofemoral bypass, 25f-26f, 27
Femoropopliteal aneurysms
   bilateral, 133f
   clinical manifestations of, 133-134
   computed tomographic angiography of, 134f
   diagnosis of, 134
   differential diagnosis of, 134
   epidemiology of, 133
   etiology of, 133
   follow-up for, 135
   imaging of, 134, 134f
   patient education about, 135
   treatment of, 134-135, 135f
Femoropopliteal angioplasty, 16
Femoropopliteal bypass, 12-13
Femoropopliteal deep venous thrombosis
   acute, 237
   balloon venoplasty and stenting for, 246-247, 248f
   complications of, 237-238
   diagnosis of, 237
   duplex ultrasound of, 237, 238f
   epidemiology of, 236
   follow-up for, 241
   imaging of, 244f
   inferior vena cava filters for, 240, 249
   intravascular ultrasound of, 248f
   low-molecular-weight heparin for, 240-241
   management of, 239-241
   natural history of, 237-239
   pathophysiology of, 237
   patient education about, 242
   percutaneous endovenous intervention for, 243-249
   pharmacomechanical therapy for, 241
   risk factors for, 236t
   thrombolytic therapy for, 241
Femoropopliteal vein
   deep venous thrombosis of. *See* Femoropopliteal deep venous
      thrombosis
   perforation of, 247, 249, 249f
Fetuin-A, 446
Fibrillin-1, 149
Fibrin D-dimer, 231
Fibromuscular dysplasia, 184, 185f
   adventitial, 187
   angiography of, 189
   atherosclerosis versus, 189

Fibromuscular dysplasia (*Cont.*):
  cervical carotid aneurysms caused by, 109
  clinical features of, 102, 388
  diagnosis of, 187, 189
  differential diagnosis of, 189, 191, 388
  epidemiology of, 102, 187
  etiology of, 102
  iliac artery, 103, 103f
  internal carotid artery, 102f-104f, 102-103
  intimal, 187, 189f
  management of, 191
  medial, 187, 188f-189f
  percutaneous transluminal balloon angioplasty for, 191
  renal artery, 102, 103f-104f, 187-191
  segmental arterial mediolysis versus, 191
  treatment of, 191
  types of, 187
  vasculitis versus, 189
Fingers, distal embolization in, 55f
Fistula
  aortoenteric, 5
  arteriovenous, 74, 85
Flexion contractures, 23
Foam sclerotherapy, 294, 297
Fondaparinux, 228
Foot orthotics, 430f, 432, 433f
Frostbite, 404-406, 405f-406f, 408, 411, 412f
Frostnip, 405, 411
Fungal infections
  aneurysmal disease caused by. *See* Mycotic aneurysmal disease
  lower extremity cellulitis caused by, 308, 308f
Fusiform aneurysms, 126

**G**
Gangrene
  digital, 360f
  forefoot, 427f
  limb, 22f-23f, 22-24, 239f
Gastric varices, 216f, 216-217
Gastrocnemius muscle
  rupture of, 312-313, 313f
  tear of, 233
Giant cell arteritis
  clinical features of, 384f, 385
  computed tomographic angiography of, 387f
  diagnosis of, 385
  epidemiology of, 384
  etiology of, 384-385
  follow-up for, 389
  imaging of, 386, 386f-387f
  laboratory studies, 385-386
  management of, 388-389
  pathophysiology of, 384-385
  patient education about, 389

    positron emission tomography, 388
    temporal artery biopsy of, 386f
Glomuvenous malformation, 74
Glucocorticoids
    giant cell arteritis treated with, 388
    Takayasu arteritis treated with, 389
Glue embolotherapy, 178
Glycosaminoglycans, 316
Goodpasture syndrome, 370
Graft infection, 4
Graft thrombosis, 4
Granulocyte-macrophage colony-stimulating factor, 442
Granuloma annulare, 442
Granulomatosis with polyangiitis
    clinical features of, 365
    computed tomography of, 364f, 366, 366f
    diagnosis of, 365-366
    differential diagnosis of, 366-367
    etiology of, 364-365
    follow-up for, 367
    histopathology of, 366
    imaging of, 365-366
    laboratory studies, 365
    management of, 367
    microscopic polyangiitis versus, 366, 370
    pathophysiology of, 364-365
    patient education about, 367
    renal biopsy of, 364f
    upper airway manifestations of, 365, 365f
Graves disease, 316-317
Great saphenous vein
    Doppler evaluation of, 297
    reflux in, 291, 296f
    superficial venous thrombosis in, 226, 227f
Grey Turner sign, 123

**H**
Hand
    circulation assessments, 79
    hypothenar hammer syndrome, 82f-83f, 82-83
    photoplethysmography of, 84, 84f-85f
    Raynaud phenomenon of. *See* Raynaud phenomenon
Hand ischemia
    after hemodialysis access placement, 84-85, 86f
    thoracic outlet syndrome and, 54f, 55
Hemangiomas
    description of, 71-73, 72f
    epidemiology of, 172, 174
    etiology of, 176
    pathophysiology of, 176
Hemodialysis access placement, hand ischemia after, 84-85, 86f
Hemodynamic insufficiency, 99
Hemolymphatic malformations, 176
Hemothorax, 42f, 44f
Henoch-Schönlein purpura, 358f, 358-362, 379

Heparin
    calf vein thrombosis treated with, 233
    deep venous thrombosis treated with, 240
    low-molecular weight
        description of, 233, 240-241
        skin necrosis induced by, 283-285
    mesenteric vein thrombosis treated with, 221, 223
    skin necrosis induced by, 283f-284f, 283-285
    unfractionated
        deep venous thrombosis treated with, 240-241
        skin necrosis induced by, 283-285
Heparin-bonded polytetrafluoroethylene conduits, 12
Heparin-induced thrombocytopenia, 241, 283, 286
Hepatic angiography, 213
Hepatitis B infection, polyarteritis nodosa associated with, 379
High-flow vascular malformations, 73-75, 74f, 77
HLA-B51, 392
HLA-DRB4, 372
Homan sign, 237
Homocystinuria, 152
Horner syndrome, 106
"Hostile" abdomen, 25
"Hostile" groin, 25
Hyperbaric oxygen therapy, 428
Hypereosinophilic syndrome, 375
Hyperkeratosis, 302, 303f
Hyperphosphatemia, 446
Hyperpigmentation, after sclerotherapy, 294
Hypersensitivity vasculitis, 359, 359t, 361t, 361-362, 379
Hypertension
    ambulatory venous, 243, 289
    in atherosclerotic renal artery stenosis, 182-183
Hyperthyroidism, 330
Hypertrophic lichen planus, 319
Hypoglossal nerve, 89f
Hypoperfusion ischemic syndrome, 85
Hypophygmia, 354
Hypothenar eminence, 82, 82f
Hypothenar hammer syndrome, 82f-83f, 82-83
Hypothyroidism, 330

I
Iliac artery
    calcified, 30f
    endofibrosis of
        angiography of, 165f
        ankle-brachial index in, 163f-164f
        claudication in, 164-165
        clinical features of, 164-165
        complications of, 166
        differential diagnosis of, 165
        endovascular treatment of, 165-166
        epidemiology of, 163
        etiology of, 163-164
        follow-up for, 166
        management of, 165-166
        pathophysiology of, 163-164
        patient education about, 166
    fibromuscular dysplasia, 103, 103f
    stenting of, 14f
Iliac-superior mesenteric artery bypass, 208f
Iliofemoral deep venous thrombosis, 252f
Immersion foot syndrome, 405, 410-412
In situ vein bypass technique, 12
Indoramin, 354
Infectious aortitis
    clinical features of, 141-142
    computed tomography of, 141f
    epidemiology of, 141
Infectious cellulitis
    follow-up for, 305
    in lymphedema, 302, 305, 305f
    patient education about, 305
    prevention of, 305
    treatment of, 305
Infectious panniculitis, 271-273
Inferior mesenteric artery, 3, 3f
Inferior vena cava filters, 240, 249
Inferior vena cava occlusion, 212f
Inflammatory bowel disease, 439
Infliximab, 439
Infrainguinal bypass, 13
Infrainguinal disease, 3
Infrarenal aortic aneurysm, 147f
Innominate artery, 46-48
Interferon-α-2a, 395t
Internal carotid artery. See also Carotid artery
    bifurcation of, 95f
    dissection of, 105-107
    fibromuscular dysplasia of, 102f-104f, 102-103
    occlusion of, 99f-101f, 99-101, 112f
    tortuosity of, 94f
Internal mammary artery, 3
Interposition vein graft, 135f
Intimal fibromuscular dysplasia, 187, 189f
Intravascular ultrasound
    femoropopliteal deep venous thrombosis, 248f
    May-Thurner syndrome, 253
Irritant contact dermatitis, 276-277
Ischemic ulcers, 426-428, 427f

K
Kasabach-Merritt syndrome, 73
Ketanserin, 354
Kikuchi disease, 269f
"Kissing" stents, 10
Klippel-Trenaunay syndrome
    capillary malformations associated with, 169f, 169-170
    clinical features of, 168f, 169

Klippel-Trenaunay syndrome (*Cont.*):
  diagnosis of, 168-169
  differential diagnosis of, 170
  epidemiology of, 168
  etiology of, 168
  follow-up for, 171
  hemolymphatic malformations and, 176
  limb hypertrophy associated with, 169f, 169-170
  lymphedema associated with, 170
  management of, 170
  pathophysiology of, 168
  ulcerative acroangiodermatitis associated with, 280f
  venous malformations associated with, 169-170
Koebnerization, 441

**L**
Large vessel arteritis, 385, 388
Laser ablation, endovenous, 291, 296-299, 298f-299f
Leg swelling, muscle rupture as cause of, 312-315.
      *See also* Edema
Leg ulcers, 288, 290, 290f
Levamisole, 367
Lichen amyloidosis, 318
Lichen simplex chronicus, 318
Limb amputation, 22-24
Limb gangrene, 22f-23f, 22-24, 239f
Limb swelling
  differential diagnosis of, 330
  medication-induced, 335-336
  muscle rupture as cause of, 312-315
Lipedema. *See also* Lipolymphedema
  age of onset, 321
  clinical features of, 321f, 322-323, 323f-324f, 325t,
      329f
  definition of, 335
  description of, 304
  diagnosis of, 322-323, 329
  differential diagnosis of, 323
  epidemiology of, 321, 328
  etiology of, 321-322
  follow-up for, 326
  grading of, 322t
  histopathology of, 323
  history-taking, 322
  imaging of, 323
  laboratory studies, 323, 329
  lymphedema versus, 325t, 330, 330t
  management of, 323, 325
  obesity versus, 323, 325t
  pathogenesis of, 321-322
  patient education about, 325
  phlebolipedema, 324f
  phlebolymphedema versus, 335
  physical examination of, 322, 322f-323f
  primary, 322

Lipodermatosclerosis, 309, 334f
Lipolymphedema. *See also* Lipedema
  clinical features of, 324f, 327f-329f
  distribution of, 329
  epidemiology of, 328
  etiology of, 328
  laboratory studies, 329-330
  management of, 331
  manual lymph drainage of, 331
  pathophysiology of, 328
  patient education about, 331
  severe, 323, 324f
Livedo racemosa
  clinical features of, 350f
  conditions associated with, 348t
  diagnosis of, 349, 349f
  differential diagnosis of, 351, 419
  distribution of, 349, 350f-351f
  erythema ab igne versus, 419
  etiology of, 348
  laboratory studies, 349
  mottling associated with, 350f
  pathophysiology of, 348
  patient education about, 351
  skin biopsy of, 351
  treatment of, 351
Livedo reticularis
  clinical features of, 348f, 350f
  conditions associated with, 348t
  diagnosis of, 349, 349f
  differential diagnosis of, 351, 419
  epidemiology of, 348
  erythema ab igne versus, 419
  etiology of, 348
  pathophysiology of, 348
  patient education about, 351
  in polyarteritis nodosa, 377f-378f
  primary, 349f
  skin biopsy of, 351
  treatment of, 351
Liver transplantation, 214
Loeys Dietz syndrome, 146
  aortic dilatation associated with, 155f
  bifid uvula associated with, 156f
  clinical features of, 155-156
  description of, 152
  differential diagnosis of, 156-157
  epidemiology of, 155
  etiology of, 155
  histopathology associated with, 156
  imaging of, 156
  management of, 157
  Marfan syndrome versus, 156
  pathophysiology of, 155
  patient education about, 157

Lower extremity cellulitis
  clinical features of, 307f, 308
  computed tomography of, 309
  diagnosis of, 308-309
  differential diagnosis of, 309-310
  epidemiology of, 307
  etiology of, 307-308
  follow-up for, 311
  imaging of, 309
  laboratory studies, 308
  magnetic resonance imaging of, 309
  management of, 310-311
  nonpurulent, 310
  pathogens that cause, 307-308
  pathophysiology of, 308
  predisposing factors, 308, 308f-309f
  purulent, 310
  recurrent, 308f
Low-flow vascular malformations, 73, 75
Low-molecular weight heparin
  description of, 233, 240-241
  skin necrosis induced by, 283-285
Lumbar arteries, 2
Lupus panniculitis, 269-273, 271f-272f
Lymphangiography, 304
Lymphangitis, 338
Lymphatic malformations, 76
Lymphedema. *See also* Phlebolymphedema
  clinical features of, 325t, 335f
  computed tomography of, 304
  congenital, 302
  diagnosis of, 302, 304
  differential diagnosis of, 233, 304
  dorsal pedal hump associated with, 302, 305f
  epidemiology of, 302
  etiology of, 302
  factitial edema versus, 338
  history-taking, 302
  infectious cellulitis associated with, 302, 305, 305f
  in Klippel-Trenaunay syndrome, 170
  lipedema versus, 325t, 330, 330t
  lipolymphedema progression of, 328
  lymphoscintigram of, 304, 305f
  magnetic resonance imaging of, 304
  management of, 304-305
  manual lymph drainage of, 331
  massive localized, 327-328
  pathophysiology of, 302
  physical examination of, 302, 303f
  secondary, 302, 330t
  signs of, 334
  skin changes associated with, 304f
  squaring of toes associated with, 302, 303f
Lymphoscintigram, 304, 305f

M
Macroemboli, 29
Magnetic resonance angiography
  aortoiliac occlusive disease evaluations, 3
  atherosclerotic renal artery stenosis evaluations, 183
  disadvantages of, 183
  giant cell arteritis evaluations, 386
  iliac artery endofibrosis evaluations, 165
  mesenteric vein thrombosis evaluations, 221, 224f
  peripheral arterial disease evaluations, 12, 15
  renal artery stenosis evaluations, 189, 191f
  subclavian steal syndrome evaluations, 64
  Takayasu arteritis evaluations, 386
  thoracic aortic aneurysm evaluations, 130
  tibioperoneal occlusive disease evaluations, 20
Magnetic resonance imaging
  congenital vascular malformations evaluations, 176
  giant cell arteritis evaluations, 386
  leg swelling evaluations, 314
  liver imaging uses of, 213
  lymphedema evaluations, 304
  splenic vein thrombosis evaluations, 217
  Takayasu arteritis evaluations, 386, 388f
Magnetic resonance lymphangiography, 330
Magnetic resonance venography
  calf vein thrombosis evaluations, 232
  May-Thurner syndrome evaluations, 253
  mesenteric vein thrombosis evaluations, 224f
  phlegmasia cerulea dolens evaluations, 265, 266f
Malperfusion, aortic dissection with, 198
Marfan syndrome, 108
  acetabulum protrusion, 153
  aortic dissection associated with, 150, 152f
  cardiovascular complications of, 150-151
  clinical features of, 149-151, 151f
  diagnosis of, 149-152, 150t
  differential diagnosis of, 151-152
  disproportionate overgrowth associated with, 149
  ectopia lentis, 149, 151f
  epidemiology of, 149
  etiology of, 149
  follow-up for, 154
  genetic counseling, 152, 154
  laboratory studies for, 151
  lifestyle modifications, 154
  Loeys Dietz syndrome versus, 156
  management of, 152-153
  mitral valve regurgitation associated with, 153
  ocular complications of, 151
  pain associated with, 151
  pathophysiology of, 149
  patient education about, 154
  pectus excavatum associated with, 149-150
  scoliosis associated with, 149
  spinal deformities in, 153

Marfan syndrome (*Cont.*):
    spontaneous pneumothorax in, 150
    thoracoabdominal aortic aneurysms in, 152f
    vascular Ehlers-Danlos syndrome versus, 146
    wrist sign in, 151f
MASS phenotype, 152
Massive localized lymphedema, 327
    diagnosis of, 329
    differential diagnosis of, 331
    distribution of, 329
    epidemiology of, 328
    etiology of, 328
    laboratory studies, 330
    management of, 331
    pathophysiology of, 328
    patient education about, 331
May-Thurner syndrome
    anatomy of, 251-252
    anticoagulation for, 253
    clinical features of, 252
    computed tomography venography of, 252
    deep venous thrombosis associated with, 251f, 251-254,
        253f-254f
    diagnosis of, 252-253
    differential diagnosis of, 252
    duplex ultrasound of, 252
    epidemiology of, 251
    factitial edema versus, 338
    follow-up for, 254
    imaging studies of, 252-253
    management of, 253
    pathophysiology of, 251-252
    patient education about, 254
Medial fibromuscular dysplasia, 187, 188f-189f
Medial hyperplasia, 187
Median arcuate ligament syndrome, 199f
Mediastinal lymphadenopathy, 263f
Medication-induced limb swelling, 335-336
Mediterranean fever gene, 392
Mesenteric angiography, 202, 206f, 221
Mesenteric bypass, for chronic mesenteric ischemia, 203
Mesenteric ischemia. *See* Acute mesenteric ischemia; Chronic
      mesenteric ischemia
Mesenteric vein thrombosis
    chronic, 220, 224
    clinical features of, 220
    computed tomography venography of, 221
    definition of, 219
    description of, 194, 198
    diagnosis of, 221
    duplex ultrasound of, 221, 222f-223f
    endovascular therapy for, 223
    epidemiology of, 220
    etiology of, 220, 221t
    heparin for, 221, 223

    hypercoagulable states, 220
    imaging of, 221, 222f-223f
    magnetic resonance angiography of, 221, 224f
    magnetic resonance venography of, 224f
    pathophysiology of, 220
    predisposing factors, 221t
    surgery for, 223-224
    warfarin for, 223
Methicillin-resistant *Staphylococcus aureus,* 141
Methotrexate, 370
Methylprednisolone, 395t, 439
Microaneurysms, 377f
Microemboli, 29-30
Microscopic polyangiitis
    chest radiographs of, 368f
    clinical features of, 369
    computed tomography of, 369f
    corticosteroids for, 370
    diagnosis of, 369-370
    differential diagnosis of, 370
    epidemiology of, 368
    etiology of, 368
    follow-up for, 371
    granulomatosis with polyangiitis versus, 366, 370
    histopathology of, 369-370
    imaging of, 369
    laboratory studies, 369
    lung biopsy of, 368f, 369
    management of, 370
    necrotizing small vessel vasculitis associated with, 368
    ocular manifestations of, 370f
    pathophysiology of, 368
    patient education about, 371
    remission of, 370
    transbronchial lung biopsy findings, 368f
Mitral valve regurgitation, 153
Modified Allen test, 79
Mondor disease, 226
Monoclonal gammopathy, 436
Motor neuropathy, 431
Mural thrombus, 59
Muscle rupture, leg swelling secondary to, 312-315
Mycophenolate mofetil, 370, 396
Mycosis fungoides, 277
Mycotic aneurysmal disease
    complications of, 142
    diagnosis of, 141-142
    epidemiology of, 141
    etiology of, 141
    management of, 142
    pathophysiology of, 141
    radiographic studies of, 142
Myxedema, pretibial, 304
    clinical features of, 316f-317f, 317, 319f
    description of, 277

diagnosis of, 317
differential diagnosis of, 318-319
distribution of, 318
epidemiology of, 316
etiology of, 316-317
follow-up for, 319
laboratory studies, 318
management of, 319
pathophysiology of, 316-317
patient education about, 319
phlebolymphedema versus, 335
workup for, 318

**N**
Nailfold capillary microscopy, 343, 345f
Necrobiosis lipoidica
    clinical features of, 440f-441f, 441
    corticosteroids for, 442
    diagnosis of, 441
    differential diagnosis of, 442
    distribution of, 441
    epidemiology of, 440
    etiology of, 440-441
    follow-up for, 442
    management of, 442-443
    pathology of, 441
    pathophysiology of, 440-441
Necrobiotic xanthogranuloma, 442
Necrotizing fasciitis, 309
Necrotizing glomerulonephritis, 364f
Neointimal hyperplasia, 247
Nephrogenic fibrosing dermopathy, 398
Nephrogenic systemic fibrosis
    clinical manifestations of, 399, 399f
    diagnosis of, 399-400
    differential diagnosis of, 400
    disease course of, 400
    epidemiology of, 398
    etiology of, 398
    gadolinium-based contrast agents for, 398
    hemodialysis for, 401
    pathogenesis of, 398-399
    pathology of, 398
    prevention of, 400
    skin manifestations of, 399, 399f-400f
    treatment of, 401
Neuropathic ulceration, 430f-433f, 430-434
Neurotrophic ulcers, 427t, 429f
Nitric oxide, 392
Nonocclusive mesenteric ischemia, 194, 198
Nuclear lymphoscintigraphy, 335

**O**
Obesity, lipedema versus, 323, 325t
Obturator artery aneurysm, 145f

Obturator bypass, 27, 27f
Occlusion
    common carotid artery, 100f
    internal carotid artery, 99f-101f, 99-101
    radial artery, 50
Orthotics, foot, 430f, 432, 433f

**P**
Paget-Schroetter syndrome
    anatomy of, 255
    catheter-directed thrombolytic therapy for, 257
    clinical features of, 256
    diagnosis of, 256
    differential diagnosis of, 256
    epidemiology of, 255
    follow-up for, 257
    imaging of, 256
    management of, 257
    pathophysiology of, 255
    patient education about, 257
    thrombolytics for, 257
    venography for, 256, 257f
Painful fat syndrome, 322
Palmar arch, 79-81, 80f
Palmaz stents, 40
Pancreatic panniculitis, 269-273
Panniculitis
    classification of, 271f
    clinical features of, 271f-272f, 271-272
    differential diagnosis of, 442
    distribution of, 272
    epidemiology of, 269
    etiology of, 270-271
    factitial, 269-273
    follow-up for, 273
    infectious, 271-273
    laboratory studies, 272-273
    lupus, 269-273, 271f-272f
    management of, 273
    pancreatic, 269-273
    pathophysiology of, 270-271
    patient education about, 273
    systemic disease associated with, 269-273
    traumatic, 269-273, 272f
Papillomatosis, 302, 304f
Parathyroid hormone, 446
Parathyroidectomy, 447
Parenchymal disease, 394
Parkes-Weber syndrome, 169-170, 176
Paroxysmal nocturnal hemoglobinuria, 212
Pathergy, 435, 435f
Peak systolic velocity, 49
Peau d'orange, 302, 303f, 317f, 400f
Pectus excavatum, 149-150
Pelvic congestion syndrome, 290

Pelvic lymphadenopathy, 264f

Penetrating carotid artery injuries
  epidemiology of, 111
  management of, 114, 114f
  screening criteria for, 112

Penile calciphylaxis, 446

Pentoxifylline, 319, 424

Percutaneous endovenous intervention, for femoropopliteal deep venous thrombosis, 243-249, 244f-246f

Percutaneous transluminal angioplasty, 64
  femoral popliteal disease treated with, 14-16
  fibromuscular dysplasia treated with, 191

Perimedial fibroplasia, 187

Peripheral arterial disease
  aortoiliac occlusive disease. See Aortoiliac occlusive disease
  brachiocephalic arteries, 47
  complications of, 13, 48
  computed tomography angiography of, 12, 15
  diagnostic evaluation of, 47
  duplex ultrasound of, 15, 47
  epidemiology of, 11, 14, 19, 46
  etiology of, 11-12, 15, 46-47
  femoropopliteal aneurysms versus, 134
  femoropopliteal bypass for, 11-13
  imaging of, 12
  incidence of, 8
  innominate artery, 46-48
  limb amputations secondary to, 22
  magnetic resonance angiography of, 15
  management of, 8, 10-13
  pathophysiology of, 11-12, 15, 46-47
  patient follow-up for, 13, 48
  postoperative management of, 48
  prevalence of, 46
  results of, 48
  risk factors for, 46-47
  subclavian artery, 46-48
  thromboangiitis obliterans versus, 381
  treatment of, 47
  vascular risk factors for, 46-47

Peripheral neuropathy, 431

Pernio, 260-261, 354, 405, 407-409, 408f, 411

Peroneal artery, 12f

Phlebolipedema, 324f

Phlebolymphedema
  clinical features of, 334, 334f
  definition of, 333
  diagnosis of, 334-335
  differential diagnosis of, 335
  duplex ultrasound of, 334-335
  epidemiology of, 333
  etiology of, 333-334
  management of, 335-336
  nuclear lymphoscintigraphy of, 335
  pathophysiology of, 333-334

patient education about, 336
  secondary, 334f

Phlegmasia cerulea dolens
  catheter-directed thrombolysis for, 266
  clinical features of, 263f, 265, 267f
  deep venous thrombosis associated with, 264
  description of, 238, 241
  diagnosis of, 265
  epidemiology of, 263-264
  etiology of, 264-265
  laboratory studies, 265
  magnetic resonance venography for, 265, 266f
  management of, 266
  pathophysiology of, 264-265
  patient education about, 267
  summary of, 267
  thrombectomy for, 266
  thrombophilia associated with, 265
  Trellis catheter for, 265f

Photoplethysmography, 84, 84f-85f

Phrenic nerve, 65f

Pigmented purpuric dermatitis, 281

Pigmented purpuric dermatoses, 442

Plantar pressures, 431

Pneumatosis, 195f

Poikiloderma atrophicans vasculare, 419-420

Polyangiitis
  granulomatosis with. See Granulomatosis with polyangiitis
  microscopic. See Microscopic polyangiitis

Polyarteritis nodosa, 366, 370
  biopsy of, 379
  clinical features of, 376, 377f-378f
  cutaneous, 379
  diagnosis of, 376, 377f-378f, 379
  differential diagnosis of, 379
  epidemiology of, 376
  etiology of, 376
  follow-up for, 379
  hepatitis B infection and, 379
  idiopathic, 379
  imaging of, 379
  laboratory studies, 376, 379
  livedo reticularis associated with, 377f-378f
  management of, 379
  pathophysiology of, 376
  patient education about, 379
  prevention of, 379

Polycythemia vera, 212

Polytetrafluoroethylene conduit, 12

Popliteal artery
  aneurysms of
    acute thrombosis of, 134
    imaging of, 133f
    repair of, 135f-136f
    thrombolytic therapy for, 136f

entrapment syndrome of
    arteriogram for, 162f
    clinical features of, 160
    diagnosis of, 160
    differential diagnosis of, 160
    duplex ultrasound of, 160, 161f-162f
    endovascular stenting of, 161
    follow-up for, 162
    management of, 161
    pathophysiology of, 160
    patient education about, 162
    types of, 160, 161f
  stenosis of, 14f-15f
Popliteal cyst, 232, 314
Portal vein thrombosis, 220f
Posterior tibial artery, 12f
Posterior uveitis, 396
Post-thrombotic syndrome, 232, 238-239, 241, 252, 252f, 304
Prednisone, 439
Pretibial myxedema
    clinical features of, 316f-317f, 317, 319f
    definition of, 335
    description of, 277
    diagnosis of, 317
    differential diagnosis of, 318-319
    distribution of, 318
    epidemiology of, 316
    etiology of, 316-317
    follow-up for, 319
    laboratory studies, 318
    management of, 319
    pathophysiology of, 316-317
    patient education about, 319
    phlebolymphedema versus, 335
    workup for, 318
Primary lipedema, 322
Primary lymphedema, 302. See also Lymphedema
Profunda femoral artery, 4
Protein C, 286
Pseudoaneurysms. See also Aneurysms
    anastomotic, 5
    anterior tibial artery, 144f
    brachial artery, 49f-50f, 51
    carotid artery traumatic injury as cause of, 115f, 116
    clinical features of, 138
    coil embolization for, 140f
    diagnosis of, 138
    epidemiology of, 138
    femoral artery, 137f
    natural history of, 138
    pathophysiology of, 138
    patient education about, 139
    postcarotid surgery, 108
    prevention of, 138

radial artery, 50f, 51-52
    risk factors for, 138
    treatment of, 138-139
    ultrasound-guided compression of, 138-139
    ultrasound-guided thrombin injection for, 138-139
Pseudo-Kaposi sarcoma
    clinical features of, 279f-280f, 280
    definition of, 276, 279
    diagnosis of, 280
    differential diagnosis of, 281
    epidemiology of, 279
    etiology of, 279-280
    histopathologic features of, 281
    imaging of, 281
    laboratory studies, 280
    management of, 281
    pathogenesis of, 279-280
    patient education about, 281
    physical examination of, 280
    stasis dermatitis versus, 281
Pseudoleukoderma angiospasticum, 351
Psoriasis, 277
Pulmonary artery aneurysm, 394
Pulmonary embolism
    description of, 23, 233
    epidemiology of, 236
    during percutaneous endovenous intervention for femoropopliteal deep venous thrombosis, 249
Pulsed dye lasers, 73, 77
Pyoderma gangrenosum
    clinical features of, 435f-437f, 436, 438
    corticosteroids for, 439
    differential diagnosis of, 438
    distribution of, 436
    epidemiology of, 435
    etiology of, 435
    follow-up for, 439
    laboratory studies, 436
    management of, 438-439
    pathergy associated with, 435, 435f
    pathophysiology of, 435
    patient education about, 439
    variants of, 436
Pyostomatitis vegetans, 436

Q
Quantitative sudomotor axon reflex test, 415, 415f

R
Radial artery
    anatomy of, 79, 83f
    aneurysm of, 51
    antegrade flow in, 86f
    perforation of, 52
    pseudoaneurysm of, 50f, 51-52

Radial artery access
  complications of
    epidemiology of, 49
    etiology of, 49-50
    follow-up, 52
    imaging of, 51
    management of, 52
    occlusion, 50
    pathophysiology of, 49-50
    patient education about, 52
    thrombosis, 50-51
    types of, 50
  uses of, 49
Radiofrequency ablation, 291, 297
*RASA1* mutations, 74
Raynaud phenomenon
  acrocyanosis versus, 354
  acro-osteolysis associated with, 342, 344f
  calcium channel blockers for, 346
  clinical features of, 342f, 345
  description of, 259f, 260
  diagnosis of, 343, 345t
  digital amputation secondary to, 344f
  epidemiology of, 342
  erythromelalgia versus, 415
  etiology of, 342-343
  follow-up for, 346
  management of, 345-346
  nailfold capillary microscopy for, 343, 345f
  nonpharmacologic treatment of, 345-346
  pathophysiology of, 342-343
  patient education about, 346
  pernio versus, 407
  pharmacologic treatment of, 346
  primary, 342-343, 345t
  refractory, 346
  scleroderma and, 344f
  secondary, 342-343, 343t
Recombinant plasminogen activator, 266f
Renal artery fibromuscular dysplasia, 102, 103f-104f
Renal artery stenosis
  atherosclerotic
    angiographic features of, 184, 184f
    arteriography of, 184f
    clinical features of, 183
    computed tomography angiography of, 183
    diagnosis of, 183-184
    differential diagnosis of, 184
    duplex ultrasound of, 182f, 183t
    epidemiology of, 182
    follow-up for, 185-186
    hypertension in, 182-183
    magnetic resonance angiography of, 183
    management of, 184-185
    natural history of, 185-186
    pathophysiology of, 182
    patient education about, 185
    stents for, 186
   computed tomography angiography of, 183, 189, 190f
   duplex ultrasound of, 182f, 187
   fibromuscular dysplasia-associated, 187-191
   magnetic resonance angiography of, 189, 191f
Reticular veins
  clinical features of, 288, 292f, 293
  diagnosis of, 293
  sclerotherapy for, 293-295
Retiform purpura, 351, 351f, 378f
Retrograde bypass, for chronic mesenteric ischemia, 205, 208f
Retroperitoneal hematoma, 122f, 146f
Reversed vein bypass technique, 12
Rheumatoid arthritis, 360, 361f
Ruptured abdominal aortic aneurysm
  clinical presentation of, 123
  endograft for, 124f
  endovascular repair of, 123
  epidemiology of, 122-123
  open surgical repair of, 123

**S**
Saddle nose deformity, 365f
Saphenous reflux, 291
Saphenous vein graft, for carotid artery aneurysm, 110f
Sarcoidosis, 442
Scimitar sign, 313, 313f
Scleredema, 319
Scleroderma, 260, 344f, 400
Scleromyxedema, 318, 400
Sclerosing lipogranuloma, 442
Sclerotherapy
  complications of, 294
  congenital vascular malformations treated with, 76-77, 77f
  foam, 294, 297
  follow-up after, 294
  hyperpigmentation after, 294
  patient education about, 294
  reticular veins treated with, 293-295
  spider veins treated with, 293-295
  varicose veins treated with, 293-295, 297
Scoliosis, in Marfan syndrome, 149
Secondary lymphedema, 302, 330t. *See also* Lymphedema
Segmental arterial mediolysis, 184, 191
Selective angiography, 113
Self-expanding stents, 40
Sensory neuropathy, 431
Skin
  necrosis of
    heparin-induced, 283f-284f, 283-285
    warfarin-induced, 284-286
  physiology of, 411
Small intestine obstruction, 224f

Small saphenous vein, 297
Small vessel vasculitis, ANCA-negative
    cryoglobulinemic vasculitis, 359, 359t, 360f
    definition of, 358
    diagnosis of, 361-362
    differential diagnosis of, 362
    follow-up for, 362
    Henoch-Schönlein purpura, 358f, 358-362, 379
    hypersensitivity vasculitis, 359, 359t, 361t, 361-362, 379
    management of, 362
    polyarteritis nodosa versus, 379
Sodium dodecyl sulphate-polyacrylamide gel electrophoresis, 146, 146f
Sodium tetradecyl sulfate, 77, 77f
Sodium thiosulfate, 447
Spider veins
    clinical features of, 288, 289f, 291f, 292f, 293
    etiology of, 293
    sclerotherapy for, 293-295
Splenectomy, 217
Splenic artery embolization, 217
Splenic vein thrombosis, 215-217
Spontaneous pneumothorax, in Marfan syndrome, 150
Squaring of toes, 302, 303f
Stanford classification, of aortic dissection, 43, 45f
Staphylococcus, 305
Stasis dermatitis
    allergic contact dermatitis with, 277f
    cellulitis and, 277, 278f
    clinical features of, 275f-277f, 275-276
    complications of, 275
    differential diagnosis of, 276-277, 318, 442
    distribution of, 275
    duplex ultrasound of, 275
    epidemiology of, 275
    etiology of, 275
    follow-up for, 277
    laboratory studies of, 275
    management of, 277
    pathophysiology of, 275
    patient education about, 277
    pretibial myxedema versus, 318
    pseudo-Kaposi sarcoma versus, 281
Statins, 127
"Steal syndrome," 26, 34
Stemmer sign, 302, 334
Stents/stenting, 16
    aortoiliac occlusive disease treated with, 9f
    atherosclerotic arch vessel disease treated with, 40
    atherosclerotic renal artery stenosis treated with, 186
    connective tissue disorders contraindications, 148
    femoral popliteal disease treated with, 14-16
    femoropopliteal deep venous thrombosis treated with, 246-247
    "kissing," 10
    thrombosis, 247

Stewart-Bluefarb syndrome, 270
Streptococcus, 305
Stroke
    cervical carotid, 88, 92
    economic costs of, 89
    epidemiology of, 88, 92
    gender differences in, 88, 92
    warfarin prophylaxis in, 98
Sturge-Weber syndrome, 76
Subclavian artery
    anatomy of, 58
    aneurysm of, 55f
    cervical ribs effect on, 54
    digital subtraction angiography of, 59f
    occlusion of, 58f
    peripheral arterial disease of, 46-48
    stenosis of, 34, 63f, 67, 69
    thrombus of, 61f
Subclavian steal syndrome
    computed tomography angiography of, 62f, 64
    coronary. See Coronary subclavian steal syndrome
    diagnosis of, 63-64
    duplex ultrasonography of, 63f
    endovascular interventions for, 64
    etiology of, 63
    extra-anatomic bypasses for, 64
    follow-up for, 64-65
    history-taking for, 62
    imaging of, 64
    medical therapy for, 64
    pathology associated with, 63
    physical examination of, 62-63
    surgery for, 64
    symptoms of, 62
    treatment of, 64
    vertebrobasilar "spells" associated with, 62
Subclavian vein, 255, 256f
Superficial femoral artery
    duplex ultrasound of, 238f
    occlusion of, 11f-12f
Superficial thrombophlebitis, 381, 382f
Superficial venous thrombosis
    anticoagulants for, 228
    calf vein thrombosis caused by, 232
    clinical findings of, 226
    diagnosis of, 226-227
    differential diagnosis of, 227
    epidemiology of, 226
    etiology of, 226
    follow-up for, 228-229
    imaging of, 226-227, 227f
    laboratory studies, 227
    lower extremity, 226
    management of, 227-228
    pathophysiology of, 226

Superficial venous thrombosis (*Cont.*):
  patient education about, 228
  prognosis for, 228
  skin staining after, 228f
  upper extremity, 226
Superior mesenteric artery
  anatomy of, 193f
  collateralization in aortoiliac occlusive disease, 3
  computed tomographic angiography of, 126f
  embolus of, 195f
  occlusion of, 210f
  stenosis of, 204f
  stenting of, 210f
  thromboembolectomy of, 196, 197f
  thromboembolism of, 193, 195, 197f
  thrombosis of, 194, 196, 197f
Superior mesenteric vein
  imaging of, 219f
  thrombosis of, 194, 198. *See also* Mesenteric vein thrombosis
Supraceliac aorta-to-iliofemoral bypass, 27
Surgery
  atherosclerotic arch vessel disease treated with, 39
  blue toe syndrome treated with, 31
  hemangiomas treated with, 73
  mesenteric vein thrombosis treated with, 223-224
  subclavian steal syndrome treated with, 64
  thoracic aortic dissection treated with, 43
  thoracic outlet syndrome treated with, 56
  thoracoabdominal aortic aneurysms treated with, 127-128
Syncope, 43
Systemic lupus erythematosus, 360

T
Takayasu arteritis
  angiography of, 388, 388f-389f
  clinical features of, 385
  diagnosis of, 385
  differential diagnosis of, 184
  duplex ultrasound of, 389f
  epidemiology of, 384
  etiology of, 385
  follow-up for, 389
  glucocorticoids for, 389
  laboratory studies, 386
  management of, 389
  pathophysiology of, 385
  patient education about, 389
Telangiectasias, 291f
Tennis leg, 312
Thalidomide, 395t
Thoracic aortic aneurysms
  ascending, 388f
  diagnosis of, 130
  endovascular repair of, 130-132, 131f-132f
  epidemiology of, 130

etiology of, 130
  imaging of, 125f, 130, 131f
  laboratory tests, 130
  management of, 130
  pathophysiology of, 130
  in Takayasu arteritis, 388f
Thoracic aortic dissection
  clinical presentation of, 43
  complications of, 44
  diagnostic evaluation of, 43
  epidemiology of, 43
  false lumens, 44, 44f
  pathology of, 42
  patient follow-up, 44
  surgical therapy for, 43
  treatment of, 43-44
Thoracic endovascular aneurysm repair, 130-132, 131f-132f
Thoracic endovascular stent grafting, 42, 44
Thoracic outlet, 256f
Thoracic outlet syndrome
  bony abnormalities associated with, 54, 54f
  cervical rib, 54, 54f, 56, 58, 60f
  clinical features of, 58
  diagnosis of, 55, 55f, 59
  differential diagnosis of, 55-56, 59
  epidemiology of, 54, 57-58
  etiology of, 58-59
  follow-up for, 56
  hand ischemia as sign of, 54f, 55
  management of, 56, 60
  pathophysiology of, 54-55, 58-59
  patient education about, 60
  physical examination findings, 54f, 57f
  thrombolytic therapy for, 60
Thoracoabdominal aortic aneurysms
  compressive symptoms associated with, 125
  computed tomographic angiography of, 125-126
  definition of, 126
  diagnostic evaluation of, 125-126
  epidemiology of, 126-127
  follow-up for, 128
  history-taking, 125
  incidence of, 127
  management of, 127
  in Marfan syndrome, 152f
  medical management of, 127
  natural history of, 127
  operative repair of, 127-128
  pathogenesis of, 127
  physical examination of, 125
  population affected, 127
  risk factors for, 127
  rupture risks, 127
  types of, 126
Thoracofemoral aorta-to-iliofemoral bypass, 27

Thromboangiitis obliterans, 260
  clinical features of, 381, 382f
  diagnosis of, 381-383, 382f
  differential diagnosis of, 383
  epidemiology of, 381
  etiology of, 381
  follow-up for, 383
  histology of, 383
  laboratory studies, 381
  management of, 383
  pathophysiology of, 381
  patient education about, 383
  peripheral arterial disease versus, 381
  radiographic studies of, 383
Thrombocytopenia, 284
Thromboembolectomy, 196, 197f
Thromboembolism
  superior mesenteric artery, 193, 195, 197f
  surgical treatment of, 195
Thrombolytic therapy
  catheter-directed, 198, 214, 257, 266
  deep venous thrombosis treated with, 241
  femoropopliteal deep venous thrombosis treated with, 241
  Paget-Schroetter syndrome treated with, 257
  in percutaneous endovenous intervention for femoropopliteal deep venous thrombosis, 246
  popliteal artery aneurysm treated with, 136f
  thoracic outlet syndrome treated with, 60
Thrombophilia, 226
Thrombophlebitis. See Superficial venous thrombosis
Thrombosis. See also Venous thromboembolism
  brachial artery, 50-51
  calf vein. See Calf vein thrombosis
  deep venous. See Deep venous thrombosis
  mesenteric vein. See Mesenteric vein thrombosis
  radial artery, 50-51
  splenic vein, 215-217
  superficial venous. See Superficial venous thrombosis
  superior mesenteric artery, 194
Tibioperoneal occlusive disease
  atherosclerosis and, 19
  claudication in, 20
  clinical features of, 20
  complications of, 21
  epidemiology of, 19
  etiology of, 19-20
  follow-up, 21
  interventions for, 21
  management of, 21
  pathophysiology of, 19-20
  patient education about, 21
Tinea pedis, 308f
Tissue plasminogen activator, 246
"Toasted skin syndrome." See Erythema ab igne
Transaminases, 241

Transaortic aortoceliac-superior mesenteric artery bypass, 207f
Transaortic mesenteric endarterectomy, for chronic mesenteric ischemia, 205, 208, 209f
Transarterial lung perfusion scintigraphy, 176
Transforming growth factor-$\beta$1, 398-399
Transient ischemic attack, 34, 92
Transthoracic echocardiography, 43
Trap door aortotomy, 208, 209f
Traumatic injuries
  carotid artery. See Carotid artery traumatic injuries
  lower extremity cellulitis secondary to, 307f, 308
Traumatic panniculitis, 269-273, 272f
Trellis device
  for axillosubclavian deep venous thrombosis, 257f
  for femoropopliteal deep venous thrombosis, 244f-245f
  in iliofemoral location, 265f
Trench foot, 405, 410f, 410-412, 413f
Truncular high-flow vascular malformations, 75
Tumor necrosis factor-alpha inhibitors, 439

U
Ulcerations/ulcers
  arterial, 425-429, 427t-428t
  ischemic, 426-428, 427f
  lower extremity cellulitis secondary to, 307f, 308
  mixed, 427t
  neuropathic, 430f-433f, 430-434
  neurotrophic, 427t, 429f
  vascular, 427t
  venous stasis, 422f-423f, 422-424
Ulcerative acroangiodermatitis, 280f
Ulcerative cervical carotid disease, 97-98
Ulnar artery
  anatomy of, 79, 83f
  antegrade flow in, 86f
  occlusion of, 83f
Ultrasound-guided compression, for pseudoaneurysms, 138-139
Ultrasound-guided thrombin injection, for pseudoaneurysms, 138-139
Ultraviolet A phototherapy, 401
Unfractionated heparin
  deep venous thrombosis treated with, 240-241
  skin necrosis induced by, 283-285
Upper extremity
  arterial aneurysm of, 54-56
  congenital vascular anomalies of. See Congenital vascular anomalies
Uterine hemorrhage, 145

V
Vagus nerve, 89f
Varicose veins
  clinical features of, 288, 288f, 292f, 296f, 296-297
  diagnosis of, 289-291, 294, 297
  differential diagnosis of, 297

Varicose veins (*Cont.*):
  endovenous laser ablation for, 291, 296-299, 298f-299f
  epidemiology of, 288
  etiology of, 293
  laboratory studies, 297
  management of, 297
  pain associated with, 288
  pathophysiology of, 289, 296
  physical examination of, 296
  risk factors for, 289
  sclerotherapy for, 293-295, 297
  treatment of, 291
Vascular Ehlers-Danlos syndrome, 145-147. *See also* Ehlers-Danlos syndrome
Vascular endothelial growth factor, 72
Vascular malformations, congenital
  arteriovenous malformation. *See* Arteriovenous malformation
  classification of, 73, 73f
  clinical presentation of, 74-76
  coil embolotherapy for, 178
  definition of, 73
  diagnosis of, 76, 176
  duplex ultrasonography of, 176
  epidemiology of, 73, 172
  ethanol sclerotherapy for, 77, 178
  etiology of, 74, 174
  fast-flow, 74f
  follow-up for, 178
  glue embolotherapy for, 178
  Hamburg classification of, 175t
  hemangiomas. *See* Hemangiomas
  high-flow, 73-75, 74f, 77
  imaging of, 176
  low-flow, 73, 75
  magnetic resonance imaging of, 176
  management of, 76-77, 177t, 177-178
  multidisciplinary approach to, 177t, 177-178
  pathogenesis of, 74
  pathophysiology of, 174
  patient education about, 77, 178

  sclerotherapy for, 76-77, 77f
  transarterial lung perfusion scintigraphy of, 176
Vasculitis
  ANCA-negative small vessel. *See* ANCA-negative small vessel vasculitis
  fibromuscular dysplasia versus, 189
  hypersensitivity, 359, 359t, 361t, 361-362, 379
Vasopressin, 147
*VEFGR3*, 74
Vein of Servelle, 169
Venous malformations, 169-170
Venous outflow obstruction, 213
Venous reflux, 289, 291
Venous stasis
  illustration of, 290f
  ulceration caused by, 422f-423f, 422-424
Venous stenosis, 246f
Venous thromboembolism
  description of, 230, 231t
  recurrence of, 238
  risk factors for, 236t
Venulectasias, 293
Vertebral artery
  duplex ultrasound of, 67f
  injury to, 105f
Vertebrobasilar insufficiency, 62, 69
Vertebrobasilar ischemia, 62
Vesiculobullous eruption, 436
Virchow's triad, 230, 237, 255

**W**
Warfarin
  deep venous thrombosis treated with, 241
  fetal malformation risks, 241
  mesenteric vein thrombosis treated with, 223
  skin necrosis induced by, 284-286
  in stroke patients, 98
Wegener granulomatosis. *See* Granulomatosis with polyangiitis
Wells score, 231, 231t
Wound healing, 19